**Textbook of Pharmacoepidemiology**

# Textbook of Pharmacoepidemiology

Third Edition

*Edited by*

**Brian L. Strom, MD, MPH**
*Chancellor, Rutgers Biomedical & Health Sciences*
*Executive Vice President for Health Affairs*
*University Professor*
*Rutgers, The State University of New Jersey*
*Newark, NJ, USA*

**Stephen E. Kimmel, MD, MSCE**
*Dean's Professor and Chair of Epidemiology*
*College of Public Health and Health Professions and College of Medicine*
*University of Florida*
*Gainesville, FL, USA*

**Sean Hennessy, PharmD, PhD**
*Professor of Epidemiology*
*Director, Center for Pharmacoepidemiology Research and Training*
*University of Pennsylvania Perelman School of Medicine*
*Philadelphia, PA, USA*

**WILEY** Blackwell

This edition first published 2022
© 2022 John Wiley & Sons Ltd

*Edition History*
*John Wiley & Sons Ltd (1e, 2006);*
*John Wiley & Sons Ltd (2e, 2013)*

The right of Brian L. Strom, Stephen E. Kimmel, Sean Hennessy to be identified as the authors of the editorial material in this work has been asserted in accordance with law.

*Registered Offices*
John Wiley & Sons, Inc., 111 River Street, Hoboken, NJ 07030, USA
John Wiley & Sons Ltd, The Atrium, Southern Gate, Chichester, West Sussex, PO19 8SQ, UK

*Editorial Office*
9600 Garsington Road, Oxford, OX4 2DQ, UK

For details of our global editorial offices, customer services, and more information about Wiley products visit us at www.wiley.com.

Wiley also publishes its books in a variety of electronic formats and by print-on-demand. Some content that appears in standard print versions of this book may not be available in other formats.

*Limit of Liability/Disclaimer of Warranty*

*Library of Congress Cataloging-in-Publication Data*

Names: Strom, Brian L., editor. | Kimmel, Stephen | Hennessy, Sean, editor.
    E., editor.
Title: Textbook of pharmacoepidemiology / edited by Brian L. Strom, Sean
    Hennessy, Stephen E. Kimmel.
Description: Third edition. | Hoboken, NJ : Wiley-Blackwell, 2021. |
    Includes bibliographical references and index.
Identifiers: LCCN 2021029285 (print) | LCCN 2021029286 (ebook) | ISBN
    9781119701071 (paperback) | ISBN 9781119701088 (adobe pdf) | ISBN
    9781119701118 (epub)
Subjects: MESH: Pharmacoepidemiology--methods
Classification: LCC RM302.5 (print) | LCC RM302.5 (ebook) | NLM QV 771 |
    DDC 615.7/042–dc23
LC record available at https://lccn.loc.gov/2021029285
LC ebook record available at https://lccn.loc.gov/2021029286

Cover Design: Wiley
Cover Image: © ShutterWorx/Getty Images r.classen/Shutterstock

Set in 9.5/12.5pt STIXTwoText by Straive, Pondicherry, India

SKYAFC2B5BC-EC13-46B5-8D90-59D73B2EB082_092021

# Contents

# List of Contributors

*Trisha Acri*
Department of Family and Community
Medicine Temple University School of
Medicine Philadelphia, PA, USA
Currently, Director of Community Research
Health Services, AIDS Care Group, AIDS Care
Group, Sharon Hill, PA, USA

*Jerry Avorn*
Harvard Medical School and Brigham and
Women's Hospital
Boston, MA, USA

*Jeffrey S. Barrett*
Critical Path Institute
Tucson, AZ, USA

*David W. Bates*
Division of General Internal Medicine and
Primary Care
Brigham and Women's Hospital and Harvard
Medical School
Boston, MA, USA

*Bernard Bégaud*
Clinical Pharmacology and
Pharmacoepidemiology, Medical School
University of Bordeaux
Bordeaux, France

*Jesse A. Berlin*
Johnson & Johnson
Titusville, NJ, USA

*Harshvinder Bhullar*
Independent Consultant London, UK

*Laura E. Bothwell*
Yale School of Public Health
New Haven, Connecticut, USA

*Adam C. Carle*
Cincinanti Children's Hospital Medical Center
Cincinnati, OH, USA
University of Cincinnati, College of Medicine
Cincinnati, OH, USA
University of Cincinnati, College of
Arts and Sciences
Cincinnati, OH, USA

*Robert T. Chen*
Brighton Collaboration, Task Force for
Global Health
Decatur, GA, USA

*Emil Cochino*
European Medicines Agency
Amsterdam, The Netherlands

*Brenda J. Crowe*
Eli Lilly and Company
Indianapolis, IN, USA

*Francesca Cunningham*
US Department of Veterans Affairs
Hines, IL, USA

*Gerald J. Dal Pan*
Office of Surveillance and Epidemiology
Center for Drug Evaluation and Research
US Food and Drug Administration
Silver Spring, MD, USA

**Rachael L. DiSantostefano**
Department of Epidemiology
Janssen Research & Development
Titusville, NJ, USA

**Scott Evans**
Biostatistics Center
The George Washington University
Rockville, MD, USA

**Stephen J.W. Evans**
The London School of Hygiene and Tropical
Medicine, London, UK

**Joshua J. Gagne**
Harvard Medical School and Brigham and
Women's Hospital, Boston, MA, USA
and
Johnson and Johnson
New Brunswick, NJ, USA

**Nicolle M. Gatto**
Aetion Inc., New York, NY, USA

**Kate Gelperin**
Division of Epidemiology Office of
Surveillance and Epidemiology
Center for Drug Evaluation and Research
US Food and Drug Administration
Silver Spring, MD, USA

**Tobias Gerhard**
Ernest Mario School of Pharmacy
Rutgers Biomedical and Health Sciences
Piscataway, NJ, USA
and
Center for Pharmacoepidemiology and
Treatment Science
Rutgers Biomedical and Health Sciences
New Brunswick, NJ, USA

**Jeremy Greene**
Johns Hopkins University
Baltimore, Maryland, MD, USA

**Robert Gross**
Center for Clinical Epidemiology and
Biostatistics

Center for Pharmacoepidemiology Research
and Training, Perelman School of Medicine
University of Pennsylvania, Philadelphia
PA, USA

**Sean Hennessy**
University of Pennsylvania Perelman School
of Medicine
Philadelphia, PA, USA

**Sonia Hernandez Diaz**
Harvard T.H. Chan School of Public Health
Boston, MA, USA

**Daniel B. Horton**
Rutgers Robert Wood Johnson
Medical School, Rutgers Center for
Pharmacoepidemiology and Treatment
Science, Rutgers School of Public Health
New Brunswick, NJ, USA

**Krista F. Huybrechts**
Brigham and Women's Hospital
Harvard Medical School
Boston, MA, USA

**Judith K. Jones**
†Formerly Principal Consultant PharmaLex,
Inc., Fairfax, VA and Adjunct Faculty
The University of Michigan School of Public
Health Summer Program
Ann Arbor, USA

**Aaron S. Kesselheim**
Harvard Medical School and Brigham and
Women's Hospital
Boston, MA, USA

**Stephen E. Kimmel**
University of Florida College of Public
Health and Health Professions & College of
Medicine
Gainesville, FL, USA

**Tamar Lasky**
US Food and Drug Administration
Silver Spring, MD, USA

**Julie Lauffenburger**
Brigham and Women's Hospital and Harvard
Medical School
Boston, MA, USA

**David Lee**
Center for Pharmaceutical Management
Management Sciences for Health
Arlington, VA, USA

**Samuel M. Lesko**
Northeast Regional Cancer Institute and
Geisinger Commonwealth School of Medicine
Scranton, PA, USA

**Bennett Levitan**
Department of Epidemiology
Janssen Research & Development
Titusville, NJ, USA

**Marie Lindquist**
Uppsala Monitoring Centre
WHO Collaborating Centre for International
Drug Monitoring
Uppsala, Sweden

**Christine Y. Lu**
Harvard Medical School and Harvard Pilgrim
Health Care Institute, Boston, MA, USA

**George Maldonado**
Division of Environmental Health Sciences
School of Public Health, University of
Minnesota, Minneapolis, MN, USA

**Claudia Manzo**
Division of Risk Management Office of
Surveillance and Epidemiology
Center for Drug Evaluation and Research
US Food and Drug Administration
Silver Spring, MD, USA

**Danica Marinac-Dabic**
Division of Epidemiology
Office of Surveillance and Biometrics Center
for Devices and Radiological Health
US Food and Drug Administration
Silver Spring, MD, USA

**Allen A. Mitchell**
Slone Epidemiology Center at Boston
University, Boston, MA, USA

**Jingping Mo**
Epidemiology, Worldwide Research &
Development, Pfizer Inc.
New York, NY, USA

**Esi M. Morgan**
Seattle Children's Hospital
Seattle, WA, USA
University of Washington
Seattle, WA, USA

**Yola Moride**
Center for Pharmacoepidemiology and
Treatment Science, Rutgers Biomedical and
Health Sciences
New Brunswick, NJ, USA

**Sharon-Lise T. Normand**
Harvard Medical School and
Harvard School of Public Health
Boston, MA, USA

**Anton Pottegård**
Clinical Pharmacology and Pharmacy
Department of Public Health
University of Southern Denmark
Odense, Denmark

**Nicole Pratt**
Quality Use of Medicines and Pharmacy
Research Centre, Clinical and Health Sciences
University of South Australia, Adelaide,
South Australia, Australia

**June Raine**
Vigilance and Risk Management of Medicine
Medicines and Healthcare Products
Regulatory Agency, London, UK

**Robert F. Reynolds**
Epidemiology, Research and Development,
GlaxoSmithKline, New York, NY, USA

**Annika Richterich**
Maastricht University
Maastricht, The Netherlands

**Mary Elizabeth Ritchey**
Med Tech Epi, LLC, Philadelphia, PA, USA
Center for Pharmacoepidemiology and
Treatment Science, Rutgers University
New Brunswick, NJ, USA

**Sebastian Schneeweiss**
Departments of Medicine and Epidemiology
Harvard Medical School and
Division of Pharmacoepidemiology
Department of Medicine
Brigham & Women's Hospital
Boston, MA, USA

**Kevin A. Schulman**
Clinical Excellence Research Center
Stanford University
Stanford, CA, USA

**Art Sedrakyan**
Department of Public Health
New York Presbyterian Hospital and
Weill Cornell Medical College
New York, NY, USA

**Hanna M. Seidling**
Head of Cooperation Unit Clinical Pharmacy
Department of Clinical Pharmacology and
Pharmacoepidemiology Cooperation Unit
Clinical Pharmacy
University of Heidelberg
Heidelberg, Germany

**Stephen B. Soumerai**
Department of Population Medicine Director
Drug Policy Research Group
Harvard Medical School and Harvard Pilgrim
Health Care Institute
Boston, MA, USA

**Brian L. Strom**
Rutgers Biomedical and Health Sciences
Newark, NJ, USA

**Samy Suissa**
McGill University and Jewish General Hospital
Montreal, Quebec, Canada

**Janet Sultana**
Mater Dei Hospital, Msida, Malta
and Exeter College of Medicine and Health
University of Exeter, Exeter, UK

**Gianluca Trifirò**
Department of Diagnostics and Public Health
University of Verona, Verona, Italy

**Shinobu Uzu**
Pharmaceuticals and Medical Devices Agency
Tokyo, Japan

**Priscilla Velentgas**
Real World Solutions, IQVIA, Inc.
Cambridge, MA, USA

**Kerstin N. Vokinger**
Harvard Medical school and Brigham and
Women's Hospital
Boston, MA, USA
and
Institute for Law University of Zurich
Zurich, Switzerland

**Suzanne L. West**
Gillings School of Global Public Health
University of North Carolina
Chapel Hill, NC, USA

**Björn Wettermark**
Disciplinary Domain of Medicine and Pharmacy
Uppsala University, Uppsala, Sweden

**H. Amy Xia**
Amgen, Thousand Oaks
CA, USA

# Preface

It was a remarkable 33 years ago that the first edition of Strom's Pharmacoepidemiology was published. The preface to that book stated that pharmacoepidemiology was a new field with a new generation of pharmacoepidemiologists arising to join the field's few pioneers. Over the ensuing 32 years, the field indeed has grown and no longer deserves to be called "new." Many of those "new generation" scientists (including two of the editors of this book) are now "middle-aged" pharmacoepidemiologists. Despite its relatively brief academic life, a short history of pharmacoepidemiology and review of its current state will set the stage for the purpose of this textbook.

Pharmacoepidemiology originally arose from the union of the fields of clinical pharmacology and epidemiology. Pharmacoepidemiology studies the use of and the effects of medical products in large numbers of people and applies the methods of epidemiology to the content area of clinical pharmacology. This field represents the science underlying post-marketing medical product surveillance, studies of the effects of medical products (i.e. drugs, biologicals, devices) performed after a product has been approved for use. In recent years, pharmacoepidemiology has expanded to include many other types of studies, as well.

The field of pharmacoepidemiology has grown enormously since the first publication of Strom. The International Society of Pharmacoepidemiology, an early idea when the first edition of this book was written, has grown into a major international scientific force, with over 1476 members from 63 countries, an extremely successful annual meeting attracting more than 1800 attendees, a large number of very active committees and scientific interest groups, and its own journal. In addition, a number of established journals have targeted pharmacoepidemiology manuscripts as desirable. As new scientific developments occur within mainstream epidemiology, they are rapidly adopted, applied, and advanced within our field as well. We have also become institutionalized as a subfield within the field of clinical pharmacology, with scientific sections of the American Society for Clinical Pharmacology and Therapeutics and with pharmacoepidemiology a required part of the clinical pharmacology board examination.

Most of the major international pharmaceutical companies have founded dedicated units to organize and lead their efforts in pharmacoepidemiology, pharmacoeconomics, and quality-of-life studies. The continuing parade of drug safety crises emphasizes the need for the field, and some foresighted manufacturers have begun to perform "prophylactic" pharmacoepidemiology studies, to have data in hand and available when questions arise, rather than waiting to begin to collect data after a crisis has developed. Pharmacoepidemiologic data are now routinely used for regulatory decisions, and many governmental agencies have been developing and expanding their own pharmacoepidemiology programs. Risk evaluation and mitigation strategies are now required by regulatory bodies with the marketing of new drugs, as a means of improving drugs' benefit/risk balance, and manufacturers are identifying ways to respond. Requirements that a drug be proven to be cost effective have been added to many national, local, and insurance health care systems, either to justify reimbursement or even to justify drug availability. A number of schools of medicine, pharmacy, and public health have established research programs in pharmacoepidemiology, and a few of them have also established pharmacoepidemiology training programs in response to a desperate need for more pharmacoepidemiology personnel. Pharmacoepidemiologic research funding is now more plentiful, and even limited support for training is available.

In the United States, drug utilization review programs are required, by law, of each of the 50 state Medicaid programs, and have been implemented as well in many managed care organizations. Now, years later, the utility of drug utilization review programs is being questioned. In addition, the Joint Commission requires that every hospital in the US have an adverse drug reaction monitoring program and a drug use evaluation program, turning every hospital into a mini-pharmacoepidemiology laboratory. Stimulated in part by the interests of the World Health Organization and the Rockefeller Foundation, there is even substantial interest in pharmacoepidemiology in the developing world. Yet, throughout the world, the increased concern by the public about privacy has made pharmacoepidemiologic research much more difficult to conduct.

In recent years, major new changes have been made in drug regulation and organization, largely in response to a series of accusations about myocardial infarction caused by analgesics, which was detected in long-term prevention trials rather than in normal use of the drugs. For example, FDA was given new regulatory authority after drug marketing. Further, the development, since 1 January 2006, of Medicare Part D, a US federal program to subsidize prescription drugs for Medicare recipients, introduced to pharmacoepidemiology a new database with a stable population approaching 50 million in what may be the largest healthcare system in the world. The US Congress has recognized the importance of the field, with the founding of the Sentinel Program, and new requirements that FDA focus on "real world evidence." A new movement has arisen in the US of "comparative effectiveness research," which in many ways learns from much longer experience in Europe, as well as decades of experience in pharmacoepidemiology. These developments portend major changes for our field.

In summary, there has been tremendous growth in the field of pharmacoepidemiology and a fair amount of maturation. With the growth and maturation of the field, Strom's *Pharmacoepidemiology* has grown and matured right along. *Pharmacoepidemiology* thus represents a comprehensive source of information about the field. As a reflection of the growth of the field, the fourth Edition of Strom was over twice as long as the first! Now, seven years after the fifth edition, the field continues to change and garner widespread interest, leading to the recent publication of the sixth edition in 2020.

So, why, one may ask, do we need a Textbook of Pharmacoepidemiology? The need arose precisely because of the growth of the field. With that, and the corresponding growth in the parent book, Strom's *Pharmacoepidemiology* has really become more of a reference book than a book usable as a textbook. Yet, there is increasing need for people to be trained in the field and an increasing number of training programs. With the maturity of the field comes therefore the necessity for both comprehensive approaches (such as Strom's *Pharmacoepidemiology*) and more focused approaches. Therefore, *Textbook of Pharmacoepidemiology* was intended as a modified and shortened version of its parent, designed to meet the need of students. We believe that students can benefit from an approach that focuses on the core of the discipline, along with learning aids.

*Textbook of Pharmacoepidemiology* attempts to fill this need, providing a focused educational resource for students. It is our hope that this book will serve as a useful textbook for students at all levels: upper-level undergraduates, graduate students, post-doctoral fellows, and others who are learning the field. To achieve our goals, we have substantially edited down from Strom's *Pharmacoepidemiology*, with a focus on what is needed by students, eliminating some chapters and shortening others. We also have provided case examples for most chapters and key points for all chapters. Each chapter is followed by a list of further reading.

So why update it? In looking at the sixth Edition of Strom, most chapters in the new edition were thoroughly revised to provide updated content. New chapters were added, along with many new authors. The second edition of the textbook was simply getting out of date in comparison to the recently published sixth edition of the parent book.

Specifically, we have tried to emphasize the methods of pharmacoepidemiology and the strengths and limitations of the field, while minimizing some of the technical specifications that are important for a reference book but not for students. Therefore, the first five chapters of Part I, "Introduction to Pharmacoepidemiology," lay out the cores of the discipline, and remain essentially unchanged from Strom's *Pharmacoepidemiology*, with the exception of the inclusion of key points and lists of further reading. We have also included a chapter on different perspectives of the field (from academia, industry, regulatory agencies, and the legal system), as a shortened form of several chapters from the reference book. Part II focuses on "Sources of Pharmacoepidemiology Data" and includes important chapters about spontaneous pharmacovigilance reporting systems, electronic databases, and other approaches to pharmacoepidemiology studies. Part III summarizes "Special Issues in Pharmacoepidemiology Methodology" that we feel are important to more advanced pharmacoepidemiology students. Although no student is likely to become an expert in all of these methods, they form a core set of knowledge that we believe all pharmacoepidemiologists should have. In addition, one never knows what one will do later in one's own career, nor when one may be called upon to help others with the use of these methods. Part IV concludes the textbook with a collection of "Special Applications" of the field, and speculation about its future, always an important consideration for new investigators in charting a career path.

Pharmacoepidemiology may be maturing, but many exciting opportunities and challenges lie ahead as the field continues to grow and respond to unforeseeable future events. It is our hope that this book can continue to serve as a useful introduction and resource for students of pharmacoepidemiology, both those enrolled in formal classes and those learning in "the real world," who will respond to the challenges that they encounter. Of course, we are always students of our own discipline, and the process of developing this textbook has been educational for us. We hope that this book will also be stimulating and educational for you.

Brian L. Strom, MD, MPH.
Stephen E. Kimmel, MD, MSCE.
Sean Hennessy, PharmD, PhD.
January 2022

# Acknowledgments

There are many individuals and institutions to whom we owe thanks for their contributions to our efforts in preparing this book. Mostly, we would like to thank all of the contributors for the work that they did in revising their book chapters and sections for this textbook and providing case examples, key points, and suggested readings. Over the years, our pharmacoepidemiology work has been supported mostly by numerous grants from government, foundations, and industry. While none of this support was specifically intended to support the development of this book, without this assistance, we would not have been able to support our careers in pharmacoepidemiology. We would like to thank our publisher, John Wiley & Sons, Ltd., for their assistance and insights, both in support of this book, and in support of the field's journal, *Pharmacoepidemiology and Drug Safety*.

John Hemphill's contributions to this book were instrumental, encompassing the role of project manager where he coordinated the entire process of contacting the authors and pulling the book together, while additionally providing editorial assistance.

BLS would like to thank Steve Kimmel and Sean Hennessy for joining him as co-editors. Steve did the bulk of the work on the first edition of this textbook, and Steve and Sean joined BLS as co-editors for the fifth and sixth edition of the parent book, *Pharmacoepidemiology*. These are two very special and talented men. It has been BLS's pleasure to help train them – now, too many years ago – help them cultivate their own careers, and see them blossom into star senior pharmacoepidemiologists. It is wonderful to be able to share with them this book, which has been an important part of BLS's life and career.

BLS would also like to thank his parents, now deceased, for the support and education that were critical to him being successful in his career. BLS would also like to thank the late Paul D. Stolley, M.D., M.P.H. and the late Kenneth L. Melmon, M.D., for their direction, guidance, and inspiration in the formative years of his career. He would also like to thank his trainees, from whom he learns at least as much as he teaches. Last, but certainly not least, BLS would like to thank his family – Lani, Shayna, and Jordi – for accepting the time demands of the book, for tolerating his endless hours working at home (on its earlier editions, for the kids), and for their ever present love and support.

SEK expresses his sincere gratitude to BLS for his almost 30 years as a mentor and colleague and for the chance to work on this book, to SH for all of his years as an amazing colleague, to his parents for providing the foundation for all of his work, and to his family – Alison, David, Benjamin, and Jonathan – for all their support and patience during the many late evenings that SEK worked on the book.

SH also thanks BLS, his longtime friend and career mentor, and all of his students, mentees, and collaborators. Finally, he thanks his parents, and his family – Kristin, Landis, and Bridget – for their love and support.

# Part I

# Introduction to Pharmacoepidemiology

# 1

# What is Pharmacoepidemiology?

*Brian L. Strom*

*Rutgers Biomedical and Health Sciences, Newark, NJ, USA*

> *"A desire to take medicine is, perhaps, the great feature which distinguishes man from other animals."*
>
> Sir William Osler, 1891

## Introduction

In recent decades, modern medicine has been blessed with a pharmaceutical armamentarium that is much more powerful now than it had had before. Although this has given health care providers the ability to provide better medical care for their patients, it has also resulted in the ability to do much greater harm. It has also generated an enormous number of product liability suits against pharmaceutical manufacturers, some appropriate and others inappropriate. In fact, the history of drug regulation parallels the history of major adverse drug reaction (ADR) "disasters." Each change in pharmaceutical law was a political reaction to an epidemic of ADRs. A 1998 study estimated that 100 000 Americans die each year from ADRs, and 1.5 million US hospitalizations each year result from ADRs; yet, 20–70% of ADRs may be preventable. The harm that drugs can cause has also led to the development of the field of pharmacoepidemiology, which is the focus of this book. More recently, the field has expanded its focus to include many issues other than adverse reactions, as well.

To clarify what is, and what is not, included within the discipline of pharmacoepidemiology, this chapter will begin by defining pharmacoepidemiology, differentiating it from other related fields. The history of drug regulation will then be briefly and selectively reviewed, focusing on the US experience as an example, demonstrating how it has led to the development of this new field. Next, the current regulatory process for the approval of new drugs will be reviewed, in order to place the use of pharmacoepidemiology and postmarketing drug surveillance into proper perspective. Finally, the potential scientific and clinical contributions of pharmacoepidemiology will be discussed.

## Definition of Pharmacoepidemiology

*Pharmacoepidemiology* is the study of the use of and the effects of drugs in large numbers of people. The term pharmacoepidemiology obviously contains two components: "pharmaco" and "epidemiology." In order to better appreciate and understand what is and what is not

*Textbook of Pharmacoepidemiology*, Third Edition. Edited by Brian L. Strom, Stephen E. Kimmel, and Sean Hennessy.
© 2022 John Wiley & Sons Ltd. Published 2022 by John Wiley & Sons Ltd.

included in this new field, it is useful to compare its scope to that of other related fields. The scope of pharmacoepidemiology will first be compared to that of clinical pharmacology, and then to that of epidemiology.

## Pharmacoepidemiology Versus Clinical Pharmacology

*Pharmacology* is the study of the effects of drugs. *Clinical pharmacology* is the study of the effects of drugs in humans (see also Chapter 4). Pharmacoepidemiology obviously can be considered, therefore, to fall within clinical pharmacology. In attempting to optimize the use of drugs, one central principle of clinical pharmacology is that therapy should be individualized, or tailored, to the needs of the specific patient at hand. This individualization of therapy requires the determination of a risk/benefit ratio specific to the patient at hand. Doing so requires a prescriber to be aware of the potential beneficial and harmful effects of the drug in question and to know how elements of the patient's clinical status might modify the probability of a good therapeutic outcome. For example, consider a patient with a serious infection, serious liver impairment, and mild impairment of his or her renal function. In considering whether to use gentamicin to treat his infection, it is not sufficient to know that gentamicin has a small probability of causing renal disease. A good clinician should realize that a patient who has impaired liver function is at a greater risk of suffering from this adverse effect than one with normal liver function. Pharmacoepidemiology can be useful in providing information about the beneficial and harmful effects of any drug, thus permitting a better assessment of the risk/benefit balance for the use of any particular drug in any particular patient.

Clinical pharmacology is traditionally divided into two basic areas: pharmacokinetics and pharmacodynamics. *Pharmacokinetics* is the study of the relationship between the dose administered of a drug and the serum or blood level achieved. It deals with drug absorption, distribution, metabolism, and excretion. *Pharmacodynamics* is the study of the relationship between drug level and drug effect. Together, these two fields allow one to predict the effect one might observe in a patient from administering a certain drug regimen. Pharmacoepidemiology encompasses elements of both of these fields, exploring the effects achieved by administering a drug regimen. It does not normally involve or require the measurement of drug levels. However, pharmacoepidemiology can be used to shed light on the pharmacokinetics of a drug when used in clinical practice, such as exploring whether aminophylline is more likely to cause nausea when administered to a patient simultaneously taking cimetidine. However, to date this is a relatively novel application of the field.

Specifically, the field of pharmacoepidemiology has primarily concerned itself with the study of adverse drug effects. Adverse reactions have traditionally been separated into those which are the result of an exaggerated but otherwise usual pharmacologic effect of the drug, sometimes called *Type A reactions*, versus those which are aberrant effects, called *Type B reactions*. Type A reactions tend to be common, dose-related, predictable, and less serious. They can usually be treated by simply reducing the dose of the drug. They tend to occur in individuals who have one of three characteristics. First, the individuals may have received more of a drug than is customarily required. Second, they may have received a conventional amount of the drug, but they may metabolize or excrete the drug unusually slowly, leading to drug levels that are too high (see also Chapter 4). Third, they may have normal drug levels, but for some reason are overly sensitive to them.

In contrast, Type B reactions tend to be uncommon, not related to dose, unpredictable, and potentially more serious. They usually require cessation of the drug. They may be due to what are known as hypersensitivity reactions or immunologic reactions. Alternatively, Type

B reactions may be some other idiosyncratic reaction to the drug, either due to some inherited susceptibility (e.g. glucose-6-phosphate dehydrogenase deficiency) or due to some other mechanism. Regardless, Type B reactions are the most difficult to predict or even detect, and represent the major focus of many pharmacoepidemiologic studies of ADRs.

One typical approach to studying ADRs has been the collection of spontaneous reports of drug-related morbidity or mortality (see Chapter 7), sometimes called pharmacovigilance (although other times that term is used to refer to all of pharmacoepidemiology). However, determining causation in case reports of adverse reactions can be problematic (see Chapter 14), as can attempts to compare the effects of drugs in the same class. Further, drug–drug interactions, predicted based on pharmacokinetic data (see Chapter 4), require massive sample sizes to confirm in people. This has led academic investigators, industry, regulatory bodies, and the legal community to turn to the field of epidemiology. Specifically, *studies of adverse effects* have been supplemented with *studies of adverse events*. In the former, investigators examine case reports of purported ADRs and attempt to make a subjective clinical judgment on an *individual* basis about whether the adverse outcome was actually caused by the antecedent drug exposure. In the latter, controlled studies are performed examining whether the adverse outcome under study occurs more often in an exposed *population* than in an unexposed population. This marriage of the fields of clinical pharmacology and epidemiology has resulted in the development of a field: pharmacoepidemiology.

## Pharmacoepidemiology Versus Epidemiology

Epidemiology is the study of the distribution and determinants of diseases in populations. Since pharmacoepidemiology is the study of the use of and effects of drugs in large numbers of people, it obviously falls within

epidemiology, as well. Epidemiology is also traditionally subdivided into two basic areas. The field began as the study of infectious diseases in large populations, i.e. epidemics. It has since been expanded to encompass the study of chronic diseases. The field of pharmacoepidemiology uses the techniques of chronic disease epidemiology to study the use of and the effects of drugs. Although application of the methods of pharmacoepidemiology can be useful in performing the clinical trials of drugs that are performed before marketing, the major application of these principles is after drug marketing. This has primarily been in the context of postmarketing drug surveillance, although in recent years the interests of pharmacoepidemiologists have broadened considerably. Now, as will be made clearer in future chapters, pharmacoepidemiology is considered of importance in the whole life cycle of a drug, from the time when it is first discovered or synthesized through when it is no longer sold as a drug.

Thus, pharmacoepidemiology is a relatively new applied field, bridging between clinical pharmacology and epidemiology. From clinical pharmacology, pharmacoepidemiology borrows its focus of inquiry. From epidemiology, pharmacoepidemiology borrows its methods of inquiry. In other words, it applies the methods of epidemiology to the content area of clinical pharmacology. In the process, multiple special logistical approaches have been developed and multiple special methodologic issues have arisen. These are the primary foci of this book.

## Historical Background

### Early Legislation

The history of drug regulation in the US is similar to that in most developed countries, and reflects the growing involvement of governments in attempting to assure that only safe and effective drug products were available and that appropriate manufacturing and marketing practices were used. The initial US law, the Pure Food and Drug Act, was passed in 1906, in response to excessive adulteration and misbranding of the food and drugs available at that time. There were no restrictions on sales or requirements for proof of the efficacy or safety of marketed drugs. Rather, the law simply gave the federal government the power to remove from the market any product that was adulterated or misbranded. The burden of proof was on the federal government.

In 1937, over 100 people died from renal failure as a result of the marketing by the Massengill Company of elixir of sulfanilimide dissolved in diethylene glycol. In response, Congress passed the 1938 Food, Drug, and Cosmetic Act. Preclinical toxicity testing was required for the first time. In addition, manufacturers were required to gather clinical data about drug safety and to submit these data to FDA before drug marketing. The FDA had 60 days to object to marketing or else it would proceed. No proof of efficacy was required.

Little attention was paid to ADRs until the early 1950s, when it was discovered that chloramphenicol could cause aplastic anemia. In 1952, the first textbook of ADRs was published. In the same year, the AMA Council on Pharmacy and Chemistry established the first official registry of adverse drug effects, to collect cases of drug-induced blood dyscrasias. In 1960, the FDA began to collect reports of ADRs and sponsored new hospital-based drug monitoring programs. The Johns Hopkins Hospital and the Boston Collaborative Drug Surveillance Program developed the use of in-hospital monitors to perform cohort studies to explore the short-term effects of drugs used in hospitals. This approach was later to be transported to the University of Florida-Shands Teaching Hospital, as well.

In the winter of 1961, the world experienced the infamous "thalidomide disaster." Thalidomide was marketed as a mild hypnotic, and had no obvious advantage over other drugs in its class. Shortly after its marketing, a dramatic increase was seen in the frequency of a previously rare birth defect, phocomelia--the absence of limbs or parts of limbs, sometimes with the presence instead of flippers. Epidemiologic studies established its cause to be in utero exposure to thalidomide. In the United Kingdom, this resulted in the establishment in 1968 of the Committee on Safety of Medicines. Later, the World Health Organization established a bureau to collect and collate information from this and other similar national drug monitoring organizations (see Chapter 7).

The US had never permitted the marketing of thalidomide and, so, was fortunately spared this epidemic. However, the "thalidomide disaster" was so dramatic that it resulted in regulatory change in the US as well. Specifically, in 1962 the Kefauver–Harris Amendments were passed. These amendments strengthened the requirements for proof of drug safety, requiring extensive preclinical pharmacologic and toxicologic testing before a drug could be tested in man. The data from these studies were required to be submitted to the US Food and Drug Administration (FDA) in an Investigational New Drug (IND) application before clinical studies could begin. Three explicit phases of clinical testing were defined, which are described in more detail below. In addition, a new requirement was added to the clinical testing, for "substantial evidence that the drug will have the effect it purports or is represented to have." "Substantial evidence" was defined as "adequate and well-controlled investigations, including clinical investigations." Functionally, this has generally been interpreted as requiring randomized clinical trials to document drug efficacy before marketing. This new procedure also delayed drug marketing until the FDA explicitly gave approval. With some modifications, these are the requirements still in place in the US today. In addition, the amendments required the review of all drugs approved between 1938 and 1962, to determine if they too were efficacious. The resulting DESI (Drug Efficacy Study

Implementation) process, conducted by the National Academy of Sciences' National Research Council with support from a contract from FDA, was not completed until years later, and resulted in the removal from the US market of many ineffective drugs and drug combinations. The result of all these changes was a great prolongation of the approval process, with attendant increases in the cost of drug development, the so-called "drug lag." However, the drugs that are marketed are presumably much safer and more effective.

## Drug Crises and Resulting Regulatory Actions

Despite the more stringent process for drug regulation, subsequent years have seen a series of major ADRs. Subacute myelo-optic-neuropathy (SMON) was found in Japan to be caused by clioquinol, a drug marketed in the early 1930s but not discovered to cause this severe neurological reaction until 1970. In the 1970s, clear cell adenocarcinoma of the cervix and vagina and other genital malformations were found to be due to in utero exposure to diethylstilbestrol two decades earlier. The mid-1970s saw the UK discovery of the oculomucocutaneous syndrome caused by practolol, five years after drug marketing. In 1980, the drug ticrynafen was noted to cause deaths from liver disease. In 1982, benoxaprofen was noted to do the same. Subsequently the use of zomepirac, another nonsteroidal anti-inflammatory drug, was noted to be associated with an increased risk of anaphylactoid reactions. Serious blood dyscrasias were linked to phenylbutazone. Small intestinal perforations were noted to be caused by a particular slow release formulation of indomethacin. Bendectin[R], a combination product indicated to treat nausea and vomiting in pregnancy, was removed from the market because of litigation claiming it was a teratogen, despite the absence of valid scientific evidence to justify this claim (see "Research on the effects of medications in pregnancy and in children" in Chapter 23). Acute flank pain and reversible acute renal failure were noted to be caused by suprofen. Isotretinoin was almost removed from the US market because of the birth defects it causes. The Eosinophilia-Myalgia syndrome was linked to a particular brand of L-tryptophan. Triazolam, thought by the Netherlands in 1979 to be subject to a disproportionate number of central nervous system side effects, was discovered by the rest of the world to be problematic in the early 1990s. Silicone breast implants, inserted by the millions in the US for cosmetic purposes, were accused of causing cancer, rheumatologic disease, and many other problems, and restricted from use except for breast reconstruction after mastectomy. Human insulin was marketed as one of the first of the new biotechnology drugs, but soon thereafter was accused of causing a disproportionate amount of hypoglycemia. Fluoxetine was marketed as a major new important and commercially successful psychiatric product, but then lost a large part of its market due to accusations about its association with suicidal ideation. An epidemic of deaths from asthma in New Zealand was traced to fenoterol, and later data suggested that similar, although smaller, risks might be present with other beta-agonist inhalers. The possibility was raised of cancer from depot-medroxyprogesterone, resulting in initial refusal to allow its marketing for this purpose in the US, then multiple studies, and ultimate approval. Arrhythmias were linked to the use of the antihistamines terfenadine and astemizole. Hypertension, seizures, and strokes were noted from postpartum use of bromocriptine. Multiple different adverse reactions were linked to temafloxacin. Other examples include liver toxicity from amoxicillin-clavulanic acid; liver toxicity from bromfenac; cancer, myocardial infarction, and gastrointestinal bleeding from calcium channel blockers; arrhythmias with cisapride interactions; primary pulmonary hypertension and cardiac valvular disease from dexfenfluramine and fenfluramine;

gastrointestinal bleeding, postoperative bleeding, deaths, and many other adverse reactions associated with ketorolac; multiple drug interactions with mibefradil; thrombosis from newer oral contraceptives; myocardial infarction from sildenafil; seizures with tramadol; anaphylactic reactions from vitamin K; liver toxicity from troglitazone; and intussusception from rotavirus vaccine.

Later drug crises have occurred due to allegations of ischemic colitis from alosetron; rhabdomyolysis from cerivastatin; bronchospasm from rapacuronium; torsades de pointes from ziprasidone; hemorrhagic stroke from phenylpropanolamine; arthralgia, myalgia, and neurologic conditions from Lyme vaccine; multiple joint and other symptoms from anthrax vaccine; myocarditis and myocardial infarction from smallpox vaccine; and heart attack and stroke from rofecoxib.

Major ADRs continue to plague new drugs, and in fact are as common if not more common in the last several decades. In total, 36 different oral prescription drug products have been removed from the US market, since 1980 alone (alosetron-2000, aprotinin-2007, astemizole-1999, benoxaprofen-1982, bromfenac-1998, cerivastatin-2001, cisapride-2000, dexfenfluramine-1997, efalizumab-2009, encainide-1991, etretinate-1998, fenfluramine-1998, flosequinan-1993, grepafloxin-1999, levomethadyl-2003, lumiracoxib-2007, mibefradil-1998, natalizumab-2005, nomifensine-1986, palladone-2005, pamoline-2005, pergolide-2010, phenylpropanolamine-2000, propoxyphene-2010, rapacuronium-2001, rimonabant-2010, rofecoxib-2004, sibutramine-2010, suprofen-1987, tegaserod-2007, terfenadine-1998, temafloxacin-1992, ticrynafen-1980, troglitazone-2000, valdecoxib-2007, zomepirac 1983). The licensed vaccines against rotavirus and Lyme were also withdrawn because of safety concerns (see "Special methodological issues in pharmacoepidemiologic studies of vaccine safety" in Chapter 23). Further, between 1990 and 2004, at least 15 non-cardiac drugs including astemizole, cisapride, droperidol, grepafloxacin, halofantrine, pimozide, propoxyphene, rofecoxib, sertindole, sibutramine terfenadine, terodiline, thioridazine, vevacetylmethadol, and ziprasidone, were subject to significant regulatory actions because of cardiac concerns.

Since 1993, trying to deal with drug safety problems, FDA morphed its extant spontaneous reporting system into the MedWatch program of collecting spontaneous reports of adverse reactions (see Chapter 7), as part of that issuing monthly notifications of label changes. Compared to the 20–25 safety-related label changes that were being made every month by mid-1999, between 19 and 57 safety-related label changes (boxed warnings, warnings, contraindications, precautions, adverse events) were made every month in 2009. From January of 2010 to July of 2016, there were 3324 safety-related label changes. The range of safety-related label changes per month was 19–87 (median of 41). Among all safety-related label changes (January of 2010 to July of 2016), 8, 13, 56, and 65% were boxed warnings, contraindications, warnings, and precautions, respectively.

According to a study from a number of years ago by the US Government Accountability Office, 51% of approved drugs have serious adverse effects not detected before approval. Further, there is recognition that the initial dose recommended for a newly marketed drug is often incorrect, and needs monitoring and modification after marketing.

In some of the examples above, the drug was never convincingly linked to the adverse reaction, yet many of these accusations led to the removal of the drug involved from the market. Interestingly, however, this withdrawal was not necessarily performed in all of the different countries in which each drug was marketed. Most of these discoveries have led to litigation, as well, and a few have even led to criminal charges against the pharmaceutical manufacturer and/or some of its employees (see Chapter 6).

## Legislative Actions Resulting from Drug Crises

Through the 1980s, there was concern that an underfunded FDA was approving drugs too slowly, and that the US suffered, compared to Europe, from a "drug lag." To provide additional resources to the FDA to help expedite the drug review and approval process, in 1992 Congress passed the Prescription Drug User Fee Act (PDUFA), allowing the FDA to charge manufacturers a fee for reviewing New Drug Applications. This legislation was reauthorized by Congress three more times: PDUFA II, also called the Food and Drug Modernization Act of 1997; PDUFA III, also called the Public Health Security and Bioterrorism Preparedness and Response Act of 2002; and PDUFA IV, also called the Food and Drug Administration Amendments (FDAAA-PL 110-85) of 2007. The goals for PDUFA I, II, III, and IV was to enable the FDA to complete the review of over 90% of priority drug applications in 6 months, and complete the review of over 90% of standard drug applications in 12 months (under PDUFA I) or 10 months (under PDUFA II, III, and IV). In addition to reauthorizing the collection of user fees from the pharmaceutical industry, PDUFA II allowed the FDA to accept a single well-controlled clinical study under certain conditions, to reduce drug development time. The result was a system where more than 550 new drugs were approved by the FDA in the 1990s.

However, whereas 1400 FDA employees in 1998 worked with the drug approval process, only 52 monitored safety; FDA spent only $2.4 million in extramural safety research. This state of affairs has coincided with the growing numbers of drug crises cited above. With successive reauthorizations of PDUFA, this markedly changed. PDUFA III allowed the FDA for the first time to use a small portion of the user fees for post-marketing drug safety monitoring, to address safety concerns.

However, there was now growing concern, in Congress and the US public, that perhaps the FDA was approving drugs too *fast*. There were also calls for the development of an independent drug safety board, analogous to the National Transportation Safety Board, with a mission much wider than FDA's regulatory mission, to complement the latter. For example, such a board could investigate drug safety crises such as those cited above, looking for ways to prevent them, and could deal with issues such as improper physician use of drugs, the need for training, and the development of new approaches to the field of pharmacoepidemiology.

Recurrent concerns about the FDA's management of postmarketing drug safety issues led to a systematic review of the entire drug risk assessment process. In 2006, the US General Accountability Office issued its report of a review of the organizational structure and effectiveness of FDA's postmarketing drug safety decision-making, followed in 2007 by the Institute of Medicine's independent assessment. Important weaknesses were noted in the current system, including the failure of the FDA's Office of New Drugs and Office of Drug Safety to communicate with each other on safety issues, the failure of the FDA to track ongoing postmarketing studies, the ambiguous role of the FDA's Office of Drug Safety in scientific advisory committees, the limited authority by the FDA to require the pharmaceutical industry to perform studies to obtain needed data, concerns about culture problems at the FDA where recommendations by members of the FDA's drug safety staff were not followed, and concerns about conflict of interest involving advisory committee members. This Institute of Medicine report was influential in shaping PDUFA IV.

Indeed, with the passage of PDUFA IV, the authority of the FDA was substantially increased, with the ability, for example, to require postmarketing studies and levy heavy fines if these requirements were not met. Further, its resources were substantially increased, with a specific charge to (i) fund epidemiology best practices and data acquisition

($7 million in fiscal 2008, increasing to $9.5 million in fiscal 2012), (ii) fund new drug trade name review ($5.3 million in fiscal 2008, rising to $6.5 million in fiscal 2012), and (iii) fund risk management and communication ($4 million in fiscal 2008, rising to $5 million in fiscal 2012) (see also "Risk management" in Chapter 23). In addition, in another use of the new PDUFA funds, the FDA plans to develop and implement agency-wide and special-purpose postmarket IT systems, including the MedWatch Plus Portal, the FDA Adverse Event Reporting System, the Sentinel System (a virtual national medical product safety system), and the Phonetic and Orthographic Computer Analysis System to find similarities in spelling or sound between proposed proprietary drug names that might increase the risk of confusion and medication errors.

FDASIA, the fifth authorization of the PDUFA, expanded the authority of the US FDA with the ability to safeguard and advance public health by: (i) "giving the authority to collect user fees from industry to fund reviews of innovator drugs, medical devices, generic drugs and biosimilar biological products"; (ii) "promoting innovation to speed patient access to safe and effective products"; (iii) "increasing stakeholder involvement in FDA processes", and (iv) "enhancing the safety of the drug supply chain." Also enacted in 2012, GDUFA permitted the FDA to assess industry user fees with the intention of increasing the predictability and timeliness of generic drug applications reviews. The Biosimilar User Fee Act (BsUFA), also enacted in 2012, authorized the FDA to collect fees directly from biosimilar drug product applicants to expedite the review of biosimilar applications. The FDA Reauthorization Act of 2017 (FDARA), reauthorized PDUFA, GDUFA, and BsUFA through fiscal year 2022.

Among other things, the twenty-first century Cures Act (enacted in December 2016 in the United States) was intended to expedite the process by which new drugs and devices are approved by easing the requirements put on drug companies looking for FDA approval on new products or new indications on existing drugs. It calls for the use of "data summaries" to support the approval of certain drugs for new indications, rather than full clinical trial data. It will also allow drug companies to promote off-label uses to insurance companies, allowing them to expand their markets. Of particular relevance to pharmacoepidemiology, it permitted the use of "real world evidence" rather than full clinical trial results. Depending on how these new rules are interpreted, this could massively change drug development in the US, and in particular the role of pharmacoepidemiology in that drug development.

## Intellectual Development of Pharmacoepidemiology Emerging from Drug Crises

Several developments of the 1960s can be thought to have marked the beginning of the field of pharmacoepidemiology. The Kefauver-Harris Amendments that were introduced in 1962 required formal safety studies for new drug applications. The DESI program that was undertaken by the FDA as part of the Kefauver-Harris Amendments required formal efficacy studies for old drugs that were approved earlier. These requirements created the demand for new expertise and new methods. In addition, the mid-1960s saw the publication of a series of drug utilization studies. These studies provided the first descriptive information on how physicians use drugs, and began a series of investigations of the frequency and determinants of poor prescribing (see also "Evaluating and improving prescribing" in Chapter 23).

In part in response to concerns about adverse drug effects, the early 1970s saw the development of the Drug Epidemiology Unit, now the Slone Epidemiology Center, which extended the hospital-based approach of the Boston Collaborative Drug Surveillance Program by collecting lifetime drug exposure histories from hospitalized patients and using these to perform hospital-based case–control studies.

The year 1976 saw the formation of the Joint Commission on Prescription Drug Use, an interdisciplinary committee of experts charged with reviewing the state of the art of pharmacoepidemiology at that time, as well as providing recommendations for the future. The Computerized Online Medicaid Analysis and Surveillance System (COMPASS®) was first developed in 1977, using Medicaid billing data to perform pharmacoepidemiologic studies (see Chapter 9). The Drug Surveillance Research Unit, now called the Drug Safety Research Trust, was developed in the United Kingdom in 1980, with its innovative system of Prescription Event Monitoring. Each of these represented major contributions to the field of pharmacoepidemiology. These and newer approaches are reviewed in Part II of this book.

In the examples of drug crises mentioned above, these were serious but uncommon drug effects, and these experiences have led to an accelerated search for new methods to study drug effects in large numbers of patients. This led to a shift from adverse effect studies to adverse event studies, with concomitant increasing use of new data resources and new methods to study adverse reactions. The American Society for Clinical Pharmacology and Therapeutics issued, in 1990, a position paper on the use of purported postmarketing drug surveillance studies for promotional purposes, and the International Society for Pharmacoepidemiology (ISPE) issued, in 1996, Guidelines for Good Epidemiology Practices for Drug, Device, and Vaccine Research in the United States, which were updated in 2007. Since the late 1990s, pharmacoepidemiologic research has also been increasingly burdened by concerns about patient confidentiality (see also Chapter 16).

There is also increasing recognition that most of the risk from most drugs to most patients occurs from known reactions to old drugs. As an attempt to address concerns about underuse, overuse, and adverse events of medical products and medical errors that may cause serious impairment to patient health, a new program of Centers for Education and Research on Therapeutics (CERTs) was authorized under the FDA Modernization Act of 1997 (as part of the same legislation that reauthorized PDUFA II described earlier). Starting in 1999 and incrementally adding more centers in 2002, 2006, and 2007, the Agency for Healthcare Research and Quality (AHRQ) that was selected to administer this program had funded up to 14 Centers for Education and Research on Therapeutics (CERTs), although this program ended in 2016 (see also Chapter 6).

The research and education activities sponsored by AHRQ through the CERTs program since the late 1990s take place in academic centers. These CERTs centers conduct research on therapeutics, exploring new uses of drugs, ways to improve the effective uses of drugs, and the risks associated with new uses or combinations of drugs. They also develop educational modules and materials for disseminating the research findings about medical products. With the development of direct-to-consumer advertising of drugs since the mid 1980s in the US, the CERTs' role in educating the public and health care professionals by providing evidence-based information has become especially important.

Another impetus for research on drugs resulted from one of the mandates (in Section 1013) of the Medicare Prescription Drug, Improvement, and Modernization Act of 2003 to provide beneficiaries with scientific information on the outcomes, comparative clinical effectiveness, and appropriateness of health care items and services. In response, the AHRQ created in 2005 the DEcIDE (Developing Evidence to Inform Decisions about Effectiveness) Network to support in academic settings the conduct of studies on effectiveness, safety, and usefulness of drugs and other treatments and services. This, too ended in 2012.

Another major new initiative of close relevance to pharmacoepidemiology is risk management. There is increasing recognition that the risk/benefit balance of some drugs can only be considered acceptable with active management of their use, to maximize their efficacy and/or minimize their risk. In response, in the late 1990s, there were new initiatives underway, ranging from FDA requirements for risk management plans, to a FDA Drug Safety and Risk Management Advisory Committee, and issuing risk minimization and management guidances in 2005 (see Chapters 6 and 23).

Another initiative closely related to pharmacoepidemiology is the Patient Safety movement. In the Institute of Medicine's report, "To Err is Human: Building a Safer Health System," the authors note that: (i) "even apparently single events or errors are due most often to the convergence of multiple contributing factors," (ii) "preventing errors and improving safety for patients requires a systems approach in order to modify the conditions that contribute to errors," and (iii) "the problem is not bad people; the problem is that the system needs to be made safer." In this framework, the concern is not about substandard or negligent care, but rather, is about errors made by even the best trained, brightest, and most competent professional health caregivers and/or patients. From this perspective, the important research questions ask about the conditions under which people make errors, the types of errors being made, and the types of systems that can be put into place to prevent errors altogether when possible. Errors that are not prevented must be identified and corrected efficiently and quickly, before they inflict harm. Turning specifically to medications, from 2.4 to 6.5% of hospitalized patients suffer ADEs, prolonging hospital stays by two days, and increase costs by $2000–2600 per patient. Over 7000 US deaths were attributed to medication errors in 1993. Although these estimates have been disputed, the overall importance of reducing these errors has not been questioned. In recognition of this problem, AHRQ launched a major new grant program of over 100 projects,

at its peak with over $50 million/year of funding. While only a portion of this is dedicated to medication errors, they are clearly a focus of interest and relevance to many (see "The pharmacoepidemiology of medication errors" in Chapter 23).

The 1990s and especially the 2000s have seen another shift in the field, away from its exclusive emphasis on drug utilization and adverse reactions, to the inclusion of other interests as well, such as the use of pharmacoepidemiology to study beneficial drug effects, the application of health economics to the study of drug effects, studies of patient engagement and patient reported outcomes, meta-analysis, etc. These new foci are discussed in more detail in Part III of this book.

Also, with the publication of the results from the Women's Health Initiative indicating that combination hormone replacement therapy causes an increased risk of myocardial infarction rather than a decreased risk, there has been increased concern about reliance solely on nonexperimental methods to study drug safety after marketing. This has led to increased use of massive randomized clinical trials as part of postmarketing surveillance (see Chapter 17). This is especially important because often the surrogate markers used for drug development cannot necessarily be relied upon to map completely to true clinical outcomes.

Finally, with the advent of the Obama administration in the US, there was enormous interest in comparative effectiveness research (CER). CER was defined in 2009 by the Federal Coordinating Council for Comparative Effectiveness Research as "the conduct and synthesis of research comparing the benefits and harms of different interventions and strategies to prevent, diagnose, treat, and monitor health conditions in "real world" settings. The purpose of this research is to improve health outcomes by developing and disseminating evidence-based information to patients, clinicians, and other decision-makers, responding to their expressed needs, about which interventions are most effective for which patients under specific circumstances." By this definition, CER includes three key elements: (i) evidence synthesis, (ii) evidence generation, and (iii) evidence dissemination. Typically, CER is conducted through observational studies of either large administrative or medical record databases (see Part II), or large naturalistic clinical trials (see Chapter 17). In many ways, the UK has been focusing on CER for years, with its National Institute for Health and Clinical Excellence (NICE), an independent organization responsible for providing national guidance on promoting good health and preventing and treating ill health. However, the Obama administration included $1.1 billion for CER in its federal stimulus package, and has plans for hundreds of millions of dollars of support per year thereafter. While CER does not overlap completely with pharmacoepidemiology, the scientific approaches are very close. Pharmacoepidemiologists evaluate the use and effects of medications. CER investigators compare, in the real world, the safety and benefits of one treatment compared to another. CER extends beyond pharmacoepidemiology in that CER can include more than just drugs; pharmacoepidemiology extends beyond CER in that it includes studies comparing exposed to unexposed patients, not just alternative exposures. However, to date, most work done in CER has been done in pharmacoepidemiology.

# The Current Drug Approval Process

## Drug Approval in the US

Since the mid-1990s, there has been a decline in the number of novel drugs approved per year, while the cost of bringing a drug to market has risen sharply. The total cost of drug development to the pharmaceutical industry increased from $24 billion in 1999, to $32 billion in 2002, and to $65.2 billion on research and development in 2008. The cost to discover

and develop a drug that successfully reached the market rose from over $800 million in 2004 to an estimated $1.3 billion to 1.7 billion currently. In addition to the sizeable costs of research and development, a substantial part of this total cost is determined also by the regulatory requirement to test new drugs during several pre-marketing and post-marketing phases, as will be reviewed next.

The current drug approval process in the US and most other developed countries includes preclinical animal testing followed by three phases of clinical testing. Phase I testing is usually conducted in just a few normal volunteers, and represents the initial trials of the drug in humans. Phase I trials are generally conducted by clinical pharmacologists, to determine the metabolism of the drug in humans, a safe dosage range in humans, and to exclude any extremely common toxic reactions which are unique to humans.

Phase II testing is also generally conducted by clinical pharmacologists, on a small number of patients who have the target disease. Phase II testing is usually the first time patients are exposed to the drug. Exceptions are drugs that are so toxic that it would not normally be considered ethical to expose healthy individuals to them, like cytotoxic drugs. For these, patients are used for Phase I testing as well. The goals of Phase II testing are to obtain more information on the pharmacokinetics of the drug and on any relatively common adverse reactions, and to obtain initial information on the possible efficacy of the drug. Specifically, Phase II is used to determine the daily dosage and regimen to be tested more rigorously in Phase III.

Phase III testing is performed by clinician-investigators in a much larger number of patients, in order to rigorously evaluate a drug's efficacy and to provide more information on its toxicity. At least one of the Phase III studies needs to be a randomized clinical trial (see Chapter 17). To meet FDA standards, at least one of the randomized clinical trials usually needs to be conducted in the US. Generally between 500 and 3000 patients are exposed to a drug during Phase III, even if drug efficacy can be demonstrated with much smaller numbers, in order to be able to detect less common adverse reactions. For example, a study including 3000 patients would allow one to be 95% certain of detecting any adverse reactions that occur in at least one exposed patient out of 1000. At the other extreme, a total of 500 patients would allow one to be 95% certain of detecting any adverse reactions which occur in six or more patients out of every 1000 exposed. Adverse reactions which occur less commonly than these are less likely to be detected in these premarketing studies. The sample sizes needed to detect drug effects are discussed in more detail in Chapter 4. Nowadays, with the increased focus on drug safety, premarketing dossiers are sometimes being extended well beyond 3000 patients. However, as one can tell from the sample size calculations in Chapter 3 and Appendix A, by itself these larger numbers gain little additional information about ADRs, unless one were to increase to perhaps 30 000 patients, well beyond the scope of most premarketing studies.

Finally, Phase IV testing is the evaluation of the effects of drugs after general marketing. The bulk of this book, is devoted to such efforts.

## Drug Approval in Other Countries

Outside the US, national systems for the regulation and approval of new drugs vary greatly, even among developed countries and especially between developed and developing countries. While in most developed countries, at least, the general process of drug development is very analogous to that in the US, the implementation varies widely. A WHO comparative analysis of drug regulation in 10 countries found that not all countries even have a written national drug policy document. Regulation of medicines in some countries is centralized in a single agency that performs the gamut of functions involving product registration, licensing, product review, approval for clinical trials, postmarketing surveillance, and inspection of manufacturing practice. Examples for this are Health Canada, the China Food and Drug Administration (CFDA), the Medicines Agency in Denmark, the Medicines Agency in Norway, the Center for Drug Administration in Singapore and the Medicines & Medical Devices Safety Authority in New Zealand. In other countries, regulatory functions are distributed among different agencies. An example of the latter is The Netherlands, where the Ministry of Health, Welfare & Sports performs the functions of licensing; the Healthcare Inspectorate checks on general manufacturing practice; and the Medicines Evaluation Board performs the functions of product assessment and registration and ADR monitoring. As another example, in Singapore, two independent agencies (the Center for Pharmaceutical Administration and the Center for Drug Evaluation) were previously responsible for medicinal regulation and evaluation, but are currently merged into a single agency (the Center for Drug Administration). Another dimension on which countries may vary is the degree of autonomy of regulatory decisions from political influence. Drug regulation in most countries is performed by a department within the executive branch (Australia, Cuba, Cyprus, Tunisia, and Venezuela are examples cited by the WHO report, and Denmark, India, and New Zealand are other examples). In other countries, this function is performed by an independent commission or board. An example of the latter arrangement is The Netherlands, where members of the Medicines Evaluation Board are appointed directly by the Crown, thereby enabling actions that are independent of interference by other government authorities, such as the Minister of Health. All 10 countries examined by the WHO require registration of pharmaceutical products, but they differ on the documentation requirements for evidence of safety and efficacy. Some countries carry out independent assessments while others, especially many developing countries, rely on WHO assessments or other sources. With the exception of Cyprus, the remaining nine countries surveyed by the WHO were found to regulate the conduct of clinical trials, but with varying rates of participation of health care professionals in reporting ADRs. Another source noted that countries also differ on the extent of emphasis on quantitative or qualitative analysis for assessing pre-and post-marketing data.

Further, within Europe, each country has its own regulatory agency, e.g. the United Kingdom's Medicines and Healthcare Products Regulatory Agency (MHRA), formed in 2003 as a merger of the Medicines Control Agency (MCA) and the Medical Devices Agency (MDA). In addition, since January 1998, some drug registration and approval within the European Union has shifted away from the national licensing authorities of the EU members to that of the centralized authority of the European Medicines Evaluation Agency (EMEA), which was established in 1993. To facilitate this centralized approval process, the EMEA pushed for harmonization of drug approvals. While the goals of harmonization are to create a single pharmaceutical market in Europe and to shorten approval times, concerns were voiced that harmonized safety standards would lower the stricter standards that were favored by some countries such as Sweden, for example, and would compromise patient safety. Now called the European Medicines Agency (EMA), the EMA is a decentralized body of the European Union, responsible for the scientific evaluation and supervision of medicines. These functions are performed by the EMA's Committee for Medicinal Products for Human Use (CHMP). EMA authorization to market a drug is valid in all European Union countries, but individual national medicines agencies are responsible for monitoring the safety of approved drugs and sharing this information with the EMA.

# Potential Contributions of Pharmacoepidemiology

The potential contributions of pharmacoepidemiology are now well recognized, even though the field is still relatively new. However, some contributions are already apparent (see Table 1.1). In fact, in the 1970s the FDA requested postmarketing research at the time of approval for about one third of drugs, compared to over 70% in the 1990s. Now, since the passage of the Food, and Drug Administration Amendments Act of 2007 (FDAAA-PL 110-85) noted above, the FDA has the right to require such studies be completed. In this section of this chapter, we will first review the potential for pharmacoepidemiologic studies to supplement the information available prior to marketing, and then review the new types of information obtainable from postmarketing

**Table 1.1** Potential contributions of pharmacoepidemiology.

---

A) Information which supplements the information available from premarketing studies – better quantitation of the incidence of known adverse and beneficial effects

1) Higher precision

2) In patients not studied prior to marketing, e.g. the elderly, children, pregnant women

3) As modified by other drugs and other illnesses

4) Relative to other drugs used for the same indications

B) New types of information not available from premarketing studies

1) Discovery of previously undetected adverse and beneficial effects

    i) Uncommon effects

    ii) Delayed effects

2) Patterns of drug utilization

3) The effects of drug overdoses

4) The economic implications of drug use

C) General contributions of pharmacoepidemiology

1) Reassurances about drug safety

2) Fulfillment of ethical and legal obligations

---

pharmacoepidemiologic studies but not obtainable prior to drug marketing. Finally, we will review the general, and probably most important, potential contributions such studies can make. In each case, the relevant information available from premarketing studies will be briefly examined first, to clarify how postmarketing studies can supplement this information.

## Supplementary Information

Premarketing studies of drug effects are necessarily limited in size. After marketing, nonexperimental epidemiologic studies can be performed, evaluating the effects of drugs administered as part of ongoing medical care. These allow the cost-effective accumulation of much larger numbers of patients than those studied prior to marketing, resulting in a more precise measurement of the incidence of adverse and beneficial drug effects (see Chapter 3). For example, at the time of drug marketing, prazosin was known to cause a dose-dependent first dose syncope, but the FDA requested the manufacturer to conduct a postmarketing surveillance study of the drug in the US to quantitate its incidence more precisely. In recent years, there has even been an attempt, in selected special cases, to release selected critically important drugs more quickly, by taking advantage of the work that can be performed after marketing. Probably the best-known early example was zidovudine. More recently, this has been the case with a number of cancer drugs, including at least one where initial expectations of efficacy were not confirmed in definitive trials after marketing, and then proven again later in a subgroup, leading to the product being removed from the market and then marketed again. As noted above, the increased sample size available after marketing also permits a more precise determination of the correct dose to be used.

Premarketing studies also tend to be very artificial. Important subgroups of patients are not typically included in studies conducted before drug marketing, usually for ethical reasons. Examples include the elderly, children, and pregnant women. Studies of the effects of drugs in these populations generally must await studies conducted after drug marketing (see also "Research on the effects of medications in pregnancy and in children" in Chapter 23).

Additionally, for reasons of statistical efficiency, premarketing clinical trials generally seek subjects who are as homogeneous as possible, in order to reduce unexplained variability in the outcome variables measured and increase the probability of detecting a difference between the study groups, if one truly exists. For these reasons, certain patients are often excluded, including those with other illnesses or those who are receiving other drugs. Postmarketing studies can explore how factors such as other illnesses and other drugs might modify the effects of the drugs, as well as looking at the effects of differences in drug regimen, adherence, etc. For example, after marketing, the ophthalmic preparation of timolol was noted to cause many serious episodes of heart block and asthma, resulting in over 10 deaths. These effects were not detected prior to marketing, as patients with underlying cardiovascular or respiratory disease were excluded from the premarketing studies.

Finally, to obtain approval to market a drug, a manufacturer needs to evaluate its overall safety and efficacy, but does not need to evaluate its safety and efficacy relative to any other drugs available for the same indication. To the contrary, with the exception of illnesses that could not ethically be treated with placebos, such as serious infections and malignancies, it is generally considered preferable, or even mandatory, to have studies with placebo controls. There are a number of reasons for this preference. First, it is easier to show that a new drug is more effective than a placebo than to show it is more effective than another effective drug. Second, one cannot actually prove that a new drug is as effective as a standard drug.

A study showing a new drug is no worse than another effective drug does not provide assurance that it is better than a placebo; one simply could have failed to detect that it was in fact worse than the standard drug. One could require a demonstration that a new drug is more effective than another effective drug, but this is a standard that does not and should not have to be met. Yet, optimal medical care requires information on the effects of a drug relative to the alternatives available for the same indication. This information must often await studies conducted after drug marketing.

## New Types of Information Not Available from Premarketing Studies

As mentioned above, premarketing studies are necessarily limited in size (see also Chapter 3). The additional sample size available in postmarketing studies permits the study of drug effects that may be uncommon, but important, such as drug-induced agranulocytosis.

Premarketing studies are also necessarily limited in time; they must come to an end, or the drug could never be marketed. In contrast, postmarketing studies permit the study of delayed drug effects, such as the unusual clear cell adenocarcinoma of the vagina and cervix, which occurred two decades later in women exposed in utero to diethylstilbestrol.

The patterns of physician prescribing and patient drug utilization often cannot be predicted prior to marketing, despite pharmaceutical manufacturers' best attempts to predict when planning for drug marketing. Studies of how a drug is actually being used, and determinants of changes in these usage patterns, can only be performed after drug marketing (see "Studies of drug utilization" and "Evaluating and improving prescribing" in Chapter 23).

In most cases, premarketing studies are performed using selected patients who are closely observed. Rarely are there any significant overdoses in this population. Thus, the study of the effects of a drug when ingested in extremely high doses is rarely possible before drug marketing. Again, this must await postmarketing pharmacoepidemiologic studies.

Finally, it is only in the past decade or two that pharmacoepidemiologists have become more sensitive to the costs of medical care, and the techniques of health economics been applied to evaluate the cost implications of drug use. It is clear that the exploration of the costs of drug use requires consideration of more than just the costs of the drugs themselves. The costs of a drug's adverse effects may be substantially higher than the cost of the drug itself, if these adverse effects result in additional medical care and possibly even hospitalizations. Conversely, a drug's beneficial effects could reduce the need for medical care, resulting in savings that can be much larger than the cost of the drug itself. As with studies of drug utilization, the economic implications of drug use can be predicted prior to marketing, but can only be rigorously studied after marketing (see Chapter 18).

## General Contributions of Pharmacoepidemiology

Lastly, it is important to review the general contributions that can be made by pharmacoepidemiology. As an academic or a clinician, one is most interested in the new information about drug effects and drug costs that can be gained from pharmacoepidemiology. Certainly, these are the findings that receive the greatest public and political attention. However, often no new information is obtained, particularly about new adverse drug effects. This is not a disappointing outcome, but in fact, a very reassuring one, and this reassurance about drug safety is one of the most important contributions that can be made by pharmacoepidemiologic studies. Related to this is the reassurance that the sponsor of the study, whether manufacturer or regulator, is fulfilling its organizational duty ethically and responsibly by looking for any undiscovered problems which may be there. In an era of product liability litigation, this is an important assurance. One cannot change whether a drug causes an adverse reaction, and the fact that it does will hopefully eventually become evident. What can be changed is the perception about whether a manufacturer did everything possible to detect it and was not negligent in its behavior.

## Key Points

- *Pharmacoepidemiology* is the study of the use of and the effects of drugs and other medical devices in large numbers of people. It uses the methods of epidemiology to study the content area of clinical pharmacology.

- The history of pharmacoepidemiology is a history of increasingly frequent accusations about ADRs, often arising out of the spontaneous reporting system, followed by formal studies proving or disproving those associations.
- The drug approval process is inherently limited, so it cannot detect before marketing adverse effects that are uncommon, delayed, unique to high risk populations, due to misuse of the drugs by prescribers or patients, etc.
- Pharmacoepidemiology can contribute information about drug safety and effectiveness that is not available from premarketing studies.

## Further Reading

Califf, R.M. (2002). The need for a national infrastructure to improve the rational use of therapeutics. *Pharmacoepidemiol. Drug Saf.* 11: 319–327.

Caranasos, G.J., Stewart, R.B., and Cluff, L.E. (1974). Drug-induced illness leading to hospitalization. *JAMA* 228: 713–717.

Cluff, L.E., Thornton, G.F., and Seidl, L.G. (1964). Studies on the epidemiology of adverse drug reactions I. Methods of surveillance. *JAMA* 188: 976–983.

Crane, J., Pearce, N., Flatt, A. et al. (1989). Prescribed fenoterol and death from asthma in New Zealand, 1981–1983: case–control study. *Lancet* 1: 917–922.

Erslev, A.J. and Wintrobe, M.M. (1962). Detection and prevention of drug induced blood dyscrasias. *JAMA* 181: 114–119.

Geiling, E.M.K. and Cannon, P.R. (1938). Pathogenic effects of elixir of sulfanilimide (diethylene glycol) poisoning. *JAMA* 111: 919–926.

Herbst, A.L., Ulfelder, H., and Poskanzer, D.C. (1971). Adenocarcinoma of the vagina: association of maternal stilbestrol therapy with tumor appearance in young women. *N. Engl. J. Med.* 284: 878–881.

ISPE (2008). Guidelines for good pharmacoepidemiology practices (GPP). *Pharmacoepidemiol. Drug Saf.* 17: 200–208.

Joint Commission on Prescription Drug Use (1980) *Final Report*. Washington, DC.

Kimmel, S.E., Keane, M.G., Crary, J.L. et al. (1999). Detailed examination of fenfluramine-phentermine users with valve abnormalities identified in Fargo, North Dakota. *Am. J. Cardiol.* 84: 304–308.

Kono, R. (1980). Trends and lessons of SMON research. In: *Drug-Induced Sufferings* (ed. T. Soda), 11. Princeton, NJ: Excerpta Medica.

Lazarou, J., Pomeranz, B.H., and Corey, P.N. (1998). Incidence of adverse drug reactions in hospitalized patients: a meta-analysis of prospective studies. *JAMA* 279: 1200–1205.

Lenz, W. (1966). Malformations caused by drugs in pregnancy. *Am. J. Dis. Child.* 112: 99–106.

Meyler, L. (1952). *Side Effects of Drugs*. Amsterdam: Elsevier.

Miller, R.R. and Greenblatt, D.J. (1976). *Drug Effects in Hospitalized Patients*. New York: John Wiley & Sons, Inc.

Rawlins, M.D. and Thompson, J.W. (1977). Pathogenesis of adverse drug reactions.

In: *Textbook of Adverse Drug Reactions* (ed. D.M. Davies), 44. Oxford: Oxford University Press.

Strom, B.L. (1990). Members of the ASCPT pharmacoepidemiology section. Position paper on the use of purported postmarketing drug surveillance studies for promotional purposes. *Clin. Pharmacol. Ther.* 48: 598.

Strom, B.L., Berlin, J.A., Kinman, J.L. et al. (1996). Parenteral ketorolac and risk of gastrointestinal and operative site bleeding: a postmarketing surveillance study. *JAMA* 275: 376–382.

Wallerstein, R.O., Condit, P.K., Kasper, C.K. et al. (1969). Statewide study of chloramphenicol therapy and fatal aplastic anemia. *JAMA* 208: 2045–2050.

Wright, P. (1975). Untoward effects associated with practolol administration. Oculomucocutaneous syndrome. *BMJ* 1: 595–598.

# 2

# Study Designs Available for Pharmacoepidemiologic Studies

*Brian L. Strom*

*Rutgers Biomedical and Health Sciences, Newark, NJ, USA*

## Introduction

Pharmacoepidemiology applies the methods of epidemiology to the content area of clinical pharmacology. Therefore, in order to understand the approaches and methodological issues specific to the field of pharmacoepidemiology, the basic principles of the field of epidemiology must be understood as well. To this end, this chapter will begin with an overview of the scientific method in general. This will be followed by a discussion of the different types of errors one can make in designing a study. Next, the chapter will review the "Criteria for the causal nature of an association," which is how one can decide whether an association demonstrated in a particular study is, in fact, a causal association. Finally, the specific study designs available for epidemiologic studies, or in fact for any clinical studies, will be reviewed. The next chapter discusses a specific methodological issue which needs to be addressed in any study, but which is of particular importance for pharmacoepidemiologic studies: the issue of sample size. These two chapters are intended to be an introduction to the field of epidemiology for the neophyte. More information on these principles can be obtained from any textbook of epidemiology or clinical epidemiology. Finally, Chapter 4 will review basic

principles of clinical pharmacology, the content area of pharmacoepidemiology.

## Overview of the Scientific Method

The scientific method to investigate a research question involves a three-stage process (see Figure 2.1). In the first stage, one selects a group of subjects for study. These subjects may be patients or animals or biologic cells and are the sources for data sought by the study to answer a question of interest. Second, one uses the information obtained in this sample of study subjects to generalize and draw a conclusion about a population in general. This conclusion is referred to as an association. Third, one generalizes again, drawing a conclusion about scientific theory or causation. Each will be discussed in turn.

Any given study is performed on a selection of individuals, who represent the *study subjects*. These study subjects should theoretically represent a random sample of some defined population. For example, one might perform a randomized clinical trial of the efficacy of enalapril in lowering blood pressure, randomly allocating a total of 40 middle aged hypertensive men to receive either enalapril or a placebo

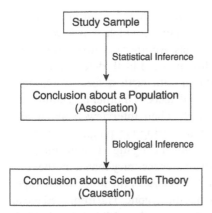

**Figure 2.1** Overview of the scientific method.

and observing their blood pressure six weeks later. One might expect to see the blood pressure of the 20 men treated with the active drug decrease more than the blood pressure of the 20 men treated with a placebo. In this example, the 40 study subjects would represent the study sample, theoretically a random sample of middle-aged hypertensive men. In reality, the study sample is almost never a true random sample of the underlying target population, because it is logistically impossible to identify every individual who belongs in the target population and then randomly choose from among them. However, the study sample is usually treated as if it were a random sample of the target population.

At this point, one would be tempted to make a generalization that enalapril lowers blood pressure in middle-aged hypertensive men. However, one must explore whether this observation could have occurred simply by chance, i.e. due to random variation. If the observed outcome in the study was simply a chance occurrence, then the same observation might not have been seen if one had chosen a different sample of 40 study subjects. Perhaps more importantly, it might not exist if one were able to study the entire theoretical population of all middle-aged hypertensive men. In order to evaluate this possibility, one can perform a statistical test, which allows an investigator to quantitate the probability that the observed outcome in this study (i.e. the difference seen between the two study groups) could have happened simply by chance. There are explicit rules and procedures for how one should properly make this determination: the science of statistics. If the results of any study under consideration demonstrate a "statistically significant difference" (i.e. ruling out the probability of a chance occurrence), then one is said to have an *association*. The process of assessing whether random variation could have led to a study's findings is referred to as *statistical inference*, and represents the major role for statistical testing in the scientific method.

If there is no statistically significant difference, then the process in Figure 2.1 stops. If there is an association, then one is tempted to generalize the results of the study even further, to state that enalapril is an antihypertensive drug, in general. This is referred to as *scientific or biological inference*, and the result is a conclusion about *causation*, that the drug really does lower blood pressure in a population of treated patients. To draw this type of conclusion, however, requires one to generalize to populations other than that included in the study, including types of people who were not represented in the study sample, such as women, children, and the elderly. Although it may be apparent in this example that this is in fact appropriate, that may well not always be the case. Unlike statistical inference, there are no precise quantitative rules for biological inference. Rather, one needs to examine the data at hand in light of all other relevant data in the rest of the scientific literature and make a subjective judgment. To assist in making that judgment, however, one can use the "Criteria for the Causal Nature of an Association," described below. First, however, we will place causal associations into a proper perspective, by describing the different types of errors that can be made in performing a study and the different types of associations that each results in.

**Table 2.1** Types of associations between factors under study.

---

1) None (independent)
2) Artifactual (spurious or false)
   a) Chance (unsystematic variation)
   b) Bias (systematic variation)
3) Indirect (confounded)
4) Causal (direct or true)

---

## Types of Errors that one Can Make in Performing a Study

There are four basic types of associations that can be observed in a study (Table 2.1). The basic purpose of research is to differentiate among them.

First, of course, one could have no association. Second, one could have an *artifactual association*, i.e. a spurious or false association. This can occur by either of two mechanisms: chance or bias. Chance is unsystematic, or random, variation. The purpose of statistical testing in science is to evaluate this, estimating the probability that the result observed in a study could have happened purely by chance.

The other possible mechanism for creating an artifactual association is bias. Epidemiologists' use of the term bias is different from that of the lay public. To an epidemiologist, *bias* is systematic variation, a consistent manner in which two study groups are treated or evaluated differently. This consistent difference can create an apparent association where one actually does not exist. Of course, it also can mask a true association.

There are many different types of potential biases. For example, consider an interview study in which the research assistant is aware of the investigator's hypothesis. Attempting to please the boss, the research assistant might probe more carefully during interviews with one study group than during interviews with the other. This difference in how carefully the

interviewer probes could create an apparent but false association, which is referred to as interviewer bias. Another example would be a study of drug-induced birth defects that compares children with birth defects to children without birth defects. A mother of a child with a birth defect, when interviewed about any drugs she took during her pregnancy, may be likely to remember drug ingestion during pregnancy with greater accuracy than a mother of a healthy child, because of the unfortunate experience she has undergone. The improved recall in the mothers of the children with birth defects may result in false apparent associations between drug exposure and birth defects. This systematic difference in recall is referred to as recall bias.

Note that biases, once present, cannot be corrected. They represent errors in the study design that can result in incorrect results in the study. It is important to note that a *statistically significant result is no protection against a bias*; one can have a very precise measurement of an incorrect answer! The only protection against biases is proper study design (See Chapter 22 for more discussion about biases in pharmacoepidemiologic studies.)

Third, one can have an indirect, or confounded, association. A *confounding variable*, or *confounder*, is a variable, other than the risk factor and other than the outcome under study, which is related independently to both the risk factor and the outcome and which may create an apparent association or mask a real one. For example, a study of risk factors for lung cancer could find a very strong association between having yellow fingertips and developing lung cancer. This is obviously not a causal association, but an indirect association, confounded by cigarette smoking. Specifically, cigarette smoking causes both yellow fingertips and lung cancer. Although this example is transparent, most examples of confounding are not. In designing a study, one must consider every variable that can be associated with the risk

**Table 2.2** Approaches to controlling confounding.

1) Random allocation
2) Subject selection
   a) Exclusion
   b) Matching
3) Data analysis
   a) Stratification
   b) Mathematical modeling

**Table 2.3** Criteria for the causal nature of an association.

1) Coherence with existing information (biological plausibility)
2) Consistency of the association
3) Time sequence
4) Specificity of the association
5) Strength of the association
   a) Quantitative strength
   b) Dose–response relationship
   c) Study design

factor under study or the outcome variable under study, in order to plan to deal with it as a potential confounding variable. Preferably, one will be able to specifically control for the variable, using one of the techniques listed in Table 2.2. (See Chapter 22 for more discussion about confounding in pharmacoepidemiologic studies.)

Fourth, and finally, there are true, causal associations.

Thus, there are three possible types of errors that can be produced in a study: random error, bias, and confounding. The probability of random error can be quantitated using statistics. Bias needs to be prevented by designing the study properly. Confounding can be controlled either in the design of the study or in its analysis. If all three types of errors can be excluded, then one is left with a true, causal association.

## Criteria for the Causal Nature of an Association

The "Criteria for the causal nature of an association" were first put forth by Sir Austin Bradford Hill, but have been described in various forms since, each with some modification. Probably the best known description of them was in the first Surgeon General's Report on Smoking and Health, published in 1964. These criteria are presented in Table 2.3, in no particular order. No one of them is absolutely necessary for an association to be a causal association. Analogously, no one of them is sufficient for an association to be considered a

causal association. Essentially, the more criteria that are present, the more likely it is that an association is a causal association. The fewer criteria that are met, the less likely it is that an association is a causal association. Each will be discussed in turn.

The first criterion listed in Table 2.3 is *coherence with existing information* or *biological plausibility*. This refers to whether the association makes sense, in light of other types of information available in the literature. These other types of information could include data from other human studies, data from studies of other related questions, data from animal studies, or data from *in vitro* studies, as well as scientific or pathophysiologic theory. To use the example provided above, it clearly was not biologically plausible that yellow fingertips could cause lung cancer, and this provided the clue that confounding was present. Using the example of the association between cigarettes and lung cancer, cigarette smoke is a known carcinogen, based on animal data. In humans, it is known to cause cancers of the head and neck, the pancreas, and the bladder. Cigarette smoke also goes down into the lungs, directly exposing the tissues in question. Thus, it certainly is biologically plausible that cigarettes could *cause* lung cancer. It is much more reassuring if an association found in a particular study makes sense, based on previously available information, and this makes one more comfortable that it might be a causal association.

Clearly, however, one could not require that this criterion always be met, or one would never have a major breakthrough in science.

The second criterion listed in Table 2.3 is the *consistency of the association*. A hallmark of science is reproducibility: if a finding is real, one should be able to reproduce it in a different setting. This could include different geographic settings, different study designs, different populations, etc. For example, in the case of cigarettes and lung cancer, the association has now been reproduced in many different studies, in different geographic locations, using different study designs. The need for reproducibility is such that one should never believe a finding reported only once: there may have been an error committed in the study, which is not apparent to either the investigator or the reader.

The third criterion listed is that of *time sequence* – a cause must precede an effect. Although this may seem obvious, there are study designs from which this cannot be determined. For example, if one were to perform a survey in a classroom of 200 medical students, asking each if he or she were currently taking diazepam and also whether he or she were anxious, one would find a strong association between the use of diazepam and anxiety, but this does not mean that diazepam causes anxiety! Although this is obvious, as it is not a biologically plausible interpretation, one cannot differentiate from this type of cross-sectional study which variable came first and which came second. In the example of cigarettes and lung cancer, obviously the cigarette smoking usually precedes the lung cancer, as a patient would not survive long enough to smoke much if the opposite were the case.

The fourth criterion listed in Table 2.3 is *specificity*. This refers to the question of whether the cause ever occurs without the presumed effect and whether the effect ever occurs without the presumed cause. This criterion is almost never met in biology, with the occasional exception of infectious diseases. Measles never occurs without the measles

virus, but even in this example, not everyone who becomes infected with the measles virus develops clinical measles. Certainly, not everyone who smokes develops lung cancer, and not everyone who develops lung cancer was a smoker. This is one of the major points the tobacco industry stresses when it attempts to make the claim that cigarette smoking has not been proven to cause lung cancer. Some authors even omit this as a criterion, as it is so rarely met. When it is met, however, it provides extremely strong support for a conclusion that an association is causal.

The fifth criterion listed in Table 2.3 is the *strength of the association*. This includes three concepts: its quantitative strength, dose–response, and the study design. Each will be discussed in turn.

The *quantitative strength* of an association refers to the effect size. To evaluate this, one asks whether the magnitude of the observed difference between the two study groups is large. A quantitatively large association can only be created by a causal association or a large error, which should be apparent in evaluating the methods of a study. A quantitatively small association may still be causal, but it could be created by a subtle error, which would not be apparent in evaluating the study. Conventionally, epidemiologists consider an association with a relative risk of less than 2.0 a weak association. Certainly, the association between cigarette smoking and lung cancer is a strong association: studies show relative risks ranging between 10.0 and 30.0.

A dose–response relationship is an extremely important and commonly used concept in clinical pharmacology and is used similarly in epidemiology. A *dose–response relationship* exists when an increase in the intensity of an exposure results in an increased risk of the disease under study. Equivalent to this is a *duration–response relationship*, which exists when a longer exposure causes an increased risk of the disease. The presence of either a dose–response relationship or a duration–response relationship strongly implies that an association is, in fact, a causal association. Certainly in the example of cigarette smoking and lung cancer, it has been shown repeatedly that an increase in either the number of cigarettes smoked each day or in the number of years of smoking increases the risk of developing lung cancer.

Finally, *study design* refers to two concepts: whether the study was well designed, and which study design was used in the studies in question. The former refers to whether the study was subject to one of the three errors described earlier in this chapter, namely random error, bias, and confounding. Table 2.4 presents the study designs typically used for epidemiologic studies, or in fact for any clinical studies. They are organized in a hierarchical fashion. As one advances from the designs at the bottom of the table to those at the top of the table, studies get progressively harder to perform, but are progressively more convincing. In other words, associations shown by studies using designs at the top of the list are more likely to be causal associations than associations shown by studies using designs at the bottom of the list. The association between cigarette smoking and lung cancer has been reproduced in multiple well-designed studies, using analyses of secular trends, case–control studies, and cohort studies. However, it has not been shown using a randomized clinical trial, which is the "cadillac" of study designs, as will be discussed below. This is the other major defense used by the tobacco industry. Of course, it would not be ethical or logistically feasible to randomly allocate individuals to smoke or not to smoke and expect this to be followed for 20 years to observe the outcome in each group.

**Table 2.4** Advantages and disadvantages of epidemiologic study designs.

| Study Design | Advantages | Disadvantages |
| --- | --- | --- |
| Randomized clinical trial (Experimental study) | Most convincing design | Most expensive |
| | Only design which controls for unknown or unmeasurable confounders | Artificial |
| | | Logistically most difficult |
| | | Ethical objections |
| Cohort study | Can study multiple outcomes | Possibly biased outcome data |
| | Can study uncommon exposures | More expensive |
| | Selection bias less likely | If done prospectively, may take years to complete |
| | Unbiased exposure data | |
| | Incidence data available | |
| Case–control study | Can study multiple exposures | Control selection problematic |
| | Can study uncommon diseases | Possibly biased exposure data |
| | Logistically easier and faster | |
| | Less expensive | |
| Analyses of secular trends | Can provide rapid answers | No control of confounding |
| Case series | Easy quantitation of incidence | No control group, so cannot be used for hypothesis testing |
| Case reports | Cheap and easy method for generating hypotheses | Cannot be used for hypothesis testing |

The issue of causation is discussed more in Chapter 7 as it relates to the process of spontaneous reporting of adverse drug reactions, and in Chapter 14 as it relates to assessing causation from case reports.

## Epidemiologic Study Designs

In order to clarify the concept of study design further, each of the designs in Table 2.4 will be discussed in turn, starting at the bottom of the list and working upwards.

### Case Reports

*Case reports* are simply reports of events observed in single patients. As used in pharmacoepidemiology, a case report describes a single patient who was exposed to a drug and experiences a particular, usually adverse, outcome. For example, one might see a published case report about a young woman who was taking oral contraceptives and who suffered a pulmonary embolism.

Case reports are useful for raising hypotheses about drug effects, to be tested with more rigorous study designs. However, in a case report one cannot know if the patient reported is either typical of those with the exposure or typical of those with the disease. Certainly, one cannot usually determine whether the adverse outcome was due to the drug exposure or would have happened anyway. As such, it is very rare that a case report can be used to make a statement about causation. One exception to this would be when the outcome is so rare and so characteristic of the exposure that one knows that it was likely to be due to the exposure, even if the history of exposure were unclear. An example of this is clear cell vaginal adenocarcinoma occurring in young women exposed in utero to diethylstilbestrol. Another exception would be when the disease course is very predictable and the treatment causes a clearly apparent change in this disease course.

An example would be the ability of penicillin to cure streptococcal endocarditis, a disease that is nearly uniformly fatal in the absence of treatment. Case reports can be particularly useful to document causation when the treatment causes a change in disease course which is reversible, such that the patient returns to his or her untreated state when the exposure is withdrawn, can be treated again, and when the change returns upon repeat treatment. Consider a patient who is suffering from an overdose of methadone, a long-acting narcotic, and is comatose. If this patient is then treated with naloxone, a narcotic antagonist, and immediately awakens, this would be very suggestive that the drug indeed is efficacious as a narcotic antagonist. As the naloxone wears off the patient would become comatose again, and then if he or she were given another dose of naloxone the patient would awaken again. This, especially if repeated a few times, would represent strong evidence that the drug is indeed effective as a narcotic antagonist. This type of challenge–rechallenge situation is relatively uncommon, however, as physicians generally will avoid exposing a patient to a drug if the patient experienced an adverse reaction to it in the past. This issue is discussed in more detail in Chapters 7 and 14.

### Case Series

*Case series* are collections of patients, all of whom have a single exposure, whose clinical outcomes are then evaluated and described. Often they are from a single hospital or medical practice. Alternatively, case series can be collections of patients with a single outcome, looking at their antecedent exposures. For example, one might observe 100 consecutive women under the age of 50 who suffer from a pulmonary embolism, and note that 30 of them had been taking oral contraceptives.

After drug marketing, case series are most useful for two related purposes. First, they can be useful for quantifying the incidence of an adverse reaction. Second, they can be useful for being certain that any particular adverse effect of concern does not occur in a population which is larger than that studied prior to drug marketing. The so-called "Phase IV" postmarketing surveillance study of prazosin was conducted for the former reason, to quantitate the incidence of first dose syncope from prazosin. The "Phase IV" postmarketing surveillance study of cimetidine was conducted for the latter reason. Metiamide was an H-2 blocker, which was withdrawn after marketing outside the US because it caused agranulocytosis. Since cimetidine is chemically related to metiamide there was a concern that cimetidine might also cause agranulocytosis. In both examples, the manufacturer asked its sales representatives to recruit physicians to participate in the study. Each participating physician then enrolled the next series of patients for whom the drug was prescribed.

In this type of study, one can be more certain that the patients are probably typical of those with the exposure or with the disease, depending on the focus of the study. However, in the absence of a control group, one cannot be certain which features in the description of the patients are unique to the exposure, or outcome. As an example, one might have a case series from a particular hospital of 100 individuals with a certain disease, and note that all were men over the age of 60. This might lead one to conclude that this disease seems to be associated with being a man over the age of 60. However, it would be clear that this would be an incorrect conclusion once one noted that the hospital this case series was drawn from was a Veterans Administration hospital, where most patients are men over the age of 60. In the previous example of pulmonary embolism and oral contraceptives, 30% of the women with pulmonary embolism had been using oral contraceptives. However, this information is not sufficient to determine whether this is higher, the same as, or even lower than would have been expected. For this reason, case series are also not very useful in determining causation, but provide clinical descriptions of a disease or of patients who receive an exposure.

## Analyses of Secular Trends

*Analyses of secular trends*, also called "ecological studies," examine trends in an exposure that is a presumed cause and trends in a disease that is a presumed effect and test whether the trends coincide. These trends can be examined over time or across geographic boundaries. In other words, one could analyze data from a single region and examine how the trend changes over time, or one could analyze data from a single time period and compare how the data differ from region to region or country to country. Vital statistics are often used for these studies. As an example, one might look at sales data for oral contraceptives and compare them to death rates from venous thromboembolism, using recorded vital statistics. When such a study was actually performed, mortality rates from venous thromboembolism were seen to increase in parallel with increasing oral contraceptive sales, but only in women of reproductive age, not in older women or in men of any age.

Analyses of secular trends are useful for rapidly providing evidence for or against a hypothesis. However, these studies lack data on individuals; they utilize only aggregated group data (e.g. annual sales data in a given geographic region in relation to annual cause-specific mortality in the same region). As such, they are unable to control for confounding variables. Thus, among exposures whose trends coincide with that of the disease, analyses of secular trends are unable to differentiate which factor is likely to be the true cause. For example, lung cancer mortality rates in the US have been increasing in women, such that lung cancer is now the leading cause of cancer mortality in women. This is certainly consistent with the increasing rates of cigarette smoking observed in women until the mid-1960s, and so appears to be supportive of the association between cigarette smoking and lung cancer. However, it would also be consistent with an association between certain occupational exposures and lung cancer, as more women in the US are now working outside the home.

## Case–Control Studies

*Case-control studies* are studies that compare cases with a disease to controls without the disease, looking for differences in antecedent exposures. As an example, one could select cases of young women with venous thromboembolism and compare them to controls without venous thromboembolism, looking for differences in antecedent oral contraceptive use. Several such studies have been performed, generally demonstrating a strong association between the use of oral contraceptives and venous thromboembolism.

Case–control studies can be particularly useful when one wants to study multiple possible causes of a single disease, as one can use the same cases and controls to examine any number of exposures as potential risk factors. This design is also particularly useful when one is studying a relatively rare disease, as it guarantees a sufficient number of cases with the disease. Using case–control studies, one can study rare diseases with markedly smaller sample sizes than those needed for cohort studies (see Chapter 3). For example, the classic study of diethylstilbestrol and clear cell vaginal adenocarcinoma required only 8 cases and 40 controls, rather than the many thousands of exposed subjects that would have been required for a cohort study of this question.

Case–control studies generally obtain their information on exposures retrospectively, i.e. by recreating events that happened in the past. Information on past exposure to potential risk factors is generally obtained by abstracting medical records or by administering questionnaires or interviews. As such, case–control studies are subject to limitations in the validity of retrospectively collected exposure information. In addition, the proper selection of controls can be a challenging task, and appropriate control selection can lead to a selection bias, which may lead to incorrect conclusions. Nevertheless, when case–control studies are done well, subsequent well-done cohort studies or randomized clinical trials, if any, will generally confirm their results. As such, the case–control design is a very useful approach for pharmacoepidemiologic studies.

## Cohort Studies

*Cohort studies* are studies that identify subsets of a defined population and follow them over time, looking for differences in their outcome. Cohort studies are generally used to compare exposed patients to unexposed patients, although they can also be used to compare one exposure to another. For example, one could compare women of reproductive age who use oral contraceptives to users of other contraceptive methods, looking for the differences in the frequency of venous thromboembolism. When such studies were performed, they in fact confirmed the relationship between oral contraceptives and thromboembolism, which had been noted using analyses of secular trends and case–control studies. Cohort studies can be performed either prospectively, that is simultaneous with the events under study, or retrospectively, that is after the outcomes under study had already occurred, by recreating those past events using medical records, questionnaires, or interviews.

The major difference between cohort and case–control studies is the basis upon which patients are recruited into the study (see Figure 2.2). Patients are recruited into

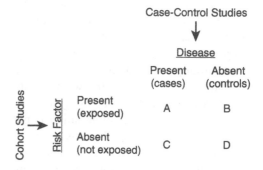

**Figure 2.2** Cohort and case–control studies provide similar information, but approach data collection from opposite directions. *Source:* Reprinted with permission from Strom (1986).

case–control studies based on the presence or absence of a disease, and their antecedent exposures are then studied. Patients are recruited into cohort studies based on the presence or absence of an exposure, and their subsequent disease course is then studied.

Cohort studies have the major advantage of being free of the major problem that plagues case–control studies: the difficult process of selecting an undiseased control group. In addition, prospective cohort studies are free of the problem of the questionable validity of retrospectively collected data. For these reasons, an association demonstrated by a cohort study is more likely to be a causal association than one demonstrated by a case–control study. Furthermore, cohort studies are particularly useful when one is studying multiple possible outcomes from a single exposure, especially a relatively uncommon exposure. Thus, they are particularly useful in postmarketing drug surveillance studies, which are looking at any possible effect of a newly marketed drug. However, cohort studies can require extremely large sample sizes to study relatively uncommon outcomes (see Chapter 3). In addition, prospective cohort studies can require a prolonged time period to study delayed drug effects.

## Analysis of Case–Control and Cohort Studies

As can be seen in Figure 2.2, both case–control and cohort studies are intended to provide the same basic information; the difference is how this information is collected. The key statistic reported from these studies is the relative risk. The *relative risk* is the ratio of the incidence rate of an outcome in the exposed group to the incidence rate of the outcome in the unexposed group. A relative risk of greater than 1.0 means that exposed subjects have a *greater* risk of the disease under study than unexposed subjects, or that the exposure appears to cause the disease. A relative risk less than 1.0 means that exposed subjects have a *lower* risk of the disease than unexposed subjects, or that the

exposure seems to protect against the disease. A relative risk of 1.0 means that exposed subjects and unexposed subjects have the same risk of developing the disease, or that the exposure and the disease appear unrelated.

One can calculate a relative risk directly from the results of a cohort study. However, in a case–control study one cannot determine the size of either the exposed population or the unexposed population that the diseased cases and undiseased controls were drawn from. The results of a case–control study do not provide information on the incidence rates of the disease in exposed and unexposed individuals. Therefore, relative risks cannot be calculated directly from a case–control study. Instead, in reporting the results of a case–control study one generally reports the *odds ratio*, which is a close estimate of the relative risk when the disease under study is relatively rare. Since case–control studies are generally used to study rare diseases, there is generally very close agreement between the odds ratio and the relative risk, and the results from case–control studies are often loosely referred to as relative risks, although they are in fact odds ratios.

Both relative risks and odds ratios can be reported with *p-values*. These p-values allow one to determine if the relative risk is statistically significantly different from 1.0, that is whether the differences between the two study groups are likely to be due to random variation or are likely to represent real associations.

Alternatively, and probably preferably, relative risks and odds ratios can be reported with *confidence intervals*, which are an indication of the range of relative risks within which the true relative risk for the entire theoretical population is most likely to lie. As an approximation, a 95% confidence interval around a relative risk means that we can be 95% confident that the true relative risk lies in the range between the lower and upper limits of this interval. If a 95% confidence interval around a relative risk excludes 1.0, then the finding is statistically significant with a p-value of less than 0.05. A confidence interval provides much more information than a p-value, however. As an example, a study that yields a relative risk (95% confidence interval) of 1.0 (0.9–1.1) is clearly showing that an association is very unlikely. A study that yields a relative risk (95% confidence interval) of 1.0 (0.1–100) provides little evidence for or against an association. Yet, both could be reported as a relative risk of 1.0 and a p-value greater than 0.05. As another example, a study that yields a relative risk (95% confidence interval) of 10.0 (9.8–10.2) precisely quantifies a 10-fold increase in risk that is also statistically significant. A study that yields a relative risk (95% confidence interval) of 10.0 (1.1–100) says little, other than an increased risk is likely. Yet, both could be reported as a relative risk of 10.0 ($p < 0.05$). As a final example, a study yielding a relative risk (95% confidence interval) of 3.0 (0.98–5.0) is strongly suggestive of an association, whereas a study reporting a relative risk (95% confidence interval) of 3.0 (0.1–30) would not be. Yet, both could be reported as a relative risk of 3.0 ($p > 0.05$).

Finally, another statistic that one can calculate from a cohort study is the *excess risk*, also called the risk difference or, sometimes, the attributable risk. Whereas the relative risk is the ratio of the incidence rates in the exposed group versus the unexposed groups, the excess risk is the arithmetic difference between incidence rates. The relative risk is more important in considering questions of causation. The excess risk is more important in considering the public health impact of an association, as it represents the increased rate of disease due to the exposure. For example, oral contraceptives are strongly associated with the development of myocardial infarction in young women. However, the risk of myocardial infarction in nonsmoking women in their 20s is so low, that even a fivefold increase in that risk would still not be of public health importance. In contrast, women in their 40s are at higher risk, especially if they are cigarette smokers as well. Thus, oral contraceptives should not be as readily used in these women.

As with relative risks, excess risks cannot be calculated from case–control studies, as incidence rates are not available. As with the other statistics, p-values can be calculated to determine whether the differences between the two study groups could have occurred just by chance. Confidence intervals can be calculated around excess risks as well, and would be interpreted analogously.

## Randomized Clinical Trials

Finally, *experimental studies* are studies in which the investigator controls the therapy that is to be received by each participant. Generally, an investigator uses that control to randomly allocate patients between or among the study groups, performing a *randomized clinical trial*. For example, one could theoretically randomly allocate sexually active women to use either oral contraceptives or no contraceptive, examining whether they differ in their incidence of subsequent venous thromboembolism. The major strength of this approach is random assignment, which is the only way to make it likely that the study groups are comparable in potential confounding variables that are either unknown or unmeasurable. For this reason, associations demonstrated in randomized clinical trials are more likely to be causal associations than those demonstrated using one of the other study designs reviewed above.

However, even randomized clinical trials are not without their problems. The randomized clinical trial outlined above, allocating women to receive contraceptives or no contraceptives, demonstrates the major potential problems inherent in the use of this study design. It would obviously be impossible to perform, ethically and logistically. In addition, randomized clinical trials are expensive and artificial. Inasmuch as they have already been performed prior to marketing to demonstrate each drug's efficacy, they tend to be unnecessary after marketing. They are likely to be used in pharmacoepidemiologic studies mainly for supplementary studies of drug efficacy. However, they remain the "gold standard" by which the other designs must be judged. Indeed, with the publication of the results from the Women's Health Initiative indicating that combination hormone replacement therapy causes an increased risk of myocardial infarction rather than a decreased risk, there has been increased concern about reliance solely on nonexperimental methods to study drug safety after marketing, and we are beginning to see the use of massive randomized clinical trials as part of postmarketing surveillance.

## Discussion

Thus, a series of different study designs are available (Table 2.4), each with respective advantages and disadvantages. Case reports, case series, analyses of secular trends, case–control studies, and cohort studies have been referred to collectively as *observational study designs* or *nonexperimental study designs*, in order to differentiate them from experimental studies. In nonexperimental study designs the investigator does not control the therapy, but simply observes and evaluates the results of ongoing medical care. Case reports, case series, and analyses of secular trends have also been referred to as *descriptive studies*. Case–control studies, cohort studies, and randomized clinical trials all have control groups, and have been referred to as *analytic studies*. The analytic study designs can be classified in two major ways, by how subjects are selected into the study and by how data are collected for the study (see Table 2.5). From the perspective of how subjects are recruited into the study, case–control studies can be contrasted with cohort studies. Specifically, case–control studies select subjects into the study based on the presence or absence of a disease, while cohort studies select subjects into the study based on the presence or absence of an exposure. From this perspective, randomized clinical trials can be

**Table 2.5** Epidemiologic study designs.

A) Classified by how subjects are recruited into the study
  1) Case–control (case-history, case-referent, retrospective, trohoc) studies
  2) Cohort (follow-up, prospective) studies
    a) Experimental studies (clinical trials, intervention studies)
B) Classified by how data are collected for the study
  1) Retrospective (historical, nonconcurrent, retrolective) studies
  2) Prospective (prolective) studies
  3) Cross-sectional studies

viewed as a subset of cohort studies, a type of cohort study in which the investigator controls the allocation of treatment, rather than simply observing ongoing medical care. From the perspective of timing, data can be collected *prospectively*, that is simultaneously with the events under study, or *retrospectively*, that is after the events under study had already developed. In the latter situation, one re-creates events that happened in the past using medical records, questionnaires, or interviews. Data can also be collected using *cross-sectional studies*, studies that have no time sense, as they examine only one point in time. In principle, either cohort or case–control studies can be performed using any of these time frames, although prospective case–control studies are unusual. Randomized clinical trials must be prospective, as this is the only way an investigator can control the therapy received.

The terms presented in this chapter, which are those that will be used throughout the book, are probably the terms used by a majority of epidemiologists. Unfortunately, however, other terms have been used for most of these study designs, as well. Table 2.5 also presents several of the synonyms that have been used in the medical literature. The same term is sometimes used by different authors to describe different concepts. For example, in this book we are reserving the use of the terms "retrospective study" and "prospective study" to refer to a time sense. As is apparent from Table 2.5, however, in the past some authors used the term "retrospective study" to refer to a case–control study and used the term "prospective study" to refer to a cohort study, confusing the two concepts inherent in the classification schemes presented in the table. Other authors use the term "retrospective study" to refer to any non-experimental study, while others appear to use the term to refer to any study they do not like, as a term of derision! Unfortunately, when reading a scientific paper, there is no way of determining which usage the author intended. What is more important than the terminology, however, are the concepts underlying the terms. Understanding these concepts, the reader can choose to use whatever terminology he or she is comfortable with.

## Conclusion

From the material presented in this chapter, it is hopefully now apparent that each study design has an appropriate role in scientific progress. In general, science proceeds from the bottom of Table 2.4 upward, from case reports and case series that are useful for suggesting an association, to analyses of trends and case–control studies that are useful for exploring these associations. Finally, if a study question warrants the investment and can tolerate the delay until results become available, then cohort studies and randomized clinical trials can be undertaken to assess these associations more definitively.

For example, regarding the question of whether oral contraceptives cause venous thromboembolism, an association was first suggested by case reports and case series, then was explored in more detail by analyses of trends and a series of case–control studies. Later, because of the importance of oral contraceptives, the number of women using them, and the fact that users were predominantly healthy women, the investment was made in

two long-term, large-scale cohort studies. This question might even be worth the investment of a randomized clinical trial, except it would not be feasible or ethical. In contrast, when thalidomide was marketed, it was not a major breakthrough; other hypnotics were already available. Case reports of phocomelia in exposed patients were followed by case–control studies and analyses of secular trends. Inasmuch as the adverse effect was so terrible and the drug was not of unique importance, the drug was then withdrawn, without the delay that would have been necessary if cohort studies and/or randomized clinical trials had been awaited. Ultimately, a retrospective cohort study was performed, comparing those exposed during the critical time period to those exposed at other times.

In general, however, clinical, regulatory, commercial, and legal decisions need to be made based on the best evidence available at the time of the decision. To quote Sir Austin Bradford Hill (1965):

> All scientific work is incomplete– whether it be observational or experimental. All scientific work is liable to be upset or modified by advancing knowledge. That does not confer upon us a freedom to ignore the knowledge we already have, or to postpone the action that it appears to demand at a given time.
>
> Who knows, asked Robert Browning, but the world may end tonight? True, but on available evidence most of us make ready to commute on the 8:30 next day.

## Key Points

- Many different types of potential biases can create artifactual associations in a scientific study. Among them are: interviewer bias, recall bias, and confounding.

- Four basic types of association can be observed in studies that examine whether there is an association between an exposure and an outcome: no association, artifactual association (from chance or bias), indirect association (from confounding), or true association.

- A series of criteria can be used to assess the causal nature of an association, to assist in making a subjective judgment about whether a given association is likely to be causal. These are: biological plausibility, consistency, time sequence, specificity, and quantitative strength.

- Study design options, in hierarchical order of progressively harder to perform but more convincing, are: case reports, case series, analyses of secular trends, case–control studies, retrospective cohort studies, prospective cohort studies, and randomized clinical trials.

- Associations between an exposure and an outcome are reported with relative risk ratios (in cohort studies), odds ratios (in case–control studies), confidence intervals, and p-values. Sometimes also as attributable (excess) risk.

## Further Reading

Bassetti, W.H.C. and Woodward, M. (2004). *Epidemiology: Study Design and Data Analysis*, 2e. Boca Raton, Florida: Chapman & Hall/CRC.

Bhopal, R.S. (2008). *Concepts of Epidemiology: Integrating the Ideas, Theories, Principles and Methods of Epidemiology*, 2e. New York: Oxford University Press.

Fletcher, R.H. and Fletcher, S.W. (2005). *Clinical Epidemiology: The Essentials*, 4e. Lippincott Williams & Wilkins.

Friedman, G. (2003). *Primer of Epidemiology*, 5e. New York: McGraw Hill.

Gordis, L. (2009). *Epidemiology*, 4e. Philadelphia, PA: Saunders.

Hennekens, C.H. and Buring, J.E. (1987). *Epidemiology in Medicine*. Boston, MA: Little Brown.

Hill, A.B. (1965). The environment and disease: association or causation? *Proc. Royal Soc. Med.* 58: 295–300.

Hulley, S.B., Cummings, S.R., Browner, W.S. et al. (2006). *Designing Clinical Research: An Epidemiologic Approach*, 3e. Baltimore, MD: Lippincott Williams & Wilkins.

Katz, D.L. (2001). *Clinical Epidemiology and Evidence-based Medicine: Fundamental Principles of Clinical Reasoning and Research*. Thousand Oaks, CA: Sage Publications.

Kelsey, J.L., Whittemore, A.S., and Evans, A.S. (1996). *Methods in Observational Epidemiology*, 2e. New York: Oxford University Press.

Lilienfeld, D.E. and Stolley, P. (1994). *Foundations of Epidemiology*, 3e. New York: Oxford University Press.

MacMahon, B. (1997). *Epidemiology: Principles and Methods*, 2e. Hagerstown MD: Lippincott-Raven.

Mausner, J.S. and Kramer, S. (1985). *Epidemiology: An Introductory Text*, 2e. Philadelphia, PA: Saunders.

Rothman, K.J. (2002). *Epidemiology: An Introduction*. New York: Oxford University Press.

Rothman, K.J., Greenland, S., and Lash, T.L. (2008). *Modern Epidemiology*, 3e. Philadelphia, PA: Lippincott Williams & Wilkins.

Sackett, D.L. (1979). Bias in analytic research. *J. Chronic Dis.* 32: 51–63.

Sackett, D.L., Haynes, R.B., and Tugwell, P. (1991). *Clinical Epidemiology: A Basic Science for Clinical Medicine*, 2e. Boston, MA: Little Brown.

Strom, B.L. (1986). Medical databases in post-marketing drug surveillance. *Trends Pharmacol. Sci.* 7: 377–380.

Szklo, M. and Nieto, F.J. (2006). *Epidemiology: Beyond the Basics*. Sudbury, MA: Jones & Bartlett.

US Public Health Service (1964). *Smoking and Health. Report of the Advisory Committee to the Surgeon General of the Public Health Service*, 20. Washington DC: Government Printing Office.

Weiss, N.S. (1996). *Clinical Epidemiology: The Study of the Outcome of Illness*, 2e. New York: Oxford University Press.

Weiss, N.S., Koepsall, T., and Koepsell, T.D. (2004). *Epidemiologic Methods: Studying the Occurrence of Illness*. New York: Oxford University Press.

# 3

# Sample Size Considerations for Pharmacoepidemiologic Studies

*Brian L. Strom*

*Rutgers Biomedical and Health Sciences, Newark, NJ, USA*

## Introduction

Chapter 1 pointed out that between 500 and 3000 subjects are usually exposed to a drug prior to marketing, in order to be 95% certain of detecting adverse effects that occur in between one and six in a thousand exposed individuals. While this seems like a reasonable goal, it poses some important problems that must be taken into account when planning pharmacoepidemiologic studies. Specifically, such studies must generally include a sufficient number of subjects to add significantly to the premarketing experience, and this requirement for large sample sizes raises logistical obstacles to cost-effective studies. This central special need for large sample sizes is what has led to the innovative approaches to collecting pharmacoepidemiologic data that are described in Section II of this book *Sources of Pharmacoepidemiology Data*.

The approach to considering the implications of a study's sample size is somewhat different depending on whether a study is already completed or is being planned. After a study is completed, if a real finding was statistically significant, then the study had a sufficient sample size to detect it, by definition. If a finding was not statistically significant, then one can use either of two approaches. First, one can examine the resulting confidence intervals in order to determine the smallest differences between the two study groups that the study had sufficient sample size to exclude. Alternatively, one can approach the question in a manner similar to the way one would approach it if one were planning the study de novo. Nomograms can be used to assist a reader in interpreting negative clinical trials in this way.

In contrast, in this chapter we will discuss in more detail how to determine a proper study sample size, from the perspective of one who is designing a study de novo. Specifically, we will begin by discussing how one calculates the minimum sample size necessary for a pharmacoepidemiologic study, to avoid the problem of a study with a sample size that is too small. We will first present the approach for cohort studies, then for case–control studies, and then for case series. For each design, one or more tables will be presented to assist the reader in carrying out these calculations.

## Sample Size Calculations for Cohort Studies

The sample size required for a cohort study depends on what you are expecting from the

*Textbook of Pharmacoepidemiology*, Third Edition. Edited by Brian L. Strom, Stephen E. Kimmel, and Sean Hennessy.

study. To calculate sample sizes for a cohort study, one needs to specify five variables (see Table 3.1).

The first variable to specify is the *alpha (α) or type I error* that one is willing to tolerate in the study. Type I error is the probability of concluding there is a difference between the groups being compared when in fact a difference does not exist. Using diagnostic tests as an analogy, a type I error is a false positive study finding. The more tolerant one is willing to be of type I error, the smaller the sample size required. The less tolerant one is willing to be of type I error, the smaller one would set alpha, and the larger the sample size that would be required. Conventionally the alpha is set at 0.05, although this certainly does not have to be the case. Note that alpha needs to be specified as either one-tailed or two-tailed. If only one of the study groups could conceivably be more likely to develop the disease and one is interested in detecting this result only, then one would specify alpha to be one-tailed. If either of the study groups may be likely to develop the disease, and either result would be of interest, then one would specify alpha to be two-tailed. To decide whether alpha should be one-tailed or two-tailed, an investigator should consider what his or her reaction would be to a result that is statistically significant in a direction opposite to the one expected. For example, what if one observed that a drug increased the frequency of dying from coronary artery disease instead of decreasing it, as expected? If the investigator's response to this would be: "Boy, what a surprise, but I believe it," then a two-tailed test should be performed. If the investigator's response would be: "I don't believe it, and I will interpret this simply as a study that does not show the expected decrease in coronary artery disease in the group treated with the study drug," then a one-tailed test should be performed. The more conservative option is the two-tailed test, assuming that the results could turn out in either direction. This is the option usually, although not always, used.

The second variable that needs to be specified to calculate a sample size for a cohort study is the *beta (β) or type II error* that one is willing to tolerate in the study. A type II error is the probability of concluding there is no difference between the groups being compared when in fact a difference does exist. In other words, a type II error is the probability of missing a real difference. Using diagnostic tests as an analogy, a type II error is a false negative study finding. The complement of beta is the power of a study, i.e. the probability of detecting a difference if a difference really exists. Power is calculated as $(1-\beta)$. Again, the more tolerant one is willing to be of Type II errors, i.e. the higher the beta, the smaller the sample size required. The beta is conventionally set at 0.1 (i.e. 90% power) or 0.2 (i.e. 80% power), although again this need not be the case. Beta is always one-tailed.

**Table 3.1** Information needed to calculate a study's sample size.

| For cohort studies | For case–control studies |
| --- | --- |
| 1) Alpha, or type I error, considered tolerable, and whether it is one-tailed or two-tailed | 1) Alpha, or type I error, considered tolerable, and whether it is one-tailed or two tailed |
| 2) Beta, or type II error, considered tolerable | 2) Beta, or type II, error considered tolerable |
| 3) Minimum relative risk to be detected | 3) Minimum relative risk to be detected |
| 4) Incidence of the disease in the unexposed control group | 4) Prevalence of the exposure in the undiseased control group |
| 5) Ratio of unexposed controls to exposed study subjects | 5) Ratio of undiseased controls to diseased study subjects |

The third variable one needs to specify in order to calculate sample sizes for a cohort study is the minimum effect size one wants to be able to detect. For a cohort study, this is expressed as a relative risk. The smaller the relative risk that one wants to detect, the larger the sample size required. Note that the relative risk often used by investigators in this calculation is the relative risk the investigator is expecting from the study. This is *not correct*, as it will lead to inadequate power to detect relative risks which are smaller than expected, but still clinically important to the investigator. In other words, if one chooses a sample size that is designed to detect a relative risk of 2.5, one should be comfortable with the thought that, if the actual relative risk turns out to be 2.2, one may not be able to detect it as a statistically significant finding.

In a cohort study one selects subjects based on the presence or absence of an exposure of interest and then investigates the incidence of the disease of interest in each of the study groups. Therefore, the fourth variable one needs to specify is the expected incidence of the study outcome in the unexposed control group. Again, the more you ask of a study (e.g. power to detect very small differences), the larger the sample size need. Specifically, the rarer the outcome of interest, the larger the sample size needed.

The fifth variable one needs to specify is the number of unexposed control subjects to be included in the study for each exposed study subject. A study has the most statistical power for a given number of study subjects if it has the same number of exposed and unexposed subjects (controls). However, sometimes the number of exposed subjects is limited and, therefore, inadequate to provide sufficient power to detect a relative risk of interest. In that case, additional power can be gained by increasing the number of controls alone. Doubling the number of controls, that is including two controls for each exposed subject, results in a modest increase in the statistical power, but it does not double it. Including

three controls for each exposed subject increases the power further. However, the increment in power achieved by increasing the ratio of control subjects to exposed subjects from 2:1 to 3:1 is smaller than the increment in power achieved by increasing the ratio from 1:1 to 2:1. Each additional increase in the size of the control group increases the power of the study further, but with progressively smaller gains in statistical power. Thus, there is rarely a reason to include greater than three or four controls per study subject. For example, one could design a study with an alpha of 0.05 to detect a relative risk of 2.0 for an outcome variable that occurs in the control group with an incidence rate of 0.01. A study with 2319 exposed individuals and 2319 controls would yield a power of 0.80, or an 80% chance of detecting a difference of that magnitude. With the same 2319 exposed subjects, ratios of control subjects to exposed subjects of 1:1, 2:1, 3:1, 4:1, 5:1, 10:1, and 50:1 would result in statistical powers of 0.80, 0.887, 0.913, 0.926, 0.933, 0.947, and 0.956, respectively.

It is important to differentiate between the number of controls (as was discussed and illustrated above) and the number of control groups. It is not uncommon, especially in case–control studies, where the selection of a proper control group can be difficult, to choose more than one control group (for example, a group of hospital controls and a group of community controls). This is done for reasons of validity, not for statistical power, and it is important that these multiple control groups not be aggregated in the analysis. In this situation, the goal is to assure that the comparison of the exposed subjects to each of the different control groups yields the same answer, not to increase the available sample size. As such, the comparison of each control group to the exposed subjects should be treated as a separate study. The comparison of the exposed group to each control group requires a separate sample size calculation.

Once the five variables above have been specified, the sample size needed for a given study can be calculated. Several different formulas have been used for this calculation, each of which gives slightly different results. The formula that is probably the most often used is modified from Schlesselman:

$$N = \frac{1}{\left[p(1-R)\right]^2}\left[Z_{1-} \sqrt{\left(1+\frac{1}{K}\right)U(1-U)} + Z_{1-} \sqrt{pR(1-Rp)+\frac{p(1-p)}{K}}\right]^2$$

where p is the incidence of the disease in the unexposed, R is the minimum relative risk to be detected, $\alpha$ is the Type I error rate which is acceptable, $\beta$ is the Type II error rate which is acceptable, $Z_{1}.\alpha$ and $Z_{1}.\beta$ refer to the unit normal deviates corresponding to $\alpha$ and $\beta$, K is the ratio of number of unexposed control subjects to the number of exposed subjects, and

$$U = \frac{Kp + pR}{K+1}.$$

$Z_{1}.\alpha$ is replaced by $Z_{1}.\alpha_{/2}$ if one is planning to analyze the study using a two-tailed alpha. Note that K does not need to be an integer.

A series of tables are presented in the Appendix, which were calculated using this formula. In Tables A1 through A4 we have assumed an alpha (two-tailed) of 0.05, a beta of 0.1 (90% power), and control to exposed ratios of 1:1, 2:1, 3:1, and 4:1, respectively. Tables A5 through A8 are similar, except they assume a beta of 0.2 (80% power). Each table presents the number of exposed subjects needed to detect any of several specified relative risks, for outcome variables that occur at any of several specified incidence rates. The total study size will be the sum of exposed subjects (as listed in the table) plus the controls.

For example, what if one wanted to investigate a new nonsteroidal anti-inflammatory drug that is about to be marketed, but premarketing data raised questions about possible hepatotoxicity? This would presumably be studied using a cohort study design and, depending upon the values chosen for alpha, beta, the incidence of the disease in the unexposed population, the relative risk one wants to be able to detect, and the ratio of control to exposed subjects, the sample sizes needed could differ markedly (see Table 3.2). For example, what if your goal was to study hepatitis that occurs, say, in 0.1% of all unexposed individuals? If one wanted to design a study with one control per exposed subject to detect a relative risk of 2.0 for this outcome variable, assuming an alpha (two-tailed) of 0.05 and a beta of 0.1, one could look in Table A1 and see that it would require 31 483 exposed subjects, as well as an equal number of unexposed controls. If one were less concerned with missing a real finding, even if it was there, one could change beta to 0.2, and the required sample size would drop to 23 518 (see Table 3.2 and Table A5). If one wanted to minimize the number of exposed subjects needed for the study, one could include up to four controls for each exposed subject (Table 3.2 and Table A8). This would result in a sample size of 13 402, with four times as many controls, a total of 67 010 subjects. Finally, if one considers it inconceivable that this new drug could *protect* against liver disease and one is not interested in that outcome, then one might use a one-tailed alpha, resulting in a somewhat lower sample size of 10 728, again with four times as many controls. Much smaller sample sizes are needed to detect relative risks of 4.0 or greater; these are also presented in Table 3.2.

In contrast, what if one's goal was to study elevated liver function tests, which, say, occur in 1% of an unexposed population? If one wants to detect a relative risk of 2 for this more common outcome variable, only 3104 subjects would be needed in each group, assuming a two-tailed alpha of 0.05, a beta of 0.1, and one control per exposed subject. Alternatively, if one wanted to detect the same relative risk for an outcome variable

**Table 3.2** Examples of sample sizes needed for a cohort study.

| Disease | Incidence rate assumed in unexposed | α | β | Relative risk to be detected | Control:exposed ratio | Sample size needed in exposed group | Sample size needed in control group |
|---|---|---|---|---|---|---|---|
| Abnormal liver function tests | 0.01 | 0.05 (2-tailed) | 0.1 | 2 | 1 | 3104 | 3104 |
| | 0.01 | 0.05 (2-tailed) | 0.2 | 2 | 1 | 2319 | 2319 |
| | 0.01 | 0.05 (2-tailed) | 0.2 | 2 | 4 | 1323 | 5292 |
| | 0.01 | 0.05 (1-tailed) | 0.2 | 2 | 4 | 1059 | 4236 |
| | 0.01 | 0.05 (2-tailed) | 0.1 | 4 | 1 | 568 | 568 |
| | 0.01 | 0.05 (2-tailed) | 0.2 | 4 | 1 | 425 | 425 |
| | 0.01 | 0.05 (2-tailed) | 0.2 | 4 | 4 | 221 | 884 |
| | 0.01 | 0.05 (1-tailed) | 0.2 | 4 | 4 | 179 | 716 |
| Hepatitis | 0.001 | 0.05 (2-tailed) | 0.1 | 2 | 1 | 31 483 | 31 483 |
| | 0.001 | 0.05 (2-tailed) | 0.2 | 2 | 1 | 23 518 | 23 518 |
| | 0.001 | 0.05 (2-tailed) | 0.2 | 2 | 4 | 13 402 | 53 608 |
| | 0.001 | 0.05 (1-tailed) | 0.2 | 2 | 4 | 10 728 | 42 912 |
| | 0.001 | 0.05 (2-tailed) | 0.1 | 4 | 1 | 5823 | 5823 |
| | 0.001 | 0.05 (2-tailed) | 0.2 | 4 | 1 | 4350 | 4350 |
| | 0.001 | 0.05 (2-tailed) | 0.2 | 4 | 4 | 2253 | 9012 |
| | 0.001 | 0.05 (1-tailed) | 0.2 | 4 | 4 | 1829 | 7316 |
| Cholestatic jaundice | 0.0001 | 0.05 (2-tailed) | 0.1 | 2 | 1 | 315 268 | 315 268 |
| | 0.0001 | 0.05 (2-tailed) | 0.2 | 2 | 1 | 235 500 | 235 500 |
| | 0.0001 | 0.05 (2-tailed) | 0.2 | 2 | 4 | 134 194 | 536 776 |
| | 0.0001 | 0.05 (1-tailed) | 0.2 | 2 | 4 | 107 418 | 429 672 |
| | 0.0001 | 0.05 (2-tailed) | 0.1 | 4 | 1 | 58 376 | 58 376 |
| | 0.0001 | 0.05 (2-tailed) | 0.2 | 4 | 1 | 43 606 | 43 606 |
| | 0.0001 | 0.05 (2-tailed) | 0.2 | 4 | 4 | 22 572 | 90 288 |
| | 0.0001 | 0.05 (1-tailed) | 0.2 | 4 | 4 | 18 331 | 73 324 |

that occurred as infrequently as 0.0001, perhaps cholestatic jaundice, one would need 315 268 subjects in each study group.

Obviously, cohort studies can require very large sample sizes to study uncommon diseases. A study of uncommon diseases is often better performed using a case–control study design, as described in the previous chapter.

## Sample Size Calculations for Case–Control Studies

The approach to calculating sample sizes for case–control studies is similar to the approach for cohort studies. Again, there are five variables that need to be specified, the values of which depend on what the investigator expects from the study (see Table 3.1). Three of these are alpha, or the type I error one is willing to tolerate; beta, or the type II error one is willing to tolerate; and the minimum odds ratio (an approximation of the relative risk) one wants to be able to detect. These are defined and described in the section on cohort studies, above.

In addition, in a case–control study one selects subjects based on the presence or absence of the disease of interest, and then investigates the prevalence of the exposure of interest in each study group. This is in contrast to a cohort study, in which one selects subjects based on the presence or absence of an exposure, and then studies whether or not the disease of interest develops in each group. Therefore, the fourth variable to be specified for a case–control study is the expected prevalence of the exposure in the undiseased control group, rather than the incidence of the disease of interest in the unexposed control group of a cohort study.

Finally, analogous to the consideration in cohort studies of the ratio of the number of unexposed control subjects to the number of exposed study subjects, one needs to consider in a case–control study the ratio of the number of undiseased control subjects to the number of diseased study subjects. The principles in deciding upon the appropriate ratio to use are similar in both study designs. Again, there is rarely a reason to include a ratio greater than 3:1 or 4:1. For example, if one were to design a study with a two-tailed alpha of 0.05 to detect a relative risk of 2.0 for an exposure which occurs in 5% of the undiseased control group, a study with 516 diseased individuals and 516 controls would yield a power of 0.80, or an 80% chance of detecting a difference of that size. Studies with the same 516 diseased subjects and ratios of controls to cases of 1:1, 2:1, 3:1, 4:1, 5:1, 10:1, and 50:1 would result in statistical powers of 0.80, 0.889, 0.916, 0.929, 0.936, 0.949, and 0.959, respectively.

The formula for calculating sample sizes for a case–control study is similar to that for cohort studies:

$$N = \frac{1}{(p-V)^2}\left[ Z_{1-\alpha}\sqrt{\left(1+\frac{1}{K}\right)U(1-U)} + Z_{(1-\beta)}\sqrt{p(1-p)/K + V(1-V)} \right]^2$$

where $R$, $\alpha$, $\beta$, $Z_{1-\alpha}$, and $Z_{1-\beta}$ are as above, $p$ is the prevalence of the exposure in the control group, and $K$ is the ratio of undiseased control subjects to diseased cases,

$$U = \left( \frac{p}{K+1}K + \frac{R}{1+p(R-1)} \right)$$

and

$$V = \frac{pR}{1+p(R-1)}.$$

Again, a series of tables that provide sample sizes for case–control studies is presented in the Appendix. In Tables A9 through A12, we have assumed an alpha (two-tailed) of 0.05, a beta of 0.1 (90% power), and control to case ratios of 1:1, 2:1, 3:1, and 4:1, respectively. Tables A13 through A16 are similar, except they assume a beta of 0.2 (80% power). Each table presents the number of diseased subjects needed to detect any of a number of specified relative risks, for a number of specified exposure rates.

For example, what if again one wanted to investigate a new nonsteroidal anti-inflammatory drug that is about to be marketed but premarketing data raised questions about possible hepatotoxicity? This time, however, one is attempting to use a case–control study design. Again, depending upon the values chosen of alpha, beta, and so on, the sample sizes needed could differ markedly (see Table 3.3). For example, what if one wanted to design a study with one control (undiseased subject) per diseased subject, assuming an alpha (two-tailed) of 0.05 and a beta of 0.1? The sample size needed to detect a relative risk of 2.0 for any disease would vary, depending on the prevalence of use of the drug being studied. If one optimistically assumed the drug will be used nearly as commonly as ibuprofen, by perhaps 1% of the population, then one could look in Table A9 and see that it would require 3210 diseased subjects and an equal number of undiseased controls. If one were less concerned with missing a real association, even if it existed, one could opt for a beta of 0.2, and the required sample size would drop to 2398 (see Table 3.3 and Table A13). If one wanted to minimize the number of diseased subjects needed for the study, one could include up to four controls for each diseased subject (Table 3.3 and Table A16). This would result in a sample size of 1370, with four times as many controls. Finally, if one considers it inconceivable that this new drug could *protect* against liver disease, then one might use a one-tailed alpha, resulting in a somewhat lower sample size of 1096, again with four times as many controls. Much smaller sample sizes are needed to detect relative risks of 4.0 or greater and are also presented in Table 3.3.

In contrast, what if one's estimates of the new drug's sales were more conservative? If one wanted to detect a relative risk of 2.0 assuming sales to 0.1% of the population, perhaps similar to tolmetin, then 31 588 subjects would be needed in each group, assuming a two-tailed alpha of 0.05, a beta of 0.1, and one control per diseased subject. In contrast, if one estimated the drug would be used in only 0.01% of the population (i.e. in controls without the study disease of interest), perhaps like phenylbutazone, one would need 315 373 subjects in each study group.

Obviously, case–control studies can require very large sample sizes to study relatively uncommonly used drugs. In addition, each disease of interest requires a separate case group and, thereby, a separate study. As such, as described in the prior chapter, studies of uncommonly used drugs and newly marketed drugs are usually better done using cohort study designs, whereas studies of rare diseases are better done using case–control designs.

## Sample Size Calculations for Case Series

As described in Chapter 2, the utility of case series in pharmacoepidemiology is limited, as the absence of a control group makes causal inference difficult. Despite this, however, this is a design that has been used repeatedly. There are scientific questions that can be addressed using this design, and the collection of a control group equivalent in size to the case series would add considerable cost to the study. Case series are usually used in pharmacoepidemiology to quantitate better the incidence of a particular disease in patients exposed to a newly marketed drug. For example, in the "Phase 4" postmarketing drug surveillance study conducted for prazosin, the investigators collected a case series of 10 000 newly exposed subjects recruited through the manufacturer's sales force, to quantitate better the incidence of first

**Table 3.3** Examples of sample sizes needed for a case–control study.

| Hypothetical drug | Prevalence rate assumed in undiseased | α | β | Odds ratio to be detected | Control: case ratio | Sample size needed in case group | Sample size needed in control group |
|---|---|---|---|---|---|---|---|
| Ibuprofen | 0.01 | 0.05 (2-tailed) | 0.1 | 2 | 1 | 3210 | 3210 |
| | 0.01 | 0.05 (2-tailed) | 0.2 | 2 | 1 | 2398 | 2398 |
| | 0.01 | 0.05 (2-tailed) | 0.2 | 2 | 4 | 1370 | 5480 |
| | 0.01 | 0.05 (1-tailed) | 0.2 | 2 | 4 | 1096 | 4384 |
| | 0.01 | 0.05 (2-tailed) | 0.1 | 4 | 1 | 601 | 601 |
| | 0.01 | 0.05 (2-tailed) | 0.2 | 4 | 1 | 449 | 449 |
| | 0.01 | 0.05 (2-tailed) | 0.2 | 4 | 4 | 234 | 936 |
| | 0.01 | 0.05 (1-tailed) | 0.2 | 4 | 4 | 190 | 760 |
| Tolmetin | 0.001 | 0.05 (2-tailed) | 0.1 | 2 | 1 | 31588 | 31588 |
| | 0.001 | 0.05 (2-tailed) | 0.2 | 2 | 1 | 23596 | 23596 |
| | 0.001 | 0.05 (2-tailed) | 0.2 | 2 | 4 | 13449 | 53796 |
| | 0.001 | 0.05 (1-tailed) | 0.2 | 2 | 4 | 10765 | 43060 |
| | 0.001 | 0.05 (2-tailed) | 0.1 | 4 | 1 | 5856 | 5856 |
| | 0.001 | 0.05 (2-tailed) | 0.2 | 4 | 1 | 4375 | 4375 |
| | 0.001 | 0.05 (2-tailed) | 0.2 | 4 | 4 | 2266 | 9064 |
| | 0.001 | 0.05 (1-tailed) | 0.2 | 4 | 4 | 1840 | 7360 |
| Phenylbutazone | 0.0001 | 0.05 (2-tailed) | 0.1 | 2 | 1 | 315373 | 315373 |
| | 0.0001 | 0.05 (2-tailed) | 0.2 | 2 | 1 | 235579 | 235579 |
| | 0.0001 | 0.05 (2-tailed) | 0.2 | 2 | 4 | 134240 | 536960 |
| | 0.0001 | 0.05 (1-tailed) | 0.2 | 2 | 4 | 107455 | 429820 |
| | 0.0001 | 0.05 (2-tailed) | 0.1 | 4 | 1 | 58409 | 58409 |
| | 0.0001 | 0.05 (2-tailed) | 0.2 | 4 | 1 | 43631 | 43631 |
| | 0.0001 | 0.05 (2-tailed) | 0.2 | 4 | 4 | 22585 | 90340 |
| | 0.0001 | 0.05 (1-tailed) | 0.2 | 4 | 4 | 18342 | 73368 |

dose syncope, which was a well-recognized adverse effect of this drug. Case series are usually used to determine whether a disease occurs more frequently than some predetermined incidence in exposed patients. Most often, the predetermined incidence of interest is zero, and one is looking for any occurrences of an extremely rare illness. As another example, when cimetidine was first marketed, there was a concern over whether it could cause agranulocytosis, since it was closely related chemically to metiamide, another H-2 blocker, which had been removed from the market in Europe because it caused agranulocytosis. This study also collected 10 000 subjects. It found only two cases of neutropenia, one in a patient also receiving chemotherapy. There were no cases of agranulocytosis.

To establish drug safety, a study must include a sufficient number of subjects to detect an elevated incidence of a disease, if it exists. Generally, this is calculated by assuming the frequency of the event in question is vanishingly small, so that the occurrence of the event follows a Poisson distribution, and then one generally calculates 95% confidence intervals around the observed results.

Table A17 in the Appendix presents a table useful for making this calculation. In order to apply this table, one first calculates the incidence rate observed from the study's results, that is the number of subjects who develop the disease of interest during the specified time interval, divided by the total number of individuals in the population at risk. For example, if three cases of liver disease were observed in a population of 1000 patients exposed to a new nonsteroidal anti-inflammatory drug during a specified period of time, the incidence would be 0.003. The number of subjects who develop the disease is the "Observed Number on Which Estimate is Based (n)" in Table A17. In this example, it is three. The lower boundary of the 95% confidence interval for the incidence rate is then the corresponding "Lower Limit Factor (L)" multiplied by the observed incidence rate. In the example above, it would be 0.206 X

0.003 = 0.000618. Analogously, the upper boundary would be the product of the corresponding "Upper Limit Factor (U)" multiplied by the observed incidence rate. In the above example, this would be $2.92 \times 0.003 = 0.00876$. In other words, the incidence rate (95% confidence interval) would be 0.003 (0.000618–0.00876). Thus, the best estimate of the incidence rate would be 30 per 10 000, but there is a 95% chance that it lies between 6.18 per 10 000 and 87.6 per 10 000.

In addition, a helpful simple guide is the so-called "rule of threes," useful in the common situation where no events of a particular kind are observed. Specifically, if no events of a particular type (i.e. the events of interest to the study) are observed in a study of X individuals, then one can be 95% certain that the event occurs no more often than 3/X. For example, if 500 patients are studied prior to marketing a drug, then one can be 95% certain that any event which does not occur in any of those patients may occur with a frequency of 3 or less in 500 exposed subjects, or that it has an incidence rate of less than 0.006. If 3000 subjects are exposed prior to drug marketing, then one can be 95% certain that any event which does not occur in this population may occur no more than three in 3000 subjects, or the event has an incidence rate of less than 0.001. Finally, if 10 000 subjects are studied in a postmarketing drug surveillance study, then one can be 95% certain that any events which are not observed may occur no more than three in 10 000 exposed individuals, or that they have an incidence rate of less than 0.0003. In other words, events not detected in the study may occur less often than one in 3333 subjects in the general population.

## Discussion

The above discussions about sample size determinations in cohort and case–control studies assume one is able to obtain information on each of the five variables that factor into these sample size calculations. Is this in fact realistic? Four of the variables are, in fact, totally in the control of the investigator, subject to his or her specification: alpha, beta, the ratio of control subjects to study subjects, and the minimum relative risk to be detected. Only one of the variables requires data derived from other sources. For cohort studies, this is the expected incidence of the disease in the unexposed control group. For case–control studies, this is the expected prevalence of the exposure in the undiseased control group. In considering this needed information, it is important to realize that the entire process of sample size calculation is approximate, despite its mathematical sophistication. There is certainly no compelling reason why an alpha should be 0.05, as opposed to 0.06 or 0.04. The other variables specified by the investigator are similarly arbitrary. As such, only an approximate estimate is needed for this missing variable. Often the needed information is readily available from some existing data source, for example vital statistics or commercial drug utilization data sources. If not, one can search the medical literature for one or more studies that have collected these data for a defined population, either deliberately or as a by-product of their data collecting effort, and assume that the population you will study will be similar. If this is not an appropriate assumption, or if no such data exist in the medical literature, one is left with two alternatives. The first, and better, alternative is to conduct a small pilot study within your population, in order to measure the information you need. The second is simply to guess. In the second case, one should consider what a reasonable higher guess and a reasonable lower guess might be, as well, to see if your sample size should be increased to take into account the imprecision of your estimate.

Finally, what if one is studying multiple outcome variables (in a cohort study) or multiple exposure variables (in a case–control study), each of which differs in the frequency you expect in the control group? In that situation, an investigator might base the study's sample size on the variable that leads to the largest requirement, and note that the study will have even more power for the other outcome (or exposure) variables. Regardless, it is usually better to have a somewhat larger than expected sample size than the minimum, to allow some leeway if any of the underlying assumptions were wrong. This also will permit subgroup analyses with adequate power. In fact, if there are important subgroup analyses that represent a priori hypotheses that one wants to be able to evaluate, one should perform separate sample size calculations for those subgroups. In this situation, one should use the incidence of disease or prevalence of exposure that occurs in the subgroups, not that which occurs in the general population.

Note that sample size calculation is often an iterative process. There is nothing wrong with performing an initial calculation, realizing that it generates an unrealistic sample size, and then modifying the underlying assumptions accordingly. What is important is that the investigator examines his or her final assumptions closely, asking whether, given the compromises made, the study is still worth undertaking.

Note that the discussion above was restricted to sample size calculations for dichotomous variables, i.e. variables with only two options: a study subject either has a disease or does not have a disease. Information was not presented on sample size calculations for continuous outcome variables, i.e. variables that have some measurement, such as height, weight, blood pressure, or serum cholesterol. Overall, the use of a continuous variable as an outcome variable, unless the measurement is extremely imprecise, will result in a marked increase in the power of a study. Details about this are omitted because epidemiologic studies unfortunately do not usually have the luxury of using such variables. Readers who are interested in more information on this can consult a textbook of sample size calculations.

All of the previous discussions have focused on calculating a minimum necessary sample size. This is the usual concern. However, two other issues specific to pharmacoepidemiology are important to consider as well. First, one of the main advantages of postmarketing pharmacoepidemiologic studies is the increased sensitivity to rare adverse reactions that can be achieved, by including a sample size larger than that used prior to marketing. Since between 500 and 3000 patients are usually studied before marketing, most pharmacoepidemiologic cohort studies are designed to include at least 10000 exposed subjects. The total population from which these 10000 exposed subjects would be recruited would need to be very much larger, of course. Case–control studies can be much smaller, but generally need to recruit cases and controls from a source population of equivalent size as for cohort studies. These are not completely arbitrary figures, but are based on the principles described above, applied to the questions which remain of great importance to address in a postmarketing setting. Nevertheless, these figures should not be rigidly accepted but should be reconsidered for each specific study. Some studies will require fewer subjects, many will require more. To accumulate these sample sizes while performing cost-effective studies, several special techniques have been developed, which are described in Section II of this book.

Second, because of the development of these new techniques and the development of large electronic data systems (see Chapters 8, 9, and 10), pharmacoepidemiologic studies have the potential for the relatively unusual problem of *too large* a sample size. It is even more important than usual, therefore, when interpreting the results of studies that use these data systems to examine their findings, differentiating clearly between statistical significance and clinical significance. With a very large sample size, one can find statistically significant differences that are clinically trivial. In addition, it must be kept in mind that subtle findings, even if statistically and clinically important, could easily have been created by biases or confounders (see Chapter 2). Subtle findings should not be ignored, but should be interpreted with caution.

## Key Points

- Premarketing studies of drugs are inherently limited in size, meaning larger studies are needed after marketing in order to detect less common drug effects.
- For a cohort study, the sample size needed is determined by specifying the Type I error one is willing to tolerate, the Type II error one is willing to tolerate, the smallest relative risk which one wants to be able to detect, the expected incidence of the outcome of interest in the unexposed control group, and the ratio of the number of unexposed control subjects to be included in the study to the number of exposed study subjects.
- For a case–control study, the needed sample size is determined by specifying the Type I error one is willing to tolerate, the Type II error one is willing to tolerate, the smallest odds ratio which one wants to be able to detect, the expected prevalence of the exposure of interest in the undiseased control group, and the ratio of the number of undiseased control subjects to be included in the study to the number of exposed study subjects.
- As a rule of thumb, if no events of a particular type are observed in a study of $X$ individuals, then one can be 95% certain that the event occurs no more often than $3/X$.

## Further Reading

Cohen, J. (1977). *Statistical Power Analysis for the Social Sciences*. New York: Academic Press.

Gifford, L.M., Aeugle, M.E., Myerson, R.M., and Tannenbaum, P.J. (1980). Cimetidine postmarket outpatient surveillance program. *JAMA* 243: 1532–1535.

Graham, R.M., Thornell, I.R., Gain, J.M. et al. (1976). Prazosin: the first dose phenomenon. *BMJ* 2: 1293–1294.

Haenszel, W., Loveland, D.B., and Sirken, M.G. (1962). Lung cancer mortality as related to residence and smoking history. I. White males. *J. Natl. Cancer Inst.* 28: 947–1001.

*Joint Commission on Prescription Drug Use* (1980) *Final Report.* Washington, DC.

Makuch, R.W. and Johnson, M.F. (1986). Some issues in the design and interpretation of "negative" clinical trials. *Arch. Intern. Med.* 146: 986–989.

Schlesselman, J.J. (1974). Sample size requirements in cohort and case–control studies of disease. *Am. J. Epidemiol.* 99: 381–384.

Stolley, P.D. and Strom, B.L. (1986). Sample size calculations for clinical pharmacology studies. *Clin. Pharmacol. Ther.* 39: 489–490.

Young, M.J., Bresnitz, E.A., and Strom, B.L. (1983). Sample size nomograms for interpreting negative clinical studies. *Ann. Intern. Med.* 99: 248–251.

# 4

# Basic Principles of Clinical Pharmacology Relevant to Pharmacoepidemiologic Studies

*Jeffrey S. Barrett*

*Critical Path Institute, Tuscon, AZ, USA*

## Introduction

*Pharmacology* deals with the study of drugs while *clinical pharmacology* deals with the study of drugs in humans. More specifically, clinical pharmacology evaluates the characteristics, effects, properties, reactions, and uses of drugs, particularly their therapeutic value in humans, including their toxicology, safety, pharmacodynamics, and pharmacokinetics. While the foundation of the discipline is underpinned by basic pharmacology (the study of the interactions that occur between a living organism and exogenous chemicals that alter normal biochemical function), the important emphasis of clinical pharmacology is the application of pharmacologic principles and methods in the care of patients. From the discovery of new target molecules and molecular targets to the evaluation of clinical utility in specific populations, clinical pharmacology bridges the gap between laboratory science and medical practice. The main objective is to promote the safe and effective use of drugs, maximizing the beneficial drug effects while minimizing harmful side effects. It is important that caregivers are skilled in the areas of drug information, medication safety, and other aspects of pharmacy practice related to clinical pharmacology.

Clinical pharmacology is an important bridging discipline that includes knowledge about the relationships between: dose and exposure at the site of action (pharmacokinetics); exposure at the site of action and clinical response (pharmacodynamics); and between clinical response and outcomes. In the process, it defines the therapeutic window (the dosage of a medication between the minimum amount that gives a desired effect and the minimum amount that gives more adverse effects than desired effects) of a drug in various patient populations. Likewise, clinical pharmacology also guides dose modifications in various patient subpopulations (e.g. pediatrics, pregnancy, elderly, and organ impairment) and/or dose adjustments for various lifestyle factors (e.g. food, time of day, drug interactions).

The discovery and development of new medicines is reliant upon clinical pharmacologic research. Scientists in academic, regulatory, and industrial settings participate in this research as part of the overall drug development process. The output from clinical pharmacologic investigation appears in the drug monograph or package insert of all new medicines and forms the basis of how drug dosing information is communicated to healthcare providers.

## Clinical Pharmacology and Pharmacoepidemiology

Pharmacoepidemiology is the study of the use and effects of drugs in large numbers of people.

To accomplish this, pharmacoepidemiology borrows from both clinical pharmacology and epidemiology. Thus, pharmacoepidemiology can also be called a bridging science. Part of the task of clinical pharmacology is to provide risk–benefit assessment for the effect of drugs in patients. Studies that estimate the probability and magnitude of beneficial effects in populations, or the probability and magnitude of adverse effects in populations, will benefit from epidemiologic methodology. Pharmacoepidemiology then can also be defined as the application of epidemiologic methods to the content area of clinical pharmacology. Figure 4.1 illustrates the relationship between clinical pharmacology and pharmacoepidemiology as well as some of the specific research areas reliant on both disciplines.

## Basics of Clinical Pharmacology

Clinical pharmacology encompasses drug composition, drug properties, interactions, toxicology, and effects (both desirable and undesirable) that can be used in pharmacotherapy of diseases. Underlying the discipline of clinical pharmacology are the fields of pharmacokinetics and pharmacodynamics, and each of these disciplines can be further defined by specific subprocesses (absorption, distribution, metabolism, elimination). Clinical pharmacology is essential to our understanding of how drugs work as well as how to guide their administration. Pharmacotherapy can be challenging because of physiologic factors that may alter drug kinetics (age, size, etc.), pathophysiologic differences that may alter pharmacodynamics, disease etiologies in studied patients that may differ from those present in the general population, and other factors that may result in great variation in safety and efficacy outcomes. The challenge is more difficult in

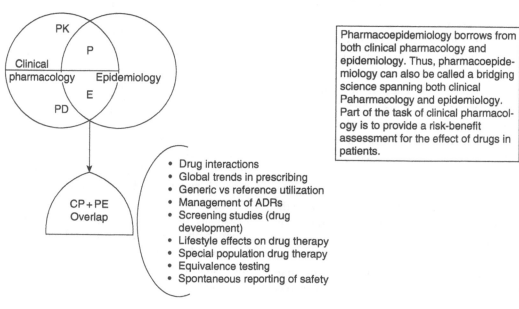

> Pharmacoepidemiology borrows from both clinical pharmacology and epidemiology. Thus, pharmacoepidemiology can also be called a bridging science spanning both clinical Paharmacology and epidemiology. Part of the task of clinical pharmacology is to provide a risk-benefit assessment for the effect of drugs in patients.

**Figure 4.1** Relationship between clinical pharmacology and pharmacoepidemiology, illustrating the overlapping areas of interest.

the critically ill given the paucity of well-controlled clinical trials in vulnerable populations.

# Pharmacokinetics

Pharmacokinetics refers to the study of the absorption and distribution of an administered drug, the chemical changes of the substance in the body (metabolism), and the effects and routes of excretion of the metabolites of the drug (elimination).

## Absorption

*Absorption* is the process of drug transfer from its site of administration to the blood stream. The rate and efficiency of absorption depend on the route of administration. For intravenous administration, absorption is complete; the total dose reaches the systemic circulation. Drugs administered enterally may be absorbed by either passive diffusion or active transport. The *bioavailability* (F) of a drug is the fraction of the administered dose that reaches the systemic circulation. If a drug is administered intravenously, then bioavailability is 100% and F = 1.0. When drugs are administered by routes other than intravenous, the bioavailability is usually less. Bioavailability is reduced by incomplete absorption, first-pass metabolism (defined below), and distribution into other tissues.

## Volume of Distribution

The *apparent volume of distribution* (Vd) is a hypothetical volume of fluid through which a drug is dispersed. A drug rarely disperses solely into the water compartments of the body. Instead, the majority of drugs disperse to several compartments, including adipose tissue and plasma proteins. The total volume into which a drug disperses if it were only fluid is called the apparent volume of distribution. This volume is not a physiologic space, but

rather a conceptual parameter. It relates the total amount of drug in the body to the concentration of drug (C) in the blood or plasma: Vd = Drug/C.

Figure 4.2 represents the fate of a drug after intravenous administration. After administration, maximal plasma concentration is achieved, and the drug is distributed. The plasma concentration then decreases over time. This initial alpha ($\alpha$) phase of drug distribution indicates the decline in plasma concentration due to the distribution of the drug. Once a drug is distributed, it undergoes metabolism and elimination. The second beta ($\beta$) phase indicates the decline in plasma concentration due to drug metabolism and clearance. The terms A and B are intercepts with the vertical axis. The extrapolation of the $\beta$ phase defines B. The dotted line is generated by subtracting the extrapolated line from the original concentration line. This second line defines $\alpha$ and A. The plasma concentration can be estimated using the formula: $C = Ae^{-\alpha t} + Be^{-\beta t}$. The distribution and elimination half lives can be determined by: $t_{1/2}\alpha = 0.693/\alpha$ and $t_{1/2}\beta = 0.693/\beta$, respectively.

For drugs in which distribution is homogenous across the various physiologic spaces, the distinction between the alpha and beta phase may be subtle and essentially a single phase best describes the decline in drug concentration.

## Metabolism

The *metabolism* of drugs is catalyzed by enzymes, and most reactions follow Michaelis Menten kinetics: V (rate of drug metabolism) = $[((V_{max})(C)/K_m) + (C)]$, where C is the drug concentration, $V_{max}$ is the maximum rate of metabolism in units of amount of product over time, typically $\mu$mol/min, and $K_m$ is the Michaelis Menten constant (substrate concentration at which the rate of conversion is half of $V_{max}$) also in units of concentration. In most situations, the drug concentration is much less than $K_m$ and the equation simplifies to:

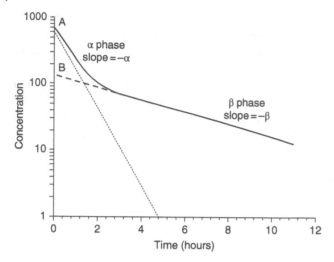

**Figure 4.2** Semi-logarithmic plot of concentration vs time after an intravenous administration of a drug that follows two-compartment pharmacokinetics.

$V = (V_{max})(C)/K_m$. In this case, the rate of drug metabolism is directly proportional to the concentration of free drug, and follows first order kinetic theory. A constant percentage of the drug is metabolized per unit time, and the absolute amount of drug eliminated per unit time is proportional to the amount of drug in the body.

Most drugs used in the clinical setting are eliminated in this manner. A few drugs, such as aspirin, ethanol, and phenytoin, are used in higher doses, resulting in higher plasma concentrations. In these situations, C is much greater than $K_m$, and the Michaelis Menten equation reduces to: $V$(rate of drug metabolism) $= (V_{max})(C)/(C) = V_{max}$. The enzyme system becomes saturated by a high free drug concentration, and the rate of metabolism is constant over time. This is called zero-order kinetics, and a constant amount of drug is metabolized per unit time. For drugs that follow zero-order elimination, a large increase in serum concentration can result from a small increase in dose.

The liver is the principal organ of drug metabolism. Other organs that display considerable metabolic activity include the gastrointestinal tract, lungs, skin, and kidneys. Following oral administration, many drugs are absorbed intact from the small intestine and transported to the liver via the portal system, where they are metabolized. This process is called first pass metabolism, and may greatly limit the bioavailability of orally administered drugs. In general, all metabolic reactions can be classified as either phase I or phase II biotransformations. Phase I reactions usually convert the parent drug to a polar metabolite by introducing or unmasking a more polar site. If phase I metabolites are sufficiently polar, they may be readily excreted. However, many phase I metabolites undergo a subsequent reaction in which endogenous substances such as glucuronic acid, sulfuric acid, or an amino acid combine with the metabolite to form a highly polar conjugate. Many drugs undergo these sequential reactions.

Phase I reactions are usually catalyzed by enzymes of the cytochrome P450 system. These drug-metabolizing enzymes are located in the lipophilic membranes of the endoplasmic reticulum of the liver and other tissues. Three gene families, CYP1, CYP2, and CYP3, are responsible for most drug biotransformations. The CYP3A subfamily accounts for greater than 50% of phase I drug metabolism, predominantly by the CYP3A4 sub-type. CYP3A4 is responsible for the metabolism of drugs commonly used in the intensive care setting, including acetaminophen, cyclosporine, methadone, midazolam, and tacrolimus. Most other drug biotransformations are performed by CYP2D6 (e.g. clozapine, codeine, flecainide, haloperidol, oxycodone), CYP2C9 (e.g. phenytoin, S-warfarin), CYP2C19 (e.g. diazepam, omeprazole, propranolol), CYP2E1 (e.g. acetaminophen, enflurane, halothane), and CYP1A2 (e.g. acetaminophen, theophylline, warfarin).

Biotransformation reactions may be enhanced or impaired by multiple factors, including age, enzyme induction or inhibition, pharmacogenetics, and the effects of other disease states. Approximately 95% of the metabolism occurs via conjugation to glucuronide (50–60%) and sulfate (25–35%). Most of the remainder of acetaminophen is metabolized via the cytochrome P450 forming N-acetyl-p-benzoquinone imine (NAPQI) thought to be responsible for hepatotoxicity. This minor but important pathway is catalyzed by CYP 2E1, and to a lesser extent, CYP 1A2 and CYP 3A4. NAPQI is detoxified by reacting with either glutathione directly or through a glutathione transferase catalyzed reaction. When hepatic synthesis of glutathione is overwhelmed, manifestations of toxicity appear, producing centrilobular necrosis. In the presence of a potent CYP 2E1 inhibitor, disulfiram, a 69% reduction in the urinary excretion of these 2E1 metabolic products is observed, supporting the major role for 2E1 in the formation of NAPQI. CYP 2E1 is unique among the CYP gene families in an ability to produce reactive oxygen radicals through a reduction of O2 and is the only CYP system strongly induced (drug molecule initiates or enhances the expression of an enzyme) by alcohol which is itself a substrate (a molecule upon which an enzyme acts). In addition to alcohol, isoniazid acts as inducer and a substrate. Ketoconazole and other imidazole compounds are inducers but not substrates. Barbiturates and phenytoin, which are nonspecific inducers, have no role

as CYP 2E1 inducers, nor are they substrates for that system. Phenytoin in fact may be hepato-protective because it is an inducer of the glucuronidation metabolic pathway for acetaminophen, thus shunting metabolism away from NAPQI production.

## Elimination

*Elimination* is the process by which drug is removed or "cleared" from the body. Clearance (CL) is the amount of blood from which all drug is removed per unit time (volume/time). The primary organs responsible for drug clearance are the kidneys and liver. The total body clearance is equal to the sum of individual clearances from all mechanisms. Typically, this is partitioned into renal and nonrenal clearance. Most elimination by the kidneys is accomplished by glomerular filtration. The amount of drug filtered is determined by glomerular integrity, the size and charge of the drug, water solubility, and the extent of protein binding. Highly protein-bound drugs are not readily filtered. Therefore, estimation of the glomerular filtration rate (GFR) has traditionally served as an approximation of renal function.

In addition to glomerular filtration, drugs may be eliminated from the kidneys via active secretion. Secretion occurs predominantly at the proximal tubule of the nephron, where active transport systems secrete primarily organic acids and bases. Organic acids include most cephalosporins, loop diuretics, methotrexate, nonsteroidal anti-inflammatories, penicillins, and thiazide diuretics. Organic bases include ranitidine and morphine. As drugs move toward the distal convoluting tubule, concentration increases. High urine flow rates decrease drug concentration in the distal tubule, decreasing the likelihood of diffusion from the lumen. For both weak acids and bases, the nonionized form is reabsorbed more readily. Altering pH can minimize reabsorption, by placing a charge on the drug and preventing diffusion. For example, salicylate is a weak acid. In case of salicylate toxicity, urine alkalinization places a charge on the molecule, and increases its elimination. The liver also contributes to elimination through metabolism or excretion into the bile. After the drug is secreted in bile, it may then be either excreted into the feces or reabsorbed via enterohepatic recirculation. The *half-life of elimination* is the time it takes to clear half of the drug from plasma. It is directly proportional to the Vd, and inversely proportional to CL: $t_{1/2}\beta = (0.693)(Vd)/CL$.

## Special Populations

The term "special populations" as applied to drug development refers to discussions in the early 1990s by industry, academic, and regulatory scientists struggling with the then current practice that early drug development was focused predominantly on young, Caucasian, male populations. Representatives from the US, Europe, and Japan jointly issued regulatory requirements for drug testing and labeling in "special populations" (namely the elderly) in 1993. In later discussions, this generalization was expanded to include four major demographic segments (women, elderly, pediatric, and major ethnic groups); despite the size of each of these subpopulations, pharmaceutical research had been limited. More importantly, these "special populations" represent diverse subpopulations of patients in whom dosing guidance is often needed and likewise targeted clinical pharmacologic research is essential.

### Elderly

Physical signs consistent with aging include wrinkles, change of hair color to gray or white, hair loss, lessened hearing, diminished eyesight, slower reaction times, and decreased agility. We are generally more concerned with how aging affects physiologic processes that dictate drug pharmacokinetics and pharmacodynamics. Advancing age is characterized by impairment in the function of the many regulatory processes that provide functional integration between cells and organs. Cardiac structure and function, renal and gastrointestinal systems, and body composition are the physiologic systems most often implicated when pharmacokinetic or pharmacodynamic differences are observed between an elderly and young population. Table 4.1 lists the primary physiologic factors affected by aging.

With respect to absorption, the impact of age is unclear and many conflicting results exist. While many studies have not shown significant age-related differences in absorption rates, the absorption of vitamin $B_{12}$, iron, and calcium is slower through reduced active transport mechanisms. A reduction in first-pass metabolism is associated with aging, most likely due to a reduction in liver mass and blood flow. Likewise, drugs undergoing significant first-pass metabolism experience an increase in bioavailability with age. This is the case for propranolol and labetalol. Conversely, prodrugs requiring activation in the liver (e.g. ACE inhibitors enalapril and perindopril) are likely to experience reduction in this phase and therefore reduced exposure to the active species.

Based on age-related changes in body composition, polar drugs that are primarily water soluble often exhibit smaller volumes of distribution, resulting in higher plasma concentrations in older patients. This is the case for agents including ethanol, theophylline, digoxin, and gentamicin. Conversely, nonpolar compounds are often lipid soluble and exhibit larger volumes of distribution in older patients. The impact of the larger Vd is prolongation of half-life with age. This is the case for drugs such as chlormethiazole and thiopentone. Conflicting results have been reported with respect to age effects on protein binding, making generalizations difficult.

Several drug classes including water-soluble antibiotics, diuretics, water-soluble beta-adrenoceptor blockers, and nonsteroidal anti-inflammatory drugs exhibit changes in

**Table 4.1** Physiologic systems affected during aging that influence drug pharmacokinetic and/or pharmacodynamic behavior.

| Physiologic system | Impact of aging |
| --- | --- |
| Cardiac structure and function | • Reduced elasticity and compliance of the aorta and great arteries (higher systolic arterial pressure, increased impedance to left ventricular hypertrophy and interstitial fibrosis)<br>• Decrease in rate of myocardial relaxation<br>• Left ventricle stiffens and takes longer to relax and fill in diastole<br>• Isotonic contraction is prolonged and velocity of shortening reduced<br>• Reduction in intrinsic heart rate and increased sinoatrial node conduction time |
| Renal system | • Renal mass decreases (reduction in number of nephrons)<br>• Reduced blood flow in the afferent arterioles in the cortex<br>• Renal plasma flow and glomerular filtration rate decline<br>• Decrease in ability to concentrate the urine during water deprivation<br>• Impaired response to water loading |
| Gastrointestinal system | • Secretion of hydrochloric acid and pepsin is decreased under basal conditions<br>• Reduced absorption of several substances in the small intestine including sugar, calcium and iron<br>• Decrease in lipase and trypsin secretion in the pancreas<br>• Progressive reduction in liver volume and liver blood flow |
| Body composition | • Progressive reduction in total body water and lean body mass, resulting in a relative increase in body fat |

clearance with age because of declining renal function. With respect to hepatic metabolism, studies have shown that significant reductions in clearance with age are observed for phase I pathways in the liver.

From the standpoint of a clinical trial, age categories are necessary to define the inclusion and exclusion criteria for the population targeted for enrollment. Pharmaceutical sponsors are increasingly encouraged to include a broader range of ages in their pivotal trials or specifically target an elderly subpopulation in a separate study, consistent with FDA guidance. The FDA guideline for studies in the elderly is directed principally toward new molecular entities likely to have significant use in the elderly, either because the disease intended to be treated is characteristically a disease of aging (e.g. Alzheimer's disease) or because the population to be treated is known to include substantial numbers of geriatric patients (e.g. hypertension).

### Pediatrics

As children develop and grow changes in body composition, development of metabolizing enzymes, and maturation of renal and liver function, all affect drug disposition.

### Renal

Renal function in the premature and full-term neonate, both glomerular filtration and tubular secretion, is significantly reduced, as compared to older children. Maturation of renal function is a dynamic process that begins during fetal life and is complete by early childhood. Maturation of tubular function is slower than that of glomerular filtration. The GFR is approximately 2–4 ml/minute/1.73 m$^2$ in full term neonates, but it may be as low as 0.6–0.8 ml/minute/1.73 m$^2$ in preterm neonates. The GFR increases rapidly during the first two weeks of life and continues to rise until adult values are reached at 8–12 months of age. For drugs that are renally eliminated, impaired renal function decreases clearance, increasing the half-life. Therefore, for drugs that are primarily eliminated by the kidney, dosing should be performed in an age-appropriate fashion that takes into account both maturational changes in kidney function.

### Hepatic

Hepatic biotransformation reactions are substantially reduced in the neonatal period. At birth, the cytochrome p450 system is 28% that of the adult. The expression of phase I enzymes such as the P-450 cytochromes changes markedly during development. CYP3A7, the predominant CYP isoform expressed in fetal liver, peaks shortly after birth and then declines rapidly to levels that are undetectable in most adults. Within hours after birth, CYP2E1 activity increases, and CYP2D6 becomes detectable soon thereafter. CYP3A4 and CYP2C appear during the first week of life, whereas CYP1A2 is the last hepatic CYP to appear, at one to three months of life. The ontogeny of phase II enzymes is less well established than the ontogeny of reactions involving phase I enzymes. Available data indicate that the individual isoforms of glucuronosyltransferase (UGT) have unique maturational profiles with pharmacokinetic consequences. For example, the glucuronidation of acetaminophen (a substrate for UGT1A6 and, to a lesser extent, UGT1A9) is decreased in newborns and young children as compared with adolescents and adults. Glucuronidation of morphine (a UGT2B7 substrate) can be detected in premature infants as young as 24 weeks of gestational age.

### Gastrointestinal

Overall, the rate at which most drugs are absorbed is slower in neonates and young infants than in older children. As a result, the time required to achieve maximal plasma levels is longer in the very young. The effect of age on enteral absorption is not uniform and is difficult to predict. Gastric emptying and intestinal motility are the primary determinants of the rate at which drugs are presented to and dispersed along the mucosal surface of the small intestine. At birth, the coordination of antral contractions improves, resulting in a marked increase in gastric emptying during the first week of life. Similarly, intestinal motor activity matures throughout early infancy, with consequent increases in the frequency, amplitude, and duration of propagating contractions. Changes in the intraluminal pH in different segments of the gastrointestinal tract can directly affect both the stability and the degree of ionization of a drug, thus influencing the relative amount of drug available for absorption. During the neonatal period, intragastric pH is relatively elevated (>4). Thus, oral administration of acid-labile compounds such as penicillin G produces greater bioavailability in neonates than in older infants and children. In contrast, drugs that are weak acids, such as phenobarbital, may require larger oral doses in the very young in order to achieve therapeutic plasma levels. Other factors that impact the rate of absorption include age-associated development of villi, splanchnic blood flow, changes in intestinal microflora, and intestinal surface area.

### Body Composition

Age-dependent changes in body composition alter the physiologic spaces into which a drug may be distributed. The percent of total body water drops from about 85% in premature infants to 75% in full-term infants to 60% in the adult. Extracellular water decreases from 45% in the infant to 25% in the adult. Total body fat in the premature infant can be as low as 1%, as compared to 15% in the normal, term infant. Many drugs are less bound to plasma proteins in the neonate and infant than in the older child. Limited data in neonates suggest that the passive diffusion of drugs into the central nervous system is age dependent, as reflected by the progressive increase in the ratios of brain phenobarbital to plasma phenobarbital from 28 to 39 weeks of gestational age, demonstrating the increased transport of phenobarbital into the brain.

## Pregnancy

The FDA classifies drugs into five categories of safety for use during pregnancy (normal pregnancy, labor, and delivery) as shown in Table 4.2. Few well-controlled studies of therapeutic drugs have been conducted in pregnant women. Most information about drug safety during pregnancy is derived from animal studies and uncontrolled assessments (e.g. post-marketing reports).

Observational studies have documented that pregnant women take a variety of medicines during pregnancy. While changes in drug exposure during pregnancy are well documented, a mechanistic understanding of these effects is not clear. The few studies conducted suggest that bioavailability is not altered during pregnancy, though increased plasma volume and protein binding changes can affect the apparent volume of distribution of some drugs. Likewise, changes in the volume of distribution and clearance during pregnancy can cause increases or decreases in the terminal elimination half-life. Renal excretion of unchanged drugs is increased during pregnancy and hence these agents may require dose increases with pregnancy. Likewise, the metabolism of drugs via select P450-mediated pathways (3A4, 2D6, and 2C9) and UGT isoenzymes are increased during pregnancy, necessitating increased dosages of drugs metabolized by these pathways. In contrast, CYP1A2 and CYP2C19 activity is decreased during pregnancy, suggesting dosing reductions for agents metabolized via these pathways. The effect of pregnancy on transport proteins is unknown. Data are limited; more clinical studies to determine the effect of pregnancy on the pharmacokinetics and pharmacodynamics of drugs commonly used in pregnancy are sorely needed.

## Organ Impairment

### Renal Dysfunction

Renal failure can influence the pharmacokinetics of drugs. In renal failure, the binding of acidic drugs to albumin is decreased, because of competition with accumulated organic acids and uremia-induced structural changes in albumin which decrease drug binding affinity, altering the Vd. Drugs that are more than 30% eliminated unchanged in the urine are likely to have significantly diminished CL in the presence of renal insufficiency.

### Hepatic Dysfunction

Drugs that undergo extensive first-pass metabolism may have a significantly higher oral bioavailability in patients with liver failure than in normal subjects. Gut hypomotility may delay the peak response to enterally administered drugs in these patients. Hypoalbuminemia or altered glycoprotein levels may affect the fractional protein binding of acidic or basic drugs, respectively. Altered plasma protein concentrations may affect the

**Table 4.2** FDA categories of drug safety during pregnancy.

| Category | Description |
| --- | --- |
| A | Controlled human studies show no fetal risks; these drugs are the safest. |
| B | Animal studies show no risk to the fetus and no controlled human studies have been conducted, or animal studies show a risk to the fetus but well-controlled human studies do not. |
| C | No adequate animal or human studies have been conducted, or adverse fetal effects have been shown in animals, but no human data are available. |
| D | Evidence of human fetal risk exists, but benefits may outweigh risks in certain situations (e.g. life-threatening disorders, serious disorders for which safer drugs cannot be used or are ineffective). |
| X | Proven fetal risks outweigh any possible benefit. |

extent of tissue distribution of drugs that normally are highly protein-bound. The presence of significant edema and ascites may alter the Vd of highly water-soluble agents, such as aminoglycoside antibiotics. The capacity of the liver to metabolize drugs depends on hepatic blood flow and liver enzyme activity, both of which can be affected by liver disease. In addition, some P450 isoforms are more susceptible than others to liver disease, impairing drug metabolism.

### Cardiac Dysfunction

Circulatory failure, or shock, can alter the pharmacokinetics of drugs frequently used in the intensive care setting. Drug absorption may be impaired because of bowel wall edema. Passive hepatic congestion may impede first-pass metabolism, resulting in higher plasma concentrations. Peripheral edema inhibits absorption by intramuscular parenteral routes. The balance of tissue hypoperfusion versus increased total body water with edema may unpredictably alter Vd. In addition, liver hypoperfusion may alter drug-metabolizing enzyme function, especially flow-dependent drugs such as lidocaine.

### Drug Interactions

Patients are often treated with more than one (often many) drug, increasing the chance of a drug–drug interaction. Pharmacokinetic interactions can alter absorption, distribution, metabolism, and clearance. Drug interactions can affect absorption through the formation of drug–drug complexes, alterations in gastric pH, and changes in gastrointestinal motility. This can have a substantial impact on the bioavailability of enterally administered agents. The volume of distribution may be altered with competitive plasma protein binding and subsequent changes in free drug concentrations.

Biotransformation reactions vary greatly among individuals and are susceptible to drug–drug interactions. Induction is the process by which enzyme activity is increased by exposure to a certain drug, resulting in an increase in metabolism of other drugs and lower plasma concentrations. Common inducers include barbiturates, carbamezapine, isoniazid, and rifampin. In contrast, inhibition is the process by which enzyme activity is decreased by exposure to a certain drug, resulting in a decrease in the metabolism of other drugs, and subsequent higher plasma concentrations. Common enzyme inhibitors include ciprofloxacin, fluconazole, metronidazole, quinidine, and valproic acid. Inducers and inhibitors of phase II enzymes have been less extensively characterized, but some clinical applications of this information have emerged, including the use of phenobarbital to induce glucuronyl transferase activity in icteric neonates. Water-soluble drugs are eliminated unchanged in the kidneys. The clearance of drugs that are excreted entirely by glomerular filtration is unlikely to be affected by other drugs. Organic acids and bases are renally secreted, and can compete with one another for elimination, resulting in unpredictable drug disposition.

## Pharmacodynamics

Pharmacodynamics characterizes what the drug does to the body (i.e. the effects or response to drug therapy). Pharmacodynamic modeling constructs quantitative relationships of measured, physiological parameters before and after drug administration, with effects defined as the changes in a physiological parameter relative to its pre-dose or baseline value. Baseline refers to un-dosed state and may be complicated in certain situations due to diurnal variations. Efficacy can be defined numerically as the expected sum of all beneficial effects following treatment. In this case, we refer to clinical and not necessarily economic benefits. Similarly, toxicity can be characterized either by the time course of a specific toxic event or the composite of toxic responses attributed to a common toxicity.

## Overview

Pharmacodynamic response to drug therapy, i.e. the concentration-effect relationship, evolves only after active drug molecules reach their intended site(s) of action. Hence, the link between pharmacokinetic and pharmacodynamic processes is implicit. Likewise, the respective factors that influence various sub-processes (absorption, distribution, tolerance, etc.) are relevant and may necessitate separate study. Differences among drug entities in pharmacodynamic time course can be considered as being direct or indirect. A direct effect is directly proportional to concentration at the site of measurement, usually the plasma. An indirect effect exhibits some type of temporal delay, either because of differences between site of action and measurement or because the effect results only after other physiologic or pharmacologic conditions are satisfied.

Direct effect relationships are easily observed with some cardiovascular agents, whose site of action is the vascular space. Pharmacologic effects such as blood pressure, ACE-inhibition, and inhibition of platelet aggregation can be characterized by direct response relationships. Such relationships can usually be defined by three typical patterns– linear, hyperbolic ($E_{max}$), and sigmoid $E_{max}$ functions. These are shown in Figure 4.3.

In each case, the plasma concentration and drug concentration at the effect site are proportional. Likewise, the concentration–effect relationship is assumed to be independent of time.

Other drugs exhibit an indirect relationship between concentration and response. In this

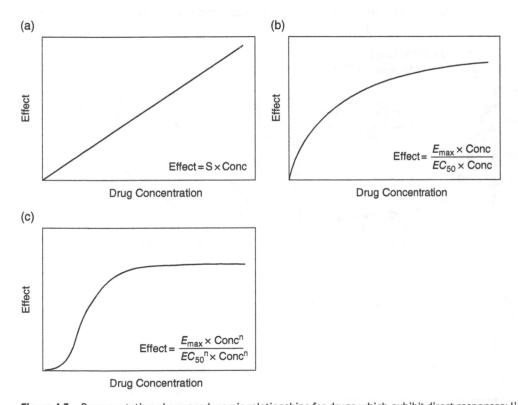

(a)

$$\text{Effect} = S \times \text{Conc}$$

(b)

$$\text{Effect} = \frac{E_{max} \times \text{Conc}}{EC_{50} \times \text{Conc}}$$

(c)

$$\text{Effect} = \frac{E_{max} \times \text{Conc}^n}{EC_{50}{}^n \times \text{Conc}^n}$$

**Figure 4.3** Representative pharmacodynamic relationships for drugs which exhibit direct responses: linear, hyperbolic and Sigmoid-$E_{max}$ relationships shown. S is the slope of the linear response; $E_{max}$ refers to the maximum effect observed; $EC_{50}$ refers to the concentration at which 50% of the maximal response is achieved, and n is the degree of sigmoidicity or shape factor (sometimes referred to as the Hill coefficient).

case, the concentration–effect relationship is time-dependent. One explanation for such effects is hysteresis. Hysteresis refers to the phenomenon where there is a time-lapse between the cause and its effect. With respect to pharmacodynamics, this most often indicates a situation in which there is a delay in equilibrium between plasma drug concentration and the concentration of active substance at the effect site (e.g. thiopental, fentanyl). Three conditions are predominantly responsible for hysteresis: the biophase (actual site of drug action) is not in the central compartment (i.e. plasma or blood compartment); the mechanism of action involves protein synthesis; and/or active metabolites are present. One can conceptualize a hypothetical effect compartment (a physical space where drug concentrations are directly correlated with drug actions) such that the relationships defined in Figure 4.4 are only observed when the effect

site concentrations (Ce) are used as opposed to the plasma concentrations (Cp). In this situation, a hysteresis loop is observed when plotting Ce versus Cp.

More complicated models (indirect-response models) have been used to express the same observations but typically necessitate a greater understanding of the underlying physiologic process (e.g. cell trafficking, enzyme recruitment, etc.). The salient point is that pharmacodynamic characterization and likewise dosing guidance derived from such investigation stands to be more informative than drug concentrations alone.

Likewise, pharmacodynamics may be the discriminating characteristic that defines dose adjustment in special populations. This is the case for the observed markedly enhanced sensitivity in infants compared with older children and adults with respect to immunosuppressive effects of cyclosporine,

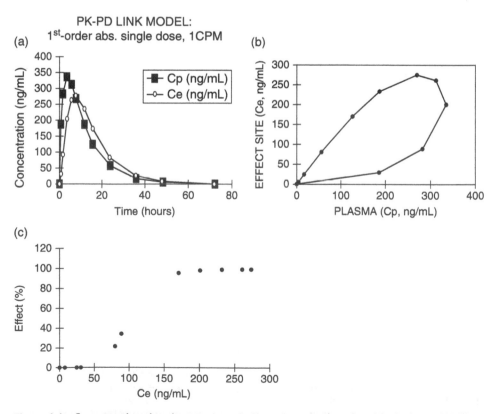

**Figure 4.4** Concentration-time, hysteresis, and effect-concentration plots (clockwise order) illustrating the use of an effect compartment to explain observed hysteresis.

and calcium channel blocking effects on the PR interval in the elderly.

## Pharmacogenomics

Pharmacogenomics is the study of how an individual's genetic inheritance affects the body's response to drugs. Pharmacogenomics holds the promise that drugs might one day be tailored to individuals and adapted to each person's own genetic makeup. Environment, diet, age, lifestyle, and state of health all can influence a person's response to medicines, but understanding an individual's genetic composition is thought to be the key to creating personalized drugs with greater efficacy and safety. Pharmacogenomics combines traditional pharmaceutical sciences, such as biochemistry, with comprehensive knowledge of genes, proteins, and single nucleotide polymorphisms. Genetic variations, or SNPs (single nucleotide polymorphisms), in the human genome can be a diagnostic tool to predict a person's drug response. For SNPs to be used in this way, a person's DNA must be sequenced for the presence of specific SNPs. SNP screenings will benefit drug development; those people whose pharmacogenomic screening shows that the drug being tested would be harmful or ineffective for them would be excluded from clinical trials. Prescreening clinical trial subjects might also allow clinical trials to be smaller, faster, and therefore less expensive. Finally, the ability to assess an individual's reaction to a drug before it is prescribed will increase confidence in prescribing the drug and the patient's confidence in taking the drug, which in turn should encourage the development of new drugs tested in a like manner.

## Model-Informed Drug Development

One of the more recent developments in the evolution of Clinical Pharmacology in the facilitation of early stage drug development is in the implementation of model-informed drug development (MIDD) principles by many pharmaceutical and Biotech companies. The approach is also endorsed by the global regulatory community including the EMA and FDA. The use of modeling and simulation approaches to de-risk decision making in drug development is not new but the systematic integration of the unique model assets in an evolving computing environment that expands with knowledge about candidate molecules and/or vaccines is still a work in progress for many pharmaceutical sponsors though feedback from early adopters suggests that the approach can reduce both time and cost in drug development when conducted in an appropriate manner. Figure 4.5 highlights many of the common early drug development decision milestones in conjunction with the various model types and methodologies that represent key stage gate milestones.

Many of these milestones represent contributions from Clinical Pharmacology and the supportive quantitative disciplines which collaborate in the MIDD effort (e.g. bioinformatics, system pharmacology, DMPK, pharmacometrics, and biostatistics). As the figure suggests, many of these milestones are not only critical to the progression of drug and/or vaccine candidates but they also represent critical go/no go criteria requiring quantitative definition around the pace of potential outcomes. The MIDD likewise is effective at generating scenarios which explore the space of potential outcomes either through direct experimentation or model-based projection (i.e. simulation).

In addition to the utility of MIDD in the decision-making process, the MIDD implementation generates modeling assets which can be used in the later stages of drug development. These can represent inputs to epidemiologic modeling and simulation exercises which explore the utility of projecting candidate attributes on target populations of interest and also accommodate the complexity of the existing standard of care, population, and subpopulation differences influenced by socioeconomic

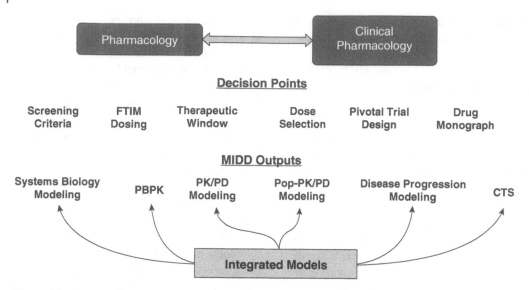

**Figure 4.5** The MIDD approach learns and confirms key characteristics of new molecular entities in a quantitative manner, with goal of providing explicit, reproducible, and predictive evidence for optimizing drug development plans and enabling critical decision.

and lifestyle factors. This represents a new frontier for these disciplines to further interact and inform each other.

## Conclusion

Clinical pharmacology serves an important role in the development of new drugs and the management of pharmacotherapy. In the context of pharmacoepidemiologic investigations, clinical pharmacology also provides a fundamental backbone for understanding the expected associations between drug therapy and clinical benefit as well as potential toxicity. The pharmacoepidemiologist must also have intimate knowledge of clinical pharmacology as the impact (clinical and economic) of a new drug once available to the marketplace can often be forecast based on how the agent's clinical pharmacologic attributes compare to existing therapies. The connection between utilization, compliance, the complexities of multimodal therapy, and the associations of drug behavior with disease- or population-specific indices must be defined relative to the known clinical pharmacologic principles that

govern how drugs behave in humans. In an era when more holistic approaches for the care of patients are sought to maintain a healthy overall well-being and avoid chronic and severe disease, clinical strategies are likely to engage more preventative approaches. Likewise, clinical pharmacology and pharmacoepidemiology will be essential disciplines that discriminate strategies that are truly beneficial from those that are not or are even harmful.

## Key Points

- There is a great need for caregivers to be skilled in the areas of drug information, medication safety, and other aspects of pharmacy practice related to clinical pharmacology.
- Clinical pharmacology defines the therapeutic window (the dosage of a medication between the minimum amount that gives a desired effect and the minimum amount that gives more adverse effects than desired effects) of a drug in various patient populations and guides dose modifications in various patient subpopulations (e.g. pediatrics, pregnancy, elderly,

and organ impairment) and/or dose adjustments for various lifestyle factors (e.g. food, time of day, drug interactions).

- Clinical pharmacology comprises all aspects of the scientific study of medicinal drugs in humans. It can be divided into pharmacokinetics (the relationship between the dose of a drug administered and the serum or blood level achieved) and pharmacodynamics (the study of the relationship between drug level and effect).

- There are many factors that affect an individual's response to a drug. These factors include sex, age, health conditions, concomitant medications, and genetic makeup. An important goal of pharmacoepidemiology is to use population research methods to characterize factors that influence individual drug response.

- Factors that influence individual drug response may do so via pharmacokinetic mechanisms, pharmacodynamic mechanisms, or both.

## Further Reading

Avorn, J. (2007). In defense of pharmacoepidemiology – embracing the yin and yang of drug research. *N. Engl. J. Med.* 357 (22): 2219–2221.

De, V.T.P. (1993). Presenting clinical pharmacology and therapeutics: a problem based approach for choosing and prescribing drugs. *Br. J. Clin. Pharmacol.* 35 (6): 581–586.

Etminan, M., Gill, S. et al. (2006). Challenges and opportunities for pharmacoepidemiology in drug-therapy decision making. *J. Clin. Pharmacol.* 46 (1): 6–9.

Etminan, M. and Samii, A. (2004). Pharmacoepidemiology I : a review of pharmacoepidemiologic study designs. *Pharmacotherapy* 24 (8): 964–969.

Evans, S.J. (2012). An agenda for UK clinical pharmacology pharmacoepidemiology. *Br. J. Clin. Pharmacol.* 73 (6): 973–978.

Guess, H.A. (1991). Pharmacoepidemiology in pre-approval clinical trial safety monitoring. *J. Clin. Epidemiol.* 44 (8): 851–857.

Hartzema, A.G. (1992). Pharmacoepidemiology- its relevance to clinical practice. *J. Clin. Pharm. Ther.* 17 (2): 73–74.

Jones, J.K. (1992). Clinical pharmacology and pharmacoepidemiology: synergistic interactions. *Int. J. Clin. Pharmacol. Ther. Toxicol.* 30 (11): 421–424.

Leake, C.D. (1948). Current pharmacology; general principles in practical clinical application. *JAMA* 138 (10): 730–737.

Lehmann, D.F. (2000). Observation and experiment on the cusp of collaboration: a parallel examination of clinical pharmacology and pharmacoepidemiology. *J. Clin. Pharmacol.* 40 (9): 939–945.

Lehmann, D.F. (2001). Improving family ties: an examination of the complementary disciplines of pharmacoepidemiology and clinical pharmacology. *Pharmacoepidemiol. Drug Saf.* 10 (1): 63–68.

Luo, X., Cappelleri, J.C. et al. (2007). A systematic review on the application of pharmacoepidemiology in assessing prescription drug-related adverse events in pediatrics. *Curr. Med. Res. Opin.* 23 (5): 1015–1024.

Royer, R.J. (1992). Clinical pharmacology and pharmacoepidemiology: future challenges for the European Community. *Int. J. Clin. Pharmacol. Ther. Toxicol.* 30 (11): 449–452.

Suissa, S. (1991). Statistical methods in pharmacoepidemiology. Principles in managing error. *Drug Saf.* 6 (5): 381–389.

Theodore, W.H. (1990). Basic principles of clinical pharmacology. *Neurol. Clin.* 8 (1): 1–13.

Tilson, H.H. (1990). Major advances in international pharmacoepidemiology. *Ann. Epidemiol.* 1 (2): 205–212.

# 5

# When Should One Perform Pharmacoepidemiologic Studies?

*Brian L. Strom*

*Rutgers Biomedical and Health Sciences, Newark, NJ, USA*

## Introduction

As discussed in the previous chapters, pharmacoepidemiologic studies apply the techniques of epidemiology to the content area of clinical pharmacology. This chapter will review when pharmacoepidemiologic studies should be performed. It will begin with a discussion of the various reasons why one might perform pharmacoepidemiologic studies. Central to many of these is one's willingness to tolerate risk. Whether one's perspective is that of a manufacturer, regulator, academician, or clinician, one needs to consider the risk of adverse reactions, which one considers tolerable. Thus, this chapter will continue with a discussion of the difference between safety and risk. It will conclude with a discussion of the determinants of one's tolerance of risk.

## Reasons to Perform Pharmacoepidemiologic Studies

The decision to conduct a pharmacoepidemiologic study can be viewed as similar to the regulatory decision about whether to approve a drug for marketing or the clinical decision about whether to prescribe a drug. In each case, decision-making involves weighing the costs and risks of a therapy against its benefits.

The main costs of a pharmacoepidemiologic study are obviously the costs (monetary, effort, time) of conducting the study itself. These costs clearly will vary, depending on the questions posed and the approach chosen to answer them. Generally, the cost per patient in a postmarketing study, with the exception of postmarketing randomized clinical trials, is likely to be at least an order of magnitude less than the cost of a premarketing study. Other costs to consider are the opportunity costs of other research that might be left undone if this research is performed.

One risk of conducting a pharmacoepidemiologic study is the possibility that it could identify an adverse outcome as associated with the drug under investigation when in fact the drug does not cause this adverse outcome. Another risk is that it could provide false reassurances about a drug's safety. Both these risks can be minimized by appropriate study designs, skilled researchers, and appropriate and responsible interpretation of the results obtained.

The benefits of pharmacoepidemiologic studies could be conceptualized in four different categories: regulatory, marketing, clinical, and legal (see Table 5.1). Each will be of

*Textbook of Pharmacoepidemiology*, Third Edition. Edited by Brian L. Strom, Stephen E. Kimmel, and Sean Hennessy.
© 2022 John Wiley & Sons Ltd. Published 2022 by John Wiley & Sons Ltd.

**Table 5.1** Reasons to perform pharmacoepidemiologic studies.

---

A) Regulatory
  1) Required
  2) To obtain earlier approval for marketing
  3) As a response to question by regulatory agency
  4) To assist application for approval for marketing elsewhere

B) Marketing
  1) To assist market penetration by documenting the safety of the drug
  2) To increase name recognition
  3) To assist in re-positioning the drug
     a) Different outcomes, e.g. quality of life and economic
     b) Different types of patients, e.g. the elderly
     c) New indications
     d) Less restrictive labeling
  4) To protect the drug from accusations about adverse effects

C) Legal
  1) In anticipation of future product liability litigation

D) Clinical
  1) Hypothesis testing
     a) Problem hypothesized on the basis of drug structure
     b) Problem suspected on the basis of preclinical or premarketing human data
     c) Problem suspected on the basis of spontaneous reports
     d) Need to better quantitate the frequency of adverse reactions
  2) Hypothesis generating–need depends on whether:
     a) it is a new chemical entity
     b) the safety profile of the class
     c) the relative safety of the drug within its class
     d) the formulation
     e) the disease to be treated, including
        i) its duration
        ii) its prevalence
        iii) its severity
        iv) whether alternative therapies are available

---

importance to different organizations and individuals involved in deciding whether to initiate a study. Any given study will usually be performed for several of these reasons. Each will be discussed in turn.

## Regulatory

Perhaps the most obvious and compelling reason to perform a postmarketing pharmacoepidemiologic study is regulatory: a plan for a postmarketing pharmacoepidemiologic study is required before the drug will be approved for marketing. Requirements for postmarketing research have become progressively more frequent in recent years. For example, in the 1970s the FDA required postmarketing research at the time of approval for about one third of drugs, a requirement which increased to over 70% in the 1990s. Many of these required studies have been randomized clinical trials, designed to clarify residual questions about a drug's efficacy. Others focus on questions of drug toxicity. Often it is unclear whether the pharmacoepidemiologic study was undertaken in response to a regulatory requirement or in response to merely a "suggestion" by the regulator, but the effect is essentially the same. Early examples of studies conducted to address regulatory questions include the "Phase IV" cohort studies performed of cimetidine and prazosin. These are discussed more in Chapter 1. Now that FDA has the authority to require such studies, such requirements are becoming more common.

Sometimes a manufacturer may offer to perform a pharmacoepidemiologic study with the hope that the regulatory agency might thereby expedite drug approval. If the agency believed that any new serious problem would be detected rapidly and reliably after marketing, it could feel more comfortable about releasing the drug sooner. Although it is difficult to assess the impact of volunteered postmarketing studies on regulatory decisions, the very large economic impact of an earlier approval has motivated some manufacturers to initiate such studies. In addition, in recent years regulatory authorities have occasionally released a particularly important drug after essentially only Phase II testing, with the understanding that additional data would be gathered during postmarketing testing. For example, zidovudine was released for marketing after only limited testing, and only later were additional data gathered on both safety and efficacy, data which indicated, among other things, that the doses initially recommended were too large.

Some postmarketing studies of drugs arise in response to case reports of adverse reactions reported to the regulatory agency. One response to such a report might be to suggest a labeling change. Often a more appropriate response, clinically and commercially, would be to propose a pharmacoepidemiologic study. This study would explore whether this adverse event in fact occurs more often in those exposed to the drug than would have been expected in the absence of the drug and, if so, how large is the increased risk of the disease. As an example, a Medicaid database was used to study hypersensitivity reactions to tolmetin, following reports about this problem to the FDA's Spontaneous Reporting System.

Finally, drugs are obviously marketed at different times in different countries. A postmarketing pharmacoepidemiologic study conducted in a country which marketed a drug relatively early could be useful in demonstrating the safety of the drug to regulatory agencies in countries which have not yet permitted the marketing of the drug. This is becoming increasingly feasible, as both the industry and the field of pharmacoepidemiology are becoming more international, and regulators are collaborating more.

## Marketing

As will be discussed below, pharmacoepidemiologic studies are performed primarily to obtain the answers to clinical questions. However, it is clear that a major underlying reason for some pharmacoepidemiologic studies is the potential marketing impact of those answers. In fact, some companies make the marketing branch of the company responsible for pharmacoepidemiology, rather than the medical branch.

Because of the known limitations in the information available about the effects of a drug at the time of its initial marketing, many physicians are appropriately hesitant to prescribe a drug until a substantial amount of experience in its use has been gathered. A formal postmarketing surveillance study can speed that process, as well as clarify advantages or disadvantages a drug has compared to its competitors.

A pharmacoepidemiologic study can also be useful to improve product name recognition. The fact that a study is underway will often be known to prescribers, as will its results once it is publicly presented and published. This increased name recognition will presumably help sales. An increase in a product's name recognition is likely to result particularly from pharmacoepidemiologic studies that recruit subjects for the study via prescribers. However, while this technique can be useful in selected situations, it is extremely expensive and less likely to be productive of scientifically useful information than most other alternatives available. In particular, the conduct of a purely marketing exercise under the guise of a postmarketing surveillance study, not designed to collect useful scientific information, is to be condemned. It is misleading and could endanger the performance of future scientifically useful studies, by resulting in prescribers who are disillusioned and, thereby, reluctant to participate in future studies.

Pharmacoepidemiologic studies can also be useful to reposition a drug that is already on the market, i.e. to develop new markets for the drug. One could explore different types of outcomes resulting from the use of the drug for the approved indication, for example, the impact of the drug on the cost of medical care (see Chapter 18) and on the patients' quality-of-life (see Chapter 19). One could also explore the use of the drug for the approved indication in types of patients other than those included in premarketing studies, for example in children, in the elderly, or in patients with multiple comorbidities and/or taking many concomitant medications. By exploring unintended beneficial effects, or even drug efficacy, one could obtain clues and supporting information for new indications for drug use. Finally, whether because of questions about efficacy or questions about toxicity, drugs are sometimes approved for initial marketing with restrictive labeling. For example, bretylium was initially approved for marketing in the US only for the treatment of life threatening arrhythmias. Approval for more widespread use requires additional data. These data can often be obtained from pharmacoepidemiologic studies.

Finally, and perhaps most importantly, pharmacoepidemiologic studies can be useful to protect the major investment made in developing and testing a new drug. When a question arises about a drug's toxicity, it often needs an immediate answer, or else the drug may lose market share or even be removed from the market. Immediate answers are often unavailable, unless the manufacturer had the foresight to perform pharmacoepidemiologic studies in anticipation of this problem. Sometimes these problems can be specifically foreseen and addressed. More commonly, they are not. However, the availability of an existing cohort of exposed patients and a control group will often allow a much more rapid answer than would have been possible if the study had to be conducted de novo. One example of this is provided by the experience of Pfizer Pharmaceuticals, when the question arose about whether piroxicam (Feldene) was more likely to cause deaths in the elderly from gastrointestinal bleeding than the other nonsteroidal anti-inflammatory drugs. Although Pfizer did not fund studies in anticipation of such a question, it was fortunate that several pharmacoepidemiologic research groups had data available on this question because of other studies that they had performed. McNeil was not as fortunate when questions were raised about anaphylactic reactions caused by zomepirac. If they had the data available at the time of the crisis which they were eventually able to have, they might not have removed the drug from the market. Later, Syntex recognized the potential benefit, and the risk, associated with the marketing of parenteral ketorolac, and chose to initiate a postmarketing surveillance cohort study at the time of the drug's launch. Indeed, the drug was accused of multiple different adverse outcomes, and it was only the existence of this study, and its subsequently published results, that saved the drug in its major markets.

## Legal

Postmarketing surveillance studies can theoretically be useful as legal prophylaxis, in anticipation of eventually having to defend against product liability suits (see Chapter 6). One often hears the phrase "What you don't know, won't hurt you." However, in pharmacoepidemiology this view is shortsighted and, in fact, very wrong. All drugs cause adverse effects; the regulatory decision to approve a drug and the clinical decision to prescribe a drug both depend on a judgment about the relative balance between the benefits of a drug and its risks. From a legal perspective, to win a product liability suit using a legal theory of negligence, a plaintiff must prove causation, damages, and negligence. A pharmaceutical manufacturer that is a defendant in such a suit cannot change whether its drug causes an adverse effect. If the drug does, this will presumably be detected at some point. Also, the manufacturer cannot change whether the plaintiff suffered legal damages from the adverse effect, that is whether the plaintiff suffered a disability or incurred expenses resulting from a need for medical attention. However, even if the drug did cause the adverse outcome in question, a manufacturer certainly can document that it was performing state-of-the-art studies to attempt to detect whatever toxic effects the drug had. In addition, such studies could make easier the defense of totally groundless suits, in which a drug is blamed for producing adverse reactions it does not cause.

## Clinical

### Hypothesis Testing

The major reason for most pharmacoepidemiologic studies is hypothesis testing. The hypotheses to be tested can be based on the structure or the chemical class of a drug. For example, the cimetidine study mentioned above was conducted because cimetidine was chemically related to metiamide, which had been removed from the market in Europe because it caused agranulocytosis. Alternatively, hypotheses can also be based on premarketing or postmarketing animal or clinical findings. For example, the hypotheses can come from spontaneous reports of adverse events experienced by patients taking the drug in question. The tolmetin, piroxicam, zomepirac, and ketorolac questions mentioned above are all examples of this. Finally, an adverse effect may clearly be due to a drug, but a study may be needed to quantitate its frequency. An example would be the postmarketing surveillance study of prazosin, performed to quantitate the frequency of first dose syncope. Of course, the hypotheses to be tested can involve beneficial drug effects as well as harmful drug effects, subject to some important methodologic limitations.

### Hypothesis Generating

Hypothesis generating studies are intended to screen for previously unknown and unsuspected drug effects. In principle, all drugs could, and perhaps should, be subjected to such studies. However, some drugs may require these studies more than others. This has been the focus of a formal study, which surveyed experts in Pharmacoepidemiology.

For example, it is generally agreed that new chemical entities are more in need of study than so-called "me too" drugs. This is because the lack of experience with related drugs makes it more likely that the new drug has possibly important unsuspected effects.

The safety profile of the class of drugs should also be important to the decision about whether to conduct a formal screening postmarketing surveillance study for a new drug. Previous experience with other drugs in the same class can be a useful predictor of what the experience with the new drug in question is likely to be. For example, with the finding that troglitazone had an increased risk of liver disease, that became a concern as well with the later thiazolidinediones, i.e. pioglitazone and rosiglitazone. Similarly, with the finding that rofecoxib was associated with myocardial infarction, that became a concern as well with celecoxib.

The relative safety of the drug within its class can also be helpful. A drug that has been studied in large numbers of patients before marketing and appears safe relative to other drugs within its class is less likely to need supplementary postmarketing surveillance studies. An extension of this approach, of course, is comparative effectiveness research.

The formulation of the drug can be considered a determinant of the need for formal screening pharmacoepidemiologic studies. A drug that will, because of its formulation, be used mainly in institutions, where there is close supervision, may be less likely to need such a study. When a drug is used under these conditions, any serious adverse effect is likely to be detected, even without any formal study.

The disease to be treated is an important determinant of whether a drug needs additional postmarketing surveillance studies. Drugs used to treat chronic illnesses are likely to be used for a long period of time. As such, it is important to know their long-term effects. This cannot be addressed adequately in the relatively brief time available for each premarketing study. Also, drugs used to treat common diseases are important to study, as many patients are likely to be exposed to these drugs.

Drugs used to treat mild or self-limited diseases also need careful study, because serious toxicity is less acceptable. This is especially true for drugs used by healthy individuals, such as contraceptives. On the other hand, when one is using a drug to treat individuals who are very ill, one is more tolerant of toxicity, assuming the drug is efficacious.

Finally, it is also important to know whether alternative therapies are available. If a new drug is not a major therapeutic advance, since it will be used to treat patients who would have been treated with the old drug, one needs to be more certain of its relative advantages and disadvantages. The presence of significant adverse effects, or the absence of beneficial effects, is less likely to be tolerated for a drug that does not represent a major therapeutic advance.

## Safety Versus Risk

Clinical pharmacologists are used to thinking about drug "safety": the statutory standard that must be met before a drug is approved for marketing in the US is that it needs to be proven to be "safe and effective under conditions of intended use." It is important, however, to differentiate safety from risk. Virtually nothing is without some risks. Even staying in bed is associated with a risk of acquiring bed sores! Certainly no drug is completely safe. Yet, the unfortunate misperception by the public persists that drugs mostly are and should be without any risk at all. Use of a "safe" drug, however, still carries some risk. It would be better to think in terms of *degrees of safety*. Specifically, a drug "is safe if its risks are judged to be acceptable." Measuring risk is an objective but probabilistic pursuit. A judgment about safety is a personal and/or social value judgment about the acceptability of that risk. Thus, assessing safety requires two extremely different kinds of activities: measuring risk and judging the acceptability of those risks. The former is the focus of much of pharmacoepidemiology and

most of this book. The latter is the focus of the following discussion.

## Risk Tolerance

Whether or not to conduct a postmarketing surveillance pharmacoepidemiologic study also depends on one's willingness to tolerate risk. From a manufacturer's perspective, one can consider this risk in terms of the risk of a potential regulatory or legal problem that may arise. Whether one's perspective is that of a manufacturer, regulator, academician, or clinician, one needs to consider the risk of adverse reactions that one is willing to accept as tolerable. There are several factors that can affect one's willingness to tolerate the risk of adverse effects from drugs (see Table 5.2). Some of these factors are related to the adverse outcome being studied. Others are related to the exposure and the setting in which the adverse outcome occurs.

**Table 5.2** Factors affecting the acceptability of risks.

A) Features of the adverse outcome
  1) Severity
  2) Reversibility
  3) Frequency
  4) "Dread disease"
  5) Immediate versus delayed
  6) Occurs in all people versus just in sensitive people
  7) Known with certainty or not
B) Characteristics of the exposure
  1) Essential versus optional
  2) Present versus absent
  3) Alternatives available
  4) Risk assumed voluntarily
  5) Drug use will be as intended versus misuse is likely
C) Perceptions of the evaluator

## Features of the Adverse Outcome

The severity and reversibility of the adverse reaction in question are of paramount importance to its tolerability. An adverse reaction that is severe is much less tolerable than one that is mild, even at the same incidence. This is especially true for adverse reactions that result in permanent harm, for example birth defects or death.

Another critical factor that affects the tolerability of an adverse outcome is the frequency of the adverse outcome in those who are exposed. Notably, this is *not* a question of the relative risk of the disease due to the exposure, but a question of the excess risk attributed to the drug of interest. Use of tampons is extraordinarily strongly linked to toxic shock: prior studies have shown relative risks between 10 and 20. However, toxic shock is sufficiently uncommon, that even a 10- to 20-fold increase in the risk of the disease still contributes an extraordinarily small excess risk of the toxic shock syndrome in those who use tampons.

In addition, the particular disease caused by the drug is important to one's tolerance of its risks. Certain diseases are considered by the public to be so-called "dread diseases," diseases that generate more fear and emotion than other diseases. Examples are AIDS and cancer. It is less likely that the risk of a drug will be considered acceptable if it causes one of these diseases.

Another relevant factor is whether the adverse outcome is immediate or delayed. Most individuals are less concerned about delayed risks than immediate risks. This is one of the factors that have probably slowed the success of anti-smoking efforts. In part, this is a function of denial; delayed risks seem as if they may never occur. In addition, an economic concept of "discounting" plays a role here. An adverse event in the future is less bad than the same event today, and a beneficial effect today is better than the same beneficial effect in the future. Something else may occur between now and then, which could make that delayed effect irrelevant or, at least, mitigate its impact. Thus, a delayed adverse event may be worth incurring if it can bring about beneficial effects today.

It is also important whether the adverse outcome is a Type A reaction or a Type B reaction. As described in Chapter 1, Type A reactions are the result of an exaggerated but otherwise usual pharmacological effect of a drug. Type A reactions tend to be common, but they are dose-related, predictable, and less serious. In contrast, Type B reactions are aberrant effects of a drug. Type B reactions tend to be uncommon, are not related to dose, and are potentially more serious. They may be due to hypersensitivity reactions, immunologic reactions, or some other idiosyncratic reaction to the drug. Regardless, Type B reactions are the more difficult to predict or even detect. If one can predict an adverse effect, then one can attempt to prevent it. For example, in order to prevent aminophylline-induced arrhythmias and seizures, one can begin therapy at lower doses and follow serum levels carefully. For this reason, all other things being equal, Type B reactions are usually considered less tolerable.

Finally, the acceptability of a risk also varies according to how well established it is. The same adverse effect is obviously less tolerable if one knows with certainty that it is caused by a drug than if it is only a remote possibility.

## Characteristics of the Exposure

The acceptability of a risk is very different, depending upon whether an exposure is essential or optional. Major adverse effects are much more acceptable when one is using a therapy that can save or prolong life, such as chemotherapy for malignancies. On the other hand, therapy for self-limited illnesses must have a low risk to be acceptable. Pharmaceutical products intended for use in healthy individuals, such as vaccines and contraceptives, must be exceedingly low in risk to be considered acceptable.

The acceptability of a risk is also dependent on whether the risk is from the presence of a treatment or its absence. One could conceptualize deaths from a disease that can be treated by a drug that is not yet on the market as an adverse effect from the absence of treatment. For example, the six-year delay in introducing beta-blockers into the US market has been blamed for resulting in more deaths than all recent adverse drug reactions combined. As a society, we are much more willing to accept risks of this type than risks from the use of a drug that has been marketed prematurely. Physicians are taught *primum non nocere* – first do no harm. This is somewhat analogous to our willingness to allow patients with terminal illnesses to die from these illnesses without intervention, while it would be considered unethical and probably illegal to perform euthanasia. In general, we are much more tolerant of sins of omission than sins of commission.

Whether any alternative treatments are available is another determinant of the acceptability of risks. If a drug is the only available treatment for a disease, particularly a serious disease, then greater risks will be considered acceptable. This was the reason zidovudine was allowed to be marketed for treatment of AIDS, despite its toxicity and the limited testing which had been performed. Analogously, studies of toxic shock syndrome associated with the use of tampons were of public health importance, despite the infrequency of the disease, because consumers could choose among other available tampons that were shown to carry different risks.

Whether a risk is assumed voluntarily is also important to its acceptability. We are willing to accept the risk of death in automobile accidents more than the much smaller risk of death in airline accidents, because we control and understand the former and accept the attendant risk voluntarily. Some people even accept the enormous risks of death from tobacco-related disease, but would object strongly to being given a drug that was a small fraction as toxic. In general, it is agreed that patients should be made aware of the possibly toxic effects of drugs that they are prescribed. When a risk is higher than it is with the usual therapeutic use of a drug, as with an invasive procedure or an investigational drug, one usually asks the patient for formal informed consent. The fact that fetuses cannot make voluntary choices about whether or not to take a drug contributes to the unacceptability of drug-induced birth defects.

Finally, from a societal perspective, one also needs to be concerned about whether a drug will be and is used as intended or whether misuse is likely. Misuse, in and of itself, can represent a risk of the drug. For example, a drug is considered less acceptable if it is addicting and, so, is likely to be abused. In addition, the potential for over-prescribing by physicians can also decrease the acceptability of the drug. For example, in the controversy about birth defects from isotretinoin, there was no question that the drug was a powerful teratogen, and that it was a very effective therapy for serious cystic acne refractory to other treatments. There also was no question about its effectiveness for less severe acne. However, that effectiveness led to its widespread use, including in individuals who could have been treated with less toxic therapies, and a larger number of pregnancy exposures, abortions, and birth defects than otherwise would have occurred.

## Perceptions of the Evaluator

Finally, much depends ultimately upon the perceptions of the individuals who are making the decision about whether a risk is acceptable. In the US, there have been more than a million deaths from traffic accidents over the past 30 years; tobacco-related diseases kill the equivalent of three jumbo jet loads every day; and 3000 children are born each year with embryopathy from their mothers' use of alcohol in pregnancy. Yet, these deaths are accepted with little concern, while the uncommon risk of an airplane crash or being struck by lightning generate fear. The decision about whether to allow isotretinoin to remain on the market hinged on whether the efficacy of the drug for a small number of people who had a disease which was disfiguring but not life-threatening was worth the birth defects that would result in some other individuals. There is no way to remove this subjective component from the decision about the acceptability of risks. Indeed, much more research is needed to elucidate patients' preferences in these matters. However, this subjective component is part of what makes informed consent so important. Most people feel that the final subjective judgment about whether an individual should assume the risk of ingesting a drug should be made by that individual, after education by their physician. However, as an attempt to assist that judgment, it is useful to have some quantitative information about the risks inherent in some other activities. Some such information is presented in Table 5.3.

## Conclusion

This chapter reviewed when pharmacoepidemiologic studies should be performed. After beginning with a discussion of the various reasons why one might perform pharmacoepidemiologic studies, it reviewed the difference between safety and risk. It concluded with a discussion of the determinants of one's tolerance of risk. Now that it is hopefully clear when one might want to perform a pharmacoepidemiologic study, the next section of this book will provide perspectives on pharmacoepidemiology from some of the different fields that use it.

**Table 5.3** Annual risks of death from some selected hazards.

| Hazard | Annual death rate (per 100 000 exposed individuals) |
| --- | --- |
| Heart disease (US, 1985) | 261.4 |
| Sport parachuting | 190 |
| Cancer (US, 1985) | 170.5 |
| Cigarette smoking (age 35) | 167 |
| Hang gliding (UK) | 150 |
| Motorcycling (US) | 100 |
| Power boat racing (US) | 80 |
| Cerebrovascular disease (US, 1985) | 51.0 |
| Scuba diving (US) | 42 |
| Scuba diving (UK) | 22 |
| Influenza (UK) | 20 |
| Passenger in motor vehicle (US) | 16.7 |
| Suicide (US, 1985) | 11.2 |
| Homicide (US, 1985) | 7.5 |
| Cave exploration (US) | 4.5 |
| Oral contraceptive user (age 25–34) | 4.3 |
| Pedestrian (US) | 3.8 |
| Bicycling (US) | 1.1 |
| Tornados (US) | 0.2 |
| Lightning (US) | 0.05 |

*Source:* data derived from O'Brien (1986), Silverberg and Lubera (1988), and Urquhart and Heilmann (1984).

## Key Points

- The decision to conduct a pharmacoepidemiologic study can be viewed as similar to the regulatory decision about whether to approve a drug for marketing or the clinical decision about whether to prescribe a drug. In each case, decision making involves weighing the costs and risks of a therapy against its benefits.

- The main costs of a pharmacoepidemiologic study are: the costs (monetary, effort, time) of conducting the study itself, the opportunity costs of other research that might be left undone if this research is performed, the possibility that it could identify an adverse outcome as associated with the drug under investigation when in fact the drug does not cause this adverse outcome, and that it could provide false reassurances about a drug's safety.
- The benefits of pharmacoepidemiologic studies could be conceptualized in four different categories: regulatory, marketing, legal, and clinical. Each will be of importance to different organizations and individuals involved in deciding whether to initiate a study. Any given study will usually be performed for several of these reasons.
- There are several factors that can affect one's willingness to tolerate the risk of adverse effects from drugs. Some of these factors are related to the adverse outcome being studied. Others are related to the exposure and the setting in which the adverse outcome occurs.

## Further Reading

Binns, T.B. (1987). Therapeutic risks in perspective. *Lancet* 2: 208–209.

O'Brien, B. (1986). *"What Are My Chances Doctor?"–A Review of Clinical Risks*. London: Office of Health Economics.

Bortnichak, E.A. and Sachs, R.M. (1986). Piroxicam in recent epidemiologic studies. *Am. J. Med.* 81: 44–48.

Feldman, H.I., Kinman, J.L., Berlin, J.A. et al. (1997). Parenteral ketorolac: the risk for acute renal failure. *Ann. Intern. Med.* 126: 193–199.

Hennessy, S., Kinman, J.L., Berlin, J.A. et al. (1997). Lack of hepatotoxic effects of parenteral ketorolac in the hospital setting. *Arch. Intern. Med.* 157: 2510–2514.

Humphries, T.J., Myerson, R.M., Gifford, L.M. et al. (1984). A unique postmarket outpatient surveillance program of cimetidine: report on phase II and final summary. *Am. J. Gastroenterol.* 79: 593–596.

Joint Commission on Prescription Drug Use (1980) *Final Report*. Washington, DC.

Lowrance, W.W. (1976). *Of Acceptable Risk*. Los Altos, CA: William Kaufmann.

Marwick, C. (1988). FDA ponders approaches to curbing adverse effects of drug used against cystic acne. *JAMA* 259: 3225.

Mattison, N. and Richard, B.W. (1987). Postapproval research requested by the FDA at the time of NCE approval, 1970–1984. *Drug Inf. J.* 21: 309–329.

Rogers, A.S., Porta, M., and Tilson, H.H. (1990). Guidelines for decision making in postmarketing surveillance of drugs. *J. Clin. Res. Pharmacol.* 4: 241–251.

Rossi, A.C. and Knapp, D.E. (1982). Tolmetin-induced anaphylactoid reactions. *N. Engl. J. Med.* 307: 499–500.

Silverberg, E. and Lubera, J.A. (1988). Cancer statistics. *CA Cancer J. Clin.* 38: 5–22.

Stallones, R.A. (1982). A review of the epidemiologic studies of toxic shock syndrome. *Ann. Intern. Med.* 96: 917–920.

Strom, B.L., Berlin, J.A., Kinman, J.L. et al. (1996). Parenteral ketorolac and risk of gastrointestinal and operative site bleeding: a postmarketing surveillance study. *JAMA* 275: 376–382.

Strom, B.L., Carson, J.L., Morse, M.L. et al. (1987). The effect of indication on hypersensitivity reactions associated with zomepirac sodium and other nonsteroidal antiinflammatory drugs. *Arthritis Rheum.* 30: 1142–1148.

Strom, B.L., Carson, J.L., Schinnar, R. et al. (1988). The effect of indication on the risk of hypersensitivity reactions associated with tolmetin sodium vs. other nonsteroidal antiinflammatory drugs. *J. Rheumatol.* 15: 695–699.

Strom, B.L. and members of the ASCPT Pharmacoepidemiology Section (1990). Position paper on the use of purported postmarketing drug surveillance studies for promotional purposes. *Clin. Pharmacol. Ther.* 48: 598.

Urquhart, J. and Heilmann, K. (1984). *Risk Watch–The Odds of Life*. New York: Facts on File.

Young, F.E. (1988). The role of the FDA in the effort against AIDS. *Public Health Rep.* 103: 242–245.

# 6

# Views from Academia, Industry, Regulatory Agencies, and the Legal System

*Joshua J. Gagne[1,2], Jerry Avorn[1], Nicolle M. Gatto[3], Jingping Mo[4], Gerald J. Dal Pan[5], June Raine[6], Shinobu Uzu[7], Aaron S. Kesselheim[1], and Kerstin N. Vokinger[1,8]*

[1] Harvard Medical School and Brigham and Women's Hospital, Boston, MA, USA
[2] Johnson and Johnson, New Brunswick, NJ, USA
[3] Aetion Inc., New York, NY, USA
[4] Epidemiology, Worldwide Research & Development, Pfizer Inc., New York, NY, USA
[5] Office of Surveillance and Epidemiology, Center for Drug Evaluation and Research, US Food and Drug Administration, Silver Spring, MD, USA
[6] Vigilance and Risk Management of Medicine, Medicines and Healthcare Products Regulatory Agency, London, UK
[7] Pharmaceuticals and Medical Devices Agency, Tokyo, Japan
[8] Institute for Law University of Zurich, Zurich, Switzerland

## The View from Academia

### Introduction

Every year prescribers and patients have more medications at their disposal, each with its own efficacy, side effects, and cost. When a new drug is introduced, its benefit-to-risk relationship is often understood in only a preliminary way, as is its cost-effectiveness. This provides a limited perspective on how it ideally should be used. High-profile withdrawals of drugs for safety reasons, along with prominent warnings about widely-used medications that remain on the market, have caused physicians, patients, and policymakers to become more aware of drug safety concerns. At the same time, health care systems all over the globe are struggling with how to provide the most appropriate care in the face of rising costs and increasingly tight fiscal constraints. Pharmacoepidemiology can serve as a key tool for helping to address all of these concerns. These issues are growing throughout the

health care system, and particularly in academic medical centers.

Once a drug is approved for marketing, it enters a complex health care system in which its prescription, its use by patients, and its outcomes often go largely unassessed. Until recently, scant attention has been paid to systematic surveillance of these actions, except for the atypical settings of some integrated health care delivery systems. The prevailing view has been that after the US Food and Drug Administration (FDA) or comparable national authority approves a drug, it is used at the discretion of the clinician, with little formal follow-up of the appropriateness or consequences of such decisions. The problem is made more acute by the fact that many regulatory agencies purposely (and often by statute) do not base their approval decisions on a medication's clinical or economic value compared to similar products; often superiority over placebo is sufficient for a drug to be approved. In addition, it is generally no one's responsibility (other than the harried prescriber) to determine how faithfully patients are adhering to the prescribed regimen. Increasingly, more attention is being paid to assessing the outcomes of medication use on a population level, considering what its useful and harmful outcomes are when it is taken by hundreds, thousands, or even millions of patients rather than by single individuals in a clinical trial or in routine practice. It is now widely appreciated that some adverse events can be identified and their risk quantified only by observing a drug's use in large numbers of patients. The best perspective on the impact of a medication on the health of the public requires measuring those outcomes in the health care system itself, rather than one person at a time. It is here that the insights of pharmacoepidemiology are playing an increasingly central role.

Driven by the pressures noted above, this situation is evolving, with growing appreciation of several important problems, each of which can be informed by the methods and tools of pharmacoepidemiology: (i) medications that seem acceptably safe on approval may prove to have important risks which were under-appreciated at the time of approval; (ii) in typical practice, clinicians often make prescribing decisions that do not reflect the best evidence-base or guideline recommendations; (iii) even this evidence base is often thinner than it should be because head-to-head comparisons of drug effectiveness or safety – either trial-based or observational – have not been done; (iv) as a result, inadequate information is available to inform decisions about which drugs work best, or most cost-effectively, for specific indications; and (v) patients frequently fail to take their medications as directed.

Pharmacoepidemiology is the core discipline required for a rigorous understanding of each of these areas, and to guide the development and evaluation of programs to address them. Many of these topics are discussed in detail in the chapters that follow; this chapter provides an overview of how the field and its methods can contribute to these larger themes in medical care delivery and health services research, from the perspective of academia.

## The Drug Approval Process

Each national health care system must grapple with the following inherent paradox of pharmacology: A new therapy must be evaluated for approval when the available data on its benefits and harms are still modest. Yet waiting until "all the evidence is in" can pose its own public health threat, if this prevents an important new treatment from being used by patients who need it. Since any medication that is effective is bound to have some adverse effect in some organ system in some patients at some doses, any approval must by definition be based on a judgment that a drug's efficacy is "worth it" in light of the known risks of the treatment. However, the trials conducted by a given drug manufacturer to win approval are often powered statistically (see Chapter 3) to demonstrate success for that single product in achieving a pre-specified therapeutic endpoint. Especially when this is demonstration of superiority over placebo, and/or when the required endpoint is reaching a surrogate outcome (e.g. a change in a laboratory test such as hemoglobin A1c or low density lipoprotein [LDL] cholesterol), the number of subjects required for these exercises, and the duration of the studies, are often inadequate to reveal important safety problems if they are present. This is exacerbated by the extensive exclusion criteria for study participation, a particular problem for high-risk populations such as the frail elderly, pregnant women, and children (see also Chapter 23).

As a result, additional methods need to be applied even to pre-approval data to aggregate adverse events from multiple study populations to provide the power needed to assess safety. Meta-analysis (see Chapter 20) of adverse effects data from multiple pre-approval trials represents the first opportunity to use these tools to inform the appropriate use of medications. This makes it possible to combine findings from different smaller studies – many of them conducted before the drug in question was approved – to produce evidence of potential harm for drugs.

These shortcomings of pre-marketing trials are likely to become even more salient as regulators move toward alternative drug approval processes. The European Medicines Agency (EMA) recently completed a pilot project to explore approval via adaptive pathways, which are intended to provide earlier and progressive patient access to new drugs. The US FDA maintains several expedited regulatory pathways. Post-approval monitoring of drugs approved through these pathways is even more critical, because safety information is more likely to emerge in the post-marketing setting for drugs approved by these pathways as compared to conventional pathways. In 2016 the US Congress enacted the 21st Century Cures Act which included, among other sections, provisions that modify the data required for FDA approval. In particular, the law promotes the use of biomarkers and surrogate measures to support the approval of new drugs as well as "real world evidence" from observational data to support supplemental indications for existing products. As these new provisions are implemented, pharmacoepidemiology will have an even greater role in generating the "real world evidence" for supplemental indications and will be increasingly relied upon to evaluate the impact on clinical outcomes, both beneficial and harmful, of new drugs approved on less rigorous evidence.

## Prescribing Practices

Once a drug has entered the health care delivery system, the tools of pharmacoepidemiology can be used to document areas in which prescribing falls short of existing knowledge. First is the issue of *underprescribing*. Studies of many important chronic diseases such as hypertension, hypercholesterolemia, and diabetes reveal that many patients with these conditions have not been diagnosed by their physicians, and when they have, they are often not prescribed an adequate regimen to control their risks, or even any regimen at all. Pharmacoepidemiology makes it possible to identify more clearly when and how prescribing falls short, insights which can then be used to shape programs to improve care (see below).

When medications are used, there is good evidence that clinicians frequently do not prescribe regimens that are optimal, based on the available clinical evidence, or prescribe medications that may interact with other drugs a patient takes, or choose more expensive drugs when comparable generic preparations would work as well and be much more affordable. Pharmacoepidemiology makes it possible to assess the distribution of drugs used for a given indication by clinician, practice, or system and can account for contraindications and compelling indications related to specific drug choices, to refine the assessment of the appropriateness of prescribing in an entire health care system, or for individual clinicians. One study assessed all hypertension-related medication use and diagnoses in one large state-funded program of medications for the elderly. The availability of clinical information made it possible to determine how well the regimen of each patient conformed to guideline recommendations. This study found that a substantial proportion of treated hypertensive patients were not receiving a regiment consistent with guidelines. Often, such suboptimal prescribing involved omissions of an indicated class (e.g. angiotensin converting enzyme inhibitors in patients with diabetes mellitus), or use of a calcium channel blocker when a beta-blocker would have been more appropriate (e.g. in a hypertensive patient who has had a myocardial infarction). Another analysis reviewed all clinical encounters of patients who had filled prescriptions for clopidogrel and found that about half did not have any evidence of conditions (such as coronary artery stenting) for which the drug had an approved indication, or any other evidence-based reasons for its use.

More sophisticated health records systems are becoming available each year that integrate pharmacy data with information from clinical laboratories, electronic health records, registries, and sources of patient-reported information to measure the adequacy of use of cholesterol-lowering agents, diabetes drugs, antihypertensives, and other drugs. This makes it possible to assess the effectiveness of prescribing outcomes for a given clinician (or practice or system), by measuring how well target metrics such as normotension or goal LDL cholesterol or hemoglobin A1c are being achieved. In all these analyses, pharmacoepidemiology makes it possible to evaluate the appropriateness of medication use in selected populations, even if it cannot with certainty determine whether a given prescription in a particular patient was the best choice.

## Evaluation of Patients' Use of Drugs in the Health Care System

Even when a medication is appropriately prescribed, patients may underuse it or use it in unsafe ways. Underuse of needed drugs by patients is one of the most common medication-related problems, and one that can be readily identified by pharmacoepidemiology (see also Chapter 21).

Because many assessments of underuse are based on pharmacy-generated data on filled prescriptions, it is sometimes difficult to know whether non-use of an indicated drug was the result of a failure of the patient to fill a prescription, or the failure of the clinician to write it. Electronic prescribing makes it possible to define this problem more precisely. One large study found that a fourth of initial prescriptions written electronically were never picked up at the pharmacy. As a result, the approximately 50% rate of non-adherence seen over time in pharmacoepidemiologic datasets based on filled prescriptions is a best-case scenario, as it does not even take into account the additional millions of regimens that are not even initiated by the patient. Terminology has evolved to define the two aspects of this problem: *secondary non-adherence* refers to the failure by a patient to continue to use a medication already begun; *primary non-adherence* occurs when a clinician writes a prescription that the patient does not even fill once. The magnitude of both primary and secondary non-adherence is substantial, and varies by drug class as well as country.

## Assessment of the Quality and Outcomes of Medication Use in Populations

Much attention is now being paid to the assessment of the outcomes of medication use in typical "real-world" populations. This perspective is based on the difference between *efficacy*, the effect of a medication in the rigorous but idealized setting of a clinical trial, compared to its *effectiveness*, a measure of its outcomes in typical practice settings. These often differ. For example, one important conventional randomized trial demonstrated convincingly that addition of spironolactone to the regimen of patients with congestive heart failure substantially improved their clinical status and reduced mortality. However, a population-based analysis later found that when these findings were applied in routine practice by typical physicians treating a much larger number of typical patients, there was a significant increase in hyperkalemia-associated morbidity and mortality. By contrast, an analysis of prescribers' response to a different study that provided new evidence about optimal management of atrial fibrillation demonstrated a more positive change in practice.

Other analyses document that despite overwhelming randomized trial evidence showing the efficacy of warfarin use in preventing stroke in patients with atrial fibrillation, population-based studies of older patients living in nursing homes revealed a surprisingly low prevalence of use of this therapy. Such underuse was found to be associated with physicians' recent experience with adverse events caused by the drug, as well as by their perceptions and attitudes about risks and benefits. This kind of real-world population research can lay the foundation for enlightened interventions to address such non-use, by taking on its underlying causes.

Pharmacoepidemiologic methods can also be used to track the diffusion of new medication classes into practice, as well as the reaction of practitioners in various settings to new information about the comparative benefits and risks of drug. Acknowledging the gap between the characteristics of clinical trial participants and those who often use a medication in practice, methods are also being developed and applied to generalize trial results to more typical patient populations. For example, the newer oral anticoagulant, dabigatran, was approved on the basis of a large randomized trial comparing it to warfarin, an older oral anticoagulant. A simulation-based approach was used to assess how the comparative benefits and risks would translate to cohorts of patients who use these drugs outside of the randomized trial and in usual routine care. Such an approach preserves the strengths of the randomized trial but makes the results more useful to patients and clinicians.

## Policy Analysis

Usually, policy changes are implemented in the health care system with no systematic plans for their evaluation, and no follow-up studies of their impact. Such changes in benefit design are often applied to medication use. However, even if a policy is changed in a way that does not anticipate an evaluation, population-based observational studies after the fact can still yield important conclusions concerning its effects, both good and bad. For example, when the Canadian province of British Columbia implemented a reference-pricing policy for antihypertensive medications in which it reimbursed only the cost of an effective generic drug in several classes, critics charged that any savings would come at the cost of increased morbidity and healthcare utilization. However, a careful time-series analysis of all medication use, physician visits, and hospital care in the province before and after policy implementation provided compelling evidence that the new reimbursement system produced no important clinical downsides, but did achieve substantial savings for the provincial health-care budget. Such observational methods have also been combined with population-based randomized policy trials, and were found to yield similar results.

## Interventional Pharmacoepidemiology

Although epidemiology is traditionally seen as a merely observational discipline, it can also be used for what might be called "interventional epidemiology" – in this case, using the tools of pharmacoepidemiology to define baseline medication use, to direct the implementation of programs to improve such use, and then to employ the same rigorous ascertainment of practice patterns and clinical events to evaluate the effectiveness of those interventions.

One example of such interventional pharmacoepidemiology has been the development, testing, and widespread deployment of the form of educational outreach known as "academic detailing." The academic detailing approach uses the engaging interactive outreach of the pharmaceutical industry, but puts in the service of transmitting messages based solely on evidence-based recommendations of optimal prescribing, developed by academic physicians. Building on pharmacoepidemiologic assessment of overall prescribing patterns in a given area, the method was then tested in several population-based randomized trials in which it was shown to be effective in improving prescribing, as well as in reducing unnecessary medication expenditures.

As computerized drug and medical data have matured, their role has expanded to support large-scale, multi-center, pragmatic randomized trials of medications themselves. In the Salford Lung Study, investigators randomized over 4000 typical patients with asthma to receive an inhaled combination of a beta-agonist and a corticosteroid or to usual care. The trial was conducted in more than six dozen general practice clinics in the UK, using an integrated electronic health record system that enabled the investigators to collect study data during the course of the trial with little additional interaction required between patients and trial staff.

## Economic Assessment of Medication-Related Issues

Using population-based datasets that contain information on expenditures as well as utilization makes it possible to assess the economic impact of such prescribing issues as well (see Chapter 18). The above study of patients treated for hypertension, for example, found that better adherence to the guideline recommendations would not only have led to more evidence-based prescribing (and therefore better clinical outcomes), it would also have resulted in savings of $1.2 billion annually if the findings were projected nationally. Similarly, the clopidogrel-use study suggested that if aspirin had been substituted in patients who lacked an evidence-based or FDA-approved indication for use of the more costly drug, it would have saved $1.5 billion at a national level.

## The Academic Medical Center

The academic medical center represents a special case of inquiry for pharmacoepidemiology, and one where the field can make particularly useful contributions. These centers are the home base for many researchers in the field, and such settings are more likely than many routine practices to have available the electronic datasets that make such analyses possible. In recent years, the Institute of Medicine

(IOM) has been promoting the idea of a Learning Healthcare System in which the data generated within a medical center are analyzed and used to improve the delivery of care within the system. The science of pharmacoepidemiology is central to the collection, analysis, and interpretation of the data generated and used in this continuous feedback loop for several reasons, including its capacity to rigorously specify treatment exposures and outcomes, and its perspective that takes into account the concept of "population at risk." For academic medical centers that evolve in the coming years to become the hubs of comprehensive accountable care organizations, the availability of such data and investigator teams will make it possible to use these epidemiologic tools to study – and improve – the patterns of use and outcomes of medications across the entire inpatient-outpatient continuum of care.

## Consortia of Academic Medical Center Programs for Pharmacoepidemiologic Research

As the field of pharmacoepidemiology matures, new collaborations are emerging to enhance the capacity of the health care delivery system and of academic centers to address important questions in medication use. Such collaborations can bring together large groups of patients for study, increasing the size of populations available for research, as well as their diversity and representativeness. Equally important, such consortia can bring together the expertise of several groups whose skills may be complementary in addressing the difficult methodologic issues inherent in observational studies of drug use and outcomes. The EMA has created ENCePP, the European Network of Centres for Pharmacoepidemiology and Pharmacovigilance. The project has developed an inventory of European research centers and data sources in pharmacoepidemiology and pharmacovigilance, and provides a public index of such resources. ENCePP has also developed an electronic register of studies that provides a publicly accessible means of identifying all registered ongoing projects in pharmacoepidemiology and pharmacovigilance. In order to be registered and receive formal ENCePP approval, study investigators must agree to a Code of Conduct, which sets forth a set of principles for such studies concerning methodologic practices and transparency; they must also agree to adhere to a checklist of methodologic standards.

Examples in the US include the FDA's Sentinel system, the Centers for Disease Control and Prevention's (CDC's) Vaccine Safety Datalink (VSD), and the Patient-Centered Outcome Research Institute's (PCORI) PCORnet. Sentinel is FDA's national monitoring system that brings together a large number of electronic health care data providers and academic investigators to conduct post-approval safety surveillance of FDA-regulated medical products. The VSD, which is a collaborative project between the CDC and health care organizations that provide data and scientific expertise, is a precursor to Sentinel that focuses on vaccine safety surveillance, such as monitoring the safety of the seasonal influenza vaccine. A product of the healthcare reform program enacted in 2010, PCORI was designed to provide funding for comparative effectiveness research (CER), which was to include the study of medications, often by means of observational studies. PCORnet is PCORI's collaborative network of health systems, clinicians, researchers, patients, and data intended to foster patient-centered research across various health systems. However, those who expected PCORI to function as a CER resource that would fund trial or observational studies comparing relevant treatment options head-to-head have been surprised at what a small proportion of its activities have supported such work.

## The Future

The continuing evolution of health care systems in both the industrialized and the developing worlds will bring about a growing role for pharmacoepidemiology in multiple settings. Many new medications have novel efficacy but also daunting risks of toxicity, and often enormous costs. Health care systems all over the world face pressures to provide only those interventions that have the best efficacy and safety, but also at a price. To accomplish this will require relying on more than manufacturers' assessments of the utility, safety, or economic value of their own products, and more than clinicians' received wisdom or traditional prescribing habits. Nor will the interest of some insurers in promoting use of the most inexpensive medications necessarily lead to optimal outcomes clinically, economically, or ethically. Pharmacoepidemiology (and its related discipline, pharmacoeconomics) can provide the tools for rigorous assessment of the good and harm that specific medications provide, and hold the promise of applying science to therapeutic decisions that are still too dominated by other forces.

## Summary Points for the View from Academia

- Pharmacoepidemiology has a growing role in providing insights into therapeutic decisions as routinely collected health care data can be analyzed by increasingly powerful software and hardware, combined with emerging sophisticated epidemiologic methods.
- Beyond defining the benefits and risks of therapeutics, these tools can point to how best to maximize benefits, reduce risks, and contain costs.

**Case Example 6.1**

The view from academia: The role of academia in developing, implementing, and evaluating innovative programs to improve medication use (Avorn 2011).

*Background*

- Practitioners have difficulty keeping up with important new findings about drug risks and benefits. As a result, there is a knowledge gap between what is known and what is practiced.
- Pharmacoepidemiology can play a more prominent role in defining prescribing patterns and their outcomes.

*Question*

How can researchers in academia improve the use of therapeutics to maximize patient benefit and minimize the likelihood of harm?

*Approach*

- Academic researchers have expertise in analyzing population-based data to identify patterns of medication use. They also have a broad grasp of the overall clinical literature; train future practitioners and researchers; develop and evaluate therapies; deliver care to patients; and include thought leaders who influence national policy.
- Such expertise can be used to understand the outcomes of medications and improve their use.
- Programs of "academic detailing" devised by academic researchers can adopt the effective outreach methods of pharmaceutical companies for noncommercial purposes by visiting physicians in their offices to promote optimal prescribing practices.

*Results*

Many randomized controlled trials have demonstrated that this approach is effective in providing prescribers with better information about benefits, risks and appropriate use of therapeutics, and changing their prescribing.

*Strengths*

- This approach enables those in academia to combine the analytic tools of pharmacoepidemiology with evidence-based medicine expertise and social marketing methods to create interventions that bridge the gap between therapeutics knowledge and practice.
- Such programs can help offset their costs by improving outcomes and reducing use of therapies that are not cost-effective.

*Limitations*

- Requires cooperation among stakeholders with different goals and perspectives within a fragmented health care system.
- Lack of cooperation among different payers can reduce incentives to operate such programs and sustain their costs.

*Key Points*

- As health care organizations become more centered on enhancing outcomes and value rather than on maximizing volume, opportunities are increasing for academic researchers to "push out" innovative user-friendly educational programs to improve medication use.
- Pharmacoepidemiology can play a central role in such work, by defining patterns of medication use, assessing risks and benefits, and evaluating changes in prescribing and outcomes in populations of patients.
- Health care organizations face pressing needs to develop data repositories and local expertise in the analysis of medication use and outcomes. Academic medical centers can set the example by organizing their own data and providing access to it to improve quality and therapeutic strategies.
- Academic medical centers can leverage their combined missions of education, health care delivery, and research to move national practice toward better use of therapeutics.
- Academic researchers are well suited to translate medical research findings on drug benefits, risks, and cost-effectiveness into educational outreach programs that can be acted upon by policy-makers, practitioners and the public.

# The View from Industry

## Note

The views expressed are those of the authors, which are not necessarily those of Aetion Inc. or Pfizer Inc.

## Introduction

Epidemiology is recognized as a key component of risk management and safety assessment activities during pre- and post-approval drug development. In addition to risk management, epidemiology contributes to several other important functions within a biopharmaceutical company, including portfolio development, the commercialization of drugs, and benefit–risk assessments. The use of epidemiology to support the appropriate marketing of drugs, including health economics, and benefit–risk assessment, are discussed elsewhere in this book (see Chapters 18 and 23). The most consistent contribution of epidemiology in the biopharmaceutical industry is arguably drug safety evaluation, including the contextualization and refinement of safety signals, and examination of specific research hypotheses. To meet these aims, epidemiologists design and implement background epidemiology studies among indicated populations, risk management interventions and evaluations, and post-approval safety studies.

Additionally, epidemiologists contribute content, expertise, and strategy to regulatory documents such as global Risk Management Plans (RMP), Pediatric Investigation Plans (PIP), and orphan drug applications, and are key contributors in interactions with regulatory authorities. This section discusses the specific application of pharmacoepidemiology to safety assessment throughout the development lifecycle from the perspective of epidemiologists working within the biopharmaceutical industry. At the end of this section, we include a case example of the epidemiology strategy implemented to support the development, approval, and post-approval activities for Xeljanz* (tofacitinib), a Janus kinase (JAK) inhibitor for treatment of rheumatoid arthritis (RA).

## Regulatory and Industry Focus on Risk Management and Epidemiology

Biopharmaceutical risk management (see also Chapter 23) is fundamentally concerned with preserving an appropriate benefit–risk balance among patients using a medicine, vaccine, or device. There are many tools by which this goal can be achieved, but *risk assessment* and *risk mitigation* are the two primary components of risk management. Epidemiologists play a vital role in the quantification and interpretation of risk. Pre-approval, they contextualize risks emerging from clinical studies by understanding the background rates of clinical outcomes of interest in the indicated population. Post-approval, they assess the safety of drugs as used in actual clinical practice. Epidemiologists' training in observational research, data analysis and interpretation, and survey and program design also contributes to effective risk mitigation program planning and assessment.

### The Evolution of Biopharmaceutical Risk Management

The guidance and regulations around risk management have evolved since the 1990s. Public pressure to speed drug approvals for HIV and cancer drugs led to the Prescription Drug User Fee Act (PDUFA) in the US. Ten years later, concern that speed might come at the expense of fully evaluating safety led to the inclusion of a risk management framework for safety assessment in PDUFA III in 2002. For the first time, dedicated funding was provided to the FDA for risk management resources. In response to this regulation, the FDA issued three guidance documents in 2005: (i) Pre-Marketing Risk Assessment, (ii) Pharmacovigilance and Pharmacoepidemiology, and (iii) Risk Minimization Action Plans (RiskMAPs).

After a number of widely used drugs were withdrawn in 2004 and 2005 for safety reasons, the public questioned the effectiveness of the FDA's methods to assess and approve drugs. The IOM was tasked with evaluating the US drug safety system and making recommendations for improvements to risk assessment, safety surveillance, and the safer use of drugs. The IOM committee made numerous recommendations, several of which pertained to epidemiologists, including: provide the FDA additional funding and staff; improve communications on drug safety, including a larger role for the drug safety staff; and most importantly, be given additional authority and enforcement tools.

As a result of the IOM report and other stakeholder research and advocacy, Congress passed the Food and Drug Administration Amendment Act (FDAAA) in 2007, which further strengthened the FDA's oversight of risk management activities. With FDAAA, the FDA was granted the ability to mandate post-approval studies (Postmarketing Requirements, or PMR) and Risk Mitigation Evaluation Strategies ("REMS"; see section later in this chapter for further information) by imposing substantial fines for noncompliance or denial/revocation of drug approval. FDAAA also allowed for voluntarily post-marketing commitments (PMC), i.e. studies that may not necessarily be required but could provide important public health information. Observational studies could be either PMRs or PMCs, and are further described in the FDA Guidance for Industry Postmarketing Studies and Clinical Trials.

Europe passed similar legislation in 2005, The Rules Governing Medicinal Products in the European Union-Volume 9A, which provide guidelines on pharmacovigilance and risk management between companies and the EMA. EU law requires companies to submit a formal RMP with each marketing authorization application (MAA). Following a review of the European system of safety monitoring as well as extensive public consultation, a Directive and Regulation (also called new EU pharmacovigilance legislation) were adopted by the European Parliament and Council of Ministers in December 2010, which became effective in July 2012, bringing about significant changes in the safety monitoring of medicines across the EU. The new EU pharmacovigilance legislation introduced a pharmacovigilance system master file (PSMF), required RMPs for all new products, enhanced post-authorization measures with legally binding post-authorization safety studies (PASS), including evaluation of the effectiveness of additional risk minimization measures (aRMMs), and post-authorization efficacy studies (PAES). The new EU pharmacovigilance legislation also introduced clarity in the oversight by the authorities for non-interventional studies: the national competent authority is responsible for nationally authorized products, EMA and its Pharmacovigilance and Risk Assessment Committee (PRAC) has the oversight responsibility when more than one member state is involved. To facilitate the performance of pharmacovigilance in accordance with the new EU legislation, the EMA developed good pharmacovigilance practices (GVP) modules. The modules that are most relevant to epidemiologists are Module VIII PASS and Module XVI Risk minimization measures: selection of tools and effectiveness.

Besides US and EU, regulations on risk management planning, including post-approval safety studies, are evolving in other parts of the world, such as Asia and Latin America. In Japan, post-marketing surveillance (PMS) is required for newly approved medicine and must be conducted in according with the good post-marketing study practice (GPSP), a set of standards unique to Japan. The GPSP ordinance mandates PMS studies, commonly known as drug use results surveys (DURSs), and defines the approach for DURS conduct. There is little flexibility in the design and format; protocol finalization and approval are usually streamlined processes. Japan's Pharmaceuticals and Medical Devices Agency (PMDA) has been working to strengthen its drug safety assessment framework. The Medical Information for Risk Assessment Initiative (MIHARI) project was initiated in 2009 with the aim of utilizing large-scale electronic health information databases as novel information sources for pharmacoepidemiologic drug safety assessments in

Japan. After conducting extensive pilot studies, the framework was implemented into practical applications in 2014 and is expected to play an important role in Japan's pharmacovigilance and risk management in the future.

In China, policies for post-approval safety studies, known as *intensive monitoring,* are still evolving, and the available guidance and overall approach are not as comprehensive as in the US, EU, or Japan. However, the basis for intensive monitoring has evolved over the past decade, and provisions for the ideas of post-marketing re-evaluation and re-registration are delineated in China's FDA regulations. In Mexico, Federal Commission for Protection against Health Risks (COFEPRIS) is the regulatory authority for pharmaceuticals. The National Center of Pharmacovigilance within COFEPRIS is responsible for the oversight of all pharmacovigilance activities, in addition to setting local policies in line with national and international pharmacovigilance guidelines. The main standard guideline governing pharmacovigilance, including PMS studies, in Mexico is the Installation and Operation of Pharmacovigilance.

Epidemiology has become increasingly important to risk management over the last three decades with evolving pharmacovigilance regulation globally, which has further solidified epidemiology's role in informing the benefit–risk of medicines throughout the development lifecycle.

## Epidemiology in Drug Safety Evaluation

### Background

The safety profile of any drug reflects an evolving body of knowledge extending from pre-clinical investigations through the post-approval lifecycle of the product. Drug manufacturers traditionally relied on two major sources for information on the safety of drugs: the clinical trials supporting the New Drug Application (NDA) and, once the drug was marketed, spontaneous reports received throughout the world

(see Chapter 7). Clinical trials and spontaneous reports are useful and have a unique place in assessing drug safety (e.g. signal detection). However, both sources have limitations that can be addressed, in part, by the proper use of observational epidemiology. Epidemiologic studies complement these two sources of data to refine the safety signals they generate and to provide a more comprehensive and pragmatic picture of the safety profile of a drug as it is used in clinical practice.

### Contributions of Pre-approval Epidemiology

Before evaluation of a potential medicine can begin, extensive pre-clinical research is conducted, involving lengthy *in vitro* and *in vivo* testing. Preclinical safety studies evaluate and identify potential toxic effects of the drug, which include assessing whether a medicine is carcinogenic, mutagenic, or teratogenic. Although the information generated from pre-clinical studies provides guidance on the selection of a safe starting dose for the first administration-to-human study, the limited predictability of animal studies to the toxicity of drugs in human is well-recognized. However, these studies can provide important information about hypothetical drug risks.

Randomized clinical trials (RCTs) provide abundant high-quality data about identified and hypothetical risks, but have limitations. Pre-approval RCTs typically involve highly selected subjects followed for a short period of time and, in the aggregate, include at most a few thousand patients. These studies are generally sufficiently large to provide evidence of a beneficial clinical effect, exclude large increases in risk of common adverse events, and identify the most common and acutely occurring adverse events. However, they are rarely large enough to detect small differences in the risk of common adverse events or to reliably estimate the risk of rare events. Using the "rule of three," where the sample size needed is roughly three times the reciprocal of the frequency of the event, at least 300 patients would be required in a trial in order to observe at least one adverse event that occurs at a rate of 1/100. Likewise, a sample of 3000 is needed to observe at least one adverse event with 95% probability if the frequency of the event is 1/1000 (see Chapter 3 for more discussion of the sample sizes needed for studies). Increasingly, preapproval studies – particularly in the rare diseases or where long-term placebo treatments are unethical – include unbalanced randomization or treatment arms with short duration of placebo or active-comparator, or use noncontemporaneous controls. While clinical trials are not intended or designed to address all potential safety issues related to a particular drug, like preclinical studies, they often give rise to signals that cannot be adequately addressed from trial data alone.

Pre-approval epidemiology complements safety data from preclinical and clinical studies and provides a context for signals arising from clinical trials. Comprehensive reviews of the epidemiologic literature are complemented by epidemiologic studies to establish the background epidemiology (e.g. incidence, prevalence, mortality) of the indication among patients expected to use the new medication (i.e. indicated populations); expected prevalence/incidence of risk factors, co-morbidities and complications; patterns of health care utilization and prescribing of currently approved treatments; and background rates of mortality and serious nonfatal events.

Epidemiologic studies conducted before or during the clinical development program are often critical to place the incidence of adverse events observed in clinical trials in perspective. Data are often lacking on the expected rates of events in the population likely to be treated. For example, studies examining the risk factors for and rates of sudden unexplained death among people with epilepsy were able to provide reassurance that the rates observed in a clinical development program were within the expected range for individuals with a comparably severe disease. Epidemiologists use information from the published literature, descriptive epidemiologic studies, and standing cohorts (i.e. open cohorts of indicated populations which are updated over time and queried for incidence of safety events and other data as needed) to support regulatory filings and to complete epidemiology sections of key regulatory documents (e.g. RMP and PIP, orphan drug applications). These background epidemiology data can also be a key component for internal decision making such as trial design, data monitoring committee decisions to stop/continue trials, decisions to move/not move to the next phase of development, risk management decisions, and risk mitigation planning.

During development, in addition to summarizing the existing relevant literature and designing and executing background epidemiology studies, industry epidemiologists are often involved in safety signal evaluation, observational analyses of RCT data (e.g. astreated or observed versus expected analyses), and designing post-approval epidemiology studies and risk minimization planning. Planning for successful post-approval epidemiology studies often begins well before approval. During the peri-approval phase, epidemiologists may conduct feasibility assessments for planned post-approval studies, start key operational aspects of post-approval studies (e.g. identifying key external partners such as contract research organizations and scientific steering committee members for the design and conduct of the study), and contribute to regulatory submissions, responses, and negotiations (e.g. responding to regulatory inquiries related to epidemiology and participating in regulatory meetings).

There are several other areas where epidemiologists are increasingly providing their expertise to support pre-approval development. In the context of risk minimization planning, the epidemiologist may conduct research to test the comprehension and utility of educational materials, evaluate the proposed risk minimization tools and processes to assess their burden on the healthcare system and patients, pilot and/or user test assessment materials such as surveys, and generally contribute to the design and implementation of these programs. Furthermore, many regulatory agencies are utilizing various benefit–risk assessment frameworks in their reviews. Epidemiologists can provide inputs or lead both quantitative and qualitative benefit-risk assessments such as multi-criteria decision analysis (MCDA), stochastic multicriteria acceptability analysis (SMAA), and the PhRMA Benefit-Risk Action Team (BRAT) framework, among others (see Chapter 23). Lastly, several accelerated/conditional approval pathways and regulations exist in the EU, and are anticipated for the US and other regions, which have requirements for Real World Data and Evidence (RWD/RWE) to complement the incomplete or uncertain data from abbreviated development programs in areas of high unmet needs. Epidemiologists' expertise in regulatory-quality RWD/RWE generation is often critical to the success of these accelerated options.

## Contributions of Post-approval Epidemiology

The need for a post-approval epidemiology study can be known and devised pre-approval or can arise once a new drug is marketed. Post-approval signals may come from clinical trial extension data (e.g. long-term extension [LTE] studies), spontaneous reports, published case-series, or signal detection of electronic healthcare data. Once a drug is marketed, epidemiologists execute post-approval commitments (e.g. epidemiology studies, active surveillance studies, other registries, REMS/aRMM evaluations, PIP observational studies, etc.); conduct studies evaluating the effectiveness of risk mitigation activities; perform signal detection in existing cohorts (e.g. via claims or electronic patient record data); and design and implement new studies as additional signals arise (e.g. from spontaneous reports, signal detection or other sources). Epidemiologists also communicate scientific findings through oral and poster presentations

at scientific conferences and peer-reviewed publications.

Spontaneous reporting systems are the most commonly used pharmacovigilance method to generate signals on new or rare adverse events not discovered in clinical trials (see Chapter 7). However, there are several important limitations in interpreting spontaneous report data. Due to the lack of complete numerator (number of cases) and the need to estimate the denominator (total number of patients actually exposed to the drug) data, it is not possible to determine the incidence of a particular event from spontaneous reports. Further evaluation of an apparent association between a drug and an adverse reaction usually requires post-approval epidemiologic studies.

Likewise, the nature of pre-approval clinical trials often necessitates further safety evaluation through post-approval epidemiology. In addition to the limited sample size and length of follow-up of pre-approval RCTs, with respect to drug safety, an additional limitation of these studies is the common strict inclusion/exclusion criteria. Patients included in pre-approval clinical studies may be the healthiest segment of that patient population. Special groups such as the elderly, pregnant women, or children are frequently excluded from trials. Patients in clinical trials also tend to be treated for well-defined indications, have limited and well-monitored concomitant drug use, and are closely followed for early signs and symptoms of adverse events which may be reversed with proper treatment.

In contrast, once a drug is marketed, it is used in a "real-world" clinical context. Patients using the drug may have multiple co-morbidities for which they are being treated simultaneously. Patients may also be taking over-the-counter medications, "natural" remedies, or illicit drugs unbeknownst to the prescribing physician. The interactions of various drugs and treatments may result in a particular drug having a different safety profile in a post-marketing setting compared to the controlled premarketing environment.

An example is the drug mibefradil, which was voluntarily withdrawn from the market by the manufacturer after less than a year as a result of new information about multiple potentially serious drug interactions. Adherence to medications also often differs between closely monitored trials and general post-approval use, as is the case with antihypertensives.

Because of the logistical complexity, high cost, and low external validity, large controlled trials have not been widely used for the post-marketing evaluation of drugs. Regulators and the medical community have communicated a desire for safety data from the populations that actually use the drugs in "real-world" clinical practice. This has led to a greater emphasis on the use of observational methods to understand the safety profile of new medications after they are marketed.

In addition to typical epidemiologic designs, depending on the specific safety research hypothesis, epidemiologists design and implement active surveillance studies, pragmatic trials (including the most naturalistic version, the large simple trial [LST]), and self-controlled designs such as the case-crossover study and self-controlled case series. Active surveillance studies can be defined as descriptive studies intended to solicit information on adverse events among a specified population, such that the numerator and denominator are as complete as possible, potentially allowing calculation of incidence.

Purely observational epidemiologic studies may not always be the most appropriate method of evaluating safety signals or comparing the safety profile of different medications, especially when there are concerns of confounding by indication. Confounding by indication occurs when the risk of an adverse event is related to the indication for medication use such that in the absence of the medication, those actually exposed are at higher or lower risk of the adverse event than those unexposed. As with any other form of confounding, one can, in theory, control for its

effects if the severity of the underlying illness (i.e. any conditions specified as labeled indications or contraindications, or included in the precautions or warnings) can be validly measured (see Chapter 22). Confounding by indication is more of an issue when a particular property of the drug is very likely to affect the type of patient it is used by or prescribed to. In these cases, studies using randomization to treatment may be necessary. A pragmatic clinical trial (PCT) is an RCT with one or more pragmatic elements and an LST is a type of PCT that combines randomization to treatment with observational follow-up of patients. The characteristics of LSTs are further described in Chapter 17.

## Epidemiology in Evaluation of Risk Mitigation Interventions

Epidemiology not only plays an important role in evaluation of the drug safety profile pre- and post-approval but, as noted earlier, also makes significant contributions to the evaluation of the effectiveness of risk mitigation intervention measures (see also Section 23.6). This component of biopharmaceutical risk management has grown considerably in the last decade, with the US, EU, Taiwan, Egypt, Australia, and a number of other countries implementing legislation that supports risk mitigation interventions.

Under FDAAA, the FDA can require a sponsor to submit a proposed Risk Evaluation and Mitigation Strategies (REMS) as part of its initial application if the FDA finds that a REMS is necessary to ensure the benefits of the drug or biological product outweigh the risks. The FDA may also require a REMS post-approval based upon new safety information. FDAAA has defined this as any information obtained during the initial review process, as a result of post-approval studies, or spontaneous reports. REMS are intended to be utilized to reduce known or hypothetical risks when traditional minimization approaches (i.e.

the product label) are insufficient. These tools generally fall into three categories: enhanced education, i.e. patient labeling (including medication guides) or communication plans such as prescriber training programs; Elements to Assure Safe Use (ETASU), e.g. requiring documentation of laboratory tests before each prescription or restricting distribution only to those who are certified prescribers; and an implementation system to monitor and evaluate the ETASU. A critical addition to this legislation that was particularly relevant to epidemiologists within industry was the requirement to perform assessments of the effectiveness of these risk minimization tools and to submit these to the Agency for review at prescribed time points, generally at 18 months, 3 years, and 7 years. The EU has similar legislation to require sponsors to implement aRMM where necessary to ensure the benefits outweigh the risks, and a similar requirement to assess the effectiveness of the aRMM, although without defined timelines. These aRMM programs and assessments are described in the EU-RMP.

Epidemiologists play a critical role in the design and implementation of these assessments because of their expertise in observational study design, survey design, data analysis, and program evaluation. For example, using an automated healthcare or claims database, assessments may measure compliance with monitoring guidelines or to measure whether a contraindicated population is prescribed the drug. Assessments may also examine the frequency of occurrence of an adverse event of interest before and after implementation of the risk minimization tool. Most commonly, however, assessments measure prescriber, pharmacist, or patient comprehension of risk information or self-reported adherence to risk minimization behaviors, and require the epidemiologist to craft cross-sectional surveys specific for each recipient, drug, and associated unique risk profile, as standardized or validated

questionnaires that measure these concepts do not exist.

The implementation of the REMS and aRMM legislation has highlighted a number of difficulties. The mandated assessments may be difficult to achieve, or achieve within the US legislative timelines, for many reasons: the need to develop and pilot knowledge/comprehension surveys unique to each drug subject to a REMS; to design, implement, and assess complex safe use programs; the scarcity of patients treated with the drug of interest; or difficulties in identifying them through automated channels. The fractured healthcare and prescription delivery system in the US and the wide variety of health systems, legal and privacy requirements, and attitudes toward these programs and research participation across Europe present a barrier to efficient distribution of educational materials, to the implementation of many safe use elements, and to the scientifically valid evaluation of these programs overall. Unfortunately, there is relatively little scholarly work published on how best to assess, how best to define success, and where necessary, how best to improve these often burdensome but important risk mitigation programs. Knowledge in these areas continues to mature as more companies and the regulatory agencies garner additional experience, and we expect that existing guidance will evolve. Risk mitigation evaluation is thus still an emerging area for epidemiologists in industry but one that complements our specialized training and expertise.

## Conclusion

Epidemiology makes a significant contribution to the development and marketing of safe and effective biopharmaceutical products worldwide. It facilitates the regulatory process and provides a rational basis for drug safety evaluation, particularly in the post-approval phase, and evaluation of risk mitigation interventions. Like any other discipline, it must be properly understood and appropriately utilized. Industry has an opportunity to contribute to the development of the field and the responsibility to do so in a manner that expands resources while assuring scientific validity. With the passage of the 2007 FDAAA legislation and the 2010 EMA Regulation on Pharmacovigilance, the need for scientists with training and research experience in pharmacoepidemiology has never been greater. To best support drug safety evaluation, epidemiology strategies must: (i) begin early in development, (ii) continue throughout the lifecycle of the drug, (iii) evolve as new safety information becomes available, and (iv) be innovative, requiring epidemiologists to be aware of new methodologies and methods specific to the disease area. Epidemiologists within industry have an opportunity to build on the successes of the last 40 years by collaborating with academics, non-profit organizations and regulators to advance the methods of drug safety evaluation and risk management.

## Summary Points for the View from Industry

- The safety profile of any drug reflects an evolving body of knowledge extending from preclinical investigations to the first use of the agent in humans and through the post-approval life cycle of the product.
- Results from clinical trials, spontaneous reports, epidemiologic studies, and where relevant, preclinical datasets, should all be evaluated for their potential to address safety questions, with close consideration given to the unique strengths and limitations of the study designs and data collection methods used.
- Epidemiology plays a central role in drug safety assessment and risk management activities within the pharmaceutical industry, whether through studies of the natural history of disease, disease progression/treatment pathways, and morbidity and mortality patterns, or in the design and implementation of post-approval safety studies or risk minimization programs.

### Case Example 6.2

View from industry: Tofacitinib pre-approval and post-approval epidemiology strategies.

*Background*
- Tofacitinib is a JAK inhibitor for the treatment of rheumatoid arthritis (RA) for adults with an inadequate response to methotrexate.
- RCTs provide high-quality data about identified and hypothesized risk but have limitations. Even though all the RCTs in the tofacitinib RA development program included at least one placebo or active control group, the size of the control groups and duration of treatment prohibited precise comparative assessments for adverse events with low frequency or long

latency. Furthermore, LTE studies, while providing greater exposure in patients taking tofacitinib, lacked control groups to allow a comparative risk assessment. Evidence of the expected rates in a concurrent and directly comparable patient population was also lacking.

*Question*
How were epidemiologic studies strategically implemented to support the safety profile of tofacitinib during the entire product lifecycle from pre-approval to post-approval activities?

*Approach*
- *Pre-approval epidemiological strategy* consisted of several distinct but complementary efforts for risk characterization for

**Case Example 6.2    (Continued)**

tofacitinib, including literature reviews, meta-analyses, and a standing cohort within a US-based registry of patients with RA. Indirect comparative methods via external patient cohorts were also used to provide evidence of expected adverse event rates, while taking into account key potential differences in the populations. The output of the analyses were used to assess the rates of identified and potential risks of interest in the tofacitinib clinical program compared with those from cohorts of RA patients treated with biologic disease modifying antirheumatic drugs (bDMARDs).

- *Post-approval epidemiology strategy* consisted of several approaches including (i) safety studies to characterize the safety of tofacitinib within the real-world or clinical practice setting, (ii) surveillance program is to evaluate any excess risk in the occurrence of known or potential adverse events, after accounting for confounding factors including disease severity and concomitant therapy, and (iii) risk mitigation activities.
  - In the US, two observational post-approval safety studies were initiated: (i) an active surveillance study within the Corrona RA registry, and (ii) a pregnancy outcome study within the Organization of Teratology Information Specialists Registry (OTIS) registry as a condition for approval of tofacitinib.
  - In the EU, four 5-year surveillance studies embedded within existing registries (ARTIS, BIOBADASER, BSRBR, and RABBIT) were proposed as a commitment to EMA to assess the safety of tofacitinib.
  - The US REMS for tofacitinib consisted of a Medication Guide, a communication plan, and a timetable for the submission of the REMS assessment (i.e. surveys at 18 months, 3 years, and 7 years). The EU aRMMs were implemented within the EU as a condition of approval within the EU consisting of an educational program intended to enhance the communication of the risks and risk minimization practices to patients and health care professionals (HCP).

*Results*

- *Pre-approval epidemiology strategy:* The data from pre-approval epidemiological analyses were articulated within regulatory documents including the NDA for FDA and the briefing document (i.e. summary of clinical safety (SCS), clinical overview (CO), etc.) for EMA and also presented at the FDA Advisory Committee Meeting for tofacitinib in May 2012. The collective body of evidence (including interim data from the US-based registry study) provided substantial additional context to rates of selected adverse events observed in the tofacitinib clinical trial program, and therefore addressed the uncertainties related to the potential risks previously expressed by the EMA.
- Tofacitinib was approved in the US in November 2012 and in the EU in March 2017.
- *Post-approval epidemiology strategy:* Several regulatory commitments, including post-approval safety studies, ongoing pharmacovigilance (i.e. spontaneous reports), and REMS and aRMM related work served to address regulatory concerns regarding drug safety among US and European patients receiving care in the real-world.
  - In the US, the FDA deemed the 18-month REMS epidemiological assessment adequate, citing that the survey data demonstrated that patients understood the

*(Continued)*

**Case Example 6.2    (Continued)**

risks associated with therapy and determined that maintaining the Medication Guide as part of the approved labeling was sufficient to address safety-related concerns.

o In the EU, the elements of the aRMM included Xeljanz HCP Brochure, Xeljanz HCP Treatment Initiation Checklist, Xeljanz HCP Treatment Maintenance Checklist, an educational website, and Xeljanz Patient Alert Card.

*Strengths*

- Data from multiple sources (i.e. observational studies, RCTs with other agents, and cohorts of patients stratified by RCT inclusion/exclusion criteria) were used to provide indirect comparisons, drawing from the strengths of each data source while balancing their weaknesses.
- Epidemiological evidence from the entire lifecycle of tofacitinib allowed regulatory agencies in the US and EU to assess and ensure the safety of the product.

*Limitations*

- All data sources have unique limitations. Limitations in clinical trials and spontaneous reports can be addressed, in part, by the proper use of observational epidemiology.

- Purely observational epidemiologic studies may not always be the most appropriate method of evaluating safety signals or comparing the safety profile of different medications, especially when there are concerns of confounding by indication.

*Key Points*

- Pre-approval epidemiology strategy complements safety data from preclinical and clinical studies and provides a context for signals arising from clinical trials.
- Post-approval epidemiology strategies may require industry epidemiologists to address regulatory-mandated post-approval commitments, such as epidemiology studies, active surveillance studies, registries, REMS/aRMM evaluations, and PIP observational studies or address post-approval safety signals arising from clinical trial extension data, spontaneous reports, published case series, or signal detection from electronic healthcare data.
- To support drug safety evaluations, epidemiologic strategies must initiate early in development, continue throughout the lifecycle of the drug, evolve as new safety information becomes available, and may require innovative methods specific to the disease area.

## The View from Regulatory Agencies

**Note**

The views expressed herein are those of the authors, and not necessarily of the US FDA, the MHRA, or the Japanese PMDA.

**Introduction**

The regulation of pharmaceuticals aims at ensuring that the public has access to

medicines that are effective, acceptably safe, and of high quality. A wide range of regulatory activities spans the entire lifecycle of a medicine, involving laboratory-based understanding of pharmacological action, animal testing, providing scientific and regulatory input to drug development programs, protection of human subjects during clinical trials, assuring the integrity of the manufacturing process, reviewing the dossier to support product approval or licensure, monitoring the safety of medicines after they enter the market, and many other activities. These regulatory activities are firmly rooted in science, have a strong public health focus, and are executed within a legal and regulatory framework.

## Assessing the Need for Medicines

Pharmacoepidemiology, along with other areas of medical epidemiology, can be used in drug development long before a medicine is licensed or even tested in humans. Pharmacoepidemiologic approaches can be used to examine patterns of utilization of existing disease treatments in order to identify and characterize disease populations and subpopulations for which unmet medical needs exist. In some cases, no available therapies may exist. In other cases, available therapy may be ineffective for or poorly tolerated by certain patients. In these cases, pharmacoepidemiologic approaches can be used to characterize the patients who experience a suboptimal response to the medicine, thus defining the target population for a drug development program. For example, population-based databases can be used to characterize the frequency and distribution of characteristics of patients with a specific disease, so that relevant populations can be included in the developmental clinical trials. Healthcare databases can be used to estimate the frequency of co-morbid conditions in the setting of the specific underlying disease to be treated, so that relevant background rates can be derived to place potential adverse events that arise during development in context. This is especially useful for clinical events that are seen more frequently in patients with the disease for which the new treatment is being tested, but which could also represent an adverse drug reaction. This situation, known as confounding by indication, is a well-known methodological problem in observational pharmacoepidemiologic studies, but can also complicate the interpretation of adverse events in clinical trials, especially if the trial is not designed or powered to analyze these events. In these situations, careful understanding of background rates can be important.

## Orphan Drugs

In the last decade, there has been substantial activity and progress in the development of drugs for rare diseases. Orphan drug programs are designed to provide incentives to pharmaceutical manufacturers who develop medicines for rare conditions, known as "orphan drugs." In the United States, an orphan drug designation is given to a drug or biologic that has shown promise as a therapy intended to treat a disease affecting fewer than 200000 persons in the United States. In Japan, orphan designation is granted for drugs or medical devices if they are intended for use in less than 50000 patients in Japan and for which there is a high medical need. In the European Union, a prevalence rate of five per 10000 persons in the EU is used. When all rare diseases are taken together, their public health impact is significant; approximately 25 million people in North America are affected by these diseases.

Medical epidemiology is central to the designation of a product as an orphan drug product, as determination of prevalence is the basis for such designation. Data sources for determining prevalence can include administrative healthcare databases, electronic medical record systems, registries, and surveys. In many cases, combining data from multiple sources will be necessary. In most cases, data from these sources, even when combined, will not cover the entire jurisdiction for which the orphan designation applies. Thus, some form of extrapolation must be performed to determine if the relevant population prevalence has been exceeded. Most orphan drug designations are for diseases or conditions whose prevalence is much lower than the 200000 prevalence threshold in the United States. A review of 25 years' experience with the orphan drug program in the United States covering 1892 orphan designations found that the median prevalence was 39000; the most common patient prevalence was 10 000 or fewer patients, with relatively few prevalence rates near the 200 000 threshold. For estimates of population prevalence near the threshold, care must be taken to ensure that the most rigorous methods have been used to estimate the population prevalence of a rare disease. The closer the estimated prevalence is to the threshold, the greater the precision needed to characterize the prevalence.

## Planning Drug Development Programs

Despite the availability of an increasing number of medicines, there remain a substantial number of unmet medical needs. Advances in understanding the molecular pathogenesis of cancers, rare diseases, and infectious diseases have led to a rapid rise in the number of drug development programs targeting these conditions. At the same time, the aging population across the globe has led to a need for improved treatments for widespread diseases such as diabetes, hypertension, ischemic heart disease, chronic obstructive pulmonary disease, Alzheimer disease, other neurodegenerative disorders, and many others. The continuing emergence of antibacterial resistance and the threat of new viral illnesses prompt the need for new antimicrobial agents. Infections with *Mycobacteria tuberculosis*, *Plasmodium falciparum*, human immunodeficiency virus, endemic parasitic diseases, and other agents contribute substantially to the global burden of disease and require new treatments.

Regulatory agencies have responded to this demand with a variety of regulatory programs and pathways designed to promote efficient development of medicines and to reduce drug development time so that these unfulfilled medical needs can be met. Some of these programs seek to optimize drug development by providing timely consultation between the regulator and the company developing a drug to clarify scientific requirements; other programs allow clinical development to be shortened by allowing the use of surrogate markers rather than clinical markers. Examples of programs to optimize drug develop include breakthrough therapy designation in the United States, the PRIME (PRIority MEdicines) initiative in the European Union, and the *SAKIGAKE* review program in Japan. "*SAKIGAKE*" is a Japanese word meaning "frontrunner" or "pioneer." In each of these situations, pharmacoepidemiologic analyses can aid in the comparison of new treatments to existing treatments, especially when data on existing treatments are derived from clinical experience and not from formal clinical trials.

The goal of a drug development program is to demonstrate that a medicine has a beneficial and meaningful effect on a clinically important outcome, generally a measure of how the patient feels, functions, or survives. Clinical trials whose primary endpoint is a direct measure of a clinically important outcome may be very long and delay access by patients to effective therapies. To allow patient access as rapidly as is feasible, and to assure that definitive evidence of effectiveness is obtained, an alternative approach allows marketing approval for a new drug product on the basis of adequate and well-controlled clinical trials establishing that the drug product has a beneficial effect on a surrogate endpoint. A surrogate endpoint is an outcome measure that is used in place of a direct measure of a clinically meaningful outcome when the effect of treatment on the surrogate endpoint is expected to reflect changes in the clinically meaningful outcome. In the context of drug development, a validated surrogate endpoint is one for which evidence exists that the effect of treatment on the surrogate endpoint predicts the effect of treatment on the clinical outcome of interest. For example, systolic blood pressure is used as a surrogate endpoint in clinical trials of antihypertensive agents because it predicts the risk of occurrence of stroke. Similarly, human immunodeficiency virus viral load is used as a surrogate endpoint in clinical trials of antiretroviral agents because it predicts the development of an acquired immunodeficiency syndrome diagnosis. The use of validated surrogate markers to support approval of medicines is widely employed.

There are, however, many serious and life-threatening conditions for which there are no validated surrogate markers, yet there is still an urgent need to bring effective therapies to patients in a timely way. For this latter situation, the concept of "accelerated approval" has been developed. Under this framework, the US FDA may grant approval to a medicine intended to treat a serious or life-threatening disease based on an unvalidated surrogate endpoint that is reasonably likely, based on epidemiologic, therapeutic, pathophysiologic, or other evidence, to predict clinical benefit on the basis of an effect on a clinical endpoint other than survival or irreversible morbidity. In these cases, postmarketing studies must be conducted to demonstrate the actual clinical benefit of the medicine.

A key regulatory tool in the EU to fulfill unmet medical needs is the conditional marketing authorization, which has reduced data requirements linked to a one-year time-limited authorization where the authorization's renewal is linked to further data submission. Under the applicable regulations, manufacturers must study the drug further once it is approved, to verify and describe its clinical benefit, where there is uncertainty as to the relationship of the surrogate endpoint to clinical benefit, or of the observed clinical benefit to ultimate outcome. At the time of approval, postmarketing studies would usually already be underway.

In Japan, the Pharmaceuticals, Medical Devices and Other Therapeutics Products Act ("PMD Act") established a system of conditional and time-limited approval for regenerative medicines based on probable benefit from early clinical trials. After obtaining such an approval, the marketing authorization holder is required to submit a standard marketing application with additional data on safety and efficacy. Similarly, since 2017 a conditional early approval program has applied to drugs offering high efficacy and clinical usefulness in the treatment of serious diseases, drugs for which conducting confirmatory studies is impracticable, and other designated drugs. One prerequisite for approval will be a commitment to complete postmarketing studies as necessary in order to reconfirm product safety and efficacy.

Understanding the relationship between a surrogate endpoint and a clinically relevant endpoint, as well as validation of the surrogate endpoint, are opportunities for pharmacoepidemiologists to contribute to drug development. Pharmacoepidemiologists can use principles of epidemiology to distinguish simple correlation between a potential endpoint and a clinically meaningful outcome, on the one hand, from a true surrogate marker. For example, a marker of disease status used in natural history studies may not be an adequate surrogate endpoint in a clinical trial because it is not related to the disease mechanisms that give rise to symptoms, morbidity, and mortality.

## Pre-approval Review of Clinical Safety Data

While the traditional role of pharmacoepidemiology, from a regulatory standpoint, has been the assessment of the safety of medicines in the post-licensing period, pharmacoepidemiology can play an important role during the pre-licensing review of safety data. The limitations of pre-licensing clinical trials in defining the full scope of adverse drug reactions are mainly related to the fact that clinical trials are relatively small in size, compared to the population of patients that will ultimately take the medicine once it is marketed. Patients who participate in clinical trials may have fewer comorbidities and take fewer concomitant medications than those treated in actual practice. Pre-licensing clinical trials generally provide relatively little data, or no data at all, in certain populations such as children, the elderly, and pregnant women, or at-risk groups such as immunosuppressed patients. These groups, however, are treated with the medicines in the course of clinical practice once the medicine is licensed.

The analytic methods of clinical trials are best suited for data arising from randomized, controlled, comparative trials. Many clinical trials of medicines intended for chronic or long-term use, including those trials in pre-approval drug development programs, may have single-arm, open-label extensions after participants have completed the randomized portion of the trial. For data generated from this portion of the clinical trial, the techniques of observational pharmacoepidemiology may be appropriate. In addition to tallying the frequencies of specific adverse events, data from long-term extension studies can be examined to characterize patterns of adverse event onset over time. If appropriate, analyses based on person-time can be performed. In this setting, the interpretations of adverse events must take into account the prior treatment received during the randomized portion of the trial, the duration of treatment, the underlying frequency of medical outcomes in the population with the disease being treated, and other factors. Pharmacoepidemiology can inform this approach.

## Planning for Post-approval Studies

At the time a medicine is approved, there are uncertainties and unknowns regarding the safety profile of the medicine. In many cases, the nature of the safety issues that will unfold post-approval cannot be predicted at the time the product is brought to market. In some cases, however, a careful review of the clinical data at the time of approval can lead to a proactive approach to obtaining more safety information.

Pharmacoepidemiology can play an important role in several specific situations. First, drug development programs based on the use of unvalidated surrogate markers, as described above, generally require postmarketing studies to demonstrate definitively the clinical

effectiveness of the product. In these situations, pharmacoepidemiologists can be involved in studies assessing the validity of the surrogate marker.

Second, pharmacoepidemiologists can be involved in the design and interpretation of postmarketing studies designed to assess the impact of new formulations of medicines developed to have a more favorable safety profile than earlier versions.

Third, pharmacoepidemiologists can be involved in planning postmarketing studies when safety signals are detected prior to approval.

## Monitoring Post-approval Safety

For the regulator, the postmarketing assessment of the safety of medicines involves both a proactive approach and, of necessity, a reactive approach. The International Council for Harmonisation of Technical Requirements for Pharmaceuticals for Human Use (ICH) has developed a useful and practical framework that summarizes the known safety issues of a product and can form the basis of ongoing monitoring and, as needed, specific studies. The ICH framework characterizes important identified risks, important potential risks, and important missing information. This framework allows pharmacoepidemiologists and others to devise proactive strategies to design observational studies or clinical trials to address unanswered questions about the safety profile of a medicine. The identification of knowledge gaps can occur at any time in the life cycle of a medicine, and can be based on data from clinical trials or observational studies of the medicine, or safety findings from other medicines in the same class. In these cases, careful review of the available data can allow the regulator, often working with the developer, to develop a thoughtful and rational approach to drug safety issues in the post-approval period.

Reactive approaches are also needed in regulatory pharmacoepidemiology because the adverse effects of medicine can become recognized at any time, sometimes many years, after approval. Because not all drug safety issues can be predicted, regulators continue to need reactive approaches. These approaches require the efficient review of the existing data, careful and timely assessment of the need for immediate or near-term regulatory action, and interaction with the product's manufacturer to plan further study. Reactive approaches become necessary, for example, when new safety issues are identified from spontaneously reported suspected adverse drug reactions, when drug safety findings are published by independent groups, and when events such as manufacturing-related product recalls result in a large number of adverse event reports that need to be reviewed in a short period of time. From the regulator's point of view, the scientific studies that form the basis of regulatory actions must be as sound and robust as possible.

## Assessing Actual Use Patterns of a Medicine

Regulators are interested not only in whether a medicine meets the relevant regulatory standards for approval, but also in how a medicine is actually used in clinical practice. Because the harms of medicines can result not only from their intrinsic pharmacological properties but also from how they are used, or misused, in actual practice, understanding the actual usage allows regulators to assess the degree to which the medicine is used in ways that are consistent with the safe use of the medicine as described in the label or marketing authorization. To do so, regulators can use a variety of pharmacoepidemiologic techniques, including administrative claims data, electronic medical records, or other public health databases.

## Assessing Impact of Regulatory Actions

Because of its public health focus, drug regulation must ensure that its actions lead to the intended public health outcomes. For serious safety issues, it is not enough simply to add a warning to a product label. Such an action is in itself an intervention, and it is thus important to understand its impact. Recognizing the fundamental importance of the need for such assessments, the Pharmacovigilance Risk Assessment Committee of the EMA developed a formal strategy to measure the impact of pharmacovigilance activities. The strategy is aimed both at informing the review of individual medicines that have been the subject of major risk minimization efforts and at determining which activities are successful and which are not, in order to optimize the pharmacovigilance system. Pharmacoepidemiology is critical to this endeavor, as it can relate regulatory activities to the outcomes which those activities are intended to impact. Pharmacoepidemiologic thinking and methodologies underpin the EMA strategy.

One domain of assessment of the impact of regulatory activities is an understanding of the effectiveness of regulatory agencies' communications about the risks of medicines. A study that examined the extent to which patients understand important information about a serious risk of a medicine that they are taking examined the results of patient-directed knowledge surveys for 66 medicines for which patients were supposed to have received a Medication Guide, a type of patient-directed labeling. For each Medication Guide, acceptable knowledge defined was 80% or more of patients correctly answering questions about the medicine's primary risk. The study found that only 20 Medication Guides (30.3%) met the 80% threshold, a finding that underscores the need for improved patient-directed information.

Analysis of the impact of regulatory actions is not limited to the assessment of actions related to individual medicines. Rather, it can look broadly at how the functioning of a drug regulatory system contributes to the system's public health mission. Because of the rapidly changing and expanding data that inform pharmacoepidemiologic studies, studies that examine overall performance are important because they can lead to system-wide improvements.

## Advancing the Science of Pharmacoepidemiology

Pharmacoepidemiology is a complex, dynamic, and changing field. It relies on the integration of epidemiology, clinical pharmacology, pharmacy, medicine, statistics, and other disciplines, for its full execution. Increasingly, the rapid advances in the availability of large, diverse, and relevant datasets have made informatics an important contributing discipline to pharmacoepidemiologic efforts. Acquiring expertise in pharmacoepidemiology thus requires an environment that provides access to experts in all the relevant disciplines. Furthermore, this discipline relies on population-based healthcare data and thus an understanding of the healthcare system in which the data were generated, which experts in the above fields may not have. As more and more drug safety questions arise that require expertise in pharmacoepidemiology as well as appropriate data, it is crucial that there be sufficient capacity, both in the form of well-trained pharmacoepidemiologists and in the availability of systems, such as networks that combine relevant data with scientific expertise, that can be used for pharmacoepidemiologic studies. Because pharmacoepidemiology is a multidisciplinary effort, there must also be appropriate mechanisms for collaboration. Regulatory agencies play a role in facilitating the reaching of these goals.

To strengthen the monitoring of marketed medicines, as noted above, EMA developed ENCePP, a network of centers with the capacity to perform post-authorization studies focusing on safety and benefit–risk.

In Japan, PMDA launched the Medical Information Database NETwork (MID-NET®) that is a distributed database compiling electronic medical records, insurance claims data, and DPC-compatible inpatient care data under a common data model. The use of the MID-NET® system will be opened to relevant members of industry and academic researchers for use in pharmacoepidemiologic studies.

FDA's Sentinel Initiative, as noted earlier, has created a linked system of electronic healthcare databases to investigate safety questions about FDA-regulated medical products, which was developed after FDA sought extensive stakeholder input as it worked with outside organizations to develop Sentinel to address important issues of governance, privacy, data standards, and public disclosure of results.

Pharmacoepidemiologic efforts such as ENCePP, MID-NET®, and Sentinel all make use of various traditional sources of healthcare data derived from existing sources that reflect current clinical practice and actual patient experiences. While these contemporary systems often rely on large datasets and, at times, integration of datasets through networks, it is important to note that pharmacoepidemiologic research has a decades-long tradition of using observational data recorded at the point of care to describe the effects of medicines in populations, though the scope of this work has largely focused on safety issues. The emergence in recent years of additional digital health-related data, such as data generated from wearable devices and health-related applications, has given rise to the notion that the expanding variety of electronic healthcare data can be used to study the effects of medicines beyond those related to safety. As methods to develop real-world evidence move forward, pharmacoepidemiologists, including those in regulatory agencies, will have an important and growing role to play, particularly in supporting timely and robust public health decisions.

## Conclusion

Pharmacoepidemiology is an essential discipline in the activities of a drug regulatory agency and is used throughout the lifecycle of a product. Clear, robust, and transparent methods of integrating data from multiple sources to arrive at sound, evidence-based conclusions are critically important. Methodologic advances in the field are needed to analyze the increasingly wide range of large data sources. These efforts depend on collaborations among regulatory agencies, academia, industry, and other stakeholders.

## Summary Points for the View from Regulatory Agencies

- Drug regulation has a public-health focus, is based in science, and is executed in the context of applicable laws and regulations.
- Pharmacoepidemiology plays an important role in drug regulation.
- Pharmacoepidemiology is important across the lifecycle of a medicine.
- Synthesis of data from multiple sources is critical for sound regulatory decisions.
- Advancing the science of pharmacoepidemiology is essential.

---

### Case Example 6.3

The view from regulatory agencies: Duration of the use of metoclopramide (Kaplan S., Staffa, J.A., Dal Pan, G.J. 2007).

*Background*
The use of long-term treatment with metoclopramide is a known risk factor for tardive dyskinesia. The product label in the United States recommended a treatment duration of no longer than 12 weeks.

*Issue*
The extent of use beyond the recommended 12 weeks of treatment had not been quantified.

*Approach*
Prescription claims data were used to estimate duration of therapy and the extent of therapy beyond the maximum time period of 12 weeks evaluated in the clinical trials and recommended in the label.

*Results*
During the study period, almost 80% of approximately 200 000 persons who had received a prescription for metoclopramide had only one episode of therapy. The length of the longest episode for most patients (85%) varied from 1 to 90 days, yet 15% of the patients appeared to have received prescriptions for metoclopramide for a period longer than 90 days. Cumulative therapy for longer than 90 days was recorded for almost 20% of the patients. These data indicate that a substantial percentage of patients were taking metoclopramide for longer than the recommended duration of treatment. The manufacturer was subsequently required to add an additional warning to the product's label, cautioning against prolonged use.

*Strengths*
The data were drawn from a reasonably large population.

*Limitations*
The data did not include information on diagnoses, so the outcome of tardive dyskinesia could not be ascertained.

*Key Points*
- Drug safety problems can emerge not only from problematic drugs, but problematic drug use
- Studies of the appropriateness of drug use in populations can identify poor drug use and lead to regulatory intervention

## The View from the Legal System

### Introduction

Pharmacoepidemiologists in their daily work encounter many different aspects of the law. Three of the most important intersections of pharmacoepidemiology and the law involve product liability law, contract law, and intellectual property law. The basic legal rules in these subject areas, and practical and ethical implications for pharmacoepidemiology, will be discussed in turn.

### Tort Law and Product Liability Lawsuits

Individuals harmed by a drug may seek damages from its manufacturer. A basic understanding of product liability law is essential for pharmacoepidemiologists, even for those who might never find themselves in a courtroom, because such lawsuits also exert substantial influence on the field itself. Tort litigation brought by government agencies and individual patients can help uncover previously unavailable data on adverse effects, questionable practices by manufacturers, and flaws in drug regulatory systems.

#### The Legal Theory of Product Liability

Product liability law is a variation of tort law that covers the principles under which consumers harmed by products sold in interstate commerce may seek redress for their injuries. Originally, consumers were required to prove four elements to make out a claim for negligence against manufacturers for creating a dangerous product: (i) that defendants had a duty to exercise reasonable care, (ii) that defendants' conduct diverged from customary practices that would be followed by other manufacturers or members of the industry, (iii) that there was a causal link between the defendants' lack of care and the outcome at issue, and (iv) that the preceding three factors led to damages.

However, some products contained a high enough inherent risk of harm that courts decided they should be held to a different legal standard. Starting in the early 1960s, judges started applying the theory of strict liability to certain product liability cases, which merely requires demonstration that the dangerous product caused the injury. As distinguished from negligence, the question of whether the defendants followed customary practices or exercised reasonable precautions is moot. For example, the product could have a "manufacturing defect," meaning that the product did not comply with the manufacturer's own standards, or a "design defect," meaning that the product was designed in a way that conferred inherently unreasonable risk for the consumer. However, courts also generally agreed that if the manufacturer of a dangerous product adequately warned about the known risks of its product, those warnings were sufficient to insulate the manufacturer from liability. Thus, strict product liability also allowed plaintiffs to bring causes of action against manufacturers based on a third principle: a "warning defect" (also called a "failure to warn").

In the pharmaceutical field, product liability cases alleging a manufacturing defect are rare, in part because of strict regulatory oversight of drug manufacturing plants. Also, cases based on a design defect theory are also difficult to win because most courts agree that all prescription drugs have some inherent risks that must be weighed against their substantial benefits. Rather, the most common bases for litigation over pharmaceutical products are warning defects about the adverse event at issue. The ultimate disposition of failure to warn cases turns on the question of whether the warning is reasonable.

#### Failure-to-Warn Claims

A failure-to-warn product liability action includes three main contentions: knowledge of the drug risk by the manufacturer, improper warning of the drug risk, and causation of damages.

## Knowledge

The plaintiff must demonstrate that a pharmaceutical manufacturer knew, or should have known, of the risk. A manufacturer of a pharmaceutical product cannot generally be held accountable for risks about which it could not have known. For example, in one case, a plaintiff brought a lawsuit claiming that her oral contraceptive medication led to her having a cerebrovascular accident. The jury found that the particular risk the plaintiff claimed could not have been known at the time the drug was prescribed, based in part on the testimony of the expert pharmacoepidemiologist who reported that "new techniques to measure these clotting effects had not then been developed" at the time of the injury. According to the court, "The warnings contained in the package inserts were adequate or that the statements contained therein were a fair representation of the medical and scientific knowledge available at the time the drug was taken by the plaintiff."

Knowledge can be actual or constructive. *Actual knowledge* is defined as literal awareness. Actual knowledge can be demonstrated by showing that the manufacturer was cognizant of reasonable information suggesting a particular risk that it did not pass on to consumers. In the case of selective serotonin reuptake inhibitors (SSRIs), used to treat depression, various manufacturers were found to have conducted clinical trials that showed an increased risk of suicidal ideation in adolescent patients taking the drug. Plaintiffs brought lawsuits charging that these findings were delayed for lengthy periods of time, not released, or the concerns not fairly represented.

*Constructive knowledge* is sometimes called "legal knowledge," because it is knowledge that the law assumes should be present, even if it is not. This knowledge could have been acquired by the exercise of reasonable care. For example, the cholesterol-lowering drug cerivastatin (Baycol) was removed from the market in 2001 after it was linked to cases of rhabdomyolysis, a potentially fatal kidney disease. The manufacturer, Bayer, was found to possess several reports from as early as 1999 suggesting a 10-fold risk of rhabdomyolysis relative to other medications in its class, but it allegedly did not process these reports and pass them along to patients or regulators. In some lawsuits, Bayer was charged with having constructive knowledge of these concerns by 1999, because the company should have processed the reports and acted on them by that time. A common legal standard used in these situations is what a reasonably prudent company with expertise in this area would have done.

## Warning

If a manufacturer has the duty to provide a warning about adverse events associated with its product, then the next question is whether an adequate warning was provided. A proper warning is relevant, timely, and accurate. For example, a relevant warning about an adverse effect is commensurate with the scope and extent of dangers associated with the drug. Warnings must not be subject to undue delay. A manufacturer must keep up with emerging scientific data and patient reports, and warn of new side effects discovered after initial approval. In the case of rosiglitazone (Avandia), a 2007 meta-analysis linked the drug to life-threatening cardiovascular adverse events. However, after a review of internal company documents, a US Senate Finance Committee report suggested that the manufacturer knew about these risks but delayed publicly warning about them and sought to limit their dissemination. Thus, a primary question in lawsuits arising from use of rosiglitazone is whether these tactics inappropriately delayed reasonable warnings about the adverse effect. Finally, warnings must be of appropriately urgent tone. In the case of rofecoxib (Vioxx), lawsuits alleged that the warning was insufficiently urgent because the risk of cardiovascular events was described in vague terms and placed in the less prominent "precautions" section of the label.

The plaintiff must also demonstrate that the inadequate warnings about the adverse effect were relevant to the plaintiff's receiving the drug. If a defendant can demonstrate that even an adequate warning would have made no difference in the decision to prescribe the drug, or to monitor the patient postprescription, the case may be dismissed for lack of a proximate cause.

According to the "learned intermediary" rule, pharmaceutical manufacturers fulfill their duties to warn by providing accurate and adequate warnings to prescribing physicians. If the manufacturer imparts an appropriate warning that physicians can sufficiently grasp, then the manufacturer can be insulated from liability. Therefore, warnings do not have to be offered about risks that should be obvious or are generally known to skilled medical practitioners. However, when the information given to physicians omits, underemphasizes, misstates, or obfuscates dangers, this deficiency is legally transferred to the patient, who maintains a right of redress against the manufacturer if those dangers materialize and cause injury.

In some special situations, pharmaceutical manufacturers may lose the ability to invoke the learned intermediary defense. If a manufacturer markets its product very aggressively and without sufficient attention to certain risks, courts may rule that it has essentially undone the physician-patient prescribing relationship. Direct-to-consumer advertising (DTCA) is one modality that can undercut the assumption that patients are largely ignorant of prescription drug risks and manufacturers lack means of interacting with patients other than through physicians. The New Jersey Supreme Court has ruled that DTCA created a limited exception to the learned intermediary defense, and in 2007 the West Virginia Supreme Court rejected the learned intermediary defense in its entirety on this basis. Nonetheless, in most jurisdictions, the learned intermediary rule still stands.

### Causation

Legal causation usually requires a clear causal chain from event to outcome, in an individual.

The legal standard for causation is therefore challenged by product liability cases, in which probabilistic evidence links drugs to injuries. Courts struggle with the question of legal causation in these cases on two distinct levels: general and specific causation.

*General causation* addresses whether a product is capable of causing a particular injury in the population of patients like the plaintiff. The basic common law standard to prove general causation is that a particular product "more likely than not" caused the damages. Some courts have held that legal causation must be demonstrated by more than an association and a mere possibility of causation, even though causal hypotheses based on such considerations are common in the scientific literature. A few courts have even gone further and defined "more likely than not" as having a relative risk of greater than 2.0, no matter how tight the confidence intervals are around a statistically significant finding of association between 1.0 and 2.0. Presumably this is based on the calculation of attributable risk in the exposed group exceeding 50%, when the relative risk exceeds 2.0. This standard has been replicated in the Federal Judicial Center's "Reference Manual on Scientific Evidence" and employed in some cases to exclude epidemiologic evidence with weaker associations.

However, all courts do not adhere rigidly to the relative risk = 2.0 rule for general causation. Both clinical trials and epidemiologic studies of the product at issue can establish general causation between a pharmaceutical product and an outcome. Animal studies, meta-analyses, case reports/case series, and secondary source materials (such as internal company documents) have also been used in court to help support establishing a causal link. Since pharmacoepidemiologic studies tend to assess the presence of an association, rather than directly addressing causation, courts sometimes apply the Bradford Hill criteria to build the bridge between an association and general causation (see Table 6.1).

To demonstrate *specific causation*, a plaintiff must show that the product in question caused

**Table 6.1** Bradford Hill criteria.

1) Strength of association
2) Consistency and replication of findings
3) Specificity with respect to both the substance and injury at issue
4) Temporal relationship
5) Biological gradient and evidence of a dose–response relationship
6) Plausibility
7) Coherence
8) Experimental removal of exposure
9) Consideration of alternative explanation

the alleged injury in the individual plaintiff. In some cases, like instantaneous allergic reactions, the causal link is clear. For more subacute or later onset responses, however, specific causation may be hard to demonstrate. For example, in one case against Merck brought by a plaintiff who suffered a myocardial infarction shortly after starting rofecoxib, the manufacturer argued that the outcome was attributable to the plaintiff's prior existing coronary artery disease. The plaintiff countered with the fact that he was in a state of stable cardiovascular health prior to initiation of rofecoxib and that he simultaneously developed two coronary artery clots after the drug's initiation (a rare presentation for ischemic heart disease). While the trial court held for the plaintiff, the decision was reversed on appeal; the appeals court ruled, "although plaintiffs were not required to establish specific causation in terms of medical certainty, nor to conclusively exclude every other reasonable hypothesis, because [the plaintiff's] preexisting cardiovascular disease was another plausible cause of his death, the plaintiffs were required to offer evidence excluding that cause with *reasonable certainty*."

### Pharmacoepidemiologic Expertise and *Daubert*

In product liability cases, pharmacoepidemiologists serve as expert witness, helping explain data about drugs and determine whether risk information was acted upon appropriately. Experts usually describe the current state of knowledge about the adverse event at issue, and may analyze available data to present before the court.

As federal Circuit Court Judge Richard Posner has explained, "the courtroom is not the place for scientific guesswork, even of the inspired sort." Pharmacoepidemiologists seeking to present expert evidence in litigation will routinely face judicial inquiry to determine whether they are fit to serve in that role. Traditionally, the judge evaluated whether expert witnesses lack qualifications or espouse scientific theories out of step with accepted knowledge. In the 1993 case of *Daubert v. Merrell Dow*, the US Supreme Court outlined a number of markers for reviewing the appropriateness of expert witness testimony, including whether the theory was current and whether it had been tested or subjected to peer review and publication. A subsequent case applied these rules and further refined them in evaluating a debate over the admissibility of expert testimony suggesting that polychlorinated biphenyls (PCBs) can cause lung cancer. The research was excluded because the experts did not validate their conclusions – the epidemiologic studies did not report a statistically significant causal link between PCBs and lung cancer, lacked proper controls, and examined substances other than PCBs. In the US, some state courts have embraced the *Daubert* guidelines, which have also been taken up by revised Federal Rules of Evidence; others adhere to a more basic doctrine that excludes testimony containing theories that do not enjoy "general acceptance in the relevant scientific community."

### Intersection Between Drug Regulation and Product Liability Litigation

In most countries, when the government regulatory authority charged with overseeing sales of pharmaceutical products approves a drug for widespread use, the drug comes with an official drug labeling. The labeling presents a description of drug's efficacy, including the trials performed in the premarket period, as well as safety concerns that have emerged during this period of testing. In the US, the labeling is usually written by the manufacturer and approved by the FDA.

In the US, the label takes on particular legal significance. The FDA requires the manufacturer to mention important warnings that are in the official labeling when marketing its product, but does not require manufacturers to mention warnings that are not in the labeling. Recently, there has been controversy over the intersection between the drug label and product liability lawsuits. For example, in one case, a man was prescribed the antidepressant sertraline (Zoloft) and immediately started experiencing agitation, confusion, and suicidal thinking, ultimately leading him to take his own life one week later. The plaintiffs claimed that the manufacturer failed to warn appropriately about the risks of suicidal behaviors. The manufacturer contended that such a claim could not be brought because the FDA had not included such a warning in the official label. That is, the claim was "preempted" by the FDA's regulatory action. However, this view was overturned by the US Supreme Court in the seminal case of *Wyeth v. Levine*, which held, "It has remained a central premise of drug regulation that the manufacturer bears responsibility for the content of its label at all times." The brand-name drug manufacturer can therefore strengthen the label at its own discretion by adding warnings to it without first notifying the FDA and receiving approval to do so. Notably, if the FDA does review all the data surrounding a particular safety issue and makes a specific statement that a strong warning is not necessary, such an action can still preempt a failure-to-warn lawsuit. The Supreme Court has also held that the responsibility to proactively update the label does not extend to generic drug manufacturers, which only must have labels that match their brand-name counterparts.

Product liability law in Europe is in many ways similar to the US. A liability action arising under the controlling EU directive includes the following contentions: (i) defective product, (ii) causation of damage, and (iii) no exclusion of liability. A product is defective if it does not provide the safety that a person is entitled to expect, taking all circumstances in account, including the presentation of the product, the use reasonably expected of the product, and the time when the product was put into circulation. Because the product liability rule is a directive, member states retain some flexibility in implementing aspects of it, such as whether they permit compensation for non-economic damages (e.g. pain and suffering) or which manufacturer defenses they seek to incorporate. As a result of this flexibility, there is substantial diversity across EU countries in how product liability cases are adjudicated. Country-specific laws outside the EU set up similar legal regimes. Like in the US, most product liability lawsuits in EU and non-EU countries in Europe are based on failure-to-warn claims about the adverse event at issue, rather than design defects. One of the exclusions of liability, as in US, is the learned intermediary defense. However, while similar product liability rules apply in Europe, fewer cases are brought to court and damage compensation is lower.

## Pharmacoepidemiology and Contract Law

Many studies in the field of pharmacoepidemiology emerge from collaborations between individuals at different institutions. Cooperative work can allow more complex research to be performed and help advance the field of pharmacoepidemiology. One type of collaborative work of particular public health importance is contract research. Contract research is undertaken by an individual, academic, or nonprofit investigator supported by a sponsor (usually an industry or governmental agency). The contract classically represents the full outline of the agreement between the parties. In countless cases, contract research in pharmacoepidemiology has led to important public health findings and changes in health care delivery.

However, contract research may pose various potential concerns, generally centering around: (i) trial design, (ii) access to data and data analysis, and (iii) publication of results. Investigators should be wary of performing contract research in which the sponsor has the right to unduly influence the design of the trial. Many sponsors prefer to retain control of the data and insert their own statistical analyses. They argue that such efforts guard against "investigators [who] want to take the data beyond where the data should go," while investigators argue that this arrangement provides the company with an opportunity to "provide the spin on the data that favors them." Examples from both government and industry abound. In the case of rosiglitazone, a clinical trial organized by the manufacturer sought to compare the product against other treatment options for diabetes, and an independent academic steering committee was organized to oversee the data analysis. Company documents suggest that the clinical trial database was exclusively controlled by the company, which provided limited access to the investigators. When members of the steering committee questioned the presentation of the results, their concerns were largely overlooked.

There have also been numerous conflicts over so-called "gag clauses" that prevent contract investigators from publishing their ultimate results. For example, after a University of Toronto physician identified safety issues related to an experimental drug used to treat iron overload in transfusion-dependent patients with thalassemia, she was not granted permission to publish her results. When she ultimately exposed her findings, she was the subject of a breach of contract lawsuit from the sponsor on the basis that her research contract provided that the published work-product was "secret and confidential" and could not be disclosed except with the manufacturer's "prior written consent."

For researchers based in academic medical centers, institutional research administration offices usually handle the details of contract negotiation with research sponsors. However, surveys of academic medical centers have found that academic institutions routinely engage in industry-sponsored research without sufficient protection for investigators. For example, improper contracts can pass through such offices that allow contract provisions permitting the research sponsor to insert its own statistical analyses and draft the manuscript, while prohibiting investigators from sharing data with third parties after a trial had ended.

Whether or not they receive support from research administration offices, pharmacoepidemiologists must thoroughly evaluate contracts guiding research for inappropriate language regarding control of design of the trial, access to data, and reporting of results (see Table 6.2). Problematic language includes overly broad confidentiality clauses, clauses that define and assign ownership of intellectual property, and clauses that require approval from a sponsor prior to publication. It may be reasonable to allow sponsors a limited amount of time to review proposed publications for inadvertent release of proprietary company information or to contribute suggestions based on their expertise. However, researchers have an ethical obligation to ensure that contracts do not unreasonably delay the publication of potentially important results. Poorly written contracts can lead to inappropriate secrecy of results, which can have public health ramifications, as well as result in litigation against researcher.

## Pharmacoepidemiology and Intellectual Property Law

A patent is a formal grant of market exclusivity authorized by the federal government, lasting for 20 years. Patents can be issued for any process, machine, manufacture, or composition of matter. To be worthy of a patent, an innovation must be useful, novel, and

**Table 6.2** Potentially objectionable language in research contracts for pharmacoepidemiologists.

| Category | Contractual terms | Critique |
| --- | --- | --- |
| Control over investigator work product | "_____ shall provide confidential information to CONSULTANT for the purpose of conducting the CONSULTANT'S professional services. All information whether written or verbal provided by, or developed for _____, and all data collected during the performance of this Agreement is deemed to be the Confidential Information of _____." | Broad definition of "confidential information" seems to cover all information. Researcher's work product becomes sponsor's confidential information. |
| Gag clauses | "No information regarding this Agreement or the interest of _____ or Client in the subject matter hereof shall be disclosed to any third party without the prior written consent of _____" | Prevents disclosure of existence of the contract as a financial source in publication. |
| Opportunity to influence outcome | Client "shall not present or publish, nor submit for publication, any work resulting from the Services without _____ prior written approval." | Contract allows sponsor to quash publication unless it approves analyses. |

All examples adapted from actual contracts offered to engage in sponsored research.

nonobvious. These criteria ensure that patents cannot be awarded for inventions that already exist, or small improvements on those inventions that are obvious to a person of ordinary skill in the field.

A patent is classically thought of as a "quid pro quo" between inventors and society. The goal of a patent is to encourage inventors to invest in the development of their ideas, because it gives them a competition-free period in which to market a successful invention. At the same time, in filing for a patent, an inventor must fully disclose the content of the claimed invention in a patent document. The government provides its police power to protect an inventor's intellectual property for a set length of time and, in exchange, inventors make their inventions available to the public and fully describes it, so that others can use it and potentially improve on it in creating subsequent innovation.

Patents have become increasingly visible in the practice of pharmacoepidemiology. Most fall into the "process" category, such as methods of analyzing claims data and comparing outcomes to identify adverse events. In recent years, numerous patents have been obtained on methods and techniques used in pharma-

coepidemiology, including investigating characteristics of drug use and adverse events. The US Supreme Court has held that patentable processes may not include fundamental principles such as "laws of nature, natural phenomena, or abstract ideas," or purely mental process. By contrast, applications of laws of nature to a particular process may still be patentable. For example, a well-known case involved a patent over a method of curing synthetic rubber that used the Arrhenius Equation to calculate the optimal cure time. The process was found to be patentable because the formula was a part of a larger inventive process for curing rubber.

There are important ethical and legal concerns related to patenting processes that provide exclusive control over various aspects of the conduct of pharmacoepidemiology and pharmacovigilance research. In one case, an HIV researcher at Stanford has faced a patent-infringement lawsuit over a publicly-available database he created to help guide antiretroviral therapy based on the resistance characteristics of the disease, because searching this database may involve a similar process to one previously patented (but never implemented) by a for-profit company.

Recently, the US Supreme Court laid down a new, strict standard for patentability of processes, excluding those that simply describe a correlation or instruct people to "gather data from which they may draw an inference." A patentable process must involve an inventive and novel application of a law of nature beyond "well-understood, routine, conventional activity, previously engaged in by those in the field." One way to operationalize this definition is using the machine-or-transformation test. That is, a process is likely to be patentable if it can be tied to a particular machine or apparatus, or if it transforms an object into a different state or thing. Notably, as pertaining to pharmacoepidemiologic patents, gathering data may not constitute a "transformation" because every algorithm inherently requires the gathering of data inputs.

In Europe, the European Patent Convention (EPC) provides the legal framework under which patents are granted. Patent lengths are the same and US and European standards with regard to the patentability for methods and techniques are also close. There are three possible routes for obtaining patent protection in Europe. One can apply for a patent directly to the national patent office of a particular country (national patent); one can apply for a patent to the EPO and designate specific EU member states where patent protection is wanted ("classical" European patent); or – as part of a new pathway intended to start in 2018 – one can apply for a patent to the EPO with the designation of a unitary patent that will be applicable for all of the EU member states where the government has ratified the Agreement on a Unified Patent Court. Decisions about which pathway is appropriate are applicant-specific and could involve considerations such as the need for broad geographical coverage vs protection in one (or a few) Member States.

## Conclusion

Legal issues intersect with the practice of pharmacoepidemiology in a number of ways.

Pharmacoepidemiologists may be involved in product liability cases brought by individuals against drug manufacturers, either as expert witnesses or on the basis of academic work they undertake. These cases traditionally involve a claim of a failure to warn, which requires proof that the manufacturer knew of the safety issue, that any provided warnings were insufficient, and that the injury received was directly caused by use of the drug. Manufacturers can invoke a "learned intermediary" defense to deflect responsibility onto the treating physician. Pharmacoepidemiologists may also be involved in contract research, but should carefully consider contractual requirements related to ownership of the work product and withholding publication. Finally, pharmacoepidemiologists may decide to try to patent their research methods, but should weigh the risks and benefits of this form of intellectual property.

## Summary Points for the View from the Legal System

- Product liability is the term for the set of principles under which consumers harmed by products sold in interstate commerce seek redress for their injuries.
- A product liability case against a manufacturer alleging failure to warn about a drug risk includes three main contentions: (i) actual or constructive knowledge of the risk, (ii) lack of a warning, or a warning that is not relevant, timely, and accurate, and (iii) causation of damages.
- Product liability cases involve two types of causation: general causation, which addresses whether the product can cause the alleged injury in patients like the plaintiff, and specific causation, which addresses whether the product caused the alleged injury in the individual plaintiff. The standard for general causation is usually that the product "more likely than not" caused the damages, which some courts have interpreted as a relative risk of greater than 2.0. The Bradford Hill criteria

can build the bridge between an association and general causation.

- Pharmaceutical manufacturers can fulfill their duties to warn by providing accurate and adequate warnings to the prescribing physician (the "learned intermediary" defense). Warnings do not have to be offered about obvious risks or risks generally known to skilled medical practitioners.
- A regulatory authority's drug label represents its best judgment about risks that warrant disclosure and how to describe those risks. In the US, the drug label does not preempt manufacturers' responsibility to monitor emerging data about adverse effects and update the label as needed.
- Contract research is central to effective pharmacoepidemiologic collaborations but problematic contract terms include overly broad confidentiality clauses, clauses that define and assign ownership of intellectual property, and clauses that require approval from a sponsor prior to publication.
- Patents offer 20-year period of government-enforced market exclusivity for novel and nonobvious processes or products. A patentable process must involve an inventive and novel application of a natural law or correlation. For example, a natural correlation may be patentable if it can be tied to a particular machine, or if it can transform an object into a different state.
- Patented processes that provide exclusive control over the conduct of pharmacoepidemiology and pharmacovigilance research can hurt the public health if they prevent sharing of data or technologies necessary for research into drug outcomes and effects.

---

**Case Example 6.4**

The view from the legal system

*Background*
An inventor seeks to patent a method of using adverse event data regarding vaccine administration to inform subsequent health care delivery. The patent claims, "A method of determining whether an immunization schedule affects the incidence or severity of a chronic immune-mediated disorder in a treatment group of mammals, relative to a control group of mammals, which comprises immunizing mammals in the treatment group of mammals with one or more doses of one or more immunogens, according to said immunization schedule, and comparing the incidence, prevalence, frequency, or severity of said chronic immune-mediated disorder or the level of a marker of such a disorder, in the treatment group, with that in the control group." Patentable methods may not include fundamental principles such as "laws of nature, natural phenomena, or abstract ideas," or purely mental processes.

By contrast, applications of laws of nature to a particular process may still be patentable.

*Question*
Is the inventor's patent valid, or does it improperly claim a "natural law"?

*Approach*
The recent Supreme Court case of *Mayo Collaborative Services v. Prometheus Laboratories* holds that processes cannot be patentable if they restate a basic scientific discovery and then instruct physicians to gather data from which they may draw an inference. That is, a patentable method cannot amount to "nothing significantly more than an instruction to doctors to apply the applicable laws when treating their patients."

*Results*
Under the *Prometheus* reasoning, the method described above likely would not reach the level of a patentable invention. The inventor here has uncovered a potentially important correlation between immunization schedules

---

**Case Example 6.4    (Continued)**

and patient outcomes, but these natural correlations are not patentable by themselves.

*Strengths*
The *Prometheus* principle prevents patents from being issued on certain fundamental discoveries related to pharmacoepidemiology. Patents in this field that are sufficiently broad could prevent others from conducting necessary research into drug outcomes and effects.

*Limitations:*
- Excluding certain discoveries from the possibility of patenting has led some observers to worry about the implications for private investment. The prospect of

patents on new pharmacoepidemiologic methods and discoveries may be essential for recouping the costs of innovation.
- Government patent offices, which are often underfunded and understaffed, will now face the task of distinguishing the development and characterization of patentable methods from other methods that simply describe natural correlations.

*Key Points*
A patentable process needs to involve an inventive and novel application of a law of nature or natural correlation beyond "well-understood, routine, conventional activity, previously engaged in by those in the field."

---

# Further Reading

## The View from Academia

Avorn, J. and Soumerai, S.B. (1983). Improving drug-therapy decisions through educational outreach. A randomized controlled trial of academically based "detailing.". *N. Engl. J. Med.* 308: 1457–1463.

Avorn, J. (2005). *Powerful Medicines: The Benefits, Risks, and Costs of Prescription Drugs.* New York: Knopf.

Avorn, J. (2011). Teaching clinicians about drugs – 50 years later, whose job is it? *N. Engl. J. Med.* 364: 1185–1187.

O'Brien, M.A., Rogers, S., Jamtvedt, G. et al. (2007). Educational outreach visits: effects on professional practice and health care outcomes. *Cochrane Database Syst. Rev.* (4): CD000409. https://doi.org/10.1002/14651858. CD000409.pub2.

Choudhry, N.K., Avorn, J., Glynn, R.J. et al. (2011). Post-myocardial infarction free Rx event and economic evaluation (MI FREEE) trial. Full coverage for preventive medications after myocardial infarction. *N. Engl. J. Med.* 365: 2088–2097.

Clancy, C. and Collins, F.S. (2010). Patient-centered outcomes research institute: the intersection of science and health care. *Sci. Transl. Med.* 2: 37.

Cutrona, S.L., Choudhry, N.K., Stedman, M. et al. (2010). Physician effectiveness in interventions to improve cardiovascular medication adherence: a systematic review. *J. Gen. Intern. Med.* 25: 1090–1096.

Fischer, M.A. and Avorn, J. (2004). Economic implications of evidence-based prescribing for hypertension: can better care cost less? *JAMA* 291: 1850–1856.

Fischer, M.A., Choudhry, N.K., and Winkelmayer, W.C. (2007). Impact of Medicaid prior authorization on angiotensin-receptor blockers: can policy promote rational prescribing? *Health Aff. (Millwood)* 26: 800–807.

Fischer, M.A., Morris, C.A., Winkelmayer, W.C., and Avorn, J. (2007). Nononcologic use of human recombinant erythropoietin therapy in hospitalized patients. *Arch. Intern. Med.* 167: 840–846.

Fischer, M.A., Stedman, M.R., Lii, J. et al. (2010). Primary medication non-adherence: analysis of 195, 930 electronic prescriptions. *J. Gen. Intern. Med.* 25: 284–290.

Jackevicius, C.A., Li, P., and Tu, J.V. (2008a). Prevalence, predictors, and outcomes of primary nonadherence after acute myocardial infarction. *Circulation* 117: 1028–1036.

Jackevicius, C.A., Tu, J.V., Demers, V. et al. (2008b). Cardiovascular outcomes after a change in prescription policy for clopidogrel. *N. Engl. J. Med.* 359: 1802–1810.

Juurlink, D.N., Mamdani, M.M., Lee, D.S. et al. (2004). Rates of hyperkalemia after publication of the randomized Aldactone evaluation study. *N. Engl. J. Med.* 351: 543–551.

Shah, N.D., Montori, V.M., Krumholz, H.M. et al. (2010). Responding to an FDA warning – geographic variation in the use of rosiglitazone. *N. Engl. J. Med.* 363: 2081–2084.

Shrank, W.H., Hoang, T., Ettner, S.L. et al. (2006). The implications of choice: prescribing generic or preferred pharmaceuticals improves medication adherence for chronic conditions. *Arch. Intern. Med.* 166: 332–337.

Solomon, D.H., Finkelstein, J.S., Katz, J.N. et al. (2003). Underuse of osteoporosis medications in elderly patients with fractures. *Am. J. Med.* 115: 398–400.

Solomon, D.H., Van Houten, L., Glynn, R.J. et al. (2001). Academic detailing to improve use of broad-spectrum antibiotics at an academic medical center. *Arch. Intern. Med.* 161: 1897–1902.

## The View from Industry

AsPEN collaborators AM, Bergman, U., Choi, N.K. et al. (2013). The Asian Pharmacoepidemiology Network (AsPEN): promoting multinational collaboration for pharmacoepidemiologic research in Asia. *Pharmacoepidemiol. Drug Saf.* 22 (7): 700–704.

Berger, M.L., Sox, H., and Willke, R. (2017). Good practices for real-world data studies of treatment and/or comparative effectiveness: recommendations from the Joint ISPOR-ISPE Special Task Force on Real-World Evidence in Healthcare Decision-Making. *Pharmacoepidemiol. Drug Saf.* 26 (9): 1033–1039.

Coplan, P., Noel, R., Levitan, B. et al. (2011). Development of a framework for enhancing the transparency, reproducibility and communication of the benefit–risk balance of medicines. *Clin. Pharmacol. Ther.* 89: 312–315.

European Medicines Agency. Guideline on the Exposure to Medicinal Products During Pregnancy: Need for Post-Authorisation Data London: Committee for Medicinal Products for Human Use (CHMP); 2005. http://www.ema.europa.eu/docs/en_GB/document_library/Regulatory_and_procedural_guideline/2009/11/WC500011303.pdf.

European Medicines Agency, Committee for Medicinal Products for Human Use (CHMP). Guideline on risk assessment of medicinal products on human reproduction and lactation: From data to labelling. 2008.

The Rules Governing Medicinal Products in the European Union-Volume 9A.

European Medicines Agency. Guideline on good pharmacovigilance practices (GVP) Module V – Risk management systems (Rev 2). 2017a.

European Medicines Agency. Guideline on good pharmacovigilance practices (GVP). Module VIII – Post-authorisation safety studies (Rev 3). 2017b.

European Medicines Agency. Guideline on good pharmacovigilance practices (GVP). Module XVI – Risk minimisation measures: selection of tools and effectiveness indicators (Rev 2). 2017c.

European Network of Centres for Pharmacoepidemiology and Pharmacovigilance (ENCePP). Guide on Methodological Standards in Pharmacoepidemiology (Revision 6) 2017. http://www.encepp.eu/standards_and_guidances/documents/ENCePPGuideofMethStandardsinPE_Rev6.pdf.

Food and Drug Administration. Guidance for Industry Postmarketing Studies and Clinical Trials 2011. https://www.federalregister.gov/documents/2011/04/01/2011-7707/guidance-for-industry-on-postmarketing-studies-and-clinical-trials-implementation-of-section-505o3.

Food and Drug Administration. Guidance for Industry and FDA Staff: Best Practices for Conducting and Reporting Pharmacoepidemiologic Safety Studies Using Electronic Healthcare Data. 2013.

Food and Drug Administration. Guidance for industry: Establishing pregnancy exposure registries Rockville 2002. http://www.fda.gov/downloads/Drugs/GuidanceComplianceRegulatoryInformation/Guidances/ucm071639.pdf.

Food and Drug Administration. Draft Guidance for Industry: FDA's Application of Statutory Factors in Determining When a REMS Is Necessary. 2016.

Institute of Medicine (IOM). The Future of Drug Safety: Promoting and Protecting the Health of the Public 2006. http://www.iom.edu/Reports/2006/The-Future-of-Drug-Safety-Promoting-and-Protecting-the-Health-of-the-Public.aspx.

International Society for Pharmacoepidemiology (2008). Guidelines for good pharmacoepidemiology practices (GPP). *Pharmacoepidemiol. Drug Saf.* 17 (2): 200–208.

Ishiguro, C.T.Y., Uyama, Y., and Tawaragi, T. (2016). The MIHARI project: establishing a new framework for pharmacoepidemiological drug safety assessments by the Pharmaceuticals and Medical Devices Agency of Japan. *Pharmacoepidemiol. Drug Saf.* 25: 854–859.

Klungel, O.H., Kurz, X., de Groot, M.C.H. et al. (2016). Multi-centre, multi-database studies with common protocols: lessons learnt from the IMI PROTECT project. *Pharmacoepidemiol. Drug Saf.* 25 (Suppl 1): 156–165.

Mussen, F., Salek, S., and Walker, S. (2007). A quantitative approach to benefit–risk assessment of medicines – part 1: the development of a new model using multi-criteria decision analysis. *Pharmacoepidemiol. Drug Saf.* 16: S2–S15.

Nyeland, M.E.L.M. and Callréus, T. (2017). Evaluating the effectiveness of risk minimisation measures: the application of a conceptual framework to Danish real-world dabigatran data. *Pharmacoepidemiol. Drug Saf.* 26 (6): 607–614.

Platt, R., Wilson, M., Chan, K.A., et al. (2009). The new sentinel network--improving the evidence of medical-product safety. *N. Engl. J. Med.* 361 (7): 645–647.

Suissa, S., Henry, D., Caetano, P., et al. (2012). CNODES: the Canadian network for observational drug effect studies. *Open Med.* 6 (4): e134–e140.

Wang, S.V., Schneeweiss, S., and On behalf of the joint ISPE-ISPOR Special Task Force on Real World Evidence in Health Care Decision Making (2017). Reporting to improve reproducibility and facilitate validity assessment for healthcare database studies V1.0. *Pharmacoepidemiol. Drug Saf.* 26 (9): 1018–1032.

## The View from Regulatory Agencies

Braun, M.M., Farag-El-Massah, S., Xu, K., and Cote, T.R. (2010). Emergence of orphan drugs in the United States: a quantitative assessment of the first 25 years. *Nat. Rev. Drug Discov.* 9: 519–522. https://doi.org/10.1038/nrd3160.

Fleming, T.R. and Powers, J.H. (2012). Biomarkers and surrogate endpoints in clinical trials. *Stat. Med.* 10: 2973–2984. https://doi.org/10.1002/sim.5403.

Goedecke, T., Morales, D., Pacarariu, A., and Kurz, X. (2017 Nov 5). Measuring the impact of medicines regulatory interventions – systematic review and methodological considerations. *Br. J. Clin. Pharmacol.* https://doi.org/10.1111/bcp.13469 [Epub ahead of print].

Hunter, N.L., Rao, G.R., and Sherman, R.E. (2017). Flexibility in the FDA approach to orphan drug development. *Nat. Rev. Drug*

Discov. 16: 737–738. https://doi.org/10.1038/nrd.2017.151.

Kaplan, S., Staffa, J.A., and Dal Pan, G.J. (2007). Duration of therapy with metoclopramide: a prescription claims data study. *Pharmacoepidemiol Drug Saf. Aug.* 16 (8): 878–881.

Knox, C., Hampp, C., Willy, M. et al. (2015). Patient understanding of drug risks: an evaluation of medication guide assessments. *Pharmacoepidemiol. Drug Saf.* 24: 518–525. https://doi.org/10.1002/pds.3762.

Schieppati, A., Henter, J.I., Daina, E., and Aperia, A. (2008). Why rare diseases are an important medical and social issue. *Lancet* 371: 2039–2041. https://doi.org/10.1016/S0140-6736(08)60872-7.

Sherman, R.E., Anderson, S.A., Dal Pan, G.J. et al. (2016). Real-world evidence – what is it and what can it tell us? *N. Engl. J. Med.* 375: 2293–2297. https://doi.org/10.1056/NEJMsb1609216.

Temple, R.J. (1995). A regulatory authority's opinion about surrogate endpoints. In: *Clinical Measurement in Drug Evaluation* (eds. W.S. Nimmo and G.T. Tucker). New York: Wiley.

## The View from the Legal System

### Drug Safety and Tort Law

Angell, M. (1997). *Science on Trial: The Clash of Medical Evidence and the Law in the Breast Implant Case.* New York: W. W. Norton & Co.

Avorn, J. (2004). *Powerful Medicines: The Benefits, Risks and Costs of Prescription Drugs.* New York, NY: Alfred A Knopf.

Brennan, T.A. (1988). Causal chains and statistical links: the role of scientific uncertainty in hazardous-substance litigation. *Cornell Law Rev.* 73: 469–533.

Federal Judicial Center (2000) *Reference Manual on Scientific Evidence* (2nd edn). http://www.fjc.gov/public/pdf.nsf/lookup/sciman00.pdf/$file/sciman00.pdf

Green, M.D. (1996). *Bendectin and Birth Defects: The Challenges of Mass Toxic Substances Litigation.* Philadelphia, PA: University of Pennsylvania Press.

Hill, A.B. (1965). The environment and disease: association or causation? *Proc. R. Soc. Med.* 58: 295–300.

Kesselheim, A.S. and Avorn, J. (2007). The role of litigation in defining drug risks. *JAMA* 297: 308–311.

Kessler, D.A. and Vladeck, D.C. (2008). A critical examination of the FDA's efforts to preempt failure-to-warn claims. *Georgetown Law J.* 96: 461–495.

Shapo, M.S. (2008). *Experimenting with the Consumer: The Mass Testing of Risky Products on the American Public.* Westport, CT: Praeger.

## Contract-Related Issues in Pharmacoepidemiology

Bodenheimer, T. (2000). Uneasy alliance – clinical investigators and the pharmaceutical industry. *New Engl. J. Med.* 342: 1539–1544.

Eichler, H.G., Kong, S.X., and Grégoire, J.P. (2006). Outcomes research collaborations between third-party payers, academia, and pharmaceutical manufacturers: what can we learn from clinical research? *Eur. J. Health Econ.* 7 (2): 129–135.

Kong, S.X. and Wertheimer, A.I. (1998). Outcomes research: collaboration among academic researchers, managed care organizations, and pharmaceutical manufacturers. *Am. J. Manag. Care* 4 (1): 28–34.

Washburn, J. and University Inc (2006). *The Corporate Corruption of Higher Education.* New York: Basic Books.

## Patent Law and Pharmacoepidemiology

Heller, M.A. and Eisenberg, R.S. (1998). Can patents deter innovation: the anticommons in biomedical research. *Science* 280: 698–701.

Jaffe, A.B. and Lerner, J. (2004). *Innovation and Its Discontents: How Our Broken Patent System Is Endangering Innovation and Progress, and*

*What To Do About It.* Princeton, NJ: Princeton University Press.

Kesselheim, A.S. and Karlawish, J. (2012). Biomarkers unbound – the supreme Court's ruling on diagnostic-test patents. *N. Engl. J. Med.* 366: 2338–2340.

Nard, C.A. and Wagner, R.P. (2007). *Patent Law: Concepts and Insights.* St. Paul, MN: Foundation Press.

National Research Council (2004). *A Patent System for the 21st Century* (eds. S.A. Merrill, R.C. Levin and M.B. Myers). Washington, DC: The National Academies Press.

Walker, A.M. (2006). More lawyers, more bureaucrats, less information on drug safety. *Pharmacoepidemiol. Drug Saf.* 15: 394–395.

**Part II**

**Sources of Pharmacoepidemiology Data**

# 7

# Postmarketing Spontaneous Pharmacovigilance Reporting Systems

*Gerald J. Dal Pan[1], Marie Lindquist[2], and Kate Gelperin[1]*

[1] Office of Surveillance and Epidemiology, Center for Drug Evaluation and Research, US Food and Drug Administration, Silver Spring, MD, USA
[2] Uppsala Monitoring Centre, WHO Collaborating Centre for International Drug Monitoring, Uppsala, Sweden

The views expressed herein are those of the authors, and not necessarily of the US Food and Drug Administration.

## Introduction

Potential signals for adverse drug reactions (ADRs) or adverse drug effects for marketed products most often arise from postmarketing spontaneous case reports, which are collated and analyzed by drug safety experts, evaluated as clinical case series, and considered for potential regulatory action. These efforts are not possible without input from dedicated health professionals and other concerned stakeholders. Adverse events (AEs) thought to be potentially drug-related may be reported by a consumer or a health professional to a drug's manufacturer, or they may be reported directly to a health authority through programs such as MedWatch or Eudravigilance. In addition, case reports and case series with valuable clinical details may be published in a peer-reviewed journal. Concerned stakeholders – health professionals as well as patients and consumers – are the source of the signals that can trigger further investigation and appropriate regulatory action when needed to protect the public from unnecessary risks or harms. At times, a causal association between a drug and an AE may seem clear due to strong temporal association between exposure to the drug and onset of an adverse effect, or when there is confirmation of positive re-challenge (i.e. signs or symptoms resolve when exposure is stopped but recur when re-introduced). But more often, causality assessment is challenging, and well-designed pharmacoepidemiology or other clinical studies are needed to assess the signal and quantify the risk.

In the United States, the Food and Drug Administration (FDA) issues Drug Safety Communications (DSCs) to alert the public about emerging safety issues, such as investigations into safety signals that may have a clinically important impact on a product's safety profile. Recently, FDA launched a new web portal that enables the public to view summary charts and listings of de-identified cases from the FDA Adverse Event Reporting System (FAERS), a compilation of all postmarketing AE reports received by FDA.

The term "pharmacovigilance" is widely used to denote postmarketing safety activities, and is defined by the World Health

*Textbook of Pharmacoepidemiology*, Third Edition. Edited by Brian L. Strom, Stephen E. Kimmel, and Sean Hennessy.
© 2022 John Wiley & Sons Ltd. Published 2022 by John Wiley & Sons Ltd.

Organization (WHO) as "the science and activities relating to the detection, assessment, understanding and prevention of adverse effects or any other possible drug-related problems."

Monitoring and understanding the safety of drug and therapeutic biologic products is a process that proceeds throughout the product's life cycle, spanning the period prior to first administration to humans through the entire marketing life of the product. Throughout the product lifecycle, astute clinical observations made at the point of care constitute an important source of information. While new technologies have enabled more thorough knowledge of a drug's actions, and computerized databases have enabled large-scale, population-based analyses of drug safety investigations, these advancements are adjuncts to, and not substitutes for, careful, well thought-out clinical observations.

Though the preapproval testing of a drug is typically rigorous, and the review of the data is thorough, there are still inevitable uncertainties about the complete safety profile of a drug when it is brought to market. Several factors contribute to these uncertainties. First, the number of patients treated with the drug prior to approval is limited, generally from several hundred to a few thousand. Second, patients in clinical trials tend to be carefully selected for inclusion in these trials, and are thus more clinically homogeneous than patients treated in the course of clinical practice once a drug is marketed. Compared to patients in clinical trials, patients treated in clinical practice may have a broader range of co-morbidities, take a wider variety of concomitant medications, and have a wider clinical severity spectrum of the underlying disease being treated. Third, additional populations of patients, such as children or older adults, who may not have been studied in large numbers in premarketing clinical trials, may be treated with the product once it is marketed. In addition, marketed drug products are often used for diseases or conditions for which they are not indicated, or at doses outside of the approved range. For these reasons, patients treated in clinical practice are more diverse than those treated in clinical trials. A postmarketing drug pharmacovigilance reporting system is therefore necessary.

## Description

### Adverse Events and Adverse Drug Reactions

A key concept in pharmacovigilance is the distinction between an *adverse event* and an *adverse drug reaction*. The International Conference on Harmonization of Technical Requirements for Registration of Pharmaceuticals for Human Use (ICH) E2D guideline on Post-Approval Safety Data Management: Definitions and Standards for Expedited Reporting, defines an AE as follows:

> An adverse event (AE) is any untoward medical occurrence in a patient administered a medicinal product and which does not necessarily have to have a causal relationship with this treatment. An adverse event can therefore be any unfavorable and unintended sign (for example, an abnormal laboratory finding), symptom, or disease temporally associated with the use of a medicinal product, whether or not considered related to this medicinal product.

The same guideline describes an ADR as follows:

> All noxious and unintended responses to a medicinal product related to any dose should be considered adverse drug reactions.

The phrase "responses to a medicinal product" means that a causal relationship between a medicinal product and an AE is at least a possibility.

A reaction, in contrast to an event, is characterized by the fact that a causal relationship between the drug and the occurrence is suspected. If an event is spontaneously reported, even if the relationship is unknown or unstated, it meets the definition of an adverse drug reaction.

The principal difference between an AE and an ADR is that a causal relationship is suspected for the latter, but is not required for the former. In this framework, ADRs are a subset of AEs. In some countries, postmarketing pharmacovigilance reporting systems are focused on ADRs, while in others data on AEs are collected. In the United States, for example, the scope of reporting requirements is "[a]ny adverse event associated with the use of a drug in humans, whether or not considered drug related . . ."

While many of the principles discussed in this chapter apply equally to AEs and ADRs, it is important to understand the distinction between these two concepts. Specifically, some databases may contain only ADRs, while others may contain AEs. These databases may behave differently when used for data mining. However, because many of the principles of drug safety surveillance apply to both AEs and ADRs, we will use the term "AE/ADR" to refer to these two terms collectively in this chapter, for convenience. When needed, we will use the individual terms if a distinction between the two is required.

## Overview of Pharmacovigilance Reporting Systems

The goal of a postmarketing, or post-approval, safety program is to identify drug-related AEs or ADRs that were not identified prior to a drug's approval, to refine knowledge of the known adverse effects of a drug, and to understand better the conditions under which the safe use of a drug can be assured.

The scope of pharmacovigilance is broad. The core activity is usually the identification of previously unrecognized AEs/ADRs with the use of the drug. However, it is not sufficient simply to note that use of a drug can lead to an AE/ADR. Rather, an investigation into not only the potential causal role of the drug in the development of the AE/ADR, but also into the conditions leading to the occurrence of the AE/ADR in one person or population and not in others must be the focus of any postmarket drug safety effort. Factors such as dose–response relationships, drug–drug interactions, drug–disease interactions, drug–food interactions, and the possibility of medication errors must be carefully considered. A full understanding of the factors that can lead to an AE/ADR may yield ideas for effective interventions to minimize the severity or occurrence of the AE/ADR, and thus enhance the safe use of the drug. For this reason, the approach to detecting and understanding clinically important AEs/ADRs in the postmarketing period must be as comprehensive as possible.

The identification of a new safety issue with a medicinal product often begins with a single observation. In the postmarketing period, such observations are usually clinical observations, often made at the point of care in the course of clinical practice. A practitioner or patient notes the development of symptoms or signs that were not present, or were present in less severe form, prior to the patient's using the medicine. If this sign or symptom is not listed in the product's approved labeling, patients and healthcare professionals may not think to attribute it to the medicine. If further evaluation reveals a clinically significant process (e.g. liver injury, rhabdomyolysis, agranulocytosis), it is important to keep in mind the possibility of a side effect due to a medication in the differential diagnosis of the event. If a medication side effect is not included in the list of possible conditions or diseases that could be causing the observed problem, the patient may not be treated appropriately.

In the postmarketing period, the investigation of AEs/ADRs is a multidisciplinary one. The analysis of a complex AE/ADR can involve the fields of medicine, pharmacology, epidemiology, statistics, pharmacy, toxicology, and others. There are several methods of clinical postmarketing safety assessment. These include the review of case reports and case series from spontaneous reporting systems and published medical literature, a wide variety of types of observational epidemiologic studies, and clinical trials. This chapter will focus on spontaneous pharmacovigilance reporting systems. No one method is a priori better than another in all settings. Rather, the choice of methods depends on the particular safety question to be answered.

## The Concept of Spontaneous AE/ADR Reporting

A core aspect of pharmacovigilance is the voluntary reporting of AEs/ADRs either directly to established national or regional centers, or alternatively to pharmaceutical manufacturers, who in turn are obligated to report the information to regulators. National reporting systems are typically run by regulatory agencies (e.g. the US FDA runs the MedWatch program) or by centers designated by the health ministry or the drug regulatory authority. In a few countries, the national pharmacovigilance center is run by a university or other scientific body. In the United States, AEs/ADRs in individual patients are generally identified at the point of care. Patients, physicians, nurses, pharmacists, or anyone else who suspects that there may be an association between an AE/ADR and a drug or therapeutic biologic product are encouraged to, but are generally not required to, report the case to either the manufacturer or to the FDA.

This system of AE/ADR reporting is often referred to as a spontaneous reporting system; "spontaneous" because the person who initially reports the AE/ADR to either the reporting center or to the manufacturer chooses whether to report an AE and what events to report. Sometimes, spontaneous reporting systems are also labeled as "passive," based on the argument that the reporting center or the manufacturer passively receives this information, rather than actively seeking it out. However, this term does not do justice to the proactive way in which many pharmacovigilance centers seek to operate, even if resource constraints often limit the ability to interact adequately with reporters. Moreover, "spontaneous reporting" does not fit well with the reporting situation of today, when most countries have introduced or enacted legislation which mandates reporting from pharmaceutical companies. For marketed products, companies often conduct planned, structured interactions with patients and practitioners (e.g. patient support programs) that have the potential to generate AE reports that may not otherwise have been communicated. Reporting may also include canvassed or stimulated reporting of suspected reactions of particular interest (see also below, in the section "National pharmacovigilance systems").

Underlying the concept of a spontaneous postmarketing AE/ADR pharmacovigilance reporting system is the notion that clinical observations made at the point of care are often valuable pieces of information in further refining the knowledge of a drug's safety profile. This is an important, though frequently underemphasized, idea. After approval, when formal study often ends and marketing of the medicine begins, there is often no further systematic way to continue the study of a medicine's safety, or even to generate drug safety hypotheses. While scientific advances and access to new data sources (e.g. electronic healthcare records) may provide some opportunity to monitor the safety of a marketed medicine, these alternative approaches to safety signal detection remain unproven.

When healthcare professionals, patients, and consumers want to make a notification of a potentially adverse effect of a medication, it is useful for this information to be systematically organized, stored, and analyzed. A reporting system fills this need. If such information were not systematically collected, potentially valuable data about medicines would be lost. This system implies an important role for healthcare professionals in postmarketing safety assessment, as the quality of reports is always dependent on the details provided by healthcare professionals.

Because most AE/ADR reporting systems rely on healthcare professionals, patients, and consumers to submit reports voluntarily, it is generally recognized that there is substantial underreporting of AEs/ADRs via current reporting systems. Two survey-based studies conducted in the US in the 1980s, one in Maryland and the other in Rhode Island, examined physician reporting to FDA, and concluded that fewer than 10% of AEs/ADRs were reported to FDA. These studies were conducted prior to the development of the current MedWatch program in 1993, and do not consider the contribution of reporting from sources other than physicians. Calculating the proportion of AE reports that a reporting system actually receives requires that the true number of AEs/ADRs in the population be known. For most AEs/ADRs, this number is not known or readily available. In some cases, however, data are available that allow an estimate of the extent of reporting to be calculated. For example, the extent of reporting to FDA of cases of hospitalized rhabdomyolysis associated with statin use was estimated using a projected estimate of the number of such cases in the United States and comparing it to the number of reports of statin-associated hospitalized rhabdomyolysis in FAERS, a database that houses FDA's postmarketing AE reports. The projected national estimate was obtained by using incidence rates from a population-based cohort study, and applying those incidence rates to national estimates of statin use. Across four statins (atorvastatin, cerivastatin, pravastatin, and simvastatin), the estimated overall extent of AE reporting was 17.7%. For individual statins, the estimated extent of reporting

ranged from 5.0% (atorvastatin) to 31.2% (cerivastatin). Further analysis revealed that the high proportion of reporting of cerivastatin cases was driven by reports received after the dissemination of a Dear Healthcare Professional letter notifying physicians of the risks of cerivastatin-associated rhabdomyolysis. The estimated extent of reporting was 14.8% before the letter and rose to 35.0% after. It is important to note that the results of this study apply only to reporting cases of statin-associated rhabdomyolysis. The extent of reporting for different drug-adverse pairs will be different, and cannot be estimated from the results of this study.

Once case reports are received by national pharmacovigilance centers, they are entered into AE/ADR databases. These databases can then be inspected for drug safety signals, which form the basis of further study, necessary regulatory action, or both.

## Report Characteristics

The individual case report is the fundamental unit of a postmarketing pharmacovigilance reporting system. The extent to which such a reporting system can address specific drug safety questions depends, in large part, on the characteristics and quality of the individual reports. Specific report formats differ across jurisdictions, though many countries and regions collect information compatible with the ICH E2B format. The standard is designed to work with a variety of national and international systems and incorporates endorsement of standards by participating Standards Development Organizations such as the International Standards Organization (ISO), Health Level Seven (HL7), European Committee for Standardization (CEN), and Clinical Data Interchange Standards Consortium (CDISC) to enable wider interoperability across the regulatory and healthcare communities. Although comprehensive in scope, the format also allows for limited data to be submitted. The principal domains of case information in the ICH E2B standard include: (i) patient characteristics, (ii) reaction(s) or event(s), (iii) results of tests and procedures relevant to the investigation of the patient, (iv) drug(s) information, and (v) a narrative case summary and further information.

Regardless of the specific formatting requirements across jurisdictions, there are some fundamental components of an individual safety report that are important for a thorough review.

Product identification, in as much detail as possible, is essential for an assessment of a case report. For pharmaceuticals, the identification of the active ingredient(s) is critical to product identification. However, other factors can also be important, depending on the specific safety question. For example, the formulation of the product can be important, as certain active ingredients may be present in a variety of formulations. For example, many opioid agents are available in oral, injectable, and transdermal formulations. Because the pharmacokinetic and other pharmaceutical properties can differ across these formulations, information about the formulation is important in determining if there are formulation specific effects, including those that may result from medication errors. Additionally, if the drug safety question involves the assessment of an AE/ADR related to a product quality defect, information on both manufacturer and lot/batch number can be very important, as product quality problems typically involve specific lots from an individual manufacturer.

Reports describing medication errors, or the potential for medication errors, ideally contain information on the product involved, the sequence of events leading up to the error, the work environment in which the error occurred, and the type of error that occurred.

Characteristics of a good quality case report include adequate information on product use, patient characteristics, medical history, and concomitant treatments, and a description of the AE/ADR, including response to treatments and clinical outcome. Our experience, based on many years of reviewing case reports, is that while a substantial amount of useful clinical information can be written in a succinct narrative, most narratives are incomplete, many to the extent that they are uninterpretable. While follow-up with the reporter is sometimes feasible for drug safety analysts to perform during case review, this has been the exception not the rule, often due to resource constraints. Incomplete and uninterpretable case reports limit the effectiveness of postmarket pharmacovigilance reporting systems. Attempts to improve the systems will need to address the problem of poor case report quality rather than merely increasing the number of reports. Unfortunately, it is not unusual for FDA to receive potentially important spontaneous reports which cannot be evaluated because of missing key information. For instance, many spontaneous reports of hypersensitivity AEs/ADRs associated with heparin administration during an investigation of tainted heparin were excluded from an FDA analysis published in 2010 because they lacked "basic or critical clinical information."

Information on product use should include the start date(s), stop date(s), dose(s), frequency of use, and indication for use. Dosage information is important in exploring dose-event relationships. Duration of use is important for characterizing the time course of AEs/ADRs relative to initiation of product use. Indication for use is also an important piece of information, as many products are used for more than one indication (either on-label or off-label).

Patient information should include age, gender, medical history, and concomitant medication usage. The presence of factors that could confound the relationship of the drug to the AE/ADR, especially elements of the medical history and concomitant medication usage, are critical to the interpretation of individual case safety reports.

A description of the AE/ADR that allows for independent medical assessment is critical. A narrative of the event that includes the temporal relationship of drug usage to the development of the AE/ADR, the clinical and diagnostic features, the clinical course, any measures instituted to treat the AE/ADR, the response to these measures, and the clinical outcome are all essential components of a high quality case report. Results of laboratory tests, imaging studies, and pathology results facilitate an independent interpretation of the report. Information on de-challenge (the course of the AE/ADR when the medication is withdrawn) and re-challenge (the determination of whether the AE/ADR recurs when the drug is re-introduced), if available, can be invaluable.

## Social Media

Social media are a range of computer-based technologies that allow the creation and sharing of information, ideas, photographs and other messages via electronic communication. User-generated content is a defining feature of social media. This content can be made available to others via computer-based networks that connect one user with other users or groups to form social networks. Depending on privacy settings, which in some cases may be chosen by the user, content may be widely available to other users or it may be restricted to only certain users or groups. Given the widespread use of the internet and, to a lesser degree, of social media, for health-related topics, there is interest in whether social media can be a source of drug safety signals or otherwise shed light on ADRs. Because social media posts describe individual experiences, they can, in theory, describe adverse reactions to medicines. The use of social media for pharmacovigilance presents both opportunities and challenges, and is an area of active research. In 2014, the Innovative Medicines Initiative (IMI), a public-private partnership between the European Union and the European Federation for Pharmaceutical Industries and Associations, launched *WEB-RADR: Recognising Adverse Drug Reactions*

(https://web-radr.eu/) to develop new technical tools to facilitate the detection and analysis of potential ADRs in social media sites. It also aimed to develop a mobile phone app for the reporting of suspected ADRs to regulatory authorities in the European Union (in the context of traditional AE reporting). One of several planned outgrowths of these efforts is the establishment of a regulatory framework for social media mining for ADRs. Preliminary recommendations from IMI WEB-RADR for a regulatory framework note that data from social media should be treated as a "secondary use of data," the use of social media for signal detection and validation should be optional, reporting of individual case safety reports of ADRs from social media sites should not be required, and that follow-up with social media users should not be required. Rather, drug manufacturers should include insights gained from social media regarding the safety of their products in the product's periodic safety update report or risk management plan. More work is needed to refine the methods of extracting and analyzing data from social media for detection of ADRs. Results of the WEB-RADR project yielded a realistic and cautionary appraisal of the current ability of social media to provide primary pharmacovigilance information.

## National Pharmacovigilance Systems

The organization of postmarketing safety reporting systems and national pharmacovigilance systems varies around the world. The fundamental feature is that health professionals, and in some cases patients or consumers, are encouraged to send reports of AEs/ADRs to one or more specified locations. These locations can be the drug regulatory authority, an academic or hospital-based pharmacovigilance center (often working with or on behalf of a drug regulatory authority), or the drug manufacturer. The roles of these institutions vary from country to country, and depend greatly on the regulatory and national drug monitoring system in the country.

In low- and middle-income countries, with varying regulatory infrastructure, the focus in pharmacovigilance has been different from that in the more affluent parts of the world. Reports can result from counterfeit and sub-standard drugs, known ADRs and drug interactions of concern to reporters, and ADRs resulting from medical error. In some countries, responding to queries about adverse reaction incidence, diagnosis, and management are a major part of the work of pharmacovigilance centers. In developing countries, there are often deficiencies in access to up-to-date information on drug safety that need remedying. On the other hand, large donations of new drugs to combat the endemic scourges of malaria, HIV/AIDS, tuberculosis, infestations, and other diseases, along with vaccines, have led to the high priority of monitoring their use for both safety and efficacy.

However, in many low- and middle-income countries there is currently not enough capacity for effective drug safety monitoring, and the improved access to new medicines adds additional strain on already overburdened or non-existent pharmacovigilance systems. A survey from 2010 of pharmacovigilance systems in low- and middle-income countries found that seven of 55 responding countries indicated that they had no designated system in place, and fewer than half of the respondents had a budget for pharmacovigilance. Consequently, lack of funding was mentioned as a hindrance to the development of pharmacovigilance, together with lack of training and a culture that does not promote AE/ADR reporting. Suggested key developments included: training for health workers and pharmacovigilance program managers; active surveillance methods, sentinel sites and registries; and better collaboration between pharmacovigilance centers and public health programs, with a designated budget for pharmacovigilance included in the latter.

The WHO is working together with major donor organizations to address the urgent need for capacity building in low- and middle-income countries. The strategy is focused on sustainable development, covering not only the implementation of reporting systems, technical support, and training of healthcare professionals, but also improvements in governance and infrastructure to support pharmacovigilance activities in the broader context of regulatory systems strengthening.

The perceived responsibility of healthcare professionals to report AEs/ADRs often varies around the world. Because the largest gaps in drug safety knowledge are believed to be for recently approved medicines, most countries emphasize the need to report AEs/ADRs, even less serious ones, for this group of medicines. For example, in the United Kingdom, recently approved drugs containing new active ingredients are marked in the British National Formulary with a black triangle, a symbol used to denote a drug product whose active ingredient has been newly licensed for use in the UK. In some cases, drug products meeting certain additional criteria are also marked with a black triangle, even if the active ingredient has been previously approved. The aim of the black triangle program is to prompt health professionals to report all suspected adverse reactions associated with the use of these products. In some countries, it is mandatory for physicians and dentists to report cases of suspected ADRs to the regulatory authority. Most countries, however, do not have such specific programs or requirements, but health professionals are encouraged to report and the national reporting centers provide general advice to health professionals on what events to report.

In a majority of countries, including countries in the ICH regions, other high income countries, and 33 of 55 low- and middle-income countries responding to a 2008 survey, pharmaceutical companies that hold marketing authorizations are obligated to report AEs or ADRs to the regulatory authority. In some countries, the event is reportable only if an attribution of causality has been made. In other countries, the event is reportable even if no attribution has been made. For example, in the United States, pharmaceutical companies are required by law to submit spontaneous reports of AEs/ADRs, regardless of attribution of causality, on an expedited basis if they are serious and unexpected. The AE/ADR is considered serious when the patient outcome is: death; life-threatening; hospitalization (initial or prolonged); disability; congenital anomaly; or, requires intervention to prevent permanent impairment or damage. Periodic reporting of other types of AEs/ADRs, such as those considered serious and expected (labeled), or nonserious, is typically required as well. The periodicity of such aggregate reports is determined by the length of time the drug has been marketed, with increased frequency for newly approved drugs, and decreased (e.g. annual) with older drugs.

While spontaneous reports of AEs/ADRs usually originate initially from the point of care, the more proximal source of reports coming into the national pharmacovigilance centers may vary, with reports most often being received from drug manufacturers or from healthcare professionals and patients. Some countries restrict reports to only those originating from physicians. Other countries also accept reports from pharmacists, nurses, and patients. There is a current trend toward encouraging direct patient or consumer reporting, replacing the notion held by many in the past that such reports would not be a reliable and useful source of information.

In most countries, the national pharmacovigilance center is part of the drug regulatory authority; in some, the monitoring is carried out jointly by the drug regulatory authority/Ministry of Health and an independent institution. In Germany, the Federal Institute for Drugs and Medical Devices (BfArM) maintains a joint database for recording reported ADRs, together with the Drug Commission of the German Medical Profession. According to the professional code of conduct of physicians in Germany, all ADRs should be reported to the Drug Commission. In the Netherlands, the practical responsibility for post-marketing surveillance is shared between the Medicines Evaluation Board (MEB) and the Netherlands Pharmacovigilance Centre (Lareb). The MEB handles communications with market authorization holders; the role of Lareb is to process and analyze reports from health professionals and patients.

Decentralized drug monitoring systems exist both within and outside the ICH region. In France, the French Medicines Agency coordinates the network of 31 regional centers that are connected to major university hospitals. In the United Kingdom, there are four regional centers connected to university hospitals, which have a special function of encouraging reporting in their regions. Since 2018, the pharmacovigilance system in China is regulated by the National Medical Products Administration (NMPA), within the State Administration for Market Regulation. In India, the Pharmacovigilance Programme of India has been in operation since 2010, with the Indian Pharmacopoeia Commission (IPC) running the National Coordinating Centre. The system is now operating nationwide, with 250 local monitoring centers in medical institutes.

## National and International Postmarketing Adverse Event Databases

Once submitted to the national drug safety monitoring program, individual case safety reports are stored in computerized postmarketing AE databases. Examples of national reporting systems and databases include the "Blue Card" system (Australia), Canada Vigilance (Canada), the Canadian Adverse Events Following Immunization Surveillance System (CAEFISS) database (Canada), the French Pharmacovigilance Spontaneous Reporting System database (France), the Adverse Drug Reaction Information Management System of the Pharmaceutical and Medication Devices Agency, Ministry of Health, Labor, and Welfare (Japan), the Lareb database (Netherlands), the BISI database (Sweden), the MHRA ADR database (United Kingdom), the FAERS database (United States), and the Vaccine Adverse Event Reporting System (VAERS) database (United States). In addition, there are two international reporting and database systems: EudraVigilance in the European Union (run by the European Medicines Agency, EMA); and VigiBase, pooling data from more than 130 member countries of the WHO International Drug Monitoring Programme (run by the Uppsala Monitoring Centre, UMC). VigiBase is also the database model used as the national database by around 70 pharmacovigilance centers around the world; reports are entered, stored and managed in an internet-based data management system, VigiFlow, from which the data is seamlessly transferred to VigiBase, and can be analyzed remotely through a search and analytical interface, VigiLyze.

To understand the results of an analysis of individual case safety reports from a postmarketing database, it is necessary to understand the unique features of the database, as each large postmarketing AE database differs from the others. It is necessary to understand if, and how, the data are coded. Many databases code drugs according to a local or national standard drug dictionary, while others use a standard international dictionary, such as WHODrug. Similarly, many databases code individual AE/ADR reporter verbatim terms which describe the AE/ADR according to a standard medical dictionary, such as the Medical Dictionary for Regulatory Activities (MedDRA). In the ICH regions, (Europe, Japan, and the United States) use of MedDRA is mandatory for coding of AEs/ADRs.

Beyond coding, several other features of the database are important to understand. First, does the database include only reports from postmarketing systems, or does it include reports from other sources, such as the medical literature or clinical trials? Second, does the

database include reports only from health professionals, or does it also include reports from patients and consumers? Third, what is the range of medical products included in the database – drugs, biologicals, blood, blood products, vaccines, dietary supplements? Fourth, does the database include reports from only one country or region, or does it include reports from regions outside the jurisdiction of the regulatory authority? Fifth, does the database include both "nonserious" and "serious" AEs/ ADRs; if so, what proportion of the reports have been classified by the health authority (or other database manager) as serious? Sixth, does the database include all AEs (i.e. events which may or may not be judged to be causally related to a medicine) or does it include only ADRs (i.e. events for which a likely causal relationship has been determined prior to entering the report into the database)? Seventh, how many individual case safety reports are in the database? Each of these factors is important in determining the utility of a particular database in answering a specific drug safety question.

## Detecting Signals from a Postmarketing Adverse Event Database

Identifying potential associations of AEs/ ADRs to drugs using only information within the database involves the detection of signals. According to the WHO, a signal is "reported information on a possible causal relationship between an adverse event and a drug, the relationship being unknown or incompletely documented previously." While there have been many definitions of a signal put forth over the years, the important underlying principle is that a signal is a hypothesis that calls for further work to be performed to evaluate that hypothesis. Signal detection is the act of looking for or identifying signals from any source.

In the setting of a relatively small number of reports, review of groups of reports or periodic summaries of reports has been a standard method of signal detection. For example, one could look at a list of all reports in which the outcome was "death" to see if this outcome was reported more frequently for some drugs than others. Summaries based on specific organ class toxicities could be reviewed to examine if reports in one system organ class were proportionately more frequent for one drug than others. These methods depend on the ability of a drug safety specialist to recognize new or unusual patterns of case reports. While an astute specialist can identify signals using this method, this manual review is often neither practical nor reproducible for detecting signals from large postmarketing AE databases, some of which contain several million records.

In an effort to address this challenge, data mining techniques have been applied to pharmacovigilance AE/ADR databases. In broad terms, data mining refers to a process of analyzing data to find patterns. In the case of AE/ADR databases, most of these patterns would not be visible without the use of statistically based, computerized algorithms. There are a variety of specific algorithms that have been applied to safety signal detection in AE/ADR databases. The fundamental feature of data mining techniques used to analyze AE databases is that each is based on finding "disproportionalities" in data, which in this context is the finding that a given AE/ADR is reported for a particular drug more often than would be expected based on the number of reports of that AE/ADR for all other drugs in the database. Several features of these methods are worth noting.

First, the methods are transparent. While the number of reports received for a drug varies over time (and may be highest in the first few years of reporting), this temporal trend will not necessarily alter the proportion of specific reactions for the drug. Thus, a given reaction may still be found to be disproportionately reported even as the total number of reports for the drug changes.

Second, these methods rely exclusively on reports within the database; no external data are needed. For this reason, understanding the characteristics of the database, as discussed above, is important. This feature has several consequences. Because the expected number of reports of a specific AE/ADR for a given drug (and thus the disproportionality of the drug–event pair) depend on the reports within the individual database, the degree of disproportionality for a given drug–event pair may vary from one database to the next. In the extreme, a given drug–event pair may have a strong signal of disproportionality in one database, and no such signal in another. A second consequence is that as the background information for all drugs in the database changes, so does the expected number of reports of a specific AE/ADR for a given drug (and again the disproportionality of the drug–event pair).

Third, a signal of disproportionality is a measure of a statistical association within a collection of AE/ADR reports (rather than in a population), and it is not a measure of causality. In this regard, it is important to underscore that *the use of data mining is for signal detection – that is, for hypothesis generation – and that further work is needed to evaluate the signal.*

Fourth, the absence of a signal of disproportionality in a postmarketing AE database is not evidence that an important AE/ADR is not associated with a particular drug.

Some of the data mining techniques used in pharmacovigilance have included the proportional reporting ratio, the reporting odds ratio, the Bayesian Confidence Propagation Neural Network (BCPNN), and the Empirical Bayes method (also known as the Gamma Poisson Shrinker or the Multi-item Gamma Poisson Shrinker). Data mining is sometimes done using a subset of an AE/ADR database. For example, a portion of the database limited to a specific class of drugs might be used to find relative differences in the frequencies of specific AEs/ADRs across the class. As part of the IMI, a public-private partnership in Europe, the EMA established the Pharmacoepidemiological Research on Outcomes of Therapeutics by a European Consortium (IMI PROTECT) with a goal of conducting research to develop and test new tools for the benefit–risk assessment of marketed drugs. A range of signal detection algorithms were compared across seven spontaneous reporting databases with no method found to be better than the others. Findings were inconsistent across databases. The choice of signaling criteria had a greater impact on signal detection performance than the choice of disproportionality methods.

## Review of Individual Case Safety Reports

The review of individual case safety reports of AEs/ADRs is a complex process. It typically begins by identifying one or more case reports with the outcome of interest. Because the case reports that form a case series often come from disparate sources, it is usually necessary to develop a case definition. The case definition centers on the clinical characteristics of the event of interest, without regard to the causal role of the medicine whose relationship to the AE is being investigated. Once a case definition is established, each report is reviewed to determine if the event meets the case definition and if the report is to be included in the case series. Depending on the specific question(s) to be answered by the case series, other exclusion criteria may also apply. For example, one would always exclude a case in which the report suggests that the patient never took the medicine of interest. In other cases, one may restrict the case series to only certain formulations of the medicine (e.g. include case reports in which an intravenous formulation, but not an oral formulation, was used, if such exclusion is appropriate for the question at hand), or to certain age groups (e.g. limit the case series to only case reports describing the suspected AEs in pediatric patients, if such exclusion is appropriate for

the question at hand), or to certain indications for use (e.g. limit the case series to case reports in which the medicine was used for a certain off-label indication, if such exclusion is appropriate to the question at hand). Exclusion criteria for a case series must be carefully considered so that potentially relevant cases are not excluded, and all available information is fully assessed. In general, if the purpose of the case series is to examine the relationship between a medicine and a suspected AE/ADR that has not been previously associated with the medicine, it is best to err on the side of inclusion to avoid missing clinically relevant, though incomplete, information about cases of interest.

Once the case series has been developed, it is next necessary to review each case report individually in order to determine if there is a plausible causal relationship between the medicine and the AE. At the level of the individual case safety report, it is often difficult to establish with certainty that the medicine caused the AE of interest. For example, if the AE/ADR of interest is one that is already common in the population that takes the medication, establishing a causal role for the medicine in the development of the condition is generally not feasible using individual case safety reports or case series. For example, the incidence of Parkinson disease is much higher in persons over the age of 60 years than it is in persons below that age. In this situation, review of a report describing a myocardial infarction in a 70-year-old patient on an anti-Parkinsonian agent will generally not be informative in determining if the agent played a causal role in the development of the myocardial infarction, as myocardial infarction occurs commonly in this age group. Similarly, review of a case report is not likely to shed light on the causal relationship between a medicine and an AE/ADR when the AE/ADR is a manifestation of the underlying illness which the medicine is treating. For example, a review of case reports of worsening asthma in patients taking an anti-asthma medication is not likely to be sufficient to establish a causal link between the worsening asthma and the medication. Review of a case series to establish a causal relationship between a drug and a AE/ADR is most straightforward when the suspected AE/ADR: (i) is rare in the population when the medication is not used, (ii) is not a manifestation of the underlying disease, (iii) has a strong temporal association with drug administration, and (iv) is biologically plausible as a drug reaction or is generally the result of a drug reaction based on other clinical experience. Examples of AEs/ADRs that often meet these criteria are acute hepatic failure, aplastic anemia, agranulocytosis, rhabdomyolysis, serious skin reactions such as Stevens-Johnson syndrome and toxic epidermal necrolysis, and certain arrhythmias, such as torsades de pointes.

The approach to assessing the causal role of a medicine in the development of an AE/ADR has evolved over the past four decades. In general, the approach relies on a systematic review of each case report to ascertain the temporal relationship between drug intake and the development of the adverse reaction, an assessment of any co-existing diseases or medications that could confound the relationship between the medicine and the AE/ADR, the clinical course after withdrawing the drug ("de-challenge"), and the clinical course after re-introduction of the drug (re-challenge), when applicable. Naranjo and colleagues described a method based on these general principles for estimating the likelihood that a drug caused an adverse clinical event. The WHO has developed a qualitative scale for categorizing causality assessments.

In the development of a case series, once the individual cases are reviewed, it is important to integrate the findings across the cases to determine patterns that may point to a relationship between the drug and the AE/ADR. For example, does the AE/ADR appear at some doses, but not at others? Does the AE/ADR appear after one or a few doses, or does it appear only after a more prolonged exposure? Is the spectrum of severity of the event homogeneous or

is it heterogeneous? Are certain co-morbidities or concomitant medications more likely to be present in patients with the event? In the review of a case series, there are no prespecified answers to these questions that establish or exclude the possibility that the drug led to the AE/ADR. Rather, the characteristics of the individual cases, taken together with the patterns observed in the case series itself, can lead the analyst to determine if the medication has a reasonable possibility of causing the condition of interest.

## Reporting Ratios

Because postmarketing safety reporting systems do not capture all cases of an event of interest, it is not possible to calculate an incidence rate for a particular drug–event pair. However, analysis of AEs/ADRs based simply on numbers of reports, even after thorough analysis of these reports, does not in itself put these reports into the context of how widely a medicine is used.

To adjust for the extent of drug utilization in a population in the analysis of AE/ADR reports, a reporting ratio can be used. A reporting ratio is defined as the number of cases of a particular AE/ADR reported to an AE database during a specific time period divided by some measure of drug utilization in the same time period. Across drugs in an AE database, the reporting ratios measure the relative frequency of the AE/ADR reports adjusting for differences in the level of drug utilization in that database. The numerator is derived from counts of AE/ADR reports associated with the drug of interest that are recorded in the postmarketing AE database during a specified time period. In the past, the denominator typically consisted of the number of dispensed prescriptions, used as a surrogate measure of drug exposure in the population over that same time period, and often estimated from proprietary drug utilization databases. The number of dispensed prescriptions was used because data on the number of unique individuals using the drug in a specified time period was generally not available. More recently, such data have become available, and reporting ratios based on persons using the medication, and not prescriptions, are being calculated. In some cases, information is available on not only the number of persons receiving the drug or the number of prescriptions dispensed, but also on the duration of use. When such data are available, the denominator for the reporting ratio may be expressed in person-time. When using denominators based on person-time, it is important to be mindful of the assumptions of the person-time method, especially the assumption that events in the numerator occur uniformly over time. Because AEs/ADRs may not occur uniformly over time after a drug is started, this assumption does not always hold.

Because the reporting ratio (sometimes referred to as "reporting rate") is not a measure of incidence or prevalence, it must be interpreted cautiously. For AEs/ADRs that are rare in the general population (e.g., aplastic anemia), reporting ratios are sometimes compared to the background rate (incidence or prevalence) of that event in a defined population. In other situations, individual reporting ratios of a particular AE/ADR across different drugs used for a similar indication or within the same class are calculated and the magnitude of the differences in reporting ratios is compared. Interpretation of the comparison of reporting ratios across drugs must be made with caution, since such comparisons are highly sensitive to variation in AE/ADR reporting and thus it is necessary to consider the differential underreporting of AEs in the postmarketing safety reporting system. The underlying assumption in estimating reporting ratios for comparison across a group of drug products is that each of the respective manufacturer's reporting practices for the drug of interest are similar over the reporting period. However, this assumption may not hold true in some cases, and a comparison of reporting ratios across drugs may not be valid.

## Strengths

### Signal Detection

The principal strength – and, arguably, the principal purpose – of a postmarketing safety reporting system is that it allows for signal detection, the further exploration of drug safety hypotheses, and appropriate regulatory decision-making and action when necessary. As noted earlier in this chapter, signals can be detected by data mining methods, reviews of individual case safety reports, or assessment of case series. In many instances, further work is needed to determine with more certainty the relationship of the drug to the AE/ADR. The capability for timely and effective signal detection is a key strength of a postmarketing pharmacovigilance reporting system.

Another key strength of a well designed and effectively utilized postmarketing pharmacovigilance reporting system is that, in certain cases, the relationship of a drug to an AE/ADR can be established with sufficient confidence, usually by a case series, that necessary regulatory action can be taken. AEs/ADRs for which the relationship to a drug can be established with reasonable certainty are generally those that have a strong temporal association with drug administration, a low or near absent frequency in the underlying population, are not part of the underlying illness being treated, are generally the result of exposure to a drug or other toxin, and have no other likely explanation. Aplastic anemia, agranulocytosis, acute liver failure, rhabdomyolysis, certain arrhythmias such as torsades de pointes, and serious skin reactions such as Stevens-Johnson syndrome are examples of AEs whose relationship to a drug can often be established by case series. However, relative to all signals detected in a postmarketing safety reporting system, those about which a reasonably firm conclusion can be made on the basis of AE/ADR reports alone are few in number.

## Opportunity for the Public to Report AEs/ADRs

Postmarketing safety reporting systems allow healthcare professionals to report suspected AEs/ADRs to national pharmacovigilance centers, drug regulatory authorities, and/or manufacturers. Such systems allow for direct engagement of healthcare professionals in the drug safety monitoring system. The advantage of this involvement is that it allows for careful clinical observations, made at the point of care, to inform drug safety surveillance. Clinicians can provide succinct but detailed accounts of relevant symptoms, signs, diagnostic test results, past medical history, concomitant medications, and clinical course of an AE/ADR, including information on de-challenge and re-challenge. Such a synthesis of clinical information is generally not available from automated data sources. For those AEs/ADRs that are serious, rare, and often the result of a medication exposure, the ability to obtain detailed information directly from the point of care is an essential feature of postmarketing pharmacovigilance reporting systems.

Postmarketing safety reporting systems also can accept reports from consumers and patients, though this practice is not a feature of all such reporting systems. In the United States, where consumers and patients can report either to the manufacturer or directly to the FDA, the percentage of reports in 2016 that originated from consumers was about 50%. When consumer and patient-generated reports do not contain sufficient medical detail for meaningful review, subsequent follow up with health professionals may be possible in potentially important cases, so that more complete clinical information (e.g. hospital discharge summary) can be obtained.

## Scope

The scope of a postmarketing safety reporting system is quite broad. The system can cover all medicines used in the population, and it can receive reports of AEs/ADRs occurring in any member of the population. Because it need not restrict the reports it receives, it can receive AE/ADR reports throughout a medicine's marketed lifecycle. Thus, AEs/ADRs recognized late in a product's lifecycle, such as those resulting from prolonged exposure to a medicine, can, in theory, be ascertained. In practice, such ascertainment is difficult to achieve, because healthcare professionals may be less likely to ascribe an AE/ADR not known to be associated with a medicine that has been marketed for several years. In addition, patients who take a medicine for several years may also receive other treatments during that time, making it difficult to conclude that there is an association between the medicine and the AE/ADR.

Despite this broad scope, a postmarketing spontaneous reporting system can be relatively inexpensive. Most of these pharmacovigilance systems rely on voluntary reporting, and those who report AEs/ADRs are generally not paid for doing so. Thus, information collection is not expensive from the perspective of an effective pharmacovigilance, given that the system has the capacity to handle all medicines and all outcomes. This is in contrast to other data used to study drug safety questions, such as data from clinical trials, registries, and electronic healthcare data, each of which is relatively expensive to operate.

## Limitations

### Quality of Reports

Perhaps the major potential limitation of a spontaneous postmarketing safety reporting system is that it depends quite heavily on the quality of individual reports. Although data mining and other informatics methods can detect signals using coded bioinformatics terms in AE databases, each individual case safety report must still be carefully reviewed by a clinical analyst to determine if there is a plausible relationship between the medicine and the development of the AE/ADR. The quality of the report, as described earlier in this chapter, is critical for an informative and meaningful review of the individual case safety report. Report quality depends on the care, effort, and judgment of the person submitting the report, as well as the diligence of the person receiving and/or transmitting the report to the health authority. Reports without sufficient information for an independent determination of the relationship between the medicine and the AE/ADR are problematic for drug safety surveillance. However, with successful follow up, sometimes even such deficient reports can yield useful information.

## Underreporting

Another well-recognized limitation of spontaneous postmarketing reporting systems is underreporting. Because most systems are voluntary, not all AEs/ADRs are reported. A consequence of underreporting of AEs/ADRs is that population-based rates of AEs/ADRs cannot be calculated, because all such occurrences in the population are not reported, and the extent of underreporting for any individual AE/ADR is not known. Reporting ratios, discussed earlier in this chapter, allow the reported number of AEs/ADRs to be put into the context of drug utilization, though this measure is not an incidence rate.

## Non-uniform Temporal Trends in Reporting

Another limitation of spontaneous reporting systems is that temporal trends in the number of AE/ADR reports for a drug–event combination may not reflect actual population-based trends for the drug–event combination. This is because multiple factors can affect the number of AE/ADR reports received for a given drug–event pair.

First, the number of reports for a medicine has been thought to peak in the second year after approval and decline thereafter, even though the drug may be used more widely. This phenomenon, known as the Weber effect, was originally described in relation to non-steroidal anti-inflammatory medicines. A more recent analysis of reporting patterns for the angiotensin II receptor blocker class of medicines revealed no discernible trend when the number of reports over time was examined. Specifically, this analysis did not confirm that the number of reports increased toward the end of the second year and declined thereafter. Rather, the analysis indicated that additional factors, such as the approval of additional indications and modifications of the firms' reporting requirements affected the total number of reports received. However, when the number of reports in a year was adjusted for the number of prescriptions dispensed in that year's period, it was found that the adjusted number of reports was highest in the first years after approval and declined thereafter. The frequency of AE/ADR reports per estimated unit of drug utilization may not be constant over time.

Second, publicity about an important new AE/ADR often gives rise to a large number of reports shortly after the publicity, with a decline in the number of reports shortly thereafter. This phenomenon is known as stimulated reporting, and was observed, for example, in the reporting pattern of statin-induced hospitalized rhabdomyolysis after there was publicity of this risk. For these reasons, changes in the number of AE/ADR reports for a given drug–event pair cannot reliably be interpreted as a change in the population-based frequency of the AE/ADR.

Another limitation of a postmarketing reporting system is that it is usually not well suited to ascertaining the relationship of a medicine to an AE/ADR that is common in the treated population, especially if the condition is a manifestation of the underlying illness. In such cases, the combined effect of confounding of patient factors and indication make causality assessment of individual cases difficult.

Finally, duplicate reports of the same AE/ADR may be received by drug manufacturers and health authorities, and if undetected as duplicates, may be entered into the database as multiple occurrences of the same event. Algorithms have been developed, and various methods can be used to identify such reports; nonetheless, this issue is a potential source of bias and limits the utility of data mining or other calculations which rely on "crude" case counts which have not been "de-duplicated."

## Particular Applications

### Case Series and Reporting Rates

Spontaneous AE/ADR reports have at times served as a necessary and sufficient basis for regulatory actions including product withdrawals. For instance, in August 2001 the manufacturer of cerivastatin withdrew that drug from marketing based on "a markedly increased reporting rate of fatal rhabdomyolysis" compared to the other drugs in the statin class. Additional confirmation of the unacceptably high risk of rhabdomyolysis with cerivastatin was eventually available three years later when results of a well-designed epidemiologic study were published. Clearly, that timeframe would have been far too long to delay decisive action, which in retrospect was soundly based on the signal from spontaneous reports. The timely detection of this signal would not have happened without the efforts of the point-of-care clinicians who took the time to report rhabdomyolysis when it occurred in their patients.

### Data Mining Signals

According to the UMC glossary of pharmacovigilance terms, a signal is "a hypothesis of a risk with a medicine, with various levels of evidence and arguments to support it." Signals are identified by UMC analysts from the WHO database (VigiBase) by applying a predefined triage algorithm (data mining) and are reported quarterly in the Signal document, which is circulated in restricted fashion to national pharmacovigilance centers for the purpose of communicating the results of UMC evaluations of potential data mining signals. The disproportionality measure used by the UMC is the Information Component (IC), originally introduced through the BCPNN, which is a logarithmic measure of the disproportionality between the observed and expected reporting of a drug-ADR pair. A positive IC value means that a particular drug–event pair is reported more often than expected, based on all the reports in the database. The following is an example of a signal identified by data mining techniques applied to VigiBase regarding the occurrence of glaucoma with topiramate. Topiramate was approved in the US in 1996 as an anticonvulsant drug. In the second quarter of 2000, reports of topiramate and glaucoma in VigiBase reached the threshold of an "association" (i.e. the lower limit of a 95% Bayesian confidence interval for the IC exceeded zero). When potential signals are identified, the available information is reviewed by the UMC staff and an expert review panel. At the time, there were six cases reported to VigiBase. After review, a summary of the findings was circulated in the Signal document in April 2001 to all national pharmacovigilance centers in the WHO Programme. Later the same year, the Market Authorization Holder issued a Dear Healthcare Professional letter warning about "an ocular syndrome that has occurred in patients receiving topiramate. This syndrome is characterized by acute myopia and secondary angle closure glaucoma." At the time, there were 23 reported cases according to the company. FDA issued a warning in the revised labeling October 1, 2001.

### Signals from Developing Countries

At the annual meetings of the WHO Programme members, country representatives are invited to share problems of current interest in their countries. Below is an example illustrating the kind of issues that have been investigated in developing countries, presented at the 2017 meeting in Uganda:

**Blindness and Retinal Disorder Associated with Clomifene Citrate: Case Series Assessment**

A case of retinal detachment with the use of clomifene citrate that caused irreversible blindness triggered an assessment by the Eritrean Pharmacovigilance Centre. A search of VigiBase identified 24 cases of blindness and retinal disorder. All cases were evaluated using Austin Bradford Hill considerations to assess the causal relation. In all cases, clomifene was reported as the sole suspected drug and in all but three cases no concomitant drugs were reported. There were two cases of blindness in which the reaction abated with sequelae following withdrawal of clomifene. The conclusion was that the findings support a causal relationship and warrant further investigation to substantiate the signal.

## The Future

Spontaneous AE/ADR reporting is an important component of drug safety surveillance. The widespread availability of electronic healthcare data may, at first, seem to undermine the importance of AE/ADR reporting. This is not likely to be the case. Because careful observation at the point of care is an essential component of pharmacovigilance, electronic systems may be able to facilitate AE/ADR reporting in the future, but will not replace it. It is technologically and administratively feasible for carefully designed systems to allow clinicians to report AEs/ADRs directly from electronic medical record systems. If designed properly, these systems could allow for the accurate, complete, and efficient inclusion of laboratory, radiologic, and other diagnostic test results, information which is often incomplete

in current AE/ADR reports. The challenge of such a system will be to encourage reporters to routinely provide a clinically meaningful narrative that concisely explains the clinical course of the AE/ADR and its relationship to medication usage. There is also interest in using modern informatics techniques to facilitate a review of AE reports, especially in large AE databases. For example, the use of natural language processing techniques is being explored to determine if it can identify individual case safety reports that warrant further evaluation, or if it can identify individual case reports that suggest a causal association between a medicine and an AE. Postmarketing safety reporting systems depend on the involvement of healthcare professionals and, in some areas, consumers and patients as well, for high quality AE/ADR reports. As new medicines become available, it will be increasingly necessary to monitor postmarketing safety. Efficient safety reporting infrastructure is particularly important in situations where compassionate use programs are utilized. Pharmacovigilance reporting systems will continue to be the cornerstone of this effort, because of their unique advantages. As social media, active surveillance, and the use of large healthcare databases begin to play a role in drug safety surveillance, demonstrate their utility, and realize their potential, they could become valuable adjuncts to existing pharmacovigilance reporting systems worldwide.

## Key Points

- AEs and ADRs are closely related, but nonetheless distinct, concepts.
- Spontaneous reporting systems are based on the notion that clinical observations made at the point of care are often valuable pieces of information in further refining knowledge of a drug's safety.
- Spontaneous reporting systems can be used to describe adverse drug events, adverse

device events, medication errors, or a combination of these.

- The characteristics and quality of individual case safety reports determine the extent to which the reports can address a drug safety question.
- The organization of national pharmacovigilance centers can vary from one country to the next.
- Data mining of spontaneous reporting databases, which allows relationships and patterns to be seen in the data which would otherwise be missed, can be used to detect drug safety signals and generate hypotheses.

- Interpretation of spontaneous reports always requires careful analysis, thought, and clear communication of results, conclusions, and limitations.
- Because postmarketing safety reporting systems do not capture all cases of an event of interest, it is not possible to calculate an incidence rate for a particular drug–event pair.
- Reporting ratios help put the number of reports of a drug-AE pair into the context of how widely a medicine is used.
- The capability for timely and effective signal detection is a key strength of a postmarketing pharmacovigilance reporting system.

---

**Case Example 7.1**

Spontaneous pharmacovigilance reporting systems: Felbamate

*Background:*
Felbamate is an anticonvulsant agent approved for use in the United States on July 29, 1993. Pre-approval studies showed no evidence of significant, nonreversible hematologic abnormalities.

*Question*
Can spontaneous postmarketing reports identify a signal for a rare event such as aplastic anemia and can safety surveillance result in a regulatory decision and labeling change that supports the safe use of this product?

*Approach*
Within about one year of approval, cases of aplastic anemia were reported to the manufacturer and to the US FDA. This finding prompted a search for and comprehensive review of all case reports of aplastic anemia in persons taking felbamate.

*Results*
- Twenty cases of aplastic anemia, three of them fatal, had been reported in the United States. Review of the case reports suggested a causal role for felbamate,

based on a careful review of the temporal relationship of the AE to use of the drug, the patients' past medical history, and concomitant medication usage.

- An estimated 100 000 patients had taken felbamate during this time. While the true incidence of aplastic anemia in patients taking felbamate cannot be calculated because case ascertainment is likely incomplete, the minimum rate is 20/100000/year, or 200/million/year.
- In contrast, the population background rate of aplastic anemia is low, about two per million per year. Thus, the observed cases of aplastic anemia suggest that aplastic anemia is at least 100 times more frequent in patients taking felbamate than in the general population.

*Outcome*
- Based on this finding, the FDA and the manufacturer recommended that patients not be treated with felbamate unless the benefits of the drug were judged to outweigh the risk of aplastic anemia.
- A subsequent review of 31 case reports of aplastic anemia in patients taking felbamate using the criteria of the International Agranulocytosis and Aplastic

*(Continued)*

**Case Example 7.1    (Continued)**

Anemia Study (IAAAS), established that felbamate was the only plausible cause in three cases, and the most likely cause in 11 cases. For the remaining nine cases, there was at least one other plausible cause. The authors concluded that the "most probable" incidence of aplastic anemia was estimated to be 127 per million.

*Strengths*
- Spontaneous reports of drug AEs can be used to identify ADRs that are rare, serious, and generally the result of a drug or toxin exposure.
- While reporting rates cannot be used to calculate incidence rates, in certain cases a reporting rate can be compared to a background incidence rate to demonstrate that the incidence of the AE in patients exposed to the drug is higher than would be expected in the absence of the drug.

*Limitations*
Formal incidence rates cannot be calculated from spontaneous reports.

*Key Points*
Because aplastic anemia is uncommon in the population and because it is generally the result of a medication or other toxin, a careful analysis of a case series can establish the relationship of a drug to aplastic anemia.

## Further Reading

Almenoff, J., Tonning, J., Gould, A. et al. (2005). Perspectives on the use of data mining in pharmacovigilance. *Drug Saf.* 28 (11): 981–1007.

Bohn, J., Kortepeter, C., Muñoz, M. et al. (2015). Patterns in spontaneous adverse event reporting among branded and generic antiepileptic drugs. *Clin. Pharmacol. Ther.* 97 (5): 508–517.

Edwards, I.R. (2017). Causality assessment in pharmacovigilance: still a challenge. *Drug Saf.* 40 (5): 365–372.

Edwards, I.R. and Lindquist, M. (2011). Social media and networks in pharmacovigilance: boon or bane? *Drug Saf.* 34 (4): 267–271.

EMA. EudraVigilance. http://www.ema.europa. eu/ema/index.jsp?curl=pages/regulation/ general/general_content_000679.jsp

ICH Harmonized Tripartite Guideline (1994). Clinical Safety Data Management: Definitions and Standards for Expedited Reporting E2A. Current Step 4 version, dated 27 October 1994. http://www.ich.org/LOB/media/ MEDIA436.pdf

ICH Harmonized Tripartite Guideline (2003). Post-approval safety data management: definitions and standards for expedited reporting. https://www.fda.gov/media/71228/ download.

Kaufman, D., Kelly, J., Anderson, T. et al. (1997). Evaluation of case reports of aplastic anemia among patients treated with felbamate. *Epilepsia* 38 (12): 1265–1269.

McAdams, M., Governale, L., Swartz, L. et al. (2008). Identifying patterns of adverse event reporting for four members of the Angiotensin II receptor blockers class of drugs: revisiting the weber effect. *Pharmacoepidemiol. Drug Saf.* 17: 882–889.

McAdams, M., Staffa, J., and Dal Pan, G. (2008). Estimating the extent of reporting to FDA: a case study of statin-associated rhabdomyolysis. *Pharmacoepidemiol. Drug Saf.* 17 (3): 229–239.

McMahon, A., Pratt, R., Hammad, T. et al. (2010). Description of hypersensitivity adverse events following administration of heparin that was potentially contaminated with oversulfated chrondroitin sulfate in early 2008. *Pharmacoepidemiol. Drug Saf.* 19 (9): 921–933.

Meyboom, R.H.B., Hekster, Y.A., Egberts, A.C.G. et al. (1997). Causal or casual? The role of causality assessment in pharmacovigilance. *Drug Saf.* 17 (6): 374–389.

Nightingale, S. (1994). Recommendation to immediately withdraw patients from treatment with felbamate. *J. Am. Med. Assoc.* 272 (13): 995.

Russmann, S. (2006). Case reports of suspected adverse drug reactions: case reports generate signals efficiently. *BMJ* 332 (7539): 488.

Sloane, R., Osanlou, O., Lewis, D. et al. (2015). Social media and pharmacovigilance: a review of the opportunities and challenges. *Br. J. Clin. Pharmacol.* 80 (4): 910–920.

Staffa, J., Chang, J., and Green, L. (2002). Cerivastatin and reports of fatal rhabdomyolysis. *N. Engl. J. Med.* 346 (7): 539–540.

van Stekelenborg, J., Ellenius, J., Maskell, S. et al. (2019). Recommendations for the use of social media in pharmacovigilance: lessons from IMI WEB-RADR. *Drug Saf.* 42 (12): 1393–1407.

US Food and Drug Administration (2005a). Guidance for Industry–E2B(M): Data Elements for Transmission of Individual Case Safety Reports. http://www.fda.gov/

RegulatoryInformation/Guidances/ ucm129428.htm.

US Food and Drug Administration (2005b). Guidance for Industry: Good Pharmacovigilance Practices and Pharmacoepidemiologic Assessment. http://www.fda.gov/downloads/ RegulatoryInformationGuidances/ UCM126834.pdf

US Food and Drug Administration (2009) 21 CFR 314.80. http://www.accessdata.fda.gov/ scripts/cdrh/cfdocs/cfcfr/CFRSearch. cfm?fr=314.80 (accessed 4 January 2009).

US Food and Drug Administration (2009). The ICH Guideline on Clinical Safety Data Management: Data Elements for Transmission of Individual Case Safety Reports.

US Food and Drug Administration (2020). MedWatch: The FDA Safety Information and Adverse Events Reporting System. https://www.fda.gov/safety/ medwatch-fda-safety-information-and-adverse-event-reporting-program.

US Food and Drug Administration (2020). Drug Safety Communications. https://www.fda.gov/ Drugs/DrugSafety/ucm199082.htm

World Health Organization (2002). *The Importance of Pharmacovigilance. Safety Monitoring of Medicinal Products.* Geneva: WHO.

# 8

# Overview of Electronic Databases in Pharmacoepidemiology

*Brian L. Strom*

*Rutgers Biomedical and Health Sciences, Newark, NJ, USA*

## Introduction

Once hypotheses about drug-induced adverse effects are generated, usually from spontaneous reporting systems (see Chapter 7), techniques are needed to test these hypotheses. Usually between 500 and 3000 patients are exposed to the drug during Phase III testing, even if drug efficacy can be demonstrated with much smaller numbers of patients. Studies of this size would be expected to observe a single case of outcomes with an incidence of one per 1000 to six per 1000 (see Chapter 3). Given this context, postmarketing studies of drug effects must then generally include at least 10 000 exposed persons in a cohort study, or enroll diseased patients from a population of equivalent size for a case–control study. Given a study of this size, the upper 95% confidence limit for the incidence of any event that is not identified would be three per 10 000 (see Chapter 3). However, prospective studies this large are expensive, and difficult to perform. Yet, such studies often need to be conducted quickly, to address acute and serious regulatory, commercial, and/or public health crises. For all of these reasons, the past decades have seen a growing use of electronic databases containing health care data, sometimes called "automated databases," as potential data sources for pharmacoepidemiologic studies.

Large electronic databases can often meet the need for a cost-effective and efficient means of conducting postmarketing surveillance studies. To meet the needs of pharmacoepidemiology, the ideal database would include records from inpatient and outpatient care, emergency care, mental health care, all laboratory and radiological tests (including pharmacogenomic tests that may not have been performed as part of clinical care), functional assessments, and all prescribed and over-the-counter medications, as well as alternative therapies. The population covered by the database would be large enough to permit discovery of rare events for the drug(s) in question, and the population would be stable over its lifetime. Although it is generally preferable for the population included in the database to be representative of the general population from which it is drawn, it may sometimes be advantageous to emphasize the more disadvantaged groups that may have been absent from premarketing testing. The drug(s) under investigation must of course be present in the formulary and must be prescribed in sufficient quantity to provide adequate power for analyses.

Other requirements of an ideal database are that all parts are easily linked by means of a patient's unique identifier, that the records are updated on a regular basis, and that the records are verifiable and are reliable. The ability to conduct medical chart review to confirm outcomes is also a necessity for most studies (unless validated algorithms for the study outcome already exist), as diagnoses entered into an electronic database may include rule-out diagnoses or interim diagnoses and recurrent/chronic, as opposed to acute, events. Information on potential confounders, such as smoking and alcohol consumption, may only be available through chart review or, more consistently, through patient interviews. With appropriate permissions and confidentiality safeguards in place, access to patients is sometimes possible and useful for assessing compliance with the medication regimen as well as for obtaining biosamples or information on other factors that may relate to drug effects. Information on drugs taken intermittently for symptom relief, over-the-counter drugs, and drugs not on the formulary must also be obtained directly from the patient.

These automated databases are the focus of this section of the book. Of course, no single database is ideal for all questions. In the current chapter, we will introduce these resources, presenting some of the general principles that apply to them all. In Chapters 9 and 10, we will present more detailed descriptions of those databases that have been used in a substantial amount of published research, along with the strengths and weaknesses of each.

## Description

So-called automated databases have existed and been used for pharmacoepidemiologic research in North America since 1980, and are primarily administrative in origin, generated by the request for payments, or claims, for clinical services and therapies. In contrast, electronic health record databases were developed for use by researchers in Europe, and similar databases have been developed in the US more recently.

### Claims and Other Administrative Databases

Claims data arise from billable interactions between patients and the health care system (see Figure 8.1). When a patient goes to a pharmacy and gets a drug dispensed, the pharmacy bills the insurance carrier for the cost of that drug, and has to identify which medication was dispensed, the milligrams per tablet, number of tablets, etc. Analogously, if a patient goes to a hospital or to a physician for medical care, the providers of care bill the insurance carrier for the cost of the medical care, and have to justify the bill with a diagnosis. If there is a common patient identification number for both the pharmacy and the medical care claims, these elements could be linked, and analyzed as a longitudinal medical record.

Since drug identity and the amount of drug dispensed affect reimbursement, and because the filing of an incorrect claim about drugs dispensed is fraud, claims are often closely audited, e.g. by Medicaid. Indeed, there have also been numerous validity checks on the drug data in claims files that showed that the drug data are of extremely high quality, i.e. confirming that the patient was dispensed exactly what the claim showed was dispensed, according to the pharmacy record. In fact, claims data of this type provide some of the best data on drug exposure in pharmacoepidemiology (see Chapter 13).

Claims Databases: Sources of Data

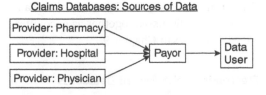

**Figure 8.1** Sources of claims data.

The quality of disease data in these databases is somewhat less perfect. If a patient is admitted to a US hospital, the hospital charges for the care and justifies that charge by assigning diagnosis codes (until recently International Classification of Diseases-Ninth Revision-Clinical Modification [ICD-9-CM] codes) and a Diagnosis Related Group (DRG). Hospital diagnosis codes are reasonably accurate diagnoses that are used for clinical purposes, based primarily on the discharge diagnoses assigned by the patient's attending physician (of course, this does not guarantee that the physician's diagnosis is correct). The amount paid by the insurer to the hospital is based on the DRG, so there is no financial incentive to provide incorrect diagnosis codes. In fact, most hospitals have mapped each set of diagnosis codes into the DRG code that generates the largest payment.

In contrast, however, outpatient diagnoses are assigned by the practitioners themselves, or by their office staff. Once again, reimbursement in the US does not usually depend on the actual diagnosis, but rather on the visit intensity during the outpatient medical encounter, and the resulting procedure codes indicate the intensity of the services provided. Thus, there is no incentive for the practitioner to provide incorrect diagnosis codes, but there is also no incentive for them to be particularly careful or complete about the diagnoses provided. For these reasons, the outpatient diagnoses are the weakest link in claims databases.

Some other databases are not made up of actual claims, but derive from other administrative processes, e.g. data from US Health Maintenance Organizations or other data sources. The characteristics of these data are similar in many ways to those of claims data, and they are discussed together as encounter-based databases in Chapter 9.

### Electronic Health Record Databases

In contrast, electronic health record databases are a more recent development, arising out of the increasing use of computerization in medical care. Initially, computers were used in Medicine primarily as a tool for literature searches. Then, they were used for billing. Now, however, there is increasing use of computers to record medical information at the point of care. In most instances, this is replacing the paper medical record as the primary medical record. As medical practices increasingly become electronic, this opens up a unique opportunity for pharmacoepidemiology, as larger and larger numbers of patients are available in such systems. The best-known and most widely used example of this approach is the UK Clinical Practice Research Database (CPRD), along with the newer database, The Health Improvement Network (THIN), both described in Chapter 10. As general practice databases, these contain primarily outpatient data. In addition, recently there are inpatient electronic health record databases available.

Electronic health record databases have unique advantages. Importantly among them is that the validity of the diagnosis data in these databases is probably better than that in claims databases, as these data are being used to document medical care rather than just for billing purposes. When performing a pharmacoepidemiologic study using these databases, there is no purpose in validating the data against the actual medical record, since one is analyzing the data from the actual medical record. However, there are also unique issues one needs to be concerned about, especially the uncertain completeness of the data from other physicians and sites of care. Any given practitioner provides only a piece of the care a patient receives, and inpatient and outpatient care are unlikely to be recorded in a common medical record.

### Strengths

Computerized databases have several important advantages. These include their potential for providing a very large sample size. This is especially important in the field of pharma-coepidemiology, where achieving an adequate sample size is uniquely problematic. In addition, these databases are relatively inexpensive to use, especially given the available sample size, as they are by-products of existing administrative systems. Studies using these data systems do not need to incur the considerable cost of data collection, other than for those subsets of the populations for whom medical records are abstracted and/or interviews are conducted. The data can be complete, i.e. for claims databases, information is available on all medical care provided for covered services, regardless of who the provider was. As indicated above, this can be a problem though for electronic health record databases, especially in the US, where primary care providers often do not serve as gatekeepers to specialty care. In addition, these databases can be population-based, they can include outpatient drugs and diseases, and there is no opportunity for recall and interviewer bias, as they do not rely on patient recall or interviewers to obtain their data. Another advantage is that these databases can potentially be linked to external other electronic databases (e.g. death records, maternal-child records, police accident records), to expand the capabilities and scope of research. This requires using common identification elements (e.g. name and date of birth) and standardized semantics to allow communication across databases.

## Weaknesses

The major weakness of such data systems is the uncertain validity of diagnosis data. This is especially true for claims databases, and for outpatient data. For these databases, access to medical record data for validation purposes is usually needed. This issue is less problematic for electronic health record databases; however, the validity of medication data from electronic health record databases in the United States is less certain than pharmacy dispensing data from claims databases. The addition of laboratory results data to these resources can assist in diagnosis validity, as well.

In addition, such databases can lack information on some potential confounding variables. For example, in claims databases there are no data on date of menopause, and diagnosis-based algorithms to identify smoking and alcohol abuse may have poor sensitivity, all of which can be of great importance to selected research questions. This argues that one either needs access to patients or access to physician records if these contain the data in question, or one needs to be selective about the research questions that one seeks to answer through these databases, avoiding questions that require data on variables which may be important potential confounders that must be controlled for.

A major other disadvantage of administrative data is the instability of the population due to job changes, employers' changes of health plans, and changes in coverage for specific employees and their family members. The opportunity for longitudinal analyses is thereby hindered by the continual enrollment and dis-enrollment of plan members. Another source of instability of the population is when patients transfer out of the system due to death or relocation. The effect of this is an inflated list with patients no longer seeking medical care. This will invalidate calculations of patient-time in studies of disease incidence, for example, because the denominator is inflated. The challenge for the investigator is to be creative in devising strategies to guard or correct for this incomplete information in the database (e.g. by performing sensitivity analysis censoring follow-up one or two years after the patient's last recorded entry in the database). Alternatively, strategies can be adopted for selecting stable populations within a particular database, and for example, by examining patterns of prescription refills for chronically used medications and by restricting the study population to include only continuously enrolled patients. Of course, the largest such data system, i.e. US Medicare, suffers much less from this problem, since it covers the elderly, so people never lose eligibility. Even there, however, patients can switch between fee-for-service plans and managed care plans, and the latter may not record all health care that is provided (see Chapter 9).

Further, by definition, such databases only include illnesses severe enough to come to medical attention. In general, this is not a problem, since illnesses that are not serious enough to come to medical attention and yet are uncommon enough for one to seek to study them in such databases, are generally of lower importance.

Some results from studies that utilize these databases may not be generalizable, e.g. on health care utilization. This is especially relevant for databases created by data from a population that is atypical in some way, e.g. US Medicaid data.

Finally, as noted briefly above, as an increasing number of electronic health record databases emerge in the US, to date all are problematic in that they do not include complete data on a defined population. In the US health system, unlike other countries, patients can, and often do, seek medical care from a variety of different health care providers at unaffiliated institutions with a non-linked electronic health record system. Thus, providers' electronic health records are inherently incomplete, and need to be linked to administrative data in order to be useful for quality research. This is different from the situation in, for example, the UK, where electronic health record databases are much more likely to be complete given the general practitioner gatekeeper paradigm and unique patient identifier for all healthcare services.

## Particular Applications

Based on these characteristics, one can identify particular situations when these databases are uniquely useful or uniquely problematic for pharmacoepidemiologic research. These databases are useful in situations: (i) when looking for uncommon outcomes because of a large sample size, (ii) when a denominator is needed to calculate incidence rates, (iii) when one is studying short-term drug effects (especially when the effects require specific drug or surgical therapy that can be used as validation of the diagnosis), (iv) when one is studying objective, laboratory-driven diagnoses, (v) when recall or interviewer bias could influence the association, (vi) when time is limited, and (vii) when the budget is limited.

Uniquely problematic situations include: (i) illnesses that do not reliably come to medical attention, (ii) inpatient drug exposures that are not included in some of these databases, (iii) outcomes that are poorly captured by the coding system, such as Stevens-Johnson Syndrome, (iv) descriptive studies, if the population studied is non-representative, (v) delayed drug effects, wherein patients can lose eligibility in the interim, and (vi) important confounders about which information cannot be obtained without accessing the patients, such as cigarette smoking, occupation, menarche, menopause, etc.

## The Future

Given the frequent use of these data resources for pharmacoepidemiologic research in the recent past, we have already learned much about their appropriate role. Inasmuch as it appears that these uses will be increasing, we are likely to continue to gain more insight in the coming years, especially with the access in the US to Medicare data, and the advent in the US of FDA's Sentinel system, exceeding 170 million individuals. However, care must be taken to ensure that all potential confounding factors of interest are available in the system or addressed in some other way, that diagnoses under study are chosen carefully, and that medical records can be obtained when needed to validate the diagnoses. In this section of the book, Chapters 9 and 10, we will review the details of a number of these databases. The databases selected for detailed review have been chosen because they have been the most widely used for published research. They are also good examples of the different types of data that are available. There are multiple others like each of them and undoubtedly many more will emerge over the ensuing years. Each has its advantages and disadvantages, but each has proven it can be useful in pharmacoepidemiologic studies.

## Key Points

- The past three decades have seen a growing use of computerized databases containing medical care data, so-called "automated databases," as potential data sources for pharmacoepidemiology studies.

- Claims data arise from a person's use of the health care system, and the submission of claims to insurance companies for payment. While claims data provide some of the best data on drug exposure in pharmacoepidemiology, the quality of disease data in these databases can be more problematic.

- Medical record databases are a more recent development, arising out of the increasing use of computerization in medical care. The validity of the diagnosis data in these databases is better than that in claims databases, as these data are being used for medical care. However, the completeness of the data from other physicians and sites of care is uncertain.

## Further Reading

Ray, W.A. and Griffin, M.R. (1989). Use of Medicaid data for pharmacoepidemiology. *Am. J. Epidemiol.* 129: 837–849.

Strom, B.L. and Carson, J.L. (1989). Automated data bases used for pharmacoepidemiology research. *Clin. Pharmacol. Ther.* 46: 390–394.

Strom, B.L. and Carson, J.L. (1990). Use of automated databases for pharmacoepidemiology research. *Epidemiol. Rev.* 12: 87–107.

# 9

# Encounter Databases

*Tobias Gerhard[1], Yola Moride[2], Anton Pottegård[3], and Nicole Pratt[4]*

[1] Ernest Mario School of Pharmacy, Rutgers Biomedical and Health Sciences, Piscataway, NJ, USA
[2] Center for Pharmacoepidemiology and Treatment Science, Rutgers Biomedical and Health Sciences, New Brunswick, NJ, USA
[3] Clinical Pharmacology and Pharmacy, Department of Public Health, University of Southern Denmark, Odense, Denmark
[4] Quality Use of Medicines and Pharmacy Research Centre, Clinical and Health Sciences, University of South Australia, Adelaide, South Australia, Australia

## Introduction

Encounter databases contain electronic records of healthcare encounters for large, defined populations. They capture information on patient characteristics, prescription fills, and medical services, as part of the routine administration or reimbursement of healthcare. This is in contrast to electronic health record (EHR) databases, described in detail in Chapter 10, which are primarily intended and maintained to support patient care. Encounter data may contain records at various levels of granularity ranging from records of individual services (fee-for-service claims) to aggregate records of care episodes (hospital discharge records). Encounter databases exist in many countries and within a number of vastly different healthcare systems. An increasing number are available for research and consequently, encounter databases have become a cornerstone of pharmacoepidemiologic research. Although they vary markedly in their specific characteristics, encounter databases share a number of defining features that warrant their discussion as a group. Rather than attempting to provide an encyclopedic description of available databases, this chapter focuses on the description of key commonalities and distinctions across encounter databases, illustrated with selected examples and supplemented by references to more comprehensive resources in the literature. The chapter also includes a dedicated discussion of the considerations faced by researchers when evaluating the appropriateness of a specific encounter database or deciding among multiple encounter databases for their research question.

## Description

Encounter data arise as part of the routine administration of a person's interactions with various sectors of the healthcare system. When combined, these data can be used to infer a longitudinal picture of a person's medical and treatment history. The quality of that picture, i.e. its usefulness for pharmacoepidemiologic and other research, depends on the completeness and validity of the information available.

*Textbook of Pharmacoepidemiology*, Third Edition. Edited by Brian L. Strom, Stephen E. Kimmel, and Sean Hennessy.
© 2022 John Wiley & Sons Ltd. Published 2022 by John Wiley & Sons Ltd.

The essential attribute of all encounter databases useful for pharmacoepidemiologic research is a defined population for which healthcare services are recorded regardless of the provider or location of care received (e.g. outpatient, inpatient, emergency department). Such databases are considered *population-based* (see Chapter 12). Precise definition of the database population avoids various forms of selection bias common in non-population-based studies (e.g. biased control selection in hospital-based case–control studies). Complete capture of all relevant healthcare services avoids bias from incomplete and potentially differential measurement of healthcare services (e.g. incomplete ascertainment of hospitalizations occurring in a non-participating healthcare system). Although representativeness of a geographic region or the general population is often desirable, it is not necessary, as long as the database population is accurately defined. While encounter databases ideally capture all healthcare services, in practice specific service types may not be captured due to the nature of the data collection process (most often due to lack of reimbursement). However, accurate qualitative description of the specific service types with lack of coverage or incomplete capture is critically important to allow evaluation of the appropriateness of the database for a given research question.

Encounter databases are maintained by a number of different entities including government agencies, insurance companies, health plans, and information services companies. The primary purpose of encounter databases is often the reimbursement of fee-for-service payment claims, and such encounter data are often referred to as claims data. In some instances, however, for example in US health plans with staff model delivery systems or capitated payment models, the purpose is purely administrative with no processing of payments for individual services. This distinction can be important as the accuracy and validity of data correspond to the purpose of the record. For example, claims records are routinely audited to prevent fraud and thus assure high accuracy of the data in instances where the information is directly relevant to the processing of the correct payment amount (e.g. quantity and dose of medications dispensed by a community pharmacy or type of procedure performed during an outpatient physician visit). In contrast, data elements that are not directly tied to the payment, for example, the specific diagnoses associated with an outpatient visit or procedure may be recorded with lower accuracy. In purely administrative databases, data characteristics depend on the specific data collection and quality assurance processes in place for each of the data elements.

While an ideal encounter database would capture all types of healthcare services, in practice, individual databases often lack coverage of certain service types depending on the purpose of the database and the nature of the data collection process. The completeness of information captured in a database is a function of the types of healthcare services (data domains) included, as well as of the comprehensiveness of data capture within each domain. Encounter databases useful for pharmacoepidemiologic research typically contain the following core data domains: (i) healthcare plan eligibility and basic demographic information, (ii) outpatient pharmacy dispensing, and (iii) medical services (typically including hospitalizations; commonly also including outpatient health services).

Data domains may be maintained in separate files within a single *integrated* database (e.g. US private and governmental databases), or in multiple autonomous databases that together function as a *federated* virtual database (e.g. Nordic healthcare databases), depending on whether the data are collected and maintained by a single or by multiple entities. Both integrated and federated databases require reliable linkage of an individual's records over time and between data domains. Table 9.1 summarizes commonly available data elements within the core data domains. The content of the core data domains often

**Table 9.1** Core data domains in encounter databases[a].

| | |
|---|---|
| **Membership** | Patient identifier, sex, age/date of birth, race/ethnicity (not universally available), zip code, dates of enrollment and disenrollment, benefits package/eligibility category (if applicable). |
| **Medical** Outpatient Services | Patient identifier, encounter date, service location (physician office, hospital outpatient, etc.), procedure codes (e.g. CPT, HCPCS), primary and secondary diagnosis codes (e.g. ICD-10-CM), provider identifier, provider profession/specialty. |
| Inpatient Services | Patient identifier, primary diagnosis, secondary diagnoses, admission and discharge dates, length of stay, patient destination, hospital identifier. Inpatient data generally do not include information on in-hospital medication use and typically represent summaries for an entire hospital stay, resulting in some lack of detail. |
| **Pharmacy** | Patient identifier, unique drug identifier (e.g. US-NDC, Nordic article number) which identifies generic name, brand name, dosage form, and strength (crosswalks may be needed for some databases while others include the individual data elements coded by the unique identifier), date dispensed, quantity dispensed, prescription duration/days supply. |
| | Typically, not recorded: Indication for the prescription, inpatient drug use, over- the-counter drugs. |

[a] adapted from Chapter 13, Strom et al. (2012); CPT, Current Procedural Terminology; HCPCS, Healthcare Common Procedure Coding System; ICD, International Classification of Diseases; NDC, National Drug Code.

varies across individual databases in terms of which types of healthcare services are captured. While some databases are limited to hospital discharge data, many also capture data on outpatient office-based physician visits, outpatient clinic visits, long-term care facilities, dental, and vision services. Another example for incomplete data capture within a data domain, is incomplete or lack of recording of over-the-counter (OTC) medication fills in prescription databases. Similar variability across databases exists in terms of access to non-encounter data, such as EHRs, laboratory test results, diagnostic examinations, provider specialty/characteristics, vital statistics, or disease registries. Lastly, profound differences also exist in data structure and coding systems.

Because the primary purpose of encounter data is administrative, any inferences about a patient's medical history made from these data have to be carefully evaluated. Validation of encounter data, ranging from the validation of individual data elements to the validation of

complex encounter data-based algorithms, is critical for rigorous pharmacoepidemiologic research with encounter databases (see Chapter 13). Validation necessitates the ability to reliably link an individual's encounter data to non-encounter data sources that serve as the external gold standard, such as electronic or paper medical records, disease registries, or survey data. Furthermore, linkage with complementary non-encounter data resources or ad hoc data collection (see Chapter 11) is also commonly implemented in order to supplement an encounter database with variables that are required to answer a specific research question but are not recorded in the database, such as lifestyle factors or disease severity.

Because of their size, population-based nature, comprehensive capture of the full spectrum of healthcare encounters, and ability to rapidly assemble cohorts and identify outcomes among them, encounter databases represent a tremendous resource for pharmacoepidemiologic studies. For some research questions, encounter data may be sufficient on their own, particularly when the outcome of interest has been previously validated and data on all important confounders are available within the database. In many instances however, validation of outcomes and supplementation with external data are necessary. In these cases, the encounter databases provide the study foundation (population base and comprehensive capture of healthcare interactions) with certain data elements critical to the study question fleshed out through linkage with additional data resources.

## Attributes of Encounter Databases

Although encounter databases share a basic set of defining characteristics, they differ in numerous attributes that deserve consideration when evaluating the fit of a database to address a specific research question. Importantly, in some databases, such as the US commercial insurance databases, these attributes can be heterogeneous across individual people, as availability of supplemental data (e.g. laboratory test results or ability to retrieve medical records) or even core data domains (e.g. pharmacy dispensing data) may be restricted to subsets of the full database population. In these instances, the suitability of the database (e.g. in terms of sample size and representativeness) should be evaluated based on the subset of the population in a given database for which the attributes required to address the question under study (i.e. key study variables) are available rather than the database population as a whole.

### Population and Coverage Period

The population captured is a critically important consideration when examining the suitability of an encounter database for the study of a specific research question of interest. The *size of the database* is typically one of the key criteria when considering an encounter database for a specific research question; both in comparison to electronic medical record databases as well as in comparison to alternative encounter databases. A large study population is generally necessary to ensure adequate statistical power when exposures or outcomes are rare (particularly when both are rare), effect sizes are small, and when subgroup effects or treatment effect heterogeneity are of interest. In addition, some common study designs and analytic methods may further increase the size of the database necessary to achieve adequate statistical power. For example, the new-user active comparator design results in study populations that often represent only a small fraction of the total number of users of a drug of interest during the study period; restriction, a common approach to reduce confounding, can substantially decrease the size of study cohorts; and instrumental variable methods are statistically inefficient compared to standard regression approaches (see Chapter 22).

In addition to the size of the database, the *characteristics of the database population* have to be carefully considered. As a general rule, the population covered by an encounter database is a function of the underlying healthcare system in the respective country during the study period. Knowledge of these systems is a prerequisite for informed consideration and use of databases for pharmacoepidemiologic research. Databases in countries or regions with universal single-payer coverage, such as Taiwan, South Korea, and the Northern European countries, generally include the entire population and do not impose eligibility restrictions. All individuals are included and membership is maintained throughout a person's life regardless of qualifying factors such as age, employment, or financial situation. Therefore, the characteristics of the population included in these databases are stable over time and closely track the characteristics of the population of the respective country or region as a whole. In contrast, database populations in countries or regions with less complete or more fragmented coverage, including the US, are heterogeneous and far more complicated. The fragmentation of the US healthcare system, in particular, leads to a complex landscape for encounter databases with different databases covering distinctly different subsets of the US population (discussed in more detail below). Furthermore, individuals may be included in different databases at different points in time based on their personal situation (e.g. employment and state of residence), resulting in short average enrollment periods (dwell times) in any specific database environment. *Dwell time* is an important consideration particularly when the research question of interest involves studying a long-term effect of a medicine. Similarly, when dwell time is short, it becomes increasing difficult to study new users of medicines as a lag time at the start of an individual's data capture is required to differentiate incident from prevalent medication exposure.

Lastly, the *time period covered by a database* often determines its usefulness for a given study question, depending on the start of data collection and recency of the latest available data. Studies examining trends in drug utilization over time or studies on the long-term effects of drugs, such as studies with cancer as an outcome, are best served by databases with long coverage periods and a stable population. Studies of newly approved medications primarily require the most current data available. The US Medicaid Analytic Extracts (MAX) data, for example, are generally not appropriate for studies of recently approved drugs, due to a two to three year lag in data availability. Importantly, when studying long-term utilization trends or long-term drug effects, it is important to be cognizant of any changes over time in health service reimbursement and administration and appreciate their impact on drug utilization.

### Services Covered and Data Completeness

For obvious reasons, medication data are a prerequisite for all encounter databases used for pharmacoepidemiologic research. Generally, these data are limited to information on medications dispensed by community pharmacies. Drugs administered during hospital stays or in long-term care units, in the emergency room, or in outpatient physician office settings are typically not included. The latter, however, can in some instances be captured through drug-specific outpatient procedure codes (e.g. drug-specific procedure codes for injection administration). OTC drug use is generally not recorded, unless OTC drugs are prescribed and specifically covered by the insurance or health system. In databases for which data capture depends on a reimbursement mechanism, drug dispensing may also be missing in cases where drugs are paid for entirely out of pocket (i.e. because the cash price is lower than the required copayment), or for non-reimbursable drugs (benzodiazepines, for example, were excluded from reimbursement by Medicare Part D prior to 2013).

Lastly, drug formularies, stepped therapy requirements, and prior authorization programs may impose restrictions on availability and copayments and thus have a significant impact on use rates of individual medications and medication classes. Individual formularies may apply to an entire database population or vary widely across individuals depending on the underlying healthcare system.

Encounter databases also vary substantially in terms of which medical services are included and importantly what information is captured about these services. Most widely used encounter databases capture hospital services including emergency departments. Hospital services are generally recorded as hospital discharge data that summarize information for an entire hospital or emergency department stay rather than provide documentation of individual services. Differences, however, exist in the granularity of these data, such as number of diagnosis fields and availability of procedure codes.

Even greater variation between databases exists in the capture of outpatient services. For example, in contrast to databases in the US, Canada, Taiwan, and South Korea, the Nordic countries do not maintain a database of outpatient office-based physician visits, though visits to outpatient hospital/specialty clinics are captured. Therefore, Nordic database studies of outcomes that do not result in hospitalizations or that require outpatient office-based diagnoses for adjustment of confounding have to rely on medication use as a proxy for outpatient office-based diagnoses. Capture of other service types, such as dental, vision, or long-term care also depend on the database and the patient's specific insurance coverage. Lastly, particularly in the US, specific benefits such as mental health or other specialty services may be excluded ("carved out") in certain benefits packages and thus not captured for individuals covered under these plans. For many databases, it is thus important to evaluate the availability of data on specific service types not only at the level of the database but at the individual level and over time using information on each person's benefit package.

Finally, databases differ in the information available about the patient and service provider. For example, data on the patient's race and ethnicity are generally not available in US administrative claims databases but available in US governmental databases. Similarly, death is reliably recorded in some databases while others require linkage to vital statistics. Databases also differ in the availability of provider specialty and identity for physician medical services as well as prescriber specialty and identity for dispensing data.

### Linkage to Non-encounter Data

Many pharmacoepidemiologic research questions cannot be answered with encounter data alone. Some questions will require randomized trials (see Chapter 17) or prospective primary data collection (see Chapter 11). However, linkages to complementary sources of data may help to overcome inherent limitations of encounter data. Commonly used sources for non-encounter data include electronic or paper medical records, laboratory test results, cause of death registries or autopsy records, disease or immunization registries, census data, biobanks, or survey data. Linkage of encounter data to complementary data sources serves two distinct purposes: (i) validation of encounter-based information against an external gold-standard, and (ii) provision of supplementary data not available in the encounter database, such as disease-specific data and symptoms. Linkage to an external gold standard, ideally the medical record, for a sample of cases is particularly critical in order to facilitate outcome validation and calculation of positive predictive values (PPVs) of encounter data-based algorithms. In absence of the medical record, validation may be performed against disease registries or patient self-report/survey. The validity of pharmacoepidemiologic drug and diagnosis data as well as approaches to the conduct of validation studies are discussed in detail in Chapter 13. The ability to retrieve medical records for outcome validation varies between databases and is often a critical factor in database selection.

Linkage to non-encounter data may also be necessary to provide supplemental information on variables that are unmeasured or poorly measured in the encounter data but necessary to adjust for confounding or appropriate restriction of the study population (e.g. indication for drug prescribing, lifestyle factors, measures of disease severity). Supplemental information such as laboratory test results or autopsy records may also be required for outcome ascertainment (e.g. HbA1c level as an outcome for a study on the comparative effectiveness of various hypoglycemic agents).

Due to privacy restrictions that prevent the sharing or use of personal identifiers, retrieval of medical records or information obtained through direct contact with physicians or patients is generally not performed by investigators, but rather facilitated through third parties (e.g. retrieval of redacted medical records for US Medicaid and Medicare) or handled internally by employees of the participating health plans (e.g. in several US commercial insurance databases). Depending on the database, encounter and non-encounter data may be available under the same umbrella organization (e.g. linkage to EHRs in many US health plans) or require linkage to outside entities (e.g. retrieval of hospital medical records for US Medicaid beneficiaries for the purpose of outcome validation), which greatly affects the feasibility, efficiency, cost, and success rates of the linkage.

Healthcare data linkages are governed by both privacy restrictions and the availability of common linkage variables in the respective databases. Privacy regulations governing the ability to link personal health information are complex and vary between countries, database owners, and over time. When these regulations do not preclude linkage, health information databases can be linked using either deterministic or probabilistic methods. Briefly, in deterministic linkage, a unique identifier or a combination of several non-unique variables available in both databases must match exactly (though the match can be implemented based on transformed versions of the variables, e.g. phonetic codes instead of names to minimize the impact of spelling errors). Deterministic linkage is most useful if reliable unique identifiers are available (e.g. US social security number) but is also achievable with combinations of multiple non-unique variables (e.g. birth dates, admission dates, and names). However, use of variables with low discriminative power and errors or missingness in the matching variable(s) will lead to a high number of overlooked (false negative) matches. Probabilistic linkage methods can reduce the number of overlooked (false negative) matches by allowing imperfect matches due to partially inaccurate or missing data but in turn may produce false positive matches. Choice of matching method thus involves a trade-off between false negative matches (i.e. missed matches) and false positive matches (i.e. incorrectly matched records). Simulation studies have suggested that deterministic linkage is an equally valid but less computationally intensive method for databases with low rates of missingness and error in the linkage variables. However, probabilistic linkage is more accurate in error prone data. Although often challenging, validation of linkage quality is critically important as all linkage methods are susceptible to error. The Nordic prescription database networks are examples of highly reliable linkage between encounter data and disease registries with unique identifiers while the Dutch PHARMO system uses probabilistic record linkage methods.

### Access

Access regulations, costs, and feasibility considerations vary widely between encounter databases and often have a major impact on database choice. Access may, for example, be restricted to certain researchers, such as those working in academia or governmental agencies. Some encounter databases facilitate direct access to either "off the shelf" or customized anonymized datasets which may be physically transferred to the researcher's institution or accessed remotely (e.g. select US commercial databases, US governmental databases, or the South Korean HIRA data), while others require in-house data analyses and thus necessitate collaborative agreements with researchers employed by the database custodian or affiliated research institutes (e.g. US health plan databases or Nordic prescription databases). Some databases are directly accessible in anonymized form but require in-house analysis performed by the database custodian when additional "custom" linkages that require personal identifiers have to be implemented (e.g. Truven MarketScan). For studies conducted through the database custodian, it is important to not only consider the attributes of the database itself, but also the data analytic capacity and track record of the in-house research collaborators. While complexity of database structure varies between databases and studies, all work with large encounter databases requires sophisticated programming skills as well as a comprehensive understanding of database-specific details. The latter consideration can be a major advantage of collaborative arrangements that include researchers or programmers from the database custodian.

Costs of data access vary across databases and often within databases depending on the specific characteristics of the study in question. Fees often vary by size (number of individuals) and complexity (number of files/data sources/number of years of data) of the requested dataset as well as by funding source (e.g. federal versus commercial funding). In-house data analysis often imposes substantial additional costs.

Application processes vary widely as well. While all databases require compliance with data privacy and security restrictions, some may also impose scientific vetting of the research plan or a justification of the benefit of the research to the public. Particularly in projects that require custom linkage with identifiable patient or provider information, close collaboration with the database custodian is needed to obtain necessary approvals and maintain confidentiality. In addition, the time required for the creation of study-specific data-cuts depends on the staffing resources and experience at the database custodian and the complexity of the required dataset. As a result, the duration from the beginning of the application process until the start of the research can vary dramatically between several weeks to multiple years.

In practice, while access considerations and familiarity with a given database are often important drivers of database choice, it is vital never to lose sight of the suitability of the database to the specific research question under study (fit-for-purpose).

## Selected Encounter Databases

A selection of widely used encounter databases and database types with their basic characteristics is presented in Table 9.2 and discussed below. Databases will be discussed by region and include US databases, Canadian databases, European databases, and Asian databases.

## Encounter Databases in the United States

US encounter databases are arguably both the largest databases available and the most fragmented worldwide. Unlike most industrialized nations, the US does not have a uniform health system or universal healthcare coverage resulting in databases with characteristics that differ markedly from databases in the rest of the world. In 2018, 324 million people, or 92% of the US population had health insurance coverage, with 27 million uninsured. 217 million people had coverage from private plans (67%), mostly employment-based plans (178 million, 55%). 111 million people (34%) had coverage from a governmental plan; 58 million by Medicaid (18%), 58 million by Medicare (18%), and 3 million had coverage from the Department of Veterans Affairs Healthcare System (1%). Note that these census data-based estimates show some inconsistencies with the reporting from the Centers for Medicare and Medicaid Services (CMS) presented later in the chapter. Broadly speaking, most employed individuals and their dependents are covered by commercial insurance, adults 65 years and older and qualifying individuals with disabilities are covered by Medicare, and the poor and other disadvantaged groups are covered by Medicaid. Furthermore, insurance coverage in the US is not mutually exclusive. In 2018, 15% of the population with health insurance had multiple coverage types either due to switches in coverage type or due to simultaneous coverage to supplement their primary insurance type.

With the exception of Medicaid programs, which generally provide prescription drug coverage for all beneficiaries, prescription drug insurance is typically provided separately from medical insurance resulting in subgroups of patients in major databases for whom only pharmacy or medical data are available. Although pharmacy claims are recorded with high accuracy, medication dispensing can be incompletely captured in patients covered by multiple insurance programs or in instances

**Table 9.2** Select database characteristics.

| Type | Government, US | Government, US | Health System Databases, US | Commercial Insurance, US | Government, Canada | Government, Northern Europe | Government, Asia |
|---|---|---|---|---|---|---|---|
| Examples | Medicare | Medicaid Analytic Extract (MAX) | Kaiser, Geisinger | HealthCore, MarketScan, Optum, Pharmetrics | Saskatchewan, Quebec | Denmark, Norway, Sweden, Netherlands | South Korea, Taiwan |
| Networks | Sentinel | Sentinel | HCSRN, Sentinel, PCORnet, VSD | Sentinel, CNODES | CNODES | PROTECT | AsPEN |
| Population | | | | | Province | Country | Country |
| Relative Size | +++ | +++ | ++ | +++ | ++ | ++ | +++ |
| Dwell time | +++ | + to ++ | + to ++ | + | +++ | ++++ | ++++ |
| Lag in availability | 3–4 years | 1–2years | <1/2 year | <1/2 year | Variable | Up to 2 years | Variable |
| Access | Direct | Direct | In-house | In-house | < 1–2years | In-house | Variable |
| Retrieval of Medical Records for Validation | Yes | Yes | Yes | Partial | No[a] | Yes | Yes for some databases |
| Coding, Drug | NDC | NDC | NDC | NDC | AHFS | ATC | ATC |
| Coding, Dx | ICD-9-CM, ICD-10-CM | ICD-9-CM, ICD-10-CM | ICD-9-CM, ICD-10-CM | ICD-9-CM, ICD-10-CM | ICD-9-CM, ICD-10-CM | ICD-8, −9 and −10 | ICD-10, ICD-9 |
| Validation | +++ | +++ | ++++ | + to +++ | ++ | ++ | ++ |
| Supplementation | +++ | ++ | ++++ | + to +++ | ++ | +++ | +++ |

[a] Apart from a few rare exceptions, one cannot retrieve medical charts of cases ascertained in a given study. However, can identify patients in medical records in institutions and link back to the database.

where the copayment is greater than the cash price of the medication. In recent years, several large US retailers have begun to offer low-cost generic medications for as little as $4 for a monthly supply, considerably less than the average tier 1 copayment ($11 in 2019). Since there is no financial incentive, pharmacies may not submit insurance claims when patients pay cash resulting in potential under-ascertainment of low cost generic medications. To date, empirical studies examining the missingness of dispensing in claims databases have reported a limited impact of such generic drug discount programs. Payments rates and modalities for medical services vary widely ranging from fee-for service to capitated arrangements in which providers receive a fixed payment per patient per unit of time for the delivery of a specified set of services. Detailed claims data are often not available for services or patients covered by such capitated payment models as the payment amount is independent from the specific services provided.

Several large US encounter databases are available and have been widely used for pharmacoepidemiologic research. These databases include markedly different groups of the population and often individuals with heterogeneous healthcare coverage are included within the same database. To complicate matters further, significant mobility exists between databases as changing life circumstances (loss of employment, change in employer, disability, reaching age 65/Medicare eligibility) result in changes in insurance coverage. This is often referred to as "churning," and substantially affects the average dwell time of individuals in US encounter databases.

US databases generally use the National Drug Code (NDC) for medication data, the Current Procedural Terminology (CPT) coding and Healthcare Common Procedure Coding System (HCPCS) for procedures, and the International Classification of Diseases, Clinical Modification (ICD-CM) system for diagnoses. The US transitioned from ICD-9-CM to ICD-10-CM on October 1, 2015, which

has important implications for pharmacoepidemiologic research conducted in US databases. Despite the existence of crosswalks, the performance characteristics of encounter-data based algorithms have to be demonstrated for the new coding system and studies that span the transition date will have to implement multiple coding systems in a single study. Data privacy and security of identifiable healthcare data in the US is governed by the Health Insurance Portability and Accountability Act of 1996 (HIPAA).

### US Private Insurance Databases

Most healthcare in the US is covered through private insurance, predominantly employer-based insurance. For-profit and not-for profit insurance companies offer a wide range of plans that vary in characteristics such as premium, copayment/coinsurance, deductibles, out of pocket limits, services covered, drug formularies, as well as provider choice. Payment systems and business models are complex and undergo continuing change over time. Because most private insurance plans are associated with the employer, many patients frequently change insurance plans due to changes in employment or when employers change their contracted insurance portfolio. Although there are hundreds of health insurance companies in the US, a relatively small number of companies provide coverage for a majority of the privately insured population. The great majority of the privately insured population are covered by insurance systems that pay for the care provided by others. Commercial insurance databases derived from these systems are some of the largest databases available for pharmacoepidemiologic research. A smaller group is covered by integrated, often not-for-profit healthcare delivery systems that assume responsibility for preventive and therapeutic health services to a defined population, often employ group or staff model delivery systems, and frequently operate their own hospitals (e.g. Kaiser Permanente). Though typically smaller in size, the databases associated with these healthcare systems offer extensive data resources that combine encounter-data with detailed clinical data resources including EHRs and direct access to patients and providers.

*Commercial insurance databases* are longitudinal collections of billable healthcare interactions. These databases are maintained by a variety of entities. This includes large insurance companies, often through health data analytics-focused subsidiaries (e.g. Optum Clinformatics/UnitedHealth Group; HealthCore Integrated Research Database/ Anthem, Comprehensive Health Insights Outcomes Data/Humana), as well as health information technology (IT) companies (e.g. Truven Health MarketScan, IQVIA PharmetricsPlus). Commercial insurance databases typically include several millions to tens of millions of individuals cross-sectionally and cumulatively often exceed 100 million unique patients over the life span of the database. Importantly however, the extremely large sizes of these databases do not necessarily translate directly into the size of pharmacoepidemiologic study cohorts. Given the approximately 30% annual churn rate in commercial insurance coverage and the fact that prescription drug coverage is often separately administered or absent, only approximately 50%, 30%, and 15%, of beneficiaries with medical coverage have continuous medical and pharmacy coverage for 1, 2, and 4+ years, respectively.

Another important and often underappreciated feature of commercial insurance databases is the large within-database heterogeneity in data availability, data completeness, data quality, and ability to link member data to non-encounter data. Within a typical commercial database, members are covered by a variety of insurance products (often from multiple insurance companies) leading to substantial differences in services captured in the database. Drug formularies, which determine coverage and out-of-pocket costs for prescription drugs, for example, vary widely between plans. Similarly, a study that requires data on dental

procedures would have to be limited to the subset of beneficiaries with a dental benefit during a specific time period. Completeness and quality of the claims data also depends on the payment model employed by the respective insurance products. As discussed earlier, completeness and accuracy with which services are captured may differ substantially depending on whether services are reimbursed through fee-for service payments or through capitated arrangements. Such capitated arrangements may apply to all medical coverage or be limited to specific services (e.g. specialist visits or mental healthcare services). The ability to validate or supplement the claims data is also often limited to subgroups of members included in the database. For example, for databases maintained by subsidies of insurance companies, data validation and supplementation may not be permitted for the (sometimes substantial) proportion of individuals in "self-funded" plans, where the employer assumes direct risk for payment and the insurance company only provides administrative services (ASO members). Similarly, the ability to identify patients and validate or supplement patient data depends on the contractual arrangements with the data sources (employers, health plans) and is generally restricted to a limited subset of the full database populations. Given the substantial heterogeneity in multiple data attributes within and between commercial databases, thoughtful consideration of detailed information on members' individual benefit packages is critical to facilitate restriction of the study population to those for whom all necessary data elements and linkages are captured or available in the database.

Several models exist to enable research access to commercial insurance databases. Some databases are directly available in their entirety through licensing arrangements (e.g. MarketScan), while others are solely accessible on a project by project basis via collaborative arrangements involving in-house programmers. Databases available for licensing are de-identified, with all personal identifiers removed and as such do not support external linkages. Studies that require such linkages for validation or supplementation of the encounter data typically require collaboration with researchers employed by the database custodian. Such collaborations have the added advantage of tapping into the often substantial experience of the custodian research team. Most major commercial insurance providers also participate as data partners for the Sentinel System.

*Integrated healthcare delivery system databases* differ from commercial insurance databases in that they include a defined population whose entire spectrum of care is under the responsibility of and provided by the integrated delivery system. Similar to commercial insurance databases, the delivery system databases include pharmacy dispensing data as well as encounter data on diagnoses and procedures from care delivered in both ambulatory and inpatient settings. However, because all care is provided by the delivery system, these databases also have access to full inpatient and outpatient electronic and paper medical records, and have the ability to interact with providers and patients. Although the latter features are also available for subsets of patients in many commercial insurance databases, the uniqueness of integrated delivery systems databases lies in the fact that these linkages cover the entire care received by the patient and is not limited to care received by specific practices or hospitals. Since many EHR systems include information on drugs prescribed, delivery system databases have often access to both prescription and dispensing data, which can be useful for a variety of research questions, such as questions of primary nonadherence. In addition, several integrated healthcare delivery systems include affiliated research centers that maintain a variety of additional data resources such as registries for cancer, diabetes, or cardiovascular disease. Integrated health delivery systems have a long track record of pharmacoepidemiologic research, and many are consortium members in the Health Care System Research Network (HCSRN, formerly known as the HMO Research Network) and data partners for the Sentinel System.

### US Government

The US government funds healthcare services through several major programs, including Medicare, and Medicaid as well as the Department of Veterans Affairs Healthcare System (VA). In contrast to the VA, which is a large provider of healthcare services operating numerous hospitals, clinics, and nursing homes, Medicaid and Medicare function as payers. Both programs pay directly for services using fee-for-service arrangements, but a large and growing proportion of beneficiaries receives Medicaid (69% in 2017) or Medicare (34% in 2018) coverage administered by private insurance companies through capitated managed care plans. For beneficiaries covered by managed-care plans, encounter data for individual services have historically been unavailable (Medicare) or were of mixed completeness and quality (Medicaid). Research with Medicaid or Medicare data has thus historically been restricted to individuals with fee-for-service coverage. Recent efforts have aimed to improve availability and quality of data for Medicare and Medicaid beneficiaries covered by managed-care plans. CMS administers Medicare and Medicaid data and facilitate access to research identifiable files for research purposes. Requests for these data files require a research protocol and data use agreement, and are reviewed by CMS's Privacy Board. The application process is managed and supported by the Research Data Assistance Center (ResDAC) at the University of Minnesota, which provides technical assistance to researchers interested in CMS Medicare and Medicaid data. Data access requires payment of fees based on the requested population size as well as the number of data files requested, which can be provided through release of data files to investigators or remotely via the CMS Virtual Research Data Center (VRDC). A mechanism to obtain inpatient hospital and emergency department medical records corresponding to Medicare and Medicaid claims has been described and implemented. Medicaid and Medicare data for select states or populations are also available from commercial entities (e.g. IBM Watson Health).

*Medicaid* is a joint state/federal program intended to provide health coverage for low-income individuals. It is administered separately by each state and state-specific eligibility rules differ within federal regulations. Traditionally, the program has provided coverage limited to certain groups of low-income individuals, including pregnant women, low-income families with children, the chronically disabled, and the elderly. Following the passage of the Affordable Care Act in 2010, about one half of US states have expanded coverage to all individuals under certain income thresholds. In 2018, the average monthly enrollment in Medicaid was 74.6 million (6.0 million aged, 10.7 million blind/disabled, 28.5 million children, 15.8 million traditionally eligible adults, and 12.2 million adults eligible through Medicaid expansion). In 38 states ≥50% of beneficiaries were covered through private managed-care plans. Medicaid coverage for eligible individuals is generally comprehensive although each state, within federally mandated parameters, administers their Medicaid program differently, resulting in variations in Medicaid coverage across the country.

Medicaid data files include enrollment and claims data for all Medicaid enrollees in the 50 states and the District of Columbia as well as for the approximately 7.0 million (2016) enrollees in the Children's Health Insurance Program (CHIP) which serves uninsured children up to age 19 in families with incomes too high to qualify them for Medicaid. Data files have been produced since 1999, available per state per year. From 1999 through 2013 exclusively as MAX files, from 2016 onward exclusively as T-MSIS Analytic Files (TAF), with a transition period in 2014 and 2015, during which, depending on the state, both file types were in

use. MAX and TAF data are both organized in 5 file types: (i) Person Summary/Demographic and Eligibility (demographic characteristics and enrollment information), (ii) Inpatient (inpatient hospital claims with one record per stay; procedure and diagnosis codes), (iii) Long-Term Care (e.g. nursing facility claims), (iv) Prescription Drug/Pharmacy (outpatient pharmacy data including NDC, quantity dispensed, days supply), and (v) other services (e.g. claims for physician, outpatient hospital, and laboratory services). Data are based on state-level data submitted through the Transformed Medicaid Statistical Information System (T-MSIS, since 2011 for some states and since October 2015 for all states) and the Medicaid Statistical Information System (MSIS; 1999 through 2015). TAF and MAX both are produced by CMS. MAX data underwent extensive editing and quality control at the federal level resulting in a substantial lag of approximately three to four years between the end of a calendar year and data availability. For TAF, more of the responsibility for data quality control has been shifted to the individual states resulting in a reduced lag in data availability (Two years or less). Once released, MAX and TAF files are final. Compared to MAX, TAF files add hundreds of additional data elements (third-party liability, provider, and managed care plan data) as well as modifications of existing data elements.

One of the intentions of the transition from MSIS to T-MSIS was to improve capture and quality of encounter data for beneficiaries covered by managed care plans. Data for these beneficiaries have historically been considered not to be up to research standards and typically have been excluded from most pharmacoepidemiologic research. Given that the majority of Medicaid enrollees are now covered under managed-care plans, availability of research quality data for this population (after extensive quality checks and validation studies) would substantially increase the potential of Medicaid data as a resource for pharmacoepidemiologic research. Gaps in data capture due to periods of ineligibility are common as eligibility is typically determined monthly and changes with income and life circumstances. This issue affects individual eligibility groups differently with more stable enrollment for those qualifying based on disability and less stable enrollment for low-income adults. Exclusion of beneficiaries without stable enrollment has been implemented based on eligibility files as well as through requirements for Medicaid encounters during specified periods before and after person time under study. Because Medicaid is administered at the state-level, state-specific policies (e.g. opioid quantity limits or prior approval requirements) have to be considered in the research design. Medicaid and Medicare data for dually eligible beneficiaries can be linked. Such linkage is important in studies of dual enrollees since Medicaid or Medicare data alone fail to document the full spectrum of care provided to such dual enrollees. Medicaid data for research are also available directly from individual states but access is often limited to researchers with established ties to the specific state Medicaid programs.

*Medicare* is the federal program that provides healthcare coverage for almost all people 65 years and over as well as for qualifying individuals with permanent disabilities. Medicare coverage consists of four parts: Medicare Part A (Hospital Insurance), Medicare Part B (Medical Insurance), Medicare Part C (Medicare Advantage), and Medicare Part D (Medicare Prescription Drug Coverage). All Parts of Medicare coverage require beneficiaries to pay deductibles and some stipulate cost sharing. Part A covers inpatient care in hospitals and skilled nursing facilities, as well as hospice. It is premium-free for the great majority of beneficiaries. Part B covers physician and other outpatient services. It is an optional program that requires monthly premiums. Approximately 90% of Medicare beneficiaries enroll in Part B. Part C allows Medicare beneficiaries to enroll in private health plans that administer Part A and B benefits. The large

majority of these so called Medicare Advantage plans also include Part D benefits (i.e. prescription drug coverage). Part C plans are optional and require premiums. In 2018, 33.6% of Medicare beneficiaries received coverage through Medicare Advantage plans. Importantly, encounter data for Medicare Advantage beneficiaries have only recently become available through CMS (to date solely for service years 2015 and 2016). Part D provides outpatient prescription drug coverage. Established in 2006, the program is administered by private companies that provide coverage through hundreds (901 in 2019) of prescription drug plans (PDPs) that differ in formulary coverage and cost sharing. Enrollment in Part D is voluntary and requires a monthly premium that varies between the individual PDPs. Medicare Part D imposes a coverage gap (doughnut hole) that requires beneficiaries to pay a substantial percentage of the cost of their medications (35% and 44% for brand name and generic drugs, respectively in 2018) until they reach the out-of-pocket spending limit ($5000 in 2018). A large proportion of Medicare beneficiaries have some type of supplemental coverage (employer sponsored, Medicaid, so-called Medigap policies) to reduce out-of-pocket costs from cost-sharing requirements. In 2018, the average monthly Medicare enrollment was 60.0 million (51.3 million aged, 8.7 million disabled). 20.2 million beneficiaries were covered through Medicare Advantage and 44.2 million had a Part D benefit, including 16 million through Medicare Advantage plans.

Medicare data are available in several file types that are linkable to each other, as well as to Medicaid data for dually-enrolled beneficiaries. File types include: MBSFs (Master Beneficiary Summary Files), which include files on demographics and enrollment, chronic conditions, and cost and utilization; Institutional Claims, which include files on inpatient services, skilled nursing facilities, and hospice; Non-institutional Claims, which include outpatient physician claims (Carrier file) and claims for durable medical equipment; and the Part D event Data file, which provides detailed prescription level outpatient pharmacy claims. Supplementary files provide information on Part D plan characteristics, pharmacies, drugs (crosswalks from First DataBank), prescribers, and formularies.

Since prescription drug data for Medicare have become available after the establishment of Medicare Part D in 2006, Medicare, due to its large and stable population, has become one of the largest and most comprehensive resources for pharmacoepidemiologic research.

### Encounter Databases in Canada

Canada, with its population of approximately 37.5 million, has a universal healthcare program covering all residents regardless of age or income. Program administration is under the responsibility of each of its 10 provinces or territories. Physician visits, diagnostic tests, procedures (in- or out-patient), and hospitalizations are provided without payment by the patient at the point of care. Encounter data are transactional and consist of billings submitted by healthcare providers on a fee-for-service basis. Similar to US encounter databases, some in-hospital services are not billed individually and a small number of physicians may have all or a portion of their activities covered by salary; hence, the services they provide may not be included in the medical services databases. In contrast, public drug coverage programs differ among provinces; programs have been available for varying lengths of time and differ with respect to eligibility criteria as well as characteristics (i.e. copayments and deductibles). Some provinces, such as Saskatchewan and Manitoba, provide coverage for the entire population while in the others, public drug programs restrict coverage to specific segments of the population, such as the elderly, welfare recipients, youth (less than 25 years of age) or those who do not have access to private insurance plans through their employers.

Within each province, three encounter databases are available: (i) beneficiary, (ii) medical services, and (iii) prescription drugs acquired through the public drug plan (with the exception of British Columbia which collects drug dispensings acquired through both public and private drug plans, as well as out-of-pocket). These databases are linkable through a unique patient identifier that remains unchanged over time. Additional linkage capacities are available to hospitalization databases, population health surveys or to province-specific disease registries. Linkage of hospital charts or outpatient charts for validation of diagnoses or collection of data that are not present in the databases requires approval from the provincial information access commissioner and may not be feasible in all provinces. A number of validation studies of Canadian databases, primarily of diagnoses codes in the medical services databases, can be found in the literature, but validation data remain far from comprehensive.

Each province maintains its own medical services encounter database, which includes all claims submitted by physicians regardless of setting (inpatient, outpatient, or emergency department) as long as the physician is paid on a fee-for-service basis. The nature of the information in the various provincial medical services databases is similar though differences exist in coding systems, such as the ICD version. For each medical service, the following information is recorded: service (date, description, location, diagnosis, and cost), provider (identifier and specialty). The vast majority of claims are submitted electronically, and the resulting medical services claims databases are populated in real-time. In a few provinces, such as Nova Scotia, Manitoba, and British Columbia, mental health services, including psychotherapy, are recorded in a distinct database.

Unlike the medical services databases, hospitalization databases are intended for the creation of health statistics rather than for reimbursement purposes. The databases contain clinical data related to hospital discharges from acute or chronic care units, or rehabilitation centers, as well as day surgeries. With the exception of Quebec, which maintains its own hospital discharge database (MED-ECHO), all provinces contribute to the Discharge Abstract Database (DAD) maintained by the Canadian Institute for Health Information (CIHI). The information is therefore homogeneous across provinces. In the hospitalization databases, diagnosis was coded with ICD-9-CM until 31 March 2006 and with ICD-10 thereafter. In the DAD database, information on mental health resources, cancer staging, and reproductive history were added in 2009–2010. Hospitalization databases are typically available six months after the end of the fiscal year (March 31st).

Province-specific prescription drug databases record all prescription drugs dispensed in an outpatient setting to individuals covered by the public drug plan. Drugs acquired out-of-pocket/OTC, in-hospital, long-term care units, not included in the formulary, or covered only by private insurance programs are not usually included in the database. One exception is PharmaNet in British Columbia that links all pharmacies to a central data system. Every prescription dispensed in the outpatient setting is recorded regardless of coverage; hence, it includes medications covered by the public drug plan, private insurance programs, as well as those acquired out-of-pocket. Drugs are coded according to the Canadian-specific Drug Information Number (DIN) as well as the American Hospital Formulary Service (AHFS). For each dispensing, the following information is recorded: drug (date of dispensing, drug name, dose per unit, mode of administration, prescribed duration [the latter is not recorded in Saskatchewan], cost including dispensing fees), pharmacist (identifier, pharmacy location), and prescriber (identifier, specialty). Indication for a drug prescription is not recorded in any of the dispensing databases. While data and coding systems are similar across provinces, inclusion of individual drugs in the formulary and type of listing (general or restricted) may vary. For each patient, the year of entry and exit from the drug program are available in the beneficiary database. This is important information for studies that include segments of the population whose membership in the drug program may be transitory, such as membership based on income or access to private insurance programs. Only 7 of the 10 Canadian provinces make prescription data available for pharmacoepidemiologic research. Approximately half of these databases are accessible through custodians located in a university setting while the other half are accessible through provincial government agencies. In addition to the drug databases, custodians also act as a repository for other provincial databases and are responsible for their linkage.

Database access varies across provinces. Some provinces (Saskatchewan, Quebec, and Nova Scotia), provide raw anonymized datasets to researchers (from academic or industry settings) while others (Ontario, BC) require data to be analyzed in-house by specific research organizations. To maintain confidentiality of the data, no patient, healthcare provider (including pharmacist), or institution identifiers are transmitted to researchers. Additional restrictions are in place in individual provinces. For example, in Quebec only a random sample of approximately 75% of the population eligible for a given study (capped at a maximum of 125 000 eligible patients) may be obtained, and no birthdates are transmitted. Exceptions can be granted through a request to the Provincial Access to Information Commission, which substantially increases the delay in data extraction. Although Canadian encounter databases are much smaller than the US encounter databases, their greatest advantage is that they include a stable population, thereby allowing longer follow-up periods. This is, for example, illustrated through a study on benzodiazepines and Alzheimer's disease by Billioti de Gage and colleagues, in which a 10 year follow-up was available. The time required for database extraction varies across provinces, ranging from 10 to 20 weeks to 1 year, more if a request to the Provincial Access to Information Commission is required.

Access to linked data (prescription, medical services, hospitalizations) is possible on a provincial basis. At a national level, the CIHI houses encounter databases from multiple prescription claims-level data, from public drug programs of British Columbia, Alberta, Saskatchewan, Manitoba, Ontario, New Brunswick, Nova Scotia, Prince Edward Island, Newfoundland and Labrador, and Yukon. These data have been linked at CIHI to the hospital discharge database (DAD), although those multi-province linked data are not accessible to external researchers. In addition, the IQVIA Private Drug Plan Database houses adjudicated prescription claims from approximately 83% of the total private (direct-pay) business in Canada. These data are useful for the conduct of drug utilization studies but are currently not linked to medical services or hospitalization data.

## Encounter Databases in Europe
### The Nordic Prescription Databases

The Nordic countries (Denmark, Iceland, Norway, Sweden, and Finland) have tax-supported universal health coverage. All citizens (a combined population of over 25 million people ranging from ~300 000 in Iceland to more than 9 million in Sweden) are provided with unrestricted access to health services including partial or complete reimbursement of medications. Pharmacies electronically submit information on dispensed prescriptions to national databases without a requirement for informed consent by the patient (available since 1994 in Finland and Denmark, since 2004 in Norway, since 2005 in Sweden, and since 2006 in Iceland). Unique civil registration codes facilitate unambiguous linkage to various national databases using a central patient router file. Linkable national databases

include but are not limited to hospital discharge databases, laboratory data including results, pathology databases, medical birth databases, cancer registries, and cause of death databases, as well as census data, health surveys, biobanks, and patient records. Together, these databases create a federated database network that provides exposure information from the prescription database as well as patient and clinical outcome data from the patient router file and multiple linked autonomous databases.

The prescription databases largely include similar data elements with slight variations between countries. Besides a patient identifier (which also encodes birth year and sex), data includes drug data (dispensing date, Nordic article number, a unique identifier similar to the NDC code used in the US, Anatomical Therapeutic Chemical [ATC] classification, quantity dispensed in defined daily doses), a prescriber identifier (which can be linked to prescriber data such as basic demographics, profession, specialty, practice site), and pharmacy data (name and location). OTC drugs are not included unless they are obtained via prescription. Importantly, some drugs that are also available OTC are used primarily via prescription, to ensure reimbursement. Besides the difference in the age of the databases, the most noticeable difference is the fact that non-reimbursed drugs are not covered by the Finnish database.

Outcome data are primarily based on national hospital discharge databases (registries). While comparable, some differences exist in the age of the patient databases with the Finnish database dating back to 1969, followed by the Danish (1977), Swedish (1987), and Norwegian registry (2008). Numerous other databases including cancer, birth, and death, together with pathology and laboratory results further complement the dataset. Importantly, no large-scale data are available that provide details regarding general practice visits or other non-hospital health services. This is often referred to as a lack of "outpatient" data. However, this term can lead to misunderstandings in the context of the Nordic health care model. All hospital databases cover activities within hospital outpatient clinics, and as such all specialized care is covered. However, in all Nordic countries, general practice physicians serve as gate keepers to specialized care (including both hospital and private practicing specialists). Detailed data, e.g. diagnoses or laboratory data, are not available. However, data on contacts (without specification for the reason for such contacts) can be obtained.

Rules governing data access vary between the Nordic countries, but generally require collaboration with local researchers. Access to Danish prescription data is particularly restrictive. Consequently, data from the Danish National Prescription Registry cannot leave the data havens provided by Danish authorities. For multinational studies involving Danish individual-level prescription data, pooled analyses require data to be transferred to e.g. Statistics Denmark or meta-analysis techniques to be applied to obtain pooled estimates. Other sources of Danish prescription data are not restricted in the same way, but only provide data on reimbursed prescriptions and either only offer local coverage or only provide data on reimbursed prescriptions and only cover more recent years.

### Other European Encounter Databases

Pharmacy-based federated database networks also exist in the Netherlands (PHARMO) and Scotland (Tayside MEMO). These networks are limited to specific regions of their respective countries and provide the ability to link to a number of databases that provide outcome and confounder information similar to those in the Nordic countries. In addition, integrated encounter databases are available in France, and select regions of Italy (Lombardy, Tuscany). The French national claims database, SNIIRAM, captures data for more than 66 million individuals (~98% of the French population) regardless of socioeconomic or employment status. It captures encounter data on outpatient visits, dispensed medication, procedures, chronic conditions, as well as hospital admission diagnoses and procedures, and date of death. Data access, however, is complex.

### Encounter Databases in Asia

There are many encounter databases available across the Asia-Pacific Region. Many of these are population-wide databases due to prominence of nationwide healthcare coverage in these countries. For example, South Korea and Taiwan both have single-payer, universal government-run health insurance systems that predominantly operate on a fee-for-service basis and have established national research databases. The National Health Insurance Databases of South Korea and Taiwan are the most well-established and widely used Asian encounter databases. Similar to encounter databases in the US, Canada, and Europe, these databases capture patient demographic information, medical (in- and outpatient) services and prescription and dispensing data. Encounter databases also exist in Australia, and Japan. In Australia, the commonwealth government maintains a dataset of dispensing of subsidized medicines under the Pharmaceutical Benefits Scheme (PBS) and medical services under the Medicare Benefits Schedule (MBS). A 10% sample of these data, linked longitudinally, is available and has been used for research. Additionally, an encounter database of services provided to Australian Veterans is maintained by the Australian Department of Veterans Affairs (DVA). These data include all prescriptions dispensed, medical services claimed and hospital visits attended by the veterans, their dependents and spouses. The DVA data have been used widely for research.

One of the advantages of databases across the Asia Pacific region is the consistency of coding systems. For example, encounter databases in South Korea, Taiwan and Australia all use ATC (Anatomical Therapeutic Chemical) codes to identify individual medicines and all but Taiwan use ICD-10 codes to identify diagnoses. This allows for comparisons of similar products across different countries without the need to map individual country-specific codes. This has allowed cross-national studies to be conducted using a distributed network approach through the Asian Pharmacoepidemiology Network (AsPEN). Pharmacoepidemiologic studies using Asian databases have historically been limited due to restrictions in the accessibility of these data. Milea and colleagues reported that of 54 encounter databases across the Asia pacific region very few allowed access to raw data. Databases in Australia, Taiwan and Japan for example were considered as having a high level of data accessibility, while South Korea had a medium level and Thailand, China, Malaysia and Singapore had a low level of accessibility. The level of accessibility can differ for individual databases within the same country, as some databases may require a local researcher to access data while others do not provide raw data with only summary level data available for researchers.

### The Taiwanese National Health Insurance Research Database (NHIRD)

Established in 1995, the National Health Insurance (NHI) program of Taiwan covers approximately 23 million individuals, more than 99% of the country's population. The NHI maintains the National Health Insurance Research Database (NHIRD), which is accessible for research. NHIRD includes but is not limited to patient demographics, prescription and dispensing data, outpatient visits, hospitalizations, and dental care. Data are updated biannually. The NHIRD can be linked to a number of external national databases through a unique and universal personal identification number. Databases available for linkage include numerous registries (birth, death, immunization, cancer, reportable infectious diseases, and suicide), population-based screening programs (various cancers, myopia,

urine, newborns) as well as regular examinations in school children. Strict procedures for data access and human subject review are in place to assure protection of confidentiality and data security.

### The South Korean Health Insurance Review and Assessment (HIRA) Data

South Korea provides universal health coverage since 1989. In 2000, all health insurance systems were integrated into a single national system creating the National Health Insurance Service (NHIS) and the Health Insurance Review and Assessment Service (HIRA). All healthcare providers are covered under the NHIS and are, with a few exceptions, reimbursed on a fee-for-service basis. Claims are electronically submitted by providers to HIRA for reimbursement and are the basis for the HIRA database, which contains healthcare utilization and prescribed medications for approximately 50 million individuals. Use of the database for research was initially limited until it became publicly available for research in 2009. HIRA research data include beneficiary ID, basic demographics, procedures, diagnostic tests, all diagnosis received by the beneficiary (coded in KCD6, the Korean Standard Classification of Disease Version 6, which is closely based on the ICD-10 system), in- and outpatient prescriptions (including brand name, generic name, prescription and dispensing date, duration, dose, and route of administration), as well as provider ID and characteristics. Validity of diagnosis data in the HIRA database has been shown to vary according to the severity of the condition (with greater validity for more severe conditions) and the care setting (with higher validity for inpatient than for outpatient diagnoses). HIRA data are available to researchers in academia and government agencies and for those in the private sector such as pharmaceutical companies and medical device companies, but access requires in person consultation at the HIRA and submission of a study proposal. Once approval is given, tailored data extracts with encrypted ID information for protection of privacy are uploaded in a remote access system accessible only by the individual researcher for the study. Importantly, HIRA data are currently available only for a five year period beginning from the current year although plans exist to expand this period to 10 years. In response to the COVID-19 pandemic, HIRA made available a de-identified COVID-19 nationwide patient dataset for researchers. The dataset contains a five year history of insurance claims for all tested cases of COVID-19. Researchers are able to download a sample datafile to develop analytic code which can then be submitted to HIRA for execution in the full dataset.

## Strengths

Encounter databases have a number of strengths in comparison to other data sources for pharmacoepidemiologic research, which explain their broad representation in the literature.

First, automated healthcare databases facilitate the rapid and cost-efficient assembly of extremely large cohorts of patients and provide data on drug exposures, health outcomes, and potential confounding factors. Encounter databases, in particular, are the largest available population-based healthcare databases. Several of the databases discussed in this chapter cumulatively include more than 100 million individuals and provide the ability to rapidly assemble cohorts that are substantially larger than analogous cohorts from EHR-databases or ad-hoc data collection. Encounter databases thus are uniquely able to address research questions that require the largest possible study sizes. The following example illustrates the differences in cohort sizes for the same study in select encounter and EHR databases. Filion and colleagues examined proton pump inhibitors and the risk of hospitalization for community-acquired pneumonia among new users of NSAIDs, aged ≥40 years in multiple databases within the Canadian Network for Observational Drug Effect Studies (CNODES). The respective sizes of study cohorts assembled using a common protocol and allowing multiple cohort entry dates for a single patient were approximately 2.2 million for MarketScan, 1.5 million for the combined Canadian provincial databases, and 0.6 million for UK General Practice Research Database (GPRD), the largest population-based EHR-database. The MarketScan cohort was more than 3.5 times larger than the GRPD cohort, despite not including data on ≥65 year olds who made up around 35% of the total study population.

Second, because encounter databases are population-based and provide a comprehensive capture of covered health care encounters regardless of the provider, they can support the full range of epidemiologic study designs including cohort, nested-case control, and self-controlled designs. While this strength is shared by a number of other population-based automated databases, it is a critical limitation to non-population based data sources such as EHR databases of individual institutions or health systems.

Third, many encounter databases facilitate systematic or ad-hoc linkage to non-encounter data resources including electronic or paper medical records, disease registries, laboratory results, or patient and provider surveys. Such linkages can support validation of study outcomes and allow supplementation of encounter-data with variables such as laboratory results or lifestyle data. In ideal circumstances, such linkages thus provide the ability to take advantage of the size and population-based nature of encounter data, while also accruing the advantages of higher data quality and greater clinical detail available from data sources such as EHRs, disease registries, or patient and provider surveys. Importantly, however, linkage ability and quality vary substantially between individual encounter databases and has to be carefully considered for each study question.

Fourth, many large encounter-databases are broadly representative of nations, regions, or particular health systems. As such, these databases can often serve an important role in facilitating health services and health policy research. Many include very stable populations that facilitate assessment of long-term safety effects and long-term trends in treatment practice and quality. Further, encounter databases from countries or regions with universal health coverage – by definition – are free from selection bias as inclusion in the database is universal.

Fifth, for encounter data generated from fee-for-service payment claims, data elements that directly pertain to the payment amount are subject to auditing and considered highly accurate. This is true for procedure claims (type of procedure performed) as well as for pharmacy claims (date, drug, and quantity dispensed). Importantly however, the accuracy of procedure data primarily relates to the occurrence of the procedure billed while the accuracy of the clinical indication associated with the procedure may be substantially lower. For example, a validation study by Wysowski and Baum that used specific surgical procedure codes in Medicaid data as part of an algorithm to identify cases of hip fracture found in medical record review that while all of the procedures billed for were actually performed, some of the procedures were used to correct orthopedic conditions other than hip fracture. A further advantage of pharmacy data compared to prescription data recorded in EHR databases (see Chapter 10) is the fact that prescription dispensings are one step closer to ingestion than what was prescribed and thus are subject to a lesser degree of exposure misclassification. The accuracy of encounter data generated by administrative processes not related to payment is less well established and likely to vary depending on the existence and rigor of quality assurance processes.

Sixth and last, data capture processes in encounter data are automated and independent of the study question and hypothesis,

greatly diminishing the likelihood of recall or assessment biases.

## Limitations

Encounter databases are primarily intended and maintained for payment or other administrative purposes, and therefore are subject to important limitations when used for research. First, one of the greatest concerns when using encounter databases for pharmacoepidemiologic research is the uncertain validity of diagnostic information (see Chapters 8 and 13). While these concerns apply to all diagnostic encounter data, they are amplified for diagnoses recorded in the outpatient setting where diagnosis is typically not directly linked to a particular level of payment. It is thus critically important for all encounter-based research to validate diagnostic data (for both outcomes and important confounders) against external gold standards such as the medical record or disease registries. These gold standards, of course, may not be correct either when compared to research grade diagnoses as employed by RCTs.

Second, encounter data lack clinical detail such as markers of disease severity (e.g. blood pressure, ejection fraction) and lifestyle factors (tobacco and alcohol use, body mass index, physical activity). Oftentimes data elements are available (e.g. diagnostic codes for obesity or smoking status) but of extremely low sensitivity. For example, a study by Lloyd and colleagues using data from the National Health and Nutrition Examination Survey to validate diagnosis of obesity in Medicare claims found that claims-based diagnostics codes fail to identify a great majority of patients with obesity (sensitivity of 18%). Though still far from perfect, clinical detail such as disease severity and lifestyle factors are generally better captured by paper or electronic medical records. Because such clinical detail is often critical for confounding adjustment, methods that minimize unmeasured or residual confounding (self-controlled designs, active comparator new-user designs, instrumental variable analyses, propensity score calibration) are of great importance to encounter-based pharmacoepidemiologic research (see Chapter 22).

Third, while limitations of encounter databases can often be overcome by facilitating linkage to non-encounter data such as EHRs, disease registries, or laboratory results, such linkages are typically time consuming and costly and, in many cases, only available to subsets of the database population. Further, when compared to population-based EHR databases the resulting linked/enriched encounter data typically remain less comprehensive, and validation is often restricted to small samples often with poor response/retrieval rates.

Fourth, in certain situations medication dispensing information may not capture data for specific drugs or drug classes. This may include drugs excluded from reimbursement, drugs that are primarily obtained OTC, as well as low-cost generic drugs that are paid for out of pocket because the cash price is lower than the required copayment. This may result in misclassification of exposure, such that some patients will appear not to be exposed to a medicine when in fact they were. Non-reimbursable drugs as well as low-cost generics are often better captured in EHR databases, which contain information on all prescriptions written. However, the disadvantage of prescription information is that not all prescriptions will be dispensed and will result in misclassification of exposure, such that some patients will appear to be exposed to a medicine when in fact they were not.

Fifth and last, due to the fragmentation of the US healthcare system, many large US encounter databases lack representativeness of the general population and feature significant turn-over and short dwell times (e.g. US private insurance databases, MAX/TAF).

## Particular Applications

Encounter databases have been used in thousands of pharmacoepidemiologic publications, many of which have shaped clinical medicine or regulatory decision-making. These databases have supported work across a wide spectrum of areas including drug safety, comparative effectiveness, drug-utilization, and health services research, methods and validation, as well as pharmacoeconomics. This section outlines some typical activities involved in encounter database studies and presents some of the considerations in choosing the optimal encounter database when multiple options are available or assessing the suitability of a specific database for a given research question.

### Typical Activities Involved in Studies Using Encounter Databases

Although encounter databases vary in data structure, coding schemes, and numerous other specifics, a number of activities are typical across all such databases. Virtually all pharmacoepidemiologic studies of encounter databases require *linkage of records between data files and over time*. Records from different data domains, such as membership, outpatient services, inpatient services, and pharmacy, are linked so that an individual's entire set of encounters over the study period can be available for analysis. Another ubiquitous step in the conduct of pharmacoepidemiologic studies involves the *aggregation of drug-, diagnosis-, and procedure codes into meaningful study variables*. Exposures, outcomes, potential confounders, and in−/exclusion criteria for study are defined via code lists using drug-, diagnosis-, and procedure codes, or combinations thereof. These code lists are typically study- and database- specific using the coding schemes utilized by the respective database and drugs approved and available for the study population during the study period. It is often desirable to use previously validated algorithms for the definition of study outcomes and important confounding variables. Such algorithms often combine diagnostic codes, drug codes, and procedure codes for more accurate measures of disease (see Chapter 13). Together with demographic information these study-specific variables (e.g. drug classes, disease states) as described above facilitate the *creation of the study population*. Study populations often consist of (new) users of specific drugs or drug classes within individuals who meet specific inclusion and exclusion criteria based on their encounter-derived medical history. Once the study population is identified in the dataset, analytic plans often specify the construction of longitudinal histories. Exposure, occurrence of outcome events, and presence of confounding factors are measured over time, typically in temporal relation to the study's index date. This facilitates the assessment of exposure periods, person-time at risk, and allows calculation of incidence rates and measures of association. If additional data not available in the encounter database are required, complementary information may be gathered through linkage to electronic medical records, data obtained directly from patients or their physicians from surveys, retrieval of paper medical records, or data routinely collected in disease, immunization, or national vital registries.

## Deciding Between Individual Encounter Databases

Database choice or evaluation of suitability of a single database should involve consideration of all database attributes relevant to the research question under study. Some of the key attributes that differentiate individual encounter databases are shown in Table 9.2 and discussed below.

*Target population:* The database should capture a large and representative sample of the target population (e.g. patients exposed to a particular drug) to adequately address the study question. For example, Stroup and colleagues aimed to examine the effectiveness of initiating treatment with either clozapine or a standard antipsychotic among adults with evidence of treatment-resistant schizophrenia using national US Medicaid data. On first glance, this might not be an obvious choice as the adult Medicaid population is highly selective and often transient. However, Medicaid covers approximately two thirds of all US adults with schizophrenia because most patients with severe schizophrenia qualify for disability. In addition, because these individuals qualify for Medicaid because of disability rather than because of their economic condition, they are typically stably enrolled without breaks in coverage. While non-US encounter databases might have provided similarly large numbers of stably-enrolled patients with schizophrenia, the authors sought a US database because of the pronounced differences in psychiatric treatment practice between US and most other countries. The study was conducted as a 1 : 1 propensity score matched cohort study and found that clozapine treated patients compared to patients treated with a standard antipsychotic had a decreased risk of psychiatric hospital admission (hazard ratio = 0.78, 95% CI = 0.69–0.88) but at an increased risk of diabetes mellitus (hazard ratio = 1.63, 95% CI = 0.98–2.70).

*Database size:* The database should be large enough to provide sufficient power to answer the research question, e.g. to detect a meaningful difference between treatment groups (should a difference truly exist). This assessment should be based not on the size of the overall database, but rather consider the size of the actual study cohort, i.e. the cohort after exclusion of individuals for whom required data elements are unavailable (e.g. after exclusion of individuals under capitated payment plans), and after application of inclusion and exclusion criteria (e.g. sufficient uninterrupted baseline period). A study by Shin et al. aimed to determine the risk of cardiovascular conditions in children and adolescents with attention deficit hyperactivity disorder (ADHD) associated with use of methylphenidate. As the outcome was rare, the South Korean HIRA database of over 50 million participants was used. From this large population database, 144 258 patients aged less than 18 with a diagnosis of ADHD were retrieved. Of these, 114 657 were new users of methylphenidate and 1224 had an incident cardiovascular event. Due to the rare outcome a self-controlled case series design was used which, compared to other designs, has the advantage of requiring fewer patients for similar power (see Chapter 22).

*Ability to validate outcomes:* Because encounter data are primarily collected for administrative purposes, the ability to validate or adjudicate outcome definitions derived from these data is essential for pharmacoepidemiologic studies. Outcome validation should generally be performed as part of any encounter-based study unless the outcome measures have previously been validated for the database. However, the ability to validate outcomes, through reliable linkage to external gold standards, such as the medical record or disease registries, varies markedly between databases and is often a major consideration for database selection. Lo Re and colleagues, for example, conducted a series of postauthorization safety studies to examine the safety (hospitalization for major adverse cardiovascular events, acute kidney injury, acute liver failure, infections, and severe hypersensitivity events) of saxagliptin compared to other oral antidiabetic drugs in patients with type 2 diabetes. The studies were conducted separately in two EHR databases (Clinical Practice Research Datalink, The Health Improvement Network) and two encounter databases (Medicare, HealthCore Integrated Research Database). One of the requirements for the choice of encounter databases in this study was the ability to obtain inpatient medical records for outcome adjudication. Using a new-user active comparator cohort design, the study found no evidence of increased risk of any of the outcome events within any of the four databases. Other outcomes are notoriously under-coded in encounter data and require development of custom algorithms. For example, using data from Quebec, Moride et al. developed and validated a case detection algorithm for suicide attempts in youth through a review of medical charts. The following algorithm was used: diagnostic code of injury or intoxication with a location of service in the ED, followed by a psychiatric consult or a psychiatric diagnosis (psychiatric diagnoses consisting of depression, eating disorder, schizophrenia, ADHD, substance abuse, others) within two days of the ED visit. This algorithm had a sensitivity of 70% and a specificity of 97.6%.

*Availability of non-standard encounter data.* While all encounter databases provide information on medical services and prescription drugs, studies often require encounter data on services that are not universally available in all databases. For example, Gupta and colleagues examined opioid prescribing practices among US dentists from 2010 to 2015 using the MarketScan database. Because dental services are not captured for all individuals in the database, the study population was appropriately restricted to those with simultaneous enrollment in a medical and a dental plan.

*Ability to supplement with non-encounter data:* Studies using encounter data may require clinical detail not available from encounter data often for the purpose of confounding adjustment or to supplement outcome identification. The ability to perform linkages that allow enrichment of the dataset with non-encounter data is thus vital and often a decisive consideration in choosing a study database. For example, Huybrechts and colleagues examined the comparative mortality risk of individual antipsychotics in elderly nursing home residents using data for US nursing home residents dually eligible for Medicaid and Medicare. Clinical variables such as cognitive function or behavioral symptoms of dementia are important potential confounders but poorly measured in encounter databases. Linkage to the Minimum Data Set (MDS, available from CMS), a federally mandated health assessment tool used in nursing homes that captures information on physical, psychological, and psychosocial functioning, active clinical diagnoses, health conditions, treatments, and services, allowed the inclusion of these important covariates into the study. Using a propensity score adjusted new-user cohort design, the authors showed that compared to initiators of risperidone, initiators of haloperidol had an increased mortality risk and initiators of quetiapine had a decreased mortality risk. As another example, a Swedish–Danish study investigated the risks associated with being admitted to an emergency department with suspected poisoning, most often psychotropics or analgesics. Leveraging the ability to link data on admissions and prescription fills to a dataset including detailed ECGs on those admitted to the hospital, they could estimate not only the occurrence of QTc prolongation within the population but also to what extent QTc prolongation as a marker was associated to 30-day mortality.

## The Future

Pharmacoepidemiologic research with encounter databases has become more and more widely used and involves an increasing number of databases in a growing number of regions of the world. This trend is expected to continue, particularly as encounter databases become available in regions for which currently no data are available. In addition, the following three major factors are likely to shape the future of encounter databases: (i) advances in IT, (ii) privacy regulations, and (iii) changing healthcare systems. Advances in IT will continue to expand the boundaries of data storage and processing, and increasingly facilitate linkages with new and more complex sources of data including biomarkers, social

media, web searches, and around the clock biometric information from wearables. In addition, automated tools for data visualization and analysis of health data are becoming more accessible. The potential for rapid development of progressively complex, detailed, and complete data resources is likely to be counteracted by increasingly strict regulations governing data privacy. These regulations will vary substantially between countries and are likely subject to rapid change. Last, and maybe most importantly, encounter-based data are a secondary byproduct of administrative systems, created to support the local healthcare system; research applications are secondary uses. As such, encounter-based healthcare data will continue to be subject to changes in the healthcare systems that generate the data. Again, these changes are likely to vary drastically between countries and over time.

For example, the US healthcare environment is undergoing enormous transformation. Historically, healthcare providers in the US have been paid using a fee-for-service approach, where providers bill health insurance companies for the cost of the services they provide, generally justifying those bills with diagnoses. These paid claims represent the core of these encounter databases. However, the net result of this approach is that the more providers do, the more they are paid which may result in over servicing and wasted resources. The result has been a large incentive to increase utilization, and rapidly increasing costs in the US for providing healthcare, made worse by an aging population. Under this model the levels of expenditure are unsustainable. This has led to a shift from a fee-for-service model to a "per patient per month" payment system, so-called "population health," which of course switches the incentive to providing less care. In order to attempt to address that, there are incentives being put in place to ensure that people are not receiving *too little* care, referred to as "value health." The US is in the middle of this transition now, varying greatly in different parts of the country.

However, in response, there has been a remarkable consolidation of physician practices, hospitals, etc., in order to achieve sufficient scale to create the needed extensive and costly data infrastructure, and to assume the large risk associated with population health. Many other initiatives are underway as well, to limit the increasing costs of medical care. The results will likely be large changes over the next few years in the data as part of US encounter databases.

Encounter-based data are an important resource for pharmacoepidemiologic research. These data are comprehensive and often have a high level of quality as they are collected for payment purposes. As these data are generated for purposes other than research, careful consideration of their applicability, completeness, and generalizability need to be carefully weighed against their convenience. As with any data source careful consideration should be given to the issues of bias and confounding (see Chapter 2) which are not problems diminished by the increased size of the database.

## Key Points

- Encounter databases are maintained in numerous countries, by a variety of entities (e.g. government agencies, insurance companies, health plans), and for a variety of purposes (e.g. reimbursement, administration).
- Encounter databases used in pharmacoepidemiology typically contain the following core data domains: (i) eligibility and basic demographic information, (ii) outpatient pharmacy dispensings, and (iii) medical services (typically including hospitalizations and emergency department services; commonly also including outpatient health services).
- A defined population for which healthcare services are recorded regardless of the provider or location of care received is critical

for the usefulness of encounter databases for pharmacoepidemiologic research. Such databases are considered *population-based*.
- Fit-for-purpose evaluation of a given encounter database should consider the following characteristics: (i) population and coverage period, (ii) services covered and data completeness, (iii) ability to link to complimentary external data sources, and (iii) access.
- Data accuracy for dispensed outpatient prescription drugs is typically high.
- The accuracy of diagnostic codes is highly variable, depending on the specific condition, the setting of care, and the purpose of the encounter database. Use of validated outcome definitions or verification of diagnoses using primary medical records is strongly encouraged.
- The US has a highly fragmented healthcare system and no single database captures a representative cross-section of its population.
- US Commercial insurance databases include some of the largest databases available. These databases typically aggregate data for members covered by a variety of insurance products.
- US integrated healthcare delivery system databases include defined populations whose entire spectrum of care is under the responsibility of and provided by the integrated delivery system. They are substantially smaller than typical commercial insurance databases but provide a more complete picture of the healthcare received by its members.
- Medicare in the US provides healthcare coverage for almost all people 65 years and over as well as for qualifying individuals with permanent disabilities. Prescription drug coverage is optional and provided under Medicare Part D by private PDPs.
- Medicaid in the US provides comprehensive hospital, medical, and prescription drug coverage for certain categories of disadvantaged individuals.

- In Canada, there is no single national linked encounter database. Owing to the structure of the healthcare system, each province and territory maintains encounter databases that include prescription and medical services claims of the public healthcare programs, which can be linked to hospital discharge data.
- All Canadian residents are covered for medical services regardless of age or income. However, drug coverage varies between provinces and access to raw data is also restricted in some provinces; these aspects are important to consider in the selection of a Canadian database.
- Owing to coverage characteristics, patients can be followed long term in Canadian databases.
- The Nordic countries provide nationwide coverage of prescription fills with easy linkage to other health registries on, e.g. hospitalizations.

- Multiple other countries throughout Europe hold data sources covering sizeable proportions of the population, e.g. Italy, Germany, France, United Kingdom, and Holland.
- Many long established databases in the Asia-Pacific region cover high proportions of the population due to single-payer, nationwide healthcare coverage.
- Despite variation in healthcare systems and languages used throughout the region many of the databases conform to world standard medical vocabularies such as the WHO ATC classification system for medicines and ICD-10 codes for diagnoses.
- Use of Asian databases have historically been limited due to restrictions in the accessibility of these data. Access to databases may only be provided to local researchers while other databases do not provide direct success to raw data with only summary level data available for researchers.

---

**Case Example 9.1    US Commercial Insurance Databases (Dave et al. 2019)**

*Background*
- Sodium–glucose cotransporter-2 inhibitors (SGLT2i) are a class of antidiabetic medications that reduce serum glucose by inhibiting its reabsorption in the proximal tubule.
- Based on their mechanism of action, they are thought to increase the risk of severe Urinary Tract Infections (UTIs); however, findings from case-reports and meta-analysis of randomized controlled trials are inconclusive.

*Question*
Are type 2 diabetes patients initiating an SGLT2i at a higher risk of developing severe UTIs compared to those initiating non-SGLT2i therapies?

*Approach*
- A retrospective cohort study was conducted using the two US based commercial claims

databases: IBM MarketScan and Optum Clinformatics Datamart between March 2013 to September 2015.
- Within each database, patients aged 18 years or older with type 2 diabetes initiating SGLT2i versus dipeptidyl peptidase-4 (DPP4i) were identified and matched using 1:1 propensity score matching using >90 baseline covariates.
- The primary outcome was a severe UTI event, defined as a composite outcome of hospitalization for primary UTI, sepsis with UTI, or pyelonephritis. Hazard ratios (HR) were estimated using Cox regression.

*Results*
- After 1:1 propensity score matching, the study identified 61876 patients in each group.
- New initiators of SGLT2i had 61 severe UTI events (incidence rate [IR] per 1000

---

**Case Example 9.1    (Continued)**

person-years, 1.76), compared with 57 events in the DPP-4 inhibitor group (IR, 1.77), corresponding to an adjusted HR of 0.98 [95% confidence interval, 0.68–1.41]).

*Strengths*
- This cohort study utilized a large, diverse cohort of patients with diabetes from two commercial insurance databases.
- The study was able to follow patients for longitudinal exposures and important clinical outcomes, including hospitalizations due to severe UTIs.

*Limitations*
The small number of outcomes precluded detailed evaluation of the associations between individual agents and the risk of

diabetes. Although the study adjusted for more than 90 potential confounders, it could not directly control for important variables such as duration of diabetes or body mass index. Hemoglobin $A_{1c}$ results were available for <15% of sample further limiting the study ability to adjust for diabetes severity.

*Key Points*
- In this large population-based cohort study of patients with type 2 diabetes, SGLT2i was not associated with an increased risk of severe UTIs. On the basis of our findings, other factors beyond the risk of severe UTIs should be considered in decisions about whether to prescribe SGLT2i for patients with diabetes in routine care settings.

---

**Case Example 9.2    Canada (Faure et al. 2020)**

*Background*
- Despite the existence of clear clinical recommendations, previous studies have shown that 19–50% of patients who experienced an acute ischemic stroke (AIS) do not receive secondary prevention, consisting mainly of antiplatelet therapy (e.g. dipyridamole, clopidogrel, acetylsalicylic acid (ASA), or ticlopidine), or anticoagulants (e.g. vitamin K antagonist (VKA) or nonvitamin K antagonist oral anticoagulants (NOAC)).
- Although the efficacy of pharmacological secondary prevention has been demonstrated in clinical trials, evidence gaps remain regarding the effectiveness of secondary prevention in the real-world clinical practice setting; available data are either not recent, involved a short-term follow-up (e.g. 30 days), or restricted to specific subpopulations.

*Questions*
- What are the patterns of secondary stroke prevention treatments in the real-world clinical practice setting?
- What is the long-term effect of secondary stroke prevention on the risk of death or AIS recurrence?

*Approach*
- Population-based cohort study of adult patients (age ≥ 18 years) who were discharged following a hospitalization for an incident AIS between January 1, 2011, and December 31, 2012 and who survived beyond the short-term period (30 days). Data sources were the linked prescription and medical services claims databases of Quebec (RAMQ databases).
- The main study outcome was the composite of death or AIS recurrence between 31 and 365 days post discharge. Cox

*(Continued)*

---

**Case Example 9.2    (Continued)**

proportional hazard models were used to compare the risk of death or AIS recurrence across treatments using no prescribed treatment as the reference. In order to account for treatment switches and discontinuation during follow-up, exposure was time-dependent.

*Results*
- In the month after discharge, 44.3% of the patients did not receive the recommended treatment and > 20% did not have any treatment.
- Untreated patients were younger, had less comorbidities, and a more severe index AIS (using hospital length of stay as a proxy for severity).
- Anticoagulants and antiplatelets were associated with a lower risk of death or recurrence (hazard ratio [HR] 0.27; 95% confidence interval [CI] 0.20–0.36 and HR 0.25; 95% CI 0.16–0.38, respectively) compared with the untreated group.

*Strengths*
- This was a population-based study that reflected current prescription patterns for secondary AIS prevention in the community practice setting.

- Compared with previous studies that were mainly limited to the short-term period after a stroke, treatment effectiveness was evaluated over a one-year period.
- The use of a time-dependent exposure variable accounted for treatment heterogeneity during follow-up.

*Limitations*
- Information on drugs acquired OTC were not available, which may have overestimated the proportion of untreated patients owing to the availability of ASA OTC. However, for cost consideration, patients chronically treated favor acquiring ASA by prescription.
- Absence of data on previous AIS events that predated the one year look back period may have resulted in misclassification of incident cases.

*Key Points*
- The risk of death or AIS recurrence was reduced by 50–75% in patients receiving a secondary prevention treatment when compared with the untreated patients.
- Findings confirm treatment benefits shown in clinical trials and emphasize the importance of AIS secondary prevention.

---

**Case Example 9.3    Encounter Databases in Asia (Roughead et al. 2015)**

*Background*
Thiazolidinediones (rosiglitazone and pioglitazone), are associated with heart failure and edema. Many of the published studies investigating these adverse events were conducted in caucasian populations. Due to the differences in metabolizing enzymes and pharmacodynamic-based variation in response to the thiazolidinediones there may be a difference in the prevalence of adverse events across different ethnic groups.

*Questions*
Do the risks of heart failure and edema associated with the thiazolidinediones vary between populations located in Asia, Australia and Canada?

*Approach*
- Sequence symmetry analysis (SSA), a signal detection method for adverse drug events utilizing administrative claims data, was used to assess the association between the thiazolidinediones and

---

**Case Example 9.3    (Continued)**

edema (as indicated by furosemide initiation) or heart failure hospitalization across countries.

- Incident dispensing of rosiglitazone, pioglitazone, metformin, and furosemide and hospitalization for heart failure were determined for each individual patient. All incident dispensing that occurred within one year of each other for the same person were included in the analysis. The crude sequence ratio (SR) was calculated by dividing the number of persons with furosemide initiated after rosiglitazone initiation with the number of persons with furosemide initiated prior to rosiglitazone.
- The SSA method uses a within-person design, making it robust toward confounders that are stable over time.

*Results*
When results were pooled across the Caucasian populations there was a significantly increased risk of furosemide initiation for rosiglitazone and pioglitazone, while in the Asian populations, the pooled risk estimates were lower for rosiglitazone and not significant for pioglitazone.

*Strengths*
- This was a large study across six different countries in eight different databases.

- Standardized analytical code and standardized data variables were used to avoid differences due to coding
- While results differed across ethic populations, results were consistent within populations

*Limitations*
- Differences in the underlying prevalence of polymorphisms in both metabolizing enzymes and pharmacodynamic receptors may have played a role; however, differences in other factors, including diet, physical activity or healthcare practice may also be contributors.
- Diagnostic information was not available in all countries which limited the strength of conclusions that could be drawn regarding the more serious outcome of heart failure hospitalization
- Not all medicines were available in all countries resulting in the exclusion of some comparisons

*Key Points*
- The risk of edema and heart failure associated with rosiglitazone was generally lower in the Asian population than in the Caucasian population.
- There is potential for differences in response to medicines by ethnicity and these differences should be investigated when considering whether regulatory action is required.

---

# Further Reading

Hall, G.C., Sauer, B., Bourke, A. et al. (2012). Guidelines for good database selection and use in pharmacoepidemiology research. *Pharmacoepidemiol. Drug Saf.* 21 (1): 1–10.

Strom, B.L., Kimmel, S.E., and Hennessy, S. (eds.) (2012). *Pharmacoepidemiology*, Fifth Edition. John Wiley and Sons.

Faure, M., Castilloux, A.M., Lillo-Le-Louet, A. et al. (2020). Secondary stroke prevention: a population-based cohort study on anticoagulation and antiplatelet treatments, and the risk of death or recurrence. *Clin. Pharmacol. Ther.* 107: 443.

Roughead, E.E., Chan, E.W., Choi, N.K. et al. (2015 Sep). Variation in association between Thiazolidinediones and heart failure across ethnic groups: retrospective analysis of large healthcare claims databases in six countries. *Drug Saf.* 38 (9): 823–831.

Dave, C.V., Schneeweiss, S., Kim, D. et al. (2019 Aug 20). Sodium-glucose cotransporter 2 inhibitors and the risk of severe urinary tract infections. *Ann Intern Med.* 171 (4): 248–256.

## US Databases

Crystal, S., Akincigil, A., Bilder, S., and Walkup, J.T. (2007). Studying prescription drug use and outcomes with Medicaid claims data: strengths, limitations, and strategies. *Med. Care* 45 (10 Supl 2): S58–S65.

Gupta, N., Vujicic, M., and Blatz, A. (2018). Opioid prescribing practices from 2010 through 2015 among dentists in the United States: what do claims data tell us? *J. Am. Dent. Assoc.* 149 (4): 237–245. e236.

Hennessy, S., Leonard, C.E., and Bilker, W.B. (2007). Researchers and HIPAA. *Epidemiology* 18 (4): 518.

Hennessy, S., Bilker, W.B., Weber, A., and Strom, B.L. (2003). Descriptive analyses of the integrity of a US Medicaid claims database. *Pharmacoepidemiol. Drug Saf.* 12 (2): 103–111.

Huybrechts, K.F., Gerhard, T., Crystal, S. et al. (2012). Differential risk of death in older residents in nursing homes prescribed specific antipsychotic drugs: population based cohort study. *BMJ* 344: e977.

Lloyd, J.T., Blackwell, S.A., Wei, I.I. et al. (2015). Validity of a claims-based diagnosis of obesity among Medicare beneficiaries. *Eval. Health Prof.* 38 (4): 508–517.

Lo Re, V., Carbonari, D.M., Saine, M.E. et al. (2017). Postauthorization safety study of the DPP.4 inhibitor saxagliptin: a large scale multinational family of cohort studies of five outcomes. *BMJ Open Diabetes Res. Care* 5 (1): e000400.

Stroup, T.S., Gerhard, T., Crystal, S. et al. (2016). Comparative effectiveness of clozapine and standard antipsychotic treatment in adults with schizophrenia. *Am. J. Psychiatry* 173 (2): 166–173.

Wysowski, D.K. and Baum, C. (1993). The validity of Medicaid diagnoses of hip fracture. *Am. J. Public Health* 83 (5): 770.

## European Databases

Bezin, J., Duong, M., Lassalle, R. et al. (2017). The national healthcare system claims databases in France, SNIIRAM and EGB: powerful tools for pharmacoepidemiology. *Pharmacoepidemiol. Drug Saf.* 26 (8): 954–962.

Furu, K., Wettermark, B., Andersen, M. et al. (2010). The Nordic countries as a cohort for pharmacoepidemiological research. *Basic Clin. Pharmacol. Toxicol.* 106 (2): 86–94.

Pottegard, A., Schmidt, S.A.J., Wallach-Kildemoes, H. et al. (2017). Data resource profile: the Danish National Prescription Registry. *Int. J. Epidemiol.* 46 (3): 798.

Schade Hansen, C., Pottegard, A., Ekelund, U. et al. (2018). Association between QTc prolongation and mortality in patients with suspected poisoning in the emergency department: a transnational propensity score matched cohort study. *BMJ Open* 8 (7): e020036.

Schmidt, M., Schmidt, S.A., Sandegaard, J.L. et al. (2015). The Danish National Patient Registry: a review of content, data quality, and research potential. *Clin. Epidemiol.* 7: 449–490.

## Canadian Databases

Billioti de Gage, S., Moride, Y., Ducruet, T. et al. (2014). Benzodiazepine use and risk of Alzheimer's disease: case–control study. *BMJ* 349: g5205.

Filion, K.B., Chateau, D., Targownik, L.E. et al. (2014). Proton pump inhibitors and the risk of hospitalisation for community-acquired pneumonia: replicated cohort studies with meta-analysis. *Gut* 63 (4): 552–558.

Moride, Y., Lynd, L.D., Ducruet, H. et al. (2014). Antidepressants and risk of suicide or self-harm in Canadian youth: a study involving common data models in Quebec and British Columbia. *Pharmacoepidemiol. Drug Saf.* 23 (S1): S10–S11.

## Asian Databases

Hsing, A.W. and Ioannidis, J.P. (2015). Nationwide population science: lessons from the Taiwan National Health Insurance Research Database. *JAMA Intern. Med.* 175 (9): 1527–1529.

Kim, J.A., Yoon, S., Kim, L.Y., and Kim, D.S. (2017). Towards actualizing the value potential of Korea Health Insurance Review and Assessment (HIRA) data as a resource for health research: strengths, limitations, applications, and strategies for optimal use of HIRA data. *J. Korean Med. Sci.* 32 (5): 718–728.

Park, B.J., Sung, J.H., Park, K.D. et al. (2003). *Report of the Evaluation for Validity of Discharged Diagnoses in Korean Health Insurance Database*, 19–52. Seoul: Seoul National University.

Shin, J.Y., Roughead, E.E., Park, B.J., and Pratt, N.L. (2016). Cardiovascular safety of methylphenidateamong children and young people with attention-deficit/hyperactivity disorder (ADHD): nationwide self controlled case series study. *BMJ* 353: i2550.

## 10

# Electronic Health Record Databases

*Daniel B. Horton[1], Harshvinder Bhullar[2], Francesca Cunningham[3], Janet Sultana[4], and Gianluca Trifirò[5]*

[1] *Rutgers Robert Wood Johnson Medical School, Rutgers Center for Pharmacoepidemiology and Treatment Science, Rutgers School of Public Health, New Brunswick, NJ, USA*
[2] *Independent Consultant, London, UK*
[3] *US Department of Veterans Affairs, Hines, IL, USA*
[4] *Mater Dei Hospital, Msida, Malta and Exeter College of Medicine and Health, University of Exeter, Exeter, UK*
[5] *Department of Diagnostics and Public Health, University of Verona, Verona, Italy*

## Introduction

Electronic health record (EHR) databases are longitudinal patient record databases that are used by clinicians in caring for their patients and anonymized for the purpose of research. They often record information unavailable in administrative databases, such as symptoms of illness, historical data, family history, smoking and alcohol use, vital signs (e.g. body mass index [BMI]), and laboratory data. Further, EHR data recorded in the provision of patient care may more accurately represent patients' true clinical states than administrative claims data, which are maintained primarily for billing or administrative purposes.

Despite their advantages, EHR databases have certain limitations. Certain available data may have high rates of missingness (e.g. race, disease severity, smoking history). The validity of diagnostic codes cannot be presumed without formal validation. Some EHR databases, including the Veterans Affairs (VA) and other US EHRs, may not capture information from out-of-system care. Other EHR databases, including some from Europe, may lack data from secondary care (e.g. hospitals and specialists) or linkage to these datasets. While EHR databases usually contain data on prescribed outpatient drugs, many lack information on drug dispensing or inpatient medications.

In this chapter, we focus on selected European primary care EHR databases and a national EHR database for United States Veterans. While there are similarities among EHR databases, there are also important differences (see Tables 10.1 and 10.2).

## Description

### Overview of Health Care Systems and Populations

**Europe**: Many European nations (e.g. Italy, Netherlands, UK) have either universal government-funded health care or universal health insurance. General practitioners (GPs), and sometimes family pediatricians, act as gatekeepers for medical care in many countries. As a result, many European primary

**Table 10.1** Overview of EHR databases.

| | BIFAP | SIDIAP | Caserta LHU | LPD Italy | Pedianet | CPRD | IMRD | IPCI | IQVIA DA | VA |
|---|---|---|---|---|---|---|---|---|---|---|
| Country (region) | Spain | Spain (Catalonia) | Italy (Caserta) | Italy | Italy | United Kingdom | United Kingdom | Netherlands | Germany, France, United Kingdom | United States |
| Initiated | 2001 | 2006 | 2000 | 1998 | 2000 | 1987 | 2002 | 1989 | 1992 | 1997 |
| Patients, follow-up time | 7.9 M patients; 49.7 M person-years | 5.6 M patients; 5.7 M person-years | 0.9 M patients, 10.2 M person-years | 1.6 M patients; 19.2 M person-years | 0.4 M pediatric patients; 1.8 M person-years | 59.5 M patients (16.4 M active); >400 M person-years | 19 M patients (3.0 M active); >90 M person-years | 2.4 M patients; >12.1 M person-years | Germany: 34 M patients (including 17.2 M German specialty patients); 54.5 M person-years France: 10.5 M patients; 6.0 M person-years UK: 4.2 M patients; 17.9 M person-years | 14.5 M patients (6.4 M active); 168 M person-years |
| Ages included (years) | All | All | All | ≥15 | ≤16 | All | All | All | All | All |
| Diagnostic coding system | ICD-9, ICPC | ICD-10 | ICD-9 | ICD-9 | ICD-9, ICD-10 | Read, ICD-10, SNOMED | Read, SNOMED | ICPC | ICD-10, Read (UK) | ICD-9, ICD-10, CPT |
| Drug coding system | ATC | ATC, NDC | ATC, NDC ATC | ATC, NDC ATC | ATC, NDC | Gemscript | Gemscript | ATC | ATC | VA Drug Classification System, NDC |
| Software used | Various, mainly OMI-AP | e-CAPTM | Saniarp, Arianna | Millewin | Junior Bit | Vision, EMIS | Vision | Various | Various | Various |

ATC, Anatomical Therapeutic Chemical; CPT, Current Procedural Terminology; ICD, International Classification of Diseases; ICPC, Classification of Primary Care; M, million; NDC, National Drug Code; NHS, National Health Service.

Table 10.2 Selected variables in EHR databases available for epidemiologic research.

| | BIFAP | SIDIAP | Caserta LHU | LPD Italy | Pedianet | CPRD | IMRD | IPCI | IQVIA DA | VA |
|---|---|---|---|---|---|---|---|---|---|---|
| Health care professional demographics | Practice location | Age, sex, professional role, performance indicators (e.g. quality of care) | Physicians' age, sex, years since graduation | Practice location | Pediatricians' age, sex, city of clinic; other information available by request | Professional role of person entering data | Professional role of person entering data | N/A | Physicians' age, sex, years in practice | Professional role of person entering prescription data |
| Types of health care professionals | Mainly GPs, other primary care professionals (e.g. pediatricians, nurses) | Primary care professionals: GPs, pediatricians, dentists, nurses, midwives | GPs; claims data from the same catchment area | GPs | Family pediatricians | GPs | GPs | GPs | Mainly GPs; IQVIA DA Germany and France also include specialists (e.g. cardiologists, dermatologists) | Primary care physicians, physician specialists (e.g. cardiologists), other clinicians (e.g. nurse practitioners, pharmacists) |
| Practice and patient demographics | Practice: Number of patients registered with GP; number of persons registered in practice available upon request. Patient: DOB, sex | Practice: Location, urban/rural, number of patients, deprivation index (MEDEA). Patient: DOB, sex, country of origin | Practice: Province. Patient: DOB, sex, healthcare exemption (based on salary, disability, chronic diseases) | Practice: Location. Patient: DOB, sex healthcare exemption (based on salary, disability) | Practice: Region, patients per practice. Patient: YOB, age, sex, region of residence, nationality, information about parents (e.g. nationality, habits, blood group, mother's educational level, SES) | Practice: Region, practice size, practice-level SES (Index of Multiple Deprivation, Townsend scores, ~60%), date of last registration, Up-to-Standard date (see text). Patient: YOB for adults, month/YOB for children; sex, ethnicity (~25% recorded; also available via census data), census-based SES; patient status (active, died, transferred out) | Practice: Region, number of patients, computerization date, Vision date, Acceptable Mortality Reporting (see text). Patient: YOB for adults, month/YOB for children; patient-level, location-based SES (Townsend deprivation scores, 95% recording), region, ethnicity, (20% recording), patient status (active, died, transferred out) | Practice: Number of employees available for some practices. Patient: DOB, sex | Practice: Region, community size, patients per practice, number of physicians, number of employees, type (e.g. GP vs specialty). Patient: Age, sex, health insurance status (e.g. private, statutory), medical insurance company, region, town size (>100000 vs. <100000) | Practice: Region, facility, type of facility (clinics at medical center vs. community-based), facility's level of complexity. Patient: DOB, sex, race, ethnicity, zip code |

| | | | | | | | | | |
|---|---|---|---|---|---|---|---|---|---|
| Vital signs and social history | Weight, BMI, BP, smoking, alcohol use | BP, BMI, smoking, alcohol use, Framingham score. Pediatric screening data (height, weight, head circumference, pubertal development) | Height, weight, BMI, smoking, alcohol use (25% of patients ≥65 since 2013); BP available (since 2016) | Gestational age, birth weight, birth height, neonatal jaundice; growth measurements (e.g. height, weight); parental smoking | Height, weight, BP, BMI (measurements may be biased toward patients with clinical indications); smoking (83–93%), obesity (61–79%), alcohol use (~80%) | Height, weight, BP, BMI (measurements may be biased toward patients with clinical indications); smoking (86–94%), obesity (73–83%), alcohol use (75–85%) | BP, weight, BMI, smoking (recorded when considered relevant) | BMI (~40%); smoking and alcohol recording unknown | BP, HR, height, weight, SES, education, marital status, smoking (>90%) |
| Referrals, procedures, results of investigations | PCPs' referrals to specialists and hospitals; results from referrals may be recorded in coded fields or as free text; self-referrals (less common) not available | Laboratory test results, diagnostic/imaging referrals; spirometry; referrals for therapeutic procedures; referrals to secondary/tertiary care (date, reason, specialty referred) | Laboratory test results (~25%); linkage to hospital discharge data, referral data, diagnostic tests orders | Apgar scores, laboratory/imaging tests ordered and reasons for request; test results sometimes unavailable | Detailed information on referrals, procedures, laboratory tests (~75%, via linkage to HES) | Electronic referrals available; most outpatient laboratory results | Often N/A; test results may be available from letters from hospitals or free text | HbA1C, blood glucose, cholesterol, LDL, HDL available; other test results variably recorded, can be requested from paper files | Specialist referrals available; all laboratory results available (require standardization) |

*(Continued)*

**Table 10.2** (Continued)

| | BIFAP | SIDIAP | Caserta LHU | LPD Italy | Pedianet | CPRD | IMRD | IPCI | IQVIA DA | VA |
|---|---|---|---|---|---|---|---|---|---|---|
| Drug data types | Drugs prescribed and dispensed in community setting; vaccine data available | Drugs prescribed and dispensed in community setting (when covered by national healthcare system); vaccine data available | Drugs prescribed in community setting; drug dispensing by linkage to claims | Drugs prescribed in community setting; vaccine data available | Drugs prescribed and dispensed in community setting; inpatient drug data available if reported to pediatrician; non-compulsory vaccine data available, remaining vaccine data identified via linked claims | Drugs prescribed in primary care; some OTC drug data available (see text); vaccine data available | Drugs prescribed in primary care; vaccine data available | Drugs prescribed in community setting; vaccine data available; drug dispensing by linkage to Dutch PHARMO database | Drugs prescribed | Drugs prescribed and dispensed in outpatient and inpatient settings; vaccine data available |
| Available drug information | Drug name, active substance, number of prescribed packages, duration, prescribed daily dose, strength, indication | ATC code, NDC, indication, profession of prescriber; prescribing data only: start/end date, drug units per day; dispensing data only: units per package, number of packages per month, month of drug dispensation | Drug ATC code, NDC (with brand, formulation, units), indication | Drug name, route, dose, frequency, duration, cost | Drug name, ATC code, indication, Italian MINSAN code, NDC (with brand, formulation, units), number of prescribed packages, dose (not available for 30%) | Drug name, route, strength, frequency, duration; immunizations including batch; cost upon request | Drug name, route, strength, frequency, duration; immunizations including batch; linkage available to cost | Drug name, quantity, strength, dose | Drug name, route, dose, frequency, duration, cost | Drug name, route, strength, dose, frequency, quantity, duration, directions; cost |

| | | | | | | | | | |
|---|---|---|---|---|---|---|---|---|---|
| Health care utilization | GP visits; referrals by GP to secondary care/ED; hospital admissions available if patients referred to GPs after discharge | PCP visits; referrals to secondary/tertiary care, sick leave (date, length, reason), hospital discharge | GP visits; hospital discharge letters, specialist referrals, ED visits by linking with claims | GP visits, hospital discharge letters, specialist referrals | Pediatrician visits, ED/ hospital admission if referred by pediatrician | GP visits, hospitalizations, consultant visits; links to HES provide detailed ward-level resource utilization (England only) | GP visits, hospitalizations entered by GP, sick leave (if issued by GP); links to HES provides detailed ward-level resource utilization (England only) | GP visits; other data not available unless hospital discharge letters sent to GP | GP visits, hospitalizations, sick leave | Outpatient visits, ED visits, hospitalization (including medical, surgical, intensive care units), Community Living Center (VA nursing home) |
| Identification of pregnancy and families | ICD-9/ICPC codes for pregnancy; cannot identify families | Pregnancy, pregnancy outcomes; mother-baby link available | ICD-9 codes for pregnancy or birth by linkage to claims; cannot identify families | N/A | May identify siblings | Pregnancy, pregnancy outcomes; family/ household identification number; mother-baby linkage | Pregnancy, pregnancy outcomes; mother-baby link via family/ household number and algorithm | Some birth-related data available through hospital discharge letters; cannot identify families | Pregnancy variable, gynecologist records; family data incomplete | ICD-9/ICD-10 codes for pregnancy |
| Identification of death and cause of death | Date of death; cause of death not available consistently | Date of death | Date of death by linkage to claims | Date of death | Date/cause of death | Date/cause of death available via CPRD data and linkage to Office for National Statistics | Death date, sometimes cause of death; death certificates available for fee | Date of death; cause of death available via free-text | Date and cause of death seldom recorded | Date of death |
| Additional data, e.g. consult records, free text, paper files | Anonymized free text notes available | Hospital discharge (30%); other data by request | N/A | N/A | Free text by request | Hospital discharge summaries, consultant letters; no free text available | Hospital discharge summaries, consultant letters; free text by request | Free text by request | N/A | Additional data (e.g. consult records, free text) by chart review |

(Continued)

Table 10.2 (Continued)

| | BIFAP | SIDIAP | Caserta LHU | LPD Italy | Pedianet | CPRD | IMRD | IPCI | IQVIA DA | VA |
|---|---|---|---|---|---|---|---|---|---|---|
| Questionnaires, investigator-initiated outcome validation | Questionnaires for GPs | Questionnaires for GPs (sample) | Questionnaires for GPs | N/A | Participating pediatricians can interview patients/families | Questionnaires for GPs and patients; response rates ~90% | Questionnaires for GPs and patients; response rates ~90% | Questionnaires for GPs (response rates low) | Questionnaires upon request | Chart review for validation |
| Settings and types of missing data | Inpatient data, most OTC drugs | Inpatient data N/A except admission/discharge data for hospitals of the Catalan Health Institute; OTC drugs, drug indications, drugs not covered by national health system | Inpatient data (except via discharge forms with main diagnoses), laboratory results for 75%, OTC drugs, vaccines | Inpatient data, OTC drugs, drug dispensing, pediatric clinical and prescribing data (any setting) | Inpatient data N/A for 60%; most OTC drug data; adult health data | Prescriptions in secondary care, many OTC drugs, drug dispensing, adherence | Prescriptions in secondary care, many OTC drugs, drug dispensing, adherence | Inpatient/specialist data, OTC drugs | Secondary care records, vaccine data, patient-level linkage between primary care and specialty clinics | Encounter/drug data from healthcare facilities outside VHA, including for local acute care (e.g. stroke); some inpatient medications administered acutely |

ATC, Anatomical Therapeutic Chemical; BP, blood pressure; DOB, date of birth; ED, emergency department; GPs, general practitioners; HES, Hospital Episode Statistics; ICD, International Classification of Diseases; ICPC, International Classification of Primary Care; N/A, not available; NDC, National Drug Code; OTC, over-the-counter; PCP, primary care professional; SES, socioeconomic status; VHA, Veterans Health Administration; YOB, year of birth.

care-based EHR databases capture most of their patients' health information, including data from specialty and secondary care (e.g. consultations, hospitalizations). European EHR databases may contain regional or nation-wide data, depending on the structure of the health care system and the database. Notably, EHR databases from countries where GPs have less of a gatekeeper role (e.g. France, Germany) have less complete records of patients' health information.

**US/VA**: The VA's Veterans Health Administration (VHA) is one of the largest integrated health care systems in the United States. Funded by the US government, the VA provides medical, surgical, and rehabilitative care to military Veterans, active duty Reservists, and National Guard across nearly 150 hospitals, >1200 outpatient clinics, and > 100 nursing homes organized within 18 regional integrated networks. In contrast to the general US population, the VA population consists of predominantly older men (87% male, 47% over age 65 as of 2017) who often have multiple chronic medical or mental health conditions, although the proportion of younger female Veterans is rising. Most medications within the VHA are prescribed by VA clinicians and dispensed by VA pharmacies. Dual-care Veterans with Medicare coverage (which covers virtually all US citizens aged 65 years and older) may receive medications through both the VA and the Medicare Part D Plan. Because the VHA is not a closed medical system, Veterans may receive out-of-network care, limiting one's ability to study certain outcomes (See "Incompleteness of Clinical Data" below).

## Overview of Databases

**Europe**: The UK was the setting of the first European EHR database, now called the Clinical Practice Research Datalink (CPRD) (formerly General Practice Research Database [GPRD]), a research service of the UK Government that was established in 1987 for conducting public health research. CPRD encompasses two datasets – CPRD Gold from practices across the UK, and CPRD Aurum predominantly from English practices – which collectively contain data from about 25% of the UK population and represent one of the largest European EHR databases. IQVIA Medical Research Data (IMRD) (formerly The Health Improvement Network [THIN]) was later established as a collaboration between software and database companies (respectively, Cegedim and Epic Database Research Company Ltd., now part of IQVIA). The same practices may contribute to both CPRD and IMRD, but the proportion of overlap changes over time as new practices join or leave each database. Information from both databases may be combined to increase sample size and improve statistical power and generalizability. Merging data between CPRD and IMRD requires identification and singular inclusion of practices contributing to both databases in a given year.

The IQVIA Disease Analyzer databases (DA, previously known as Mediplus) contain anonymized patient records from primary care practices and office-based specialists (e.g. cardiologists, dermatologists, gynecologists, orthopedists) in France, Germany, and the UK. To preserve confidentiality, patients who see both GPs and specialists have different database identity codes, making it challenging to track patients across settings of care.

Italy's Health Search Longitudinal Patient Database (LPD Italy from IQVIA) is the country's largest EHR database. The Caserta Local Health Unit (LHU) database contains EHR data from approximately 60% of inhabitants in a province of southern Italy and represents the only Italian database that systematically links EHR and administrative claims data, including drug dispensing and hospital discharge data. Caserta LHU data may also be linked to comprehensive, multi-dimensional geriatric assessments for almost three-quarters of the local elderly population, making it valuable for geriatric research. Another Italian database,

Pedianet, contains data on over 400 000 children throughout Italy.

In Spain, Base de Datos para la Investigación Farmacoepidemiológica en Atención Primaria (BIFAP) contains primary care data from 9 of 17 autonomous communities representing nearly 20% of the Spanish population. Sistema de Información para el Desarrollo de la Investigación en Atención Primaria (SIDIAP) contains data from 85% of the population of a single autonomous community, Catalonia.

GPs across the Netherlands contribute data to Integrated Primary Care Information (IPCI, previously Interdisciplinary Processing of Clinical Information), which contains data from approximately 14% of the Dutch population.

**US/VA**: The VA database contains demographic, clinical, and administrative data since 1997 along with prescription data since 1999 and laboratory data starting in 2000. In 2017, the number of Veterans in the VA database was about 2% of the US population and 32% of US Veterans.

## Data Collection and Structure

**Europe**: Primary care practitioners use EHRs to document clinical information about their patients, which can then be electronically extracted for research purposes, examined for completeness and accuracy, and anonymized. Some EHR databases receive frequent data updates (e.g. Pedianet, CPRD, IMRD) while others receive data updates just one to two times per year (e.g. BIFAP, IPCI, LPD Italy). Primary care EHR databases generally contain a minimum common set of patient information, including demographics, medical diagnoses, and drug prescriptions, but they differ from one another in types of variables and data included (see Table 10.2).

European EHR databases record diagnoses using a variety of standardized coding systems: Read codes (IMRD, CPRD); International Classification of Diseases, 9th edition (ICD-9) (Caserta LHU Caserta, one autonomous region in BIFAP, LPD Italy, Pedianet); ICD-10 (IQVIA DA, SIDIAP, Pedianet, Hospital Episode

Statistics [HES] data linked with CPRD and IMRD); and the International Classification of Primary Care (ICPC) (IPCI, most autonomous regions in BIFAP) (see Table 10.1).

The European EHR databases also vary in how they record drug data. CPRD and IMRD employ British National Formulary (BNF) codes through the Gemscript system. Non-UK European databases record medications using Anatomical Therapeutic Chemical (ATC) classification codes; most countries also have national drug codes. All European EHR databases discussed contain data on prescribed medications. Caserta LHU, BIFAP, Pedianet, and SIDIAP also contain drug dispensing data. Additionally, Caserta LHU, BIFAP, Pedianet, and (for roughly half of drugs) DA databases specify drug indications.

All the above databases are generally representative of their underlying populations in terms of age/sex distribution and prevalence of most diseases and drugs used. However, certain diseases may vary in frequency across databases depending on local or disease-specific patterns of clinical care. BIFAP, CPRD, DA France and Germany, IPCI, Pedianet, LPD Italy, and IMRD include most regions of their respective countries.

Hospitalizations, referrals, and the resulting consultation letters are recorded to varying degrees in European EHR databases (see Table 10.2). Data from social history, including smoking and alcohol usage, is available to varying extents in most EHR databases See "Data Quality: Accuracy and Completeness" below and Table 10.2). Substance exposure information is less consistently recorded in DA databases and IPCI. Pedianet contains information on parental smoking habits.

In most European EHR databases, data are more commonly recorded using structured (coded) fields rather than unstructured free text. BIFAP and IPCI also contain large volumes of unstructured data. These and certain other databases (e.g. Pedianet, SIDIAP) make information from anonymized free text entries available to researchers for outcome validation and supplemental data extraction. Several databases (e.g. BIFAP, CPRD, DA Germany, Pedianet, SIDIAP, IMRD) also allow researchers to administer questionnaires directly to clinicians or patients for a fee.

**US/VA**: Local VA medical centers record outpatient and inpatient clinical and administrative data within the Veterans Health Information Systems Technology and Architecture (VistA) system. Data from VistA are available for research within the Corporate Data Warehouse (CDW), which contains a wide range of data elements from outpatient and inpatient settings, including demographics, diagnoses (ICD-9 and ICD-10 codes), vital signs, laboratory and radiology results, surgical procedures, free text notes, consults, and social history (e.g. smoking). The VA Vital Status File contains death data from multiple sources that are regularly cross-checked with the Social Security Administration Death Master File. In addition, VA has several disease-specific registries used for patient care and research (e.g. cancer, diabetes, severe mental illness, amyotrophic lateral sclerosis, rheumatoid arthritis).

The VA database contains information on both prescribing and dispensing of drugs in both outpatient and inpatient settings. Drug data may be found within several databases: the CDW; Pharmacy Benefit Management (PBM) database, which contains information on nonprescription medication dispensing and medical supplies; and the Bar Code Medication Administration (BCMA) database, which contains records of inpatient administrations of medications to patients. The VHA also maintains its own adverse drug and vaccine event reporting system (see Chapter 7).

Investigators may also extract data for research directly from the EHR through manual chart review or natural language processing. Primary data collection from unstructured data fields, such as reports or free text notes, can facilitate outcome ascertainment or validation. In addition to EHR data, surveys of Veterans or clinicians permit access to additional information.

## Data Quality: Accuracy and Completeness

**Europe**: Data quality checks are performed periodically by European EHR databases on three levels: (i) practitioner recording, (ii) data extraction; and (iii) database maintenance.

In the UK, national quality improvement initiatives and advances in software have increased overall capture and accuracy of data. For example, the UK Quality and Outcomes Framework (QOF) used financial incentives to improve documentation for >100 quality indicators for 10 chronic diseases. UK GPs contributing to IMRD or CPRD receive software training and regular evaluation of their data recording and prescribing behavior, including feedback reports with tips on improving recording. Other database-directed quality measures include audits of newly added practices and comparison of data to national databases (e.g. mortality, hospitalizations, cancer and cardiovascular registries).

CPRD only provides data from practices meeting quality standards (~90% of practices). The Up-to-Standard date is a practice-based quality marker based on death rates and gaps in recording, corresponding to when a practice in CPRD is considered to have continuous, complete recording of data. For IMRD, IQVIA employs a practice-specific quality measure known as Acceptable Mortality Reporting (AMR), denoting the first year that mortality reporting was deemed complete. Other European EHR databases have their own standards for ensuring quality and completeness.

With regards to specific variables, data completeness varies among databases (See "Incompleteness of Clinical Data" and Table 10.2). Pregnancy, family structure, mortality, and cause of death are heterogeneously recorded and may be difficult to ascertain. CPRD offers a probabilistic mother–baby link algorithm and is linkable to mortality records from the Office for National Statistics to improve death estimates and confirm cause of death. In IMRD, researchers may also use data algorithms to link family members or determine cause-specific mortality.

US/VA: The CDW, a non-transformed mirror of the medical record, is updated nightly. Updates of the Vital Status File occur monthly. The accuracy and completeness of data reflect the EHR and beneficiary claims they source. Earlier years of demographic race and ethnicity data can have up to 20% missing data.

The PBM prescription database undergoes daily quality assurance processes to ensure completeness and accuracy. As with medications obtained through Medicaid (see Chapter 9), low or nil co-payments produce strong financial incentives for Veterans to obtain outpatient prescriptions through the VA.

### Data Access for Researchers

Europe: Research performed using European EHR databases must generally first be reviewed by the local institutional review board (IRB) and the respective database's ethics board. Given researchers' inability to identify individual patients in anonymized databases, most studies meet criteria for IRB exemption. Several European databases are available for licensing by investigators in government, academia, and industry, while access to certain European databases (Caserta LHU, IPCI, LPD Italy, Pedianet) requires collaboration with affiliated researchers.

US/VA: To use VA data, researchers must first receive approval by the local or central VA IRB. Access to VA data is limited to VA-affiliated researchers and their collaborators.

## Strengths

### Population-Based Data, Sample Size, and Length of Follow-up

Population-based data from European EHRs draw subjects from the general population, minimizing selection bias and improving validity and generalizability of pharmacoepidemiologic studies. These data sources are ideal for nested case–control and cohort studies. EHRs generally have a longer follow-up period compared to claims data. These characteristics, along with the large populations covered by EHRs, make these data sources particularly ideal to study rare diseases and rare outcomes.

### Validity of Clinical Information

Epidemiologic studies in EHR databases involve use of lists of codes, and sometimes coding algorithms, for identifying specific medical conditions, drugs/other exposures of interest, and covariates. The validity of such code lists and algorithms has often been studied in many of these databases. If a proposed outcome has not previously been validated, researchers should strongly consider validating that outcome to ensure that diagnostic codes or algorithms reflect patients' true conditions.

### Accuracy of Drug Information

EHR databases contain information on name, strength, and quantity of prescribed drugs, which can be used to estimate prescription coverage. In the UK, unlike in other countries, the prescription is the payment document. Refills can be accurately identified from prescriptions in IMRD. The concordance between issued prescriptions and dispensed drugs in IMRD is generally high, with some exceptions. Caserta LHU, BIFAP, Pedianet, SIDIAP, and VA data contain information on outpatient drug prescribing and dispensing. VA data also capture inpatient drug dispensing and administration.

### Ability to Access Original Health Records

Some EHRs provide access to original anonymized healthcare records, such as free text data (e.g. IMRD, IPCI), anonymized copies of paper records (e.g. IMRD), or the entire

EHR (e.g. VA), as well as access to clinicians or patients via surveys (Table 10.2). Such access can be useful for validation purposes.

### Linkage to External Patient-Level Data

Many EHR databases may be linked to other health-related, patient-level information, thus extending the utility of EHR data. The data source most commonly linked to CPRD and IMRD is HES, which contain data on hospitalizations, accident and emergency episodes, and specialized testing, including imaging. The combination of data from primary care and HES facilitates research on conditions managed across multiple healthcare settings. Linkage to official death records may improve the accuracy of mortality studies and validate mortality data from general practice. Researchers can link EHR data with other data sources, including disease (e.g. cancer and COVID-19) registries, mental health datasets, and socioeconomic and deprivation indices. EHR data may also be linked to individual patient-generated data, including patient-reported outcomes, environmental data, drug diaries, and biospecimens. EHR databases outside the UK also permit linkages to other data sources: Caserta LHU EHR to claims data; VA data to Medicare and Medicaid claims data and to genetic information from the Million Veteran Program biobank.

## Limitations

### Incompleteness of Clinical Data

The accuracy and completeness of EHR data rely heavily on the quality of the recording from physicians during routine care. Human errors as well as systematic recording errors may occur, with the latter leading to bias. For example, geriatric data in EHRs are likely to be selectively recorded for frailer patients. Another example is that clinicians may be more likely to record laboratory or radiologic findings that are abnormal, while normal and some abnormal results may not be documented reliably.

Because European EHR databases are designed to capture health information from primary care settings, they typically lack information from specialists. Researchers using IMRD or CPRD may access more extensive and reliable data from other settings through linkage with HES data and other sources. Similarly, as mentioned above, EHR data from Caserta LHU can be linked with claims data.

The nature of illness can affect the pattern of data recording. Unlike in claims databases, codes for chronic diseases may be entered only once into some EHR databases. For this reason, episodes of care involving acute events may be better recorded than chronic diseases.

While many EHR databases capture information about race and ethnicity, smoking and alcohol use, BMI, socioeconomic status, employment status, and occupation, these fields may be missing for many individuals (see Table 10.2). UK EHR databases may miss many pediatric growth measurements that are instead recorded locally on paper. Recording of pediatric growth measurements is more comprehensive in Pedianet.

Veterans in the VHA may receive health care outside the VHA either by choice (especially older Veterans with Medicare coverage) or by necessity (e.g. emergent care). As a result, occurrences of acute conditions may be generally missed in inpatient data from VA hospitals, potentially resulting in missing outcome data. The frequent omission of acute inpatient outcomes is a major limitation of the VA database; among veterans aged 65 and older, this limitation can be overcome by linking VA data to Medicare claims data.

### Incompleteness of Drug Data

Information on medication days' supply and daily dosage may not be explicitly recorded in EHR data but can be imputed. Additionally, algorithms have been developed to determine daily dosage and other drug data (e.g. frequency) from unstructured text. Only a few databases (BIFAP, Caserta LHU, Pedianet, and to some extent DA) specifically link prescribed drugs to the specific indication of use. Without this information, one can refer to diagnoses recorded in or around encounters that correspond to prescribed drugs.

Prescribing records do not indicate whether prescriptions were filled. Only BIFAP, Caserta LHU, SIDIAP, and the VA also contain drug dispensing data. Data on over-the-counter (OTC) drugs are frequently missing from EHR databases, but exceptions exist where health care systems pay for OTC drugs (e.g. long-term use of aspirin and nonsteroidal anti-inflammatory drugs in UK databases) and where OTC drugs are prescribed (e.g. Caserta LHU, Pedianet, VA). SIDIAP captures prescribing and dispensing of drugs irrespective of coverage by the national health system, leading to comprehensive recording of OTC medications.

In European EHR databases, data on medications restricted to specialist care, dispensed from hospital pharmacies (e.g. biologics), and given during hospitalization or upon hospital discharge may be missing. In the UK, patients generally receive a limited quantity of medications upon hospital discharge. In the VA, certain medications are recorded in the EHR but not the prescription databases, e.g. medications obtained from floor stock or administered acutely in emergencies. Other drug administrations may occasionally be incomplete in VA prescription databases.

## The Future

Through interoperable platforms, health information exchanges, patient portals with patient-generated data, and other technologic advances, EHR databases continue to evolve and expand in pursuit of delivering high-quality, high-value health care. Such advances enable clinicians and researchers to have greater access to increasing volumes of data. As EHR systems evolve, systems administrators, clinical informatics specialists, and end users must address important challenges, including missing data and variable recording. To optimize clinical care and facilitate high-quality research, health care systems must implement approaches to ensure consistent and complete clinical documentation within the EHR. The vital need to maintain individuals' privacy and confidentiality must be balanced with the potential societal benefits of enhanced linkage and sharing of data across disparate platforms and data sources.

The many advancements in EHR systems have important implications for the conduct of research. Technologic advances, such as natural language processing and machine learning, enable researches to use complex EHR data in novel ways. Large international research networks, such as TEDDY (Teddy European Network of Excellence for Paediatric Research) and OHDSI (Observational Health Data Sciences and Informatics), have demonstrated the capacity and power of international collaborations to use EHR databases for large-scale research on drug use and outcomes, including during the COVID-19 pandemic. Such collaborations lead to more generalizable research with increased statistical power to study rare diseases, uncommon drugs, and rare outcomes. Linkage of EHRs with hospital data, administrative claims, and other data sources (e.g. patient registries) helps maximize the advantages of each data source and minimize their respective limitations. Furthermore, linkage of EHR data to patient-generated data and biospecimens enhances discovery through population-representative, patient-centered research and molecular pharmacoepidemiology. Researchers can also use EHR systems to conduct large pragmatic trials. In addition, expansion of EHRs in low- and middle-income countries facilitates research in areas of great need.

High-quality research conducted within EHR databases can favorably influence public policy and public health. EHR databases also have an important regulatory role in post-market evaluation, pharmacovigilance, and risk minimization. With rapid, nearly real-time analyses of recent population-based data, EHR databases are useful settings to conduct post-authorization safety studies as well as research addressing emergent health crises, such as COVID-19. Through high-quality clinical and translational research and pharmacovigilance, EHR systems of the future will continue to serve as key platforms for answering important questions and improving the health of patients, communities, and populations.

## Summary Points for Electronic Health Record Databases

- European EHRs databases contain anonymized, population-based data collected in the context of patient care (e.g. diagnoses, prescribed drugs, health-related behaviors, vital signs, referrals) predominantly from outpatient settings by primary care practitioners.
- The United States Veterans Affairs databases contain a wide range of clinical data (e.g. diagnoses, prescribed and dispensed drugs, health-related behaviors, vital signs, laboratory data, mortality, free-text data) on US Veterans from outpatient and inpatient settings.
- EHR databases vary widely in characteristics, including data structure and coding systems; location, size, and proportion of population covered; population of focus (e.g. general, children, Veterans); types of data included

(e.g. laboratory results, socioeconomic data, dispensed drugs, mortality, free text); ability to link to other data sources (e.g. claims data, inpatient data); and modes of access.
- With long durations of follow-up and often large populations, EHR databases are suitable settings for studying a wide variety of medical conditions, including rare diseases and rare outcomes, using numerous study designs. Validation of key outcomes improves study validity.
- Incomplete information about certain types of data (e.g. health-related behaviors, data from specialists or hospitals) can lead to bias or other study limitations when using EHR databases. With some databases, investigators may obtain additional information by linking to other datasets (e.g. secondary care, disease registries), reviewing free text, or sending questionnaires to physicians or patients.
- Research using EHR databases can contribute meaningfully to efforts related to public health, public policy, and pharmacovigilance.

## Acknowledgment

The authors wish to thank Alexis Ogdie for her contributions along with the following individuals who provided information about specific databases: BIFAP: Miguel Gil García, Miguel Angel Maciá Martínez, Dolores Montero Corominas; Caserta LHU: Valentina Ientile and Michele Tari; CPRD: Lucy Carty; LPD Italy: Alessandro Pasqua, Iacopo Cricelli, Francesco Lapi; IPCI: Marcel de Wilde; Pedianet: Carlo Giaquinto, Luigi Cantarutti, Anna Cantarutti; SIDIAP: Bonaventura Bolíbar, Eduardo Hermosilla Pérez, Maria del Mar García Gil, Talita Duarte Salles; VA: Lucy Pandey, Kwan Hur.

---

**Case Example 10.1    Electronic Health Record Database in Spain (see de Abajo et al., Lancet, 2020)**

---

*Background*
- Angiotensin-converting enzyme 2 (ACE2) is the molecular receptor used by severe acute respiratory syndrome coronavirus 2 (SARS-CoV-2) to enter cells and cause infection.
- Renin–angiotensin–aldosterone system (RAAS) inhibitors (e.g. ACE inhibitors, angiotensin-receptor blockers [ARBs]) increase ACE2 expression in some animal models and may reduce angiotensin II-associated lung injury, raising questions about the role of RAAS inhibitors in increasing or decreasing the risk of SARS-CoV-2 infection and severity of coronavirus disease-2019 (COVID-19).
- Early in the COVID-19 pandemic, associations between certain comorbidities (e.g. diabetes, hypertension) and severe COVID-19 led to questions about the safety of continuing RAAS inhibitors.

*Issue*
Using BIFAP and another local EHR database (HORUS), a population-based study was conducted to evaluate the association between use of RAAS inhibitors and severe COVID-19 in Madrid, Spain.

*Approach*
- A case-population design was used.
- Cases were adults consecutively admitted in March 2020 to hospitals in Madrid with a diagnosis of COVID-19, stratified by severity; patients with severe COVID-19 required intensive care unit (ICU) admission or died.
- Each case was matched by age, sex, and index date (day and month of hospital admission) to 10 random controls in Madrid using 2018 data from BIFAP

(2019–2020 BIFAP data were not available).
- Exposure was defined as a prescription for RAAS inhibitors lasting until one month before the index date (current use), compared with current use of other antihypertensives (e.g. calcium channel blockers, beta blockers, diuretics).
- Potential confounders were a history of diabetes, hyperlipidemia (defined as use of lipid-lowering drugs), atrial fibrillation, heart failure, ischemic heart disease, thromboembolic disease, cerebrovascular accident, asthma, cancer, chronic kidney disease, or chronic obstructive pulmonary disease; underlying cardiovascular disease (composite of comorbidities); cardiovascular risk factors (composite of comorbidities including hypertension).
- Associations were estimated using multivariable conditional logistic regression, adjusted for confounders. Potential effect modification by age, sex, and comorbidity (e.g. hypertension, diabetes) was examined. Models were also stratified by COVID-19 severity.
- Secondary analyses considered associations for individual drug classes (e.g. ACE inhibitors versus calcium channel blockers).
- Sensitivity analyses considered impact of secular trends of RAAS use (given the two-year gap between case and control data) and media alerts about the safety of RAAS inhibitors, among others.

*Results*
- Data were collected from 1139 cases and 11 390 matched controls. Comorbidities and use of antihypertensives were more prevalent among cases than controls.

---

**Case Example 10.1    (Continued)**

- Current use of RAAS inhibitors was 43.6% in cases and 33.6% in controls, compared with current use of other antihypertensives in 13.6% of cases and 9.9% of controls.
- Adjusting for covariates, the odds ratio for the risk of COVID-19 requiring hospitalization among users of RAAS inhibitors was 0.94 (95% CI: 0.77, 1.15).
- Most secondary analyses based on drug class (ACE inhibitors, ARBs) and COVID-19 severity were similar; larger associations were seen with aldosterone antagonists (adjusted OR 1.68, 95% CI 0.97, 2.91) and short-term use of RAAS inhibitor (adjusted OR 1.39, 95% CI 0.92, 2.10).
- Stratified analyses suggested potential effect modification by diabetes, with adjusted OR of 0.53 (95% CI 0.34, 0.80) in patients diagnosed with diabetes.
- Sensitivity analyses yielded similar results.

*Strengths*
- Population-based data, active-comparator design, and covariate adjustment reduced bias from confounding and enhanced the generalizability of the findings.
- Most secondary and sensitivity analyses were consistent with the findings of a null

association between use of RAAS inhibitors and hospitalized/severe COVID-19.

*Limitations*
- Cases and controls were drawn from different databases (albeit from the same underlying population and source data) and different years, but sensitivity analyses considering the influence of secular trends in use of RAAS inhibitors were similar.
- No adjustment for smoking, other lifestyle habits, or other potential unmeasured confounders.
- Analyses considered drug prescription data, not accounting for consumption or adherence.
- No consideration of dose effects of medications.
- Certain secondary analyses suggested possible elevated risk with certain patterns of RAAS inhibitor use, of unclear significance.

*Key Points*
- Current use of RAAS inhibitors was not appreciably associated with altered risk of hospitalized or severe COVID-19.
- These findings did not support the practice of either stopping or starting RAAS inhibitors during the COVID-19 pandemic.

---

# Further Readings

de Abajo, F.J., Rodríguez-Martín, S., Lerma, V. et al. (2020). Use of renin-angiotensin-aldosterone system inhibitors and risk of COVID-19 requiring admission to hospital: a case-population study. *Lancet* 395 (10238): 1705–1714.

Becher, H., Kostev, K., and Schroder-Bernhardi, D. (2009). Validity and representativeness of the disease analyzer patient database for use in pharmacoepidemiological and

pharmacoeconomic studies. *Int. J. Clin. Pract.* 47 (10): 617–626.

Cai, B., Xu, W., Bortnichak, E., and Watson, D.J. (2012). An algorithm to identify medical practices common to both the general practice research database and the health improvement network database. *Pharmacoepidemiol. Drug Saf.* 21 (7): 770–774.

Carbonari, D.M., Saine, M.E., Newcomb, C.W. et al. (2015). Use of demographic and pharmacy data to identify patients included within both the Clinical Practice Research Datalink (CPRD) and The Health Improvement Network (THIN). *Pharmacoepidemiol. Drug Saf.* 24 (9): 999–1003.

Dave, S. and Peterson, I. (2009). Creating medical and drug code lists to identify cases in primary care databases. *Pharmacoepidemiol. Drug Saf.* 18: 704–707.

Evans, R.S. (2016). Electronic health records: then, now, and in the future. *Yearb. Med. Inform.* 1: S48–S61.

Garvin, J.H., Kalsy, M., Brandt, C. et al. (2017). An evolving ecosystem for natural language processing in Department of Veterans Affairs. *J. Med. Syst.* 41 (2): 32.

Gellad, W.F. (2016). The veterans choice act and dual health system use. *J. Gen. Intern. Med.* 31 (2): 153–154.

Hall, G.C., Sauer, B., Bourke, A. et al. (2012). Guidelines for good database selection and use in pharmacoepidemiology research. *Pharmacoepidemiol. Drug Saf.* 21 (1): 1–10.

Haynes, K., Bilker, W.B., Tenhave, T.R. et al. (2011). Temporal and within practice variability in The Health Improvement Network. *Pharmacoepidemiol. Drug Saf.* 20 (9): 948–955.

Herrett, E., Thomas, S., Schoonen, S. et al. (2010). Validation and validity of diagnoses in the general practice research database: a systematic review. *Br. J. Clin. Pharmacol.* 69 (1): 4–14.

Herrett, E., Gallagher, A.M., Bhaskaran, K. et al. (2015). Data resource profile: Clinical Practice Research Datalink (CPRD). *Int. J. Epidemiol.* 44 (3): 827–836.

Khan, N., Perera, R., Harper, S., and Rose, P. (2010). Adaptation and validation of the Charlson index for read/OXMIS coded databases. *BMC Family Prac.* 5 (11): 1.

Lester, H. (2008). The UK quality and outcomes framework. *BMJ* 337: a2095.

Lewis, J.D., Schinnar, R., Bilker, W.B. et al. (2007). Validation studies of The Health Improvement Network (THIN) database for pharmacoepidemiology research. *Pharmacoepidemiol. Drug Saf.* 16: 393–401.

Lewis, J., Bilker, W., Weinstein, R., and Strom, B. (2005). The relationship between time since registration and measured incidence rates in the general practice research database. *Pharmacoepidemiol. Drug Saf.* 14: 443–451.

Lum, K.J., Newcomb, C.W., Roy, J.A. et al. (2017). Evaluation of methods to estimate missing days' supply within pharmacy data of the Clinical Practice Research Datalink (CPRD) and The Health Improvement Network (THIN). *Eur. J. Clin. Pharmacol.* 73 (1): 115–123.

Maguire, A., Blak, B., and Thompson, M. (2009). The importance of defining periods of complete mortality reporting for research using automated data from primary care. *Pharmacoepidemiol. Drug Saf.* 18: 76–83.

Marston, L., Carpenter, J.R., Walters, K.R. et al. (2014). Smoker, ex-smoker or non-smoker? The validity of routinely recorded smoking status in UK primary care: a cross-sectional study. *BMJ Open* 4 (4): e004958.

Oyinlola, J.O., Campbell, J., and Kousoulis, A.A. (2016). Is real world evidence influencing practice? A systematic review of CPRD research in NICE guidances. *BMC Health Serv. Res.* 16: 299.

Robb, M.A., Racoosin, J.A., Worrall, C. et al. (2012). Active surveillance of postmarket medical product safety in the Federal Partners' collaboration. *Med. Care* 50 (11): 948–953.

Smith, M.W. and Joseph, G.J. (2003). Pharmacy data in the VA health care system. *Med. Care Res. Rev.* 60 (3 Suppl): 92S–123S.

Sohn, M., Arnold, N., Maynard, C., and Hynes, D. (2006). Accuracy and completeness of mortality data in the Department of Veterans Affairs. *Popul. Health Metrics* 4: 2–8.

Trifiro, G., Sultana, J., and Bate, A. (2018). From big data to smart data for pharmacovigilance:

the role of healthcare databases and other emerging sources. *Drug Saf.* 41 (2): 143–149.

van Staa, T.P., Dyson, L., McCann, G. et al. (2014). The opportunities and challenges of pragmatic point-of-care randomised trials using routinely collected electronic records:

evaluations of two exemplar trials. *Health Technol. Assess.* 18 (43): 1–146.

Wolf, A., Dedman, D., Campbell, J. et al. (2019). Data resource profile: Clinical Practice Research Datalink (CPRD) aurum. *Int. J. Epidemiol.* 48 (6): 1740–1740g.

## 11

# Primary Data Collection for Pharmacoepidemiology

*Priscilla Velentgas*

*Real World Solutions, IQVIA, Inc., Cambridge, MA, USA*

## Introduction

Primary data collection refers to data that are collected specifically for a given research study or program, while secondary data are data that were collected to meet needs other than the research for which they are being used. Primary data collection can be used in all types of pharmacoepidemiologic study designs, both interventional and non-interventional, cohort, and case–control studies, as well as patient registries. Registries are conceptually a data collection structure for disease or product related studies, and in practice may closely resemble observational cohort study designs. Registry-based studies generally address effectiveness and safety of various medical treatments, and also are used to characterize diseases including progression over time.

### Research Questions that Require Primary Data

The nature of the research question(s) and accompanying study design determine the need for collection of primary data from clinicians, patients, and/or others to address a study's aims, and are generally weighed against the availability of the required information in existing data sources (see Chapter 12). Some

"hybrid or enriched" studies may combine existing data with primary data collection for critical aspects of the patient or health care provider (HCP) experience (see "Hybrid or enriched designs" below).

Research questions that may require primary data include the following:

*Designs involving randomization* – pragmatic as well as explanatory randomized clinical trial designs (see Chapter 17) necessitate at least minimal site and/or patient contact for screening to determine eligibility and consent to participate in the trial. While randomized studies frequently involve extensive primary data collection to meet the trial objectives, these considerations overlap with those of observational designs and will be addressed further in that context.

*Outcome assessment/adjudication* – studies may require collection of detailed primary data for outcome assessment and/or for outcome adjudication. Collection of primary data for outcome assessment becomes important when study outcomes are not consistently recorded in available health care data, or are not recorded with the reliability, timing or frequency needed to meet study aims. Additional primary data may also be collected to validate or confirm outcomes collected through secondary data or patient self-report. Outcome

*Textbook of Pharmacoepidemiology*, Third Edition. Edited by Brian L. Strom, Stephen E. Kimmel, and Sean Hennessy.

validation can also be important for safety studies that use the patient as the primary reporter of potential adverse events (AEs), and clinical validation may be needed to confirm the endpoint of interest. For example, in the European PROTECT (Pharmacoepidemiological Research on Outcomes of Therapeutics) Consortium, funded by the Innovative Medicines Initiative, data were collected directly from pregnant women recruited online from the UK, Denmark, The Netherlands and Poland. Researchers learned that women could accurately report serious birth defects, but there were many reports of potential abnormalities that were difficult to classify without more clinical information.

Some observational as well as interventional studies, especially those designed to meet post-marketing requirements with safety or effectiveness outcomes that require an additional level of rigor, may include a full or modified approach to clinical outcome review or adjudication by a central committee over and above the reporting by individual study sites. Reasons supporting the need for additional outcome adjudication include concerns regarding investigator bias, if they hold strong opinions as to the benefit or harm associated with a treatment under study, the need to apply consistent standard definitions given variability in diagnostic criteria in usual practice, and lack of detail or inconsistent use of standard coding practices in accessible secondary data sources.

*Clinical assessments not consistently captured in secondary data* – Even as the collection of health care data from routine care is increasingly recorded and available from electronic as well as paper medical records, substantial variability in performing assessments on the part of HCPs according to individual and local practice, magnified by patients' variability in coming in for recommended routine visits, limits the extent to which clinical data from secondary sources can be used to address some research questions. See section on "Clinician or site-reported outcomes" below.

Commonly, prospective studies including planned analysis of laboratory data or imaging studies over time may incorporate primary data collection to ensure complete collection of assessments and that timing of assessments is aligned with the study follow-up period. Additionally, use of a central lab to reduce variability in laboratory measures may be considered to further increase the validity of study results. The PROVALID study, (PROspective cohort study in patients with type 2 diabetes [T2D] mellitus for VALIDation of biomarkers), launched in 5 EU countries (Austria, Hungary, Netherlands, Poland and Scotland), will obtain laboratory measurements on 4000 enrolled patients with type-2 diabetes treated in the primary care setting to examine the impact of medication and predict the clinical course of disease, including renal and cardiovascular events. Sites that participate in PROVALID are required to collect a minimum set of clinical data parameters, with the option to collect many additional laboratory and medical history characteristics on enrolled patients.

*Characterization of patient-reported outcomes not captured in secondary data* – It is often important to evaluate the burden of disease on patients and how that burden is affected by various treatments. Burden can include measures of disease related or general quality of life, ability to complete activities or attend work, assessment of pain or symptoms related to the underlying condition. Additional detail is provided in the section on "Patient-Generated Data" below.

*Studies of rare populations* – when necessary to assemble as large and representative a sample as possible from a rare population, one or more existing data sources may not capture enough of the patient population of interest to address study aims. Registries of rare disease and of pregnancy exposures commonly face the challenge of a small number of patients with the condition or exposure of interest, distributed over many countries, for which no single existing data source likely includes enough patients to address research aims.

Registries of rare diseases have been utilized in a number of ways to support the assessment of potential treatments. These include providing information on the natural history of disease to inform the design of studies and trials, serving as historical comparators for single arm trials, and for identification of patients for studies of treatment effectiveness, including registry-based randomized trials. The validity of conclusions that may be drawn from analyses of registry data depend on the degree to which subjects in the registry are not selectively included because of their treatments and outcomes, and the degree to which follow up and capture of necessary clinical data is sufficiently complete.

Pregnancy exposure registries are post-approval studies of the safety of drugs or vaccines, which women may use during pregnancy. Depending on the product and indication, the number of exposed pregnant women may be very small and geographically dispersed. Recent draft FDA guidance for pregnancy registries states that ". . .pregnancy registries remain an important tool for safety data collection in the post-marketing setting because of the prospective design and the ability to collect detailed patient level data." Such data include detail of timing of exposures and clinical detail around pregnancy and offspring outcomes, with requirements determined by the research question and outcomes of interest for each registry.

**Vaccine safety** – When conducting studies of vaccine safety, detailed information on vaccine brand and formulation as well as batch or lot numbers may not be readily available in secondary data, and some AEs of interest may not be routinely captured in existing data sources (see "Special Methodological Issues in Pharmacoepidemiologic Studies of Vaccine Safety" in Chapter 23).

Beginning in 2014, the European Medicines Agency (EMA) has required annual enhanced safety surveillance for all seasonal influenza vaccines. The interim guidance from the Pharmacovigilance Risk Assessment Committee included the requirement to collect data that would support the identification of any significant change in frequency or severity of reactogenicity in comparison with previous years' experience with the same vaccine composition. Reactogenicity AEs of interest include vaccination site reactions, headache, malaise, myalgia, shivering, rash, vomiting, nausea, arthralgia, decreased appetite, irritability and crying (in pediatric vaccinees less than five years of age). Such symptoms, especially when mild or moderate in severity, are not commonly reported to HCPs and thus medical records are not a useful source of data to study these outcomes following vaccination. Instead, studies and surveillance activities to implement the requirements for enhanced safety surveillance have incorporated patient (and adult proxy for pediatric patients) self-report of occurrence of symptoms to obtain this information in a systematic manner, for example through distribution of Safety Report Cards allowing patients to report these symptoms by telephone or mail. Enrollment of vaccinated subjects at the point of vaccination allows for capture of the specific vaccine brand and batch or lot number, either through investigators' knowledge that only specific vaccines are being distributed at the site, or through direct collection of this information from staff administering the vaccines.

**Studies of medical devices** – As with vaccines, device studies may require information on batch and manufacture location that are not available in existing data sources (see "Epidemiologic Studies of Implantable Medical Devices" in Chapter 23). Additional information on the "operator" or HCP implanting or administering the device may also help to provide a full characterization of product safety and effectiveness.

For example, data collected through the National Cardiovascular Data Registry (NCDR) has been utilized for studies that compares the effectiveness of different types of devices on cardiovascular outcomes, as well as allowing for examination of the role of manufacturing site in device failure. In a 2017 report comparing safety of the Mynx vascular closure device to other similar devices using the NCDR CathPCI Registry, a safety signal was observed in both the full identified analysis population and a subset of centers with greater experience with the device.

*Special requirements, controlled distribution products* – some products are approved by regulatory authorities with special requirements for safety reporting. Often such requirements necessitate data collection specific to the product and the safety concern to ensure robust monitoring of these concerns.

Several active mandated safety registries and an example of a multi-sponsor pediatric safety registry were described in a 2009 publication entitled, "Registries Rising: FDA Looking at TNF Inhibitors; AHRQ Updates Standards." These examples included a pregnancy registry for milnacipran; a pregnancy registry as part of a restricted distribution program for eltrombopag, a thrombopoeitin receptor agonist for treatment of idiopathic thrombocytopenia purpura; and a safety registry for teriparatide, an anabolic treatment for osteoporosis and an expanded indication of glucocorticoid-induced osteoporosis. In a 2018 review of FDA post-market requirements for new drugs and biologics approved from 2009 to 2012, 97 out of 110 new drugs or biologics had at least one post-market requirement; of these nearly one-third were for prospective cohort studies, registries, or clinical trials.

### Hybrid or Enriched Designs

The terms "hybrid or enriched" are frequently used to describe study designs that draw upon both primary and secondary data, with some data collected de novo, specifically for the purposes of the study, and other study-specific data collected via probabilistic or deterministic linkage with other data sources, such as electronic health records, administrative claims and billing data, vital records or existing registries. The DISCOVER study is an example of an enriched study. The study objective was to characterize and describe the global variation in management of patients initiating second line therapy for T2D; data were collected from patients at sites in 38 countries, with linkage of electronic health records where feasible.

## Methods of Primary Data Collection

### Site-Based Data Collection

Often primary data collection for pharmacoepidemiologic studies begins with the identification of sites or HCPs who agree to participate in the study and then for those HCPs to recruit patients following agreed upon inclusion and exclusion criteria as described in the protocol. Traditionally, data collection was performed on paper, but now most such data collection is electronic through case report forms, which are data collection forms designed specifically for the study purposes as part of an electronic data capture system. This model requires institutional board review (ethical review) and site contracts with each investigator. Generally, investigators expect some payment for data collection, and such payments must be proportional to time spent.

### Clinician or Site-Reported Outcomes (ClinROs)

Clinician-reported outcome measures, or clinician or site-reported outcomes (ClinROs), are standardized, usually validated assessment tools, used to measure disease severity or progression, and often incorporated as endpoints for pharmacoepidemiologic studies. While some are recommended for use in routine clinical practice, the consistency of uptake and timing of administration is often not complete enough to robustly address specific research questions of interest without additional requirements for study-specific collection. For example, in rheumatoid arthritis, a number of disease activity measures have been endorsed by the American College of Rheumatology, most requiring assessment by a physician of 28 joints for tenderness and swelling. Although use of disease activity measures is strongly recommended to assess treatment effectiveness and prevent or slow progression, regular use of such measures in clinical practice remains low because of barriers in implementing assessments as part of the workflow in routine visits.

### Patient-Generated Data

Patients are increasingly contacted directly to provide a wide range of information for research studies including medical history, exposures and outcomes, as well as being contacted through devices that monitor their clinical status, behaviors such as medication adherence, and physical activity. Studies may be designed more flexibly with options to collect some data directly from patients either during an in-office study visit or electronically, outside of study visits.

Multiple studies have established the validity of patient-reported prescription medication use, laying a foundation for its reliability as well as supporting the value of additional information that can be obtained from patients that is not typically available through secondary data, such as non-prescription medication use, recreational drug use, smoking and alcohol intake. There are a large number of validated patient reported outcome measures that can provide important insights on the patient experience, including treatment satisfaction, quality of life, burden of disease, ability to care for oneself, work, etc. and new tools are constantly in development.

An expanding array of wearable devices and connected digital products may be used to directly track physiologic and behavioral measures from patients without the involvement of a HCP or study investigator. Researchers have reviewed mention of digital connected devices in studies registered with http://clinicaltrials.

gov from 2000 to 2017, and showed a 34% annual increase in use of these devices. Continued quantification of the validity and reliability of wearable sensors that collect information about physical activity and other clinically useful data will encourage greater use in longitudinal observational studies and randomized trials.

### Registries as Means of Data Collection

As previously mentioned, registries may be established to fill a need for data collection that may support multiple research and/or public health surveillance objectives.

Population-based state, regional, and national cancer registries have played a major role in cancer surveillance, by quantifying cancer incidence and mortality, and trends over time throughout the world, and in pharmacoepidemiology, by providing data on prognostic factors, treatment, and outcomes for analysis within single or across linked databases. In the United States, the Surveillance, Epidemiology, and End Results (SEER) program of the National Cancer Institute works from a network of 17 active cancer registries in 14 states, that actively collect information on all reported cancers diagnosed in their coverage areas.

Pharmacoepidemiologic studies using cancer registries have included case–control studies of hormonal contraception and breast, ovarian, and endometrial cancer, and patterns of care studies of the dissemination of advanced cancer treatment modalities throughout different population groups and into community practice. With approval, researchers may be granted access to the SEER-Medicare linked data files, which include Medicare claims prior to, during, and following cancer diagnosis and treatment. Topics studied include influences of treatment, facility, and provider characteristics and interventions on survival and cost outcomes, as well as disparities in care.

## Biobanks/Specimen Banks

Clinical data may be linked with biorepository data to guide researchers in the identification of biomarkers that are predictive of clinical outcomes and support the development of targeted therapies, e.g. by identifying patients whose tumors harbor a genomic variant that can potentially be targeted by a new drug. Some biobanks have been established internationally, such as the EuroBioBank network, developed to support research on rare diseases. The UK Biobank is another example of an international long-term registry accessible for research, which is following around 500 000 volunteers for at least 25 years to investigate the contributions of genetic predisposition and environmental exposure (including nutrition and lifestyle) in the disease development, and gain valuable insights to support advances in the development of new medicines. An additional area of data collection for the UK Biobank to support the inclusion of objective measures of physical activity in large scale observational studies has been to obtain measures of physical activity from accelerometers from over 100 000 participants. Forty-five percent of those invited to wear accelerometers for seven days accepted the invitations; from these over 93% provided sufficient valid data for analysis.

## Guidelines on the Quality of Data Collection

There are a variety of guidelines that address principles for pharmacoepidemiologic studies that use primary data collection, such as the Guidelines for Good Pharmacoepidemiologic Practice developed by the International Society for Pharmacoepidemiology, the checklist for study protocols developed by the European Network of Centers for Pharmacoepidemiology and Pharmacovigilance, and principles of good epidemiologic methods and practice. The GRACE (Good Research for Comparative Effectiveness) Principles for conducting and evaluating observational studies of comparative

effectiveness are also applicable to studies that use primary data collection and may help guide the actual study design. Extensive detail and guidance regarding operational and scientific considerations for primary data collection can be found in the Registries for Evaluating Patient Outcomes: a User's Guide.

## Strengths

A notable strength of primary data collection is that it can address research objectives that require information that is not accessible or not consistently recorded in available secondary data sources including detail of vaccine and medical device exposures, clinical outcomes, and patient reported outcomes. This type of information can be particularly meaningful to clinicians, patients, regulators, payers and those involved in drug development, and can be more robust than inferences derived from billing data and incomplete or inconsistent electronic health data.

Studies that use collect data directly from patients also provide the opportunity to follow patients over long periods of time and to evaluate a range of outcomes including those of greatest priority to patients themselves. For chronic diseases, patients may be followed for years by their treating physicians, regardless of whether a patient's health insurance program changes – an important limitation of health insurance claims data. It is often the patient's relationship with the physician, and the physician's relationship with the research program that play an important role in long-term retention. Direct-to-patient data collection approaches also offer flexibility in study design and potential for further efficiencies in data collection and reduced study burden.

## Limitations

Primary data collection requires cooperation of data contributors, often over long periods of time (follow-up). While it would seem that altruism should be a sufficient motivation, experience has shown that successful primary data collection requires an infrastructure supporting patient and/or physician enrollment and retention, as well as an active program of data curation to assure that the data that are collected are accurate and reliable. Further, investigators need to consider the validity of patient-centered endpoints, especially pertaining to general and disease-specific quality of life assessments and to detailed information on past exposures, such as in case–control studies where the study outcome is known to the patients at the time of the assessment. Like all data, the contribution to be made by patients in recall of past medical diagnoses and exposures of interest to pharmacoepidemiologic studies must be considered carefully in view of their strengths and limitations.

Maintaining high subject retention in a study over time can be difficult to achieve when using primary data collection. Retention rates are often higher for studies that are both (i) responsive to the needs of patients and physicians so they are motivated to continue participating (a special concern for pregnancy registries and other vulnerable populations), and (ii) parsimonious in their data collection. Operational challenges relate to the need to deploy primary data collection systems that are easy to use, and that are simple enough to encourage steady reporting but which do not result in reporting fatigue. Multiple methods of data entry such as internet, text messaging, and/or mail, can be an advantage, considering the demographics of the target population. Many researchers believe that consistent personal interactions from study staff to clinical investigators and/or patients improves retention, and this approach is often used in pregnancy registries.

While there is some optimism that newer technologies and the nearly universal adoption of smartphones would support the use of text messaging and internet-based patient surveys, results from the PROTECT study raised a cautionary note. Researchers noted that internet-based recruitment of pregnant women was surprisingly difficult and study retention was low, speculating that although it was relatively easy to send questionnaires frequently, participants appeared to tire quickly of responding to the same questions over time.

## Particular Applications

To provide further illustration of some of the applications of primary data collection in modern pharmacoepidemiologic research, several examples are described in further detail in this section. These include a prospective comparative effectiveness research study incorporating collection of clinical endpoints and PROs, a novel hybrid study intended to provide data in support of a label expansion with FDA, use of large registry data as framework for conduct of multiple observational studies, and incorporation of measures of physical activity through accelerometry as part of the UK Biobank effort.

The Registry in Glaucoma Outcomes Research (RiGOR) study, funded by the US Agency for Healthcare Research and Quality, was a prospective observational study that used primary data collection to address which treatment strategy for open-angle glaucoma was associated with the greatest improvement in patient outcomes. The study found that patients treated with incisional surgery after failing at least one course of medication were twice as likely as patients treated with additional medication to achieve a 15% reduction in intraocular pressure (IOP) at 12 months, while patients treated with laser surgery had similar results to those who were treated with additional medication. While IOP is routinely recorded when glaucoma patients see their ophthalmologists, in order to ensure complete assessment of IOP at around 6 and 12 months of follow-up, it was a required element in the study's case report form, along with a vast array of other detailed clinical information. The RiGOR study also included several validated PROs assessments as secondary endpoints, which further required patients to complete these questionnaires at the time of a study visit or at home through mail or electronic means.

The Bioventus Exogen* device registry is an example of a hybrid or enriched design involving both primary and secondary data. This study was planned following extensive discussions with the US Food and Drug Administration Center for Drug Evaluation and Research (FDA CDER) regarding this novel design for a label expansion. The study utilizes a prospective direct-to-patient product registry linked with a propensity score matched comparator group from a commercial claims database for a study of a device used to treat bone fracture non-union, currently used broadly outside of labeled indications to treat fracture.

Two European cancer registries provide examples of registry infrastructure created to address innumerable current and future research questions pertaining to cancer incidence and survival. The EUROCARE (European Cancer Registry Based Study On Survival And Care Of Cancer Patients) registry is a very large collaborative research project on cancer survival. The registry started in 1989, aiming to provide updated descriptions of cancer survival time trends and differences across European countries, to measure cancer prevalence, and to study patterns of care of cancer patients. In its fifth and current edition, EUROCARE-5 includes data on more than 21 million cancer diagnoses provided by 116 Cancer Registries in 30 European countries. At least 171 publications have been generated from EUROCARE1-5, covering trends in survival across a very broad range of cancer types as well as patterns of care, and predictors of survival and other outcomes.

## Conclusions

Despite the growing availability of large amount of data on treatments and patients' clinical experience as recorded in existing health records and billing data, it is unlikely that such data will ever contain all information needed for every study purpose; thus, the need for primary data collection will remain. Traditionally, HCPs have been the primary reporters/recorders of data for studies that use primary data collection, although data is increasingly collected directly from patients as well. While methods for primary data collection can and will change over time, it is likely that researchers will always need to invest time in data curation to assure that the data are accurately represented and to check for critical data that are systematically missing. Primary data collection will continue to be a mainstay of pharmacoepidemiologic research, either as the sole method of data collection or as a key component of research that uses multiple modes of data collection or a mix of primary and secondary data sources.

## Key Points

- Primary data collection is needed for most pharmacoepidemiologic studies that require detailed clinical outcomes assessment, patient-reported outcomes, or physiological measures.
- Sources of primary data include assessments and measures taken by an HCP or study site, patient generated data, and connected digital devices.
- Primary data may be linked with secondary data sources such as billing data, electronic health records, or existing registries utilizing "hybrid" or "enriched" approaches.
- Studies utilizing primary data must incorporate data quality monitoring that reflects the nature of the data collection and potential errors and the nature of the evidence need.
- Long term follow-up of patients is both a potential strength of study designs that utilize primary data collection in that there are no limits on the follow-up period imposed by a database, and a challenge to maintain HCP and patient engagement over long periods of time.

**Case Example 11.1**

**European Cohort Study of Biomarkers in Type 2 Diabetes**

*Source:* Eder S et al. 2018, Heinzel A et al. 2018.

*Background*

The prevalence of T2D with and without chronic kidney disease (CKD) varies substantially between European countries.

*Question*

The PROVALID study will use biomarkers and other detailed clinical and demographic data to predict the course of disease among patients and subgroups and to explain regional differences in outcomes such as rate of loss of estimated glomerular filtration rate (eGFR) and renal and cardiovascular outcomes.

*Approach*

- Prospective cohort study conducted in five European countries (Austria, Hungary, Netherlands, Poland and Scotland). Four thousand T2D patients were enrolled from primary care setting between 2011 and 2015.
- Baseline clinical measures and laboratory measures corresponding to a minimal dataset as well as optional items were collected for all enrollees.
- Annual blood and urine samples are collected to allow for validation of potential biomarkers for renal disease diagnosis and progression, with central laboratory analysis of lab parameters during the study period.
- Medication histories were obtained by interview of the patients or family members.
- Standard descriptive statistics with comparisons between groups using Chi2-tests or Kruskal-Wallis tests for baseline descriptive analyses.
- Univariate and multivariate linear mixed models for analyses of relationship of clinical risk factors and protein biomarkers on outcome of rate of change in eGFR (slope) over follow-up period.

*Results*

- The 4000 patients recruited for PROVALID had a mean age of 63 years old and duration of diabetes of eight years. Mean values for baseline renal function showed renal function not indicative of CKD as measured by eGFR and albumin levels. Using the KDIGO grading system, 81% of patients were in stages G1 or G2 for eGFR and 78% were in stage A1 for albumin creatinine ratio at enrollment, indicating most had not yet advanced to CKD or were in mild stages, which was expected given the population was identified from primary care. (Eder 2018).
- From a longitudinal analysis of the relationship of 17 plasma protein biomarkers to a rate of progression of eGFR among 481 patients mostly at an early stage of CKD, univariable analysis showed that nine biomarkers differed significantly between patients with stable eGFR and fast progression of eGFR decline, and 14 biomarkers were significant predictors of rate of progression of eGFR. However, results of multivariate analysis showed that no biomarkers remained significant predictors of eGFR decline over time after adjustment for baseline eGFR. (Heinzel 2018).

*Strengths*

- Large cohort representing 5 EU countries.
- Prospective collection of biomarkers and annual blood and urine samples to be able to investigate and validate future candidate markers for prediction of renal and cardiovascular disease outcomes.

*Limitations*

- Potential for attrition bias over time.
- Results will be most generalizable to T2D patients with no or early stage CKD.

*Key points*

The PROVALID cohort can make a potentially strong contribution to understanding of predictors of progression of CKD and cardiovascular disease among T2D patients and validation of potential biomarkers within this population.

# Further Reading

Coleman, A., Lum, F., Velentgas, P. et al. (2016). RiGOR: a prospective observational study comparing the effectiveness of treatment strategies for open-angle glaucoma. *J. Comp. Eff. Res.* 5 (1): 65–78.

Doherty, A., Jackson, D., Hammerla, N. et al. (2017). Large scale population assessment of physical activity using wrist worn accelerometers: the UK Biobank study. *PLoS One* 12 (2): e0169649. https://doi.org/10.1371/journal.pone.0169649.

Dreyer, N.A., Blackburn, S.C.F., Mt-Isa, S. et al. (2015 Jul-Dec). Direct-to-patient research: piloting a new approach to understanding drug safety during pregnancy. *JMIR Public Health Surveill.* 1 (2): e22.

Eder, S., Leirer, J., Kershbaum, J. et al. (2018). A prospective cohort study in patients with type 2 diabetes mellitus for validation of biomarkers (PROVALID) – study design and baseline characteristics. *Kidney Blood Press. Res.* 43: 181–190.

EuroBioBank Network. http://www.eurobiobank.org

Gliklich RE, Leavy MB, Dreyer NA (sr eds). Registries for Evaluating Patient Outcomes: A User's Guide. 4th ed. (Prepared by L&M Policy Research, LLC, under Contract No. 290–2014-00004-C with partners OM1 and IQVIA) AHRQ Publication No. 19(20)-EHC020. Rockville, MD: Agency for Healthcare Research and Quality; September 2020. Posted final reports are located on the Effective Health Care Program search page. DOI: 10.23970/AHRQEPCREGISTRIES4.

Heinzel, A., Kammer, M., Mayer, G. et al. (2018 Sep). Validation of plasma biomarker candidates for the prediction of eGFR decline in patients with type 2 diabetes. *Diabetes Care* 41 (9): 1947–1954. https://doi.org/10.2337/dc18-0532.

Hobbs MN. "Registries Rising: FDA Looking At TNF Inhibitors; AHRQ Updates Standards." The Pink Sheet. August 2009;71(34):8–9.

Pharmacoepidemiological Research on Outcomes of Therapeutics by a European ConsorTium (PROTECT). http://www.imi-protect.eu accessed 13 October 2020.

Jansen-van der Weide, M.C., Gaasterland, C.M.W., Roes, K.C.B. et al. (2018). Rare disease registries: potential applications towards impact on development of new drug treatments. *Orphanet J. Rare Dis.* 13: 154. https://doi.org/10.1186/s13023-018-0836-0.

Mack C, Pavesio A, Kelly K, Wester T, Jones J, Maislin G, Irwin D, Brinkley E, Zura RD. Breaking News: Study of Fracture Healing in Patients at Risk of Non-Union. Poster. 33rd ICPE: International Conference on Pharmacoepidemiology & Therapeutic Risk Management, Montreal, Canada, August 23–27, 2017.

Marra, C., Chen, J.L., Coravos, A. et al. (2020). Quantifying the use of connected digital products in clinical research. *NPJ Digit. Med.* 3: 50. https://doi.org/10.1038/s41746-020-0259-x.

National Cancer Institute, Surveillance, Epidemiology, and End Results Program. Overview of the SEER Program (web page). Available at http://seer.cancer.gov/about accessed 13 October 2020.

Pharmacovigilance Risk Assessment Committee (PRAC) [Internet] Interim guidance on enhanced safety surveillance for seasonal influenza vaccines in the EU. London: European Medicines Agency (EMA) 2014. Available at: http://www.ema.europa.eu/docs/en_GB/document_library/Scientific_guideline/2014/04/WC500165492.pdf accessed 13 October 2020.

Resnic, F.S., Majithia, A., Marinac-Dabic, D. et al. (2017). Registry-based prospective, active surveillance of medical-device safety. *N. Engl. J. Med.* 376: 526–535. https://doi.org/10.1056/NEJMoa1516333.

Seltzer, J.H., Heise, T., Carson, P. et al. (2017). Use of endpoint adjudication to improve the quality and validity of endpoint assessment for medical device development and post marketing evaluation: rationale and best practices. A report from the cardiac safety research consortium. *Am. Heart J.* 190: 76–85.

Singh, J.A., Saag, K.G., Bridges, S.L. Jr. et al. (January 2016). 2015 American College of Rheumatology Guideline for the treatment of rheumatoid arthritis. *Arthritis Care Res.* 68 (1): 1–26. https://doi.org/10.1002/art.39480.

The DISCOVER study. http://www.discoverdiabetes.com/DISCOVER-study.html Accessed October 13, 2020.

UK Biobank. www.ukbiobank.ac.uk accessed 13 October 2020.

US Food and Drug Administration. Postapproval Pregnancy Safety Studies Guidance for Industry: Draft Guidance. May 2019. https://www.fda.gov/media/124746/download accessed 13 October 2020.

Wallacj, J.D., Egilman, A.C., Dhruva, S.S. et al. (2018). Postmarket studies required by the US Food and Drug Administration for newdrugs and biologics approved between 2009 and 2012: cross sectional analysis. *BMJ* k2031: 361.

World Health Organization. International Agency for Research on Cancer. Eurocare study: Survival of cancer patients in Europe. http://www.eurocare.it/Home/tabid/36/Default.aspx accessed 13 October 2020.

# 12

## How Should One Perform Pharmacoepidemiologic Studies? Choosing Among the Available Alternatives

*Brian L. Strom*

*Rutgers Biomedical and Health Sciences, Newark, NJ, USA*

## Introduction

As discussed in the previous chapters, pharmacoepidemiologic studies apply the techniques of epidemiology to the content area of clinical pharmacology. Between 500 and 3000 individuals are usually studied prior to drug marketing. Most postmarketing pharmacoepidemiologic studies need to include at least 10 000 subjects, or draw from an equivalent population for a case–control study, in order to contribute sufficient new information to be worth their cost and effort (see Chapter 3). This large sample size raises logistical challenges. Chapters 7 through 11 presented many of the different data collection approaches and data resources that have been developed to perform pharmacoepidemiologic studies efficiently, meeting the need for these very large sample sizes. This chapter is intended to synthesize this material, to assist the reader in choosing among the available approaches.

## Choosing Among the Available Approaches to Pharmacoepidemiologic Studies

Once one has decided to perform a pharmacoepidemiologic study, one needs to decide which of the data collection approaches or data resources described in the earlier chapters of this book should be used. Although, to some degree, the choice may too often be based upon a researcher's familiarity with given data resources and/or the investigators who have been using them, it is very important to tailor the choice of pharmacoepidemiologic resource to the question to be addressed. One often may want to use more than one data collection strategy or resource, in parallel or in combination. If no single resource is optimal for addressing a question, it can be useful to use a number of approaches that complement each other. Indeed, this is probably the preferable approach for addressing important questions. Regardless, investigators are often left with a difficult and complex choice.

In order to explain how to choose among the available pharmacoepidemiologic data resources, it is useful to synthesize the information from the previous chapters on the relative strengths and weaknesses of each of the available pharmacoepidemiologic approaches, examining the comparative characteristics of each (see Table 12.1). One can then examine the characteristics of the research question at hand, in order to choose the pharmacoepidemiologic approach best suited to addressing that question (see Table 12.2). The assessment and weights provided in this discussion and in the accompanying tables are arbitrary. They

**Table 12.1** Comparative characteristics of pharmacoepidemiologic data resources[a].

| Pharmacoepidemiologic approach | Relative size | Relative cost[a] | Relative speed | Representativeness | Population-based | Cohort studies possible | Case–control studies possible |
|---|---|---|---|---|---|---|---|
| Spontaneous reporting | ++++ | + | ++++ | ++ | − | − | + (with external controls) |
| Health maintenance organizations/ health plans | ++ | +++ | +++ | +++ | ++ | ++++ | ++++ |
| Commercial insurance databases | ++ | +++ | +++ | +++ | ++ | ++++ | ++++ |
| US Government claims databases | +++ | ++ | ++ | variable | ++++ | ++++ | ++++ |
| UK medical record databases | ++ | ++ | +++ | +++ | +++ | ++++ | ++++ |
| In-hospital databases | + | ++ | +++ | ++ | − | ++ | ++ |
| Canadian provincial databases | ++ | ++ | +++ | ++++ | ++++ | ++++ | ++++ |
| Pharmacy-based medical record linkage systems | ++ | ++ | +++ | ++++ | ++++ | ++++ | ++++ |
| Ad hoc studies | variable | +++ | + | variable | − | − | ++++ |
| Case–control surveillance | | | | | | | |
| Prescription-event monitoring | +++ | +++ | + | +++ | ++ | ++++ | + (nested) |
| Registries | variable | +++ | + | variable | variable | +++ | ++ |
| Field studies | as feasible +++ | +++ | + | as desired | as desired | − | ++++ |
| Ad hoc case–control studies | | | | | | | |
| Ad hoc cohort studies | as feasible ++++ | ++++ | − | as desired | as desired | +++ | ++ (nested) |
| Randomized trials | as feasible ++++ | ++++ | − | − | − | ++++ | ++ (nested) |

| Pharmacoepidemiologic approach | Validity of exposure data | Validity of outcome data | Control of confounding | Inpatient drug exposure data | Outpatient diagnosis data | Loss to follow-up |
|---|---|---|---|---|---|---|
| Spontaneous reporting | +++ | ++ | − | +++ | +++ | N/A |
| Health maintenance organizations/health plans | ++++ | +++ | ++ | − | ++ | 3–15%/yr |
| Commercial insurance databases | ++++ | +++ | ++ | − | ++ | about 25%/yr |
| US Government claims databases | ++++ | +++ | ++ | − | ++ | variable |
| UK medical record databases | +++ | ++++ | ++ | − | ++ | Nil |
| In-hospital databases | ++++ | +++ | ++ | ++++ | − | Nil |
| Canadian provincial databases | ++++ | +++ | ++ | − | ++ | Nil |
| Pharmacy-based medical record linkage systems | ++++ | + | + | − | − | Nil |
| Ad hoc studies | ++ | ++++ | +++ | − | + | N/A |
| Case–control surveillance | | | | | | |
| Prescription-event monitoring | +++ | +++ | ++ | − | +++ | variable |
| Registries | +++ | +++ | ++ | + | Variable | N/A |
| Field studies | ++ | ++++ | +++ | ++ | + | N/A |
| Ad hoc case–control studies | | | | | | |
| Ad hoc cohort studies | +++ | +++ | +++ | ++ | ++++ | Variable |
| Randomized trials | ++++ | +++ | ++++ | ++ | ++++ | N/A |

[a] See the text of this chapter for descriptions of the column headings, and previous chapters for descriptions of the data resources.

**Table 12.2** Characteristics of research questions and their impact on the choice of pharmacoepidemiologic data resources[a].

| Pharmacoepidemiologic approach | Hypothesis generating | Hypothesis strengthening | Hypothesis testing[d] | Study of benefits (versus risk) | Incidence rates desired | Low incidence outcome | Low prevalence exposure |
| --- | --- | --- | --- | --- | --- | --- | --- |
| Spontaneous reporting | +++ | + | − | − | − | ++++ | ++++ |
| Health maintenance organizations/ health plans | ++ | ++++ | +++ | ++ | +++ | +++ | +++ |
| Commercial insurance databases | ++ | ++++ | +++ | ++ | +++ | +++ | +++ |
| US Government claims databases | ++ | ++++ | +++ | ++ | +++ | ++++ | ++++ |
| UK medical record databases | ++ | ++++ | +++ | ++ | ++++ | +++ | +++ |
| In-hospital databases | + | ++++ | +++ | ++ | +++ | + | + |
| Canadian provincial databases | ++ | ++++ | +++ | ++ | +++ | +++ | +++ |
| Pharmacy-based medical record linkage systems | + | ++ | ++ | ++ | +++ | +++ | +++ |
| Ad hoc Studies | +++ | +++ | +++ | +++ | − | ++++ | + |
| Case–control surveillance | | | | | | | |
| Prescription-event monitoring | ++ | ++ | +++ | +++ | +++ | +++ | +++ |
| Registries | + | +++ | +++ | +++ | +++ | +++ | +++ |
| Field Studies | + | ++ | +++ | +++ | + | ++++ | + |
| Ad hoc case–control studies | | | | | | | |
| Ad hoc cohort studies | + | ++ | +++ | +++ | ++++ | ++ | +++ |
| Randomized trials | + | + | ++++ | ++++ | ++++ | + | ++++ |
| Pharmacoepidemiologic approach | Important confounders | Drug use inpatient (versus outpatient) | Outcome does not result in hospitalization | Outcome does not result in medical attention | Outcome a delayed effect new drug | Exposure a new drug | Urgent question |
| Spontaneous reporting | − | +++ | ++++ | + | + | ++++ | ++++ |

| Data resource / study type | | | | | | | |
|---|---|---|---|---|---|---|---|
| Health maintenance organizations/health plans | +++ | − | +++ | − | + | ++ | +++ |
| Commercial insurance databases | ++ | − | +++ | − | + | +++ | +++ |
| US Government claims databases | ++ | − | +++ | − | + to +++ | ++ | ++ |
| UK medical record databases | +++ | − | +++ | − | +++ | +++ | +++ |
| In-hospital databases | ++ | ++++ | − | − | − | +++ | +++ |
| Canadian provincial databases | ++ | − | +++ | − | +++ | ++ | +++ |
| Pharmacy-based medical record linkage systems | + | − | − | − | ++ | +++ | +++ |
| Ad hoc studies | +++ | + | − | − | ++ | + | + |
| Case–control surveillance | ++ | + | ++++ | + | + | ++++ | + |
| Prescription-event monitoring | ++ | + | +++ | ++ | ++ | +++ | + |
| Registries | ++ | ++ | + | ++ | ++ | +++ | + |
| Field studies | +++ | ++++ | ++ | − | ++ | + | + |
| Ad hoc case–control studies | +++ | ++++ | +++ | +++ | + | ++++ | + |
| Ad hoc cohort studies | +++ | ++++ | +++ | + | + | ++++ | + |
| Randomized trials | +++ | ++++ | ++++ | ++++ | + | ++++ | + |

[a] See the text of this chapter for descriptions of the column headings, and previous chapters for descriptions of the data resources.

[b] Hypothesis-generating studies are studies designed to raise new questions about possible unexpected drug effects, whether adverse or beneficial.

[c] Hypothesis-strengthening studies are studies designed to provide support for, although not definitive evidence for, existing hypotheses.

[d] Hypothesis-testing studies are studies designed to evaluate in detail hypotheses raised elsewhere.

are not being represented as a consensus of the pharmacoepidemiologic community, but represent the judgment of this author alone, based on the material presented in earlier chapters of this book. Nevertheless, I think that most would agree with the general principles presented, and even many of the relative ratings. My hope is that this synthesis of information, despite some of the arbitrary ratings inherent in it, will make it easier for the reader to synthesize the large amount of information presented in the prior chapters.

Note that there are a number of other data sources not discussed here, some of which have been, or in the future may be of importance to pharmacoepidemiologic research. Examples include the old Boston Collaborative Drug Surveillance data, MEMO, Pharmetrics, Aetna, Humana, and many others, many reviewed in prior editions of this book. Given the wonderful proliferation of pharmacoepidemiologic data resources, we are making no attempt to include them all. Instead, we will discuss them in categories of type of data, as we did in the chapters themselves.

## Comparative Characteristics of Pharmacoepidemiologic Data Resources

Table 12.1 lists each of the different pharmacoepidemiologic data resources that were described in earlier chapters, along with some of their characteristics.

The *relative size* of the database refers to the population it covers. Only spontaneous reporting systems, US Medicare, some of the pharmacy-based medical record linkage systems, and Prescription Event Monitoring in the UK cover entire countries or large fractions thereof. Of course, population databases differ considerably in size, based on the size of their underlying populations. Aggregations of Medicaid databases are the next largest, with the commercial databases approaching that. The UK electronic health record databases would be next in size, as would the health

maintenance organizations, depending on how many are included. The Canadian provincial databases again could be equivalently large, depending in part on how many are included in a study. The other data resources are generally smaller. Case–control surveillance, as formerly conducted by the Slone Epidemiology Unit, can cover a variable population, depending on the number of hospitals and metropolitan areas they include in their network for a given study. The population base of registry-based case–control studies depends on the registries used for case finding. Ad hoc studies can be whatever size the researcher desires and can marshal resources for.

As to *relative cost*, studies that collect new data are most expensive, especially randomized trials and cohort studies, for which sample sizes generally need to be large and follow-up may need to be prolonged. In the case of randomized trials, there are additional logistical complexities. Studies that use existing data are least expensive, although their cost increases when they gather primary medical records for validation. Studies that use existing data resources to identify subjects but then collect new data about those subjects are intermediate in cost.

With regard to the *relative speed* of study completion, studies that collect new data take longer, especially randomized trials and cohort studies. Studies that use existing data are able to answer a question most quickly, although considerable additional time may be needed to obtain primary medical records for validation. Studies that use existing data resources to identify subjects but then collect new data about those subjects are intermediate in speed.

*Representativeness* refers to how well the subjects in the data resource represent the population at large or a more specific population of interest. US Medicare, Prescription Event Monitoring in the UK, the provincial health databases in Canada, and the pharmacy-based medical record linkage systems each include entire countries, provinces, or states and, so, are typical populations. Spontaneous reporting systems are drawn from entire populations, but of course the selective nature of their reporting could lead to less certain representativeness. Medicaid programs are limited to the disadvantaged, and include a population that is least representative of a general population. Analogously, randomized trials include populations limited by the various selection criteria plus their willingness to volunteer for the study. The CPRD and THIN use a non-random large subset of the total UK population, and may be representative of the overall UK population. Health plans and commercial databases are closer to representative populations than a Medicaid population would be, although they include a largely working population and, so, include few patients of low socioeconomic status and fewer than normal elderly. Some of the remaining data collection approaches or resources are characterized in Table 12.1 as "variable," meaning their representativeness depends on which hospitals are recruited into the study. Ad hoc studies are listed in Table 12.1 "as desired," because they can be designed to be representative or not, as the investigator wishes.

Whether a database is *population-based* refers to whether there is an identifiable population (which is not necessarily based in geography), all of whose medical care would be included in that database, regardless of the provider. This allows one to measure incidence rates of diseases, as well as being more certain that one knows of all medical care that any given patient receives. As an example, assuming little or no out-of-plan care, the Kaiser programs are population-based. One can use Kaiser data, therefore, to study medical care received in and out of the hospital, as well as diseases which may result in repeat hospitalizations. For example, one could study the impact of the treatment initially received for venous thromboembolism on the risk of subsequent disease recurrence. In contrast, hospital-based case–control studies conducted outside a closed network like Kaiser are not population-based: they include only the specific hospitals

that belong to the system and do not capture all healthcare services a patient may receive. Thus, a patient diagnosed with and treated for venous thromboembolism in a participating hospital could be readmitted to a different, non-participating hospital if the disease recurred. This recurrence would not be detected in a study using such a system. The data resources that are population-based are those which use data from organized health care delivery or payment systems. Registry-based and ad hoc case–control studies can occasionally be conducted as population-based studies, if all cases in a defined geographic area are recruited into the study, but this is unusual (see also Chapter 11).

*Whether cohort studies are possible* within a particular data resource would depend on whether individuals can be identified by whether or not they were exposed to a drug of interest. This would be true in any of the population-based systems, as well as any of the systems designed to perform cohort studies.

*Whether case–control studies are possible* within a given data resource depends on whether patients can be identified by whether or not they suffered from a disease of interest. This would be true in any of the population-based systems. Data from spontaneous reporting systems can be used for case finding for case–control studies, although this has been done infrequently.

The *validity of the exposure data* is most certain in hospital-based settings, where one can be reasonably certain of both the identity of a drug and that the patient actually ingested it. Exposure data in spontaneous reporting systems come mostly from health care providers and, so, are probably valid. However, one cannot be certain of patient adherence in spontaneous reporting data. Exposure data from claims data and from pharmacy-based medical record linkage systems are unbiased data recorded by pharmacies, often for billing purposes, a process that is closely audited as it impacts reimbursement. These data are likely to be accurate with regard to medication possession, although, again, one cannot assure adherence. Refill adherence though has been found to correlate closely with adherence measured using microchips embedded in medication bottles (see Chapter 21). However, there are drugs that may fall beneath a patient's deductibles or co-payments, or not be on formularies, so dispensed by the pharmacy but paid for in cash. In claims databases, these scenarios may result in misclassification of a true medication exposure as the patient would falsely appear unexposed. Also, since drug benefits vary depending on the plan, pharmacy files may not capture all prescribed drugs if beneficiaries reach the drug benefit limit or pay for the prescription out-of-pocket. In the UK medical record systems, drugs prescribed by physicians other than the general practitioner could be missed, although continued prescribing by the general practitioner would be detected. Adhoc case–control studies generally rely on patient histories for exposure data. These may be very inaccurate, as patients often do not recall correctly the medications they are taking. However, this would be expected to vary, depending on the condition studied, type of drug taken, the questioning technique used, etc. (see Chapter 13).

The *validity of the outcome data* is also most certain in hospital-based settings, in which the patient is subjected to intensive medical surveillance. It is least certain in outpatient data from organized systems of medical care. There are, however, methods of improving the accuracy of these data, such as using drugs, laboratory data, and procedures as markers of the disease and obtaining primary medical records (see Chapter 13). The outcome data from automated databases are listed as variable, therefore, depending on exactly which data are being used, and how. The UK medical record systems analyze the actual medical record, rather than claims, and can access additional questionnaire data from the general practitioner, as well. Thus, their outcome data may be more accurate.

*Control of confounding* refers to the ability to control for confounding variables. Randomization is the most convincing way of controlling for unknown, unmeasured, or unmeasurable confounding variables. Approaches that collect sufficient information to control for known and measurable variables are next most effective. These include health plans, the UK medical record systems, case–control surveillance, ad hoc case–control studies, and ad hoc cohort studies. Users of health databases in Canada, commercial databases, and Medicaid (sometimes) can obtain primary medical records, but not all information necessary is always available in those records. They are generally unable to contact patients directly to obtain supplementary information that might not be in a medical record. Finally, spontaneous reporting systems do not provide enough systematically collected information for control of confounding.

Relatively few of the data systems have data on *inpatient drug use*. The exceptions include spontaneous reporting systems, the in-hospital databases, and some ad hoc studies if designed to collect such.

Only a few of the data resources have sufficient *data on outpatient diagnoses* available without special effort, to be able to study them as outcome variables. Ad hoc studies can be designed to be able to collect such information. In the case of ad hoc randomized clinical trials, this data collection effort could even include tailored laboratory and physical examination measurements. In some of the resources, the outpatient outcome data are collected observationally, but directly via the physician, and so are more likely to be accurate. Included are spontaneous reporting systems, the UK medical record systems, HMOs, Prescription Event Monitoring, and some ad hoc cohort studies. Other outpatient data come via physician claims for medical care, including Medicaid databases, commercial databases, and the provincial health databases in Canada. Finally, other data resources can access outpatient diagnoses only via the patient, and so they are less likely to be complete; although the diagnosis can often be validated using medical records, it generally needs to be identified by the patient. These include most ad hoc case–control studies.

The degree of *loss to follow-up* differs substantially among the different resources. They are specified in Table 12.1.

## Characteristics of Research Questions and their Impact on the Choice of Pharmacoepidemiologic Data Resources

Once one is familiar with the characteristics of the pharmacoepidemiologic resources available, one must then examine more closely the research question, to determine which resources can best be used to answer it (see Table 12.2).

Pharmacoepidemiologic studies can be undertaken to generate hypotheses about drug effects, to strengthen hypotheses, and/or to test a priori hypotheses about drug effects. *Hypothesis-generating studies* are studies designed to raise new questions about possible unexpected drug effects, whether adverse or beneficial. Virtually all studies can and do raise such questions, through incidental findings in studies performed for other reasons. In addition, virtually any case–control study could be used, in principle, to screen for possible drug causes of a disease under study, and virtually any cohort study could be used to screen for unexpected outcomes from a drug exposure under study. In practice, however, the only settings in which this has been attempted systematically have been health plans, case–control surveillance, Prescription Event Monitoring, and Medicaid databases. To date, the most productive source of new hypotheses about drug effects has been spontaneous reporting. However, this is the goal of Sentinel, a Congressionally mandated data system of over 100 million US lives, initially built primarily for hypothesis strengthening as "Mini-Sentinel," although now being used for hypothesis

generation as well, in addition to the traditional approach of using such data for hypothesis testing. In the future, new approaches using the internet (e.g. health websites with consumer posting boards and other social media) could potentially be used for hypothesis generation of events, including those not coming to medical attention.

*Hypothesis-strengthening studies* are studies designed to provide support for, although not definitive evidence for, existing hypotheses. The objective of these studies is to provide sufficient support for, or evidence against, a hypothesis to permit a decision about whether a subsequent, more definitive, study should be undertaken. As such, hypothesis-strengthening studies need to be conducted rapidly and inexpensively. Hypothesis-strengthening studies can include crude analyses conducted using almost any dataset, evaluating a hypothesis which arose elsewhere. Because not all potentially confounding variables would be controlled, the findings could not be considered definitive. Examples would be the modular studies conducted within Sentinel. Alternatively, hypothesis-strengthening studies can be more detailed studies, controlling for confounding, conducted using the same data resource that raised the hypothesis. In this case, because the study is not specifically undertaken to test an a priori hypothesis, the hypothesis-testing type of study can only serve to strengthen, not test, the hypothesis. Spontaneous reporting systems are useful for raising hypotheses, but are not very useful for providing additional support for those hypotheses. Conversely, randomized trials can certainly strengthen hypotheses, but are generally too costly and logistically too complex to be used for this purpose (Post-hoc analyses of randomized trials can obviously be re-analyzed, for the purposes of generating or strengthening hypotheses, but then they are really being analyzed as cohort studies). Of the remaining approaches, those that can quickly access, in computerized form, both exposure data and outcome data are most useful. Those that can rapidly access only one of these data types, only exposure or only outcome data, are next most useful, while those that need to gather both data types are least useful, because of the time and expense that would be entailed.

*Hypothesis-testing studies* are studies designed to evaluate in detail hypotheses raised elsewhere. Such studies must be able to have simultaneous comparison groups and must be able to control for most known potential confounding variables. For these reasons, spontaneous reporting systems cannot be used for this purpose, as they cannot be used to conduct studies with simultaneous controls (with rare exception). The most powerful approach, of course, is a randomized clinical trial, as it is the only way to control for unknown or unmeasurable confounding variables. Instrumental variable analyses can approximate a randomized clinical trial, but only in the to-date limited circumstances that all the underlying assumptions are met. (On the other hand, studies of dose–response, duration-response, drug–drug interactions, determinants of response, etc. are more readily done in non-randomized than randomized studies.) Techniques which allow access to patients and their medical records are the next most powerful, as one can gather information on potential confounders that might only be reliably obtained from one of those sources or the other. Techniques which allow access to primary records but not the patient are next most useful.

The research implications of questions about the *beneficial effects* of drugs are different, depending upon whether the beneficial effects of interest are expected or unexpected effects. Studies of *unexpected beneficial effects* are exactly analogous to studies of unexpected adverse effects, in terms of their implications to one's choice of an approach; in both situations one is studying side effects. Studies of *expected beneficial effects*, or drug efficacy, raise the special methodologic problem of confounding by the indication: patients who receive a drug are different from those who do

not in a way which usually is related to the outcome under investigation in the study. It *is* sometimes possible to address these questions using nonexperimental study designs. Generally, however, the randomized clinical trial is far preferable, when feasible.

In order to address questions about the *incidence of a disease* in those exposed to a drug, one must be able to quantify how many people received the drug. This information can be obtained using any resource that can perform a cohort study. Techniques that need to gather the outcome data de novo may miss some of the outcomes if there is incomplete participation and/or reporting of outcomes, such as with Prescription Event Monitoring, ad hoc cohort studies, and outpatient pharmacy-based cohort studies. On the other hand, ad hoc data collection is the only way of systematically collecting information about outcomes that need not come to medical attention (see below). The only approaches that are free from either of these problems are the hospital-based approaches. Registry-based case–control studies and ad hoc case–control studies can occasionally be used to estimate incidence rates, if one obtains a complete collection of cases from a defined geographic area. The other approaches listed cannot be used to calculate incidence rates.

To address a question about a *low incidence outcome*, one needs to study a large population (see Chapter 3). This can best be done using spontaneous reporting, US Medicare, Prescription Event Monitoring, or the pharmacy-based medical record linkage systems, which can or do cover entire countries. Alternatively, one could use commercial databases, health plans, or aggregates of Medicaid databases, which cover a large proportion of the United States, or the medical record systems in the UK. Canadian provincial databases can also be fairly large, and one can perform a study in multiple such databases. Ad hoc cohort studies could potentially be expanded to cover equivalent populations. Case–control studies, either ad hoc studies, studies using registries, or studies using case–control surveillance, can also be expanded to cover large populations, although not as large as the previously-mentioned approaches. Because case–control studies recruit study subjects on the basis of the patients suffering from a disease, they are more efficient than attempting to perform such studies using analogous cohort studies. Finally, randomized trials could, in principle, be expanded to achieve very large sample sizes, especially large simple trials (see Chapter 17), but this can be very difficult and costly.

To address a question about a *low prevalence exposure*, one also needs to study a large population (see Chapter 3). Again this can best be done using spontaneous reporting, US Medicare, the pharmacy-based medical record linkage systems, or Prescription Event Monitoring, which cover entire countries. Alternatively, one could use commercial databases, large health plans, or aggregates of Medicaid databases, which cover a large proportion of the United States, or the medical record databases in the UK. Ad hoc cohort studies could also be used to recruit exposed patients from a large population. Analogously, randomized trials, which specify exposure, could assure an adequate number of exposed individuals. Case–control studies, either ad hoc studies, studies using registries, or studies using case–control surveillance, could theoretically be expanded to cover a large enough population, but this would be difficult and expensive.

When there are *important confounders* that need to be taken into account in order to answer the question at hand, then one needs to be certain that sufficient and accurate information is available on those confounders. Spontaneous reporting systems cannot be used for this purpose. The most powerful approach is a randomized trial, as it is the most convincing way to control for unknown or unmeasurable confounding variables. Techniques which allow access to patients and their medical records are the next most powerful, as one can

gather information on potential confounders that might only be reliably obtained from one of those sources or the other. Techniques which allow access to primary records but not the patient are the next most useful.

If the research question involves *inpatient* drug use, then the data resource must obviously be capable of collecting data on inpatient drug exposures. The number of approaches that have this capability are limited, and include: spontaneous reporting systems and inpatient database systems. Ad hoc studies could also, of course, be designed to collect such information in the hospital.

When the *outcome under study does not result in hospitalization, but does result in medical attention*, the best approaches are randomized trials and ad hoc studies which can be specifically designed to be sure this information can be collected. Prescription Event Monitoring and the UK medical record systems, which collect their data from general practitioners, are excellent sources of data for this type of question. Reports of such outcomes are likely to come to spontaneous reporting systems, as well. Medicaid databases and commercial databases can also be used, as they include outpatient data, although one must be cautious about the validity of the diagnosis information in outpatient claims. Canadian provincial databases are similar, as are health plans. Finally, registry-based case–control studies could theoretically be performed, if they included outpatient cases of the disease under study.

When the *outcome under study does not result in medical attention at all*, the approaches available are much more limited. Only randomized trials and prospective cohort studies can be specifically designed to be certain this information is collected. Finally, occasionally one could collect information on such an outcome in a spontaneous reporting system, if the report came from a patient or if the report came from a health care provider who became aware of the problem while the patient was visiting for medical care for some other problem.

In the future, as noted above, new approaches using the internet (e.g. health websites with consumer posting boards) could potentially be used for hypothesis generation of events not coming to medical attention.

When the *outcome under study is a delayed drug effect*, then one obviously needs approaches capable of tracking individuals over a long period of time. The best approach for this are some of the provincial health databases in Canada. Drug data are available in some for more than 25 years, and there is little turnover in the population covered. Thus, this is an ideal system within which to perform such long-term studies. Some health plans have even longer follow-up time available. However, as health plans, they suffer from substantial turnover, albeit more modest after the first few years of enrollment. Commercial databases are similar. Any of the methods of conducting case–control studies can address such questions, although one would have to be especially careful about the validity of the exposure information collected many years after the exposure. Medicaid databases have been available since 1973. However, the large turnover in Medicaid programs, due to changes in eligibility with changes in family and employment status, makes studies of long-term drug effects problematic. Similarly, one could conceivably perform studies of long-term drug effects using Prescription Event Monitoring, the pharmacy-based medical record linkage systems, ad hoc cohort studies, or randomized clinical trials, but these approaches are not as well-suited to this type of question as the previously-discussed techniques. Theoretically, one also could identify long-term drug effects in a spontaneous reporting system. This is unlikely, however, as a physician is unlikely to link a current medical event with a drug exposure long ago.

When *the exposure under study is a new drug*, then one is, of course, limited to data sources that collect data on recent exposures, and preferably those that can collect a significant number of such exposures quickly. Ad hoc cohort studies or a randomized clinical trial are ideal for this, as they recruit patients into the study on the basis of their exposure. Spontaneous reporting is similarly a good approach for this, as new drugs are automatically and immediately covered, and in fact reports are much more common in the first three years after a drug is marketed. The major databases are next most useful, especially the commercial databases, as their large population base will allow one to accumulate a sufficient number of exposed individuals rapidly, so one can perform a study sooner. In some cases, there is a delay until the drug is available on the program's formulary; however, that especially can be an issue with HMOs. The US government claims databases (Medicare and Medicaid) have a delay in availability of their data, which makes them less useful for the newest drugs. Ad hoc case–control studies, by whatever approach, must wait until sufficient drug exposure has occurred that it can affect the outcome variable being studied.

Finally, if *one needs an answer to a question urgently*, potentially the fastest approach, if the needed data are included, is a spontaneous reporting system; drugs are included in these systems immediately, and an extremely large population base is covered. Of course, one cannot rely on any adverse reaction being detected in a spontaneous reporting system. The computerized databases are also useful for these purposes, depending on the speed with which the exposures accumulate in that database; of course, if the drug in question is not on the formulary in question, it cannot be studied. Modular analyses in Sentinel were designed for exactly this purpose. The remaining approaches are of limited use, as they take too long to address a question. One exception to this is Prescription Event Monitoring, if the drug in question happens to have been a subject of one of its studies. The other, and more likely exception, is case–control surveillance if the disease under study is available in adequate numbers in its database, either because it was the topic of a prior study or because there were a sufficient number of individuals with the disease collected to be included in control groups for prior studies.

## Examples

As an example, one might want to explore whether nonsteroidal anti-inflammatory drugs (NSAIDs) cause upper gastrointestinal bleeding and, if so, how often. One could examine the manufacturer's premarketing data from clinical trials, but the number of patients included is not likely to be large enough to study clinical bleeding, and the setting is very artificial. Alternatively, one could examine premarketing studies using more sensitive outcome measures, such as endoscopy. However, these are even more artificial. Instead, one could use any of the databases to address the question quickly, as they have data on drug exposures that preceded the hospital admission. Some databases could only be used to investigate gastrointestinal bleeding resulting in hospitalization (e.g. Kaiser Permanente, except via chart review). Others could be used to explore inpatient or outpatient bleeding (e.g. Medicare, Medicaid, Canadian provincial databases). Because of confounding by cigarette smoking, alcohol, etc. which would not be well measured in these databases, one also might want to address this question using case–control or cohort studies, whether conducted ad hoc or using any of the special approaches available, for example case–control surveillance or Prescription Event Monitoring. If one wanted to be able to calculate incidence rates, one would need to restrict these studies to cohort studies, rather than case–control studies. One would be unlikely to be able to use registries, as there are no registries, known to this author at least, which record patients with upper gastrointestinal bleeding. One would not be able to perform analyses of secular trends, as upper gastrointestinal bleeding would not appear in vital statistics data, except as a cause of hospitalization or death. Studying death from upper gastrointestinal bleeding is problematic, as it is a disease from which patients usually do not die. Rather than studying determinants of upper gastrointestinal bleeding, one would really be studying determinants of complications from upper gastrointestinal bleeding, diseases for which upper gastrointestinal bleeding is a complication, or determinants of physicians' decisions to withhold supportive transfusion therapy from patients with upper gastrointestinal bleeding, for example: age, terminal illnesses, etc.

Alternatively, one might want to address a similar question about nausea and vomiting caused by NSAIDs. Although this question is very similar, one's options in addressing it would be much more limited, as nausea and vomiting often do not come to medical attention. Other than a randomized clinical trial, for a drug that is largely used on an outpatient basis one is limited to systems which request information from patients, or ad hoc cohort studies.

As another example, one might want to follow-up on a signal generated by the spontaneous reporting system, designing a study to investigate whether a drug, which has been on the market for, say, five years, is a cause of a relatively rare condition, such as allergic hypersensitivity reactions. Because of the infrequency of the disease, one would need to draw on a very large population. The best alternatives would be Medicare or Medicaid databases, health plans, commercial databases, case–control studies, or Prescription Event Monitoring. To expedite this hypothesis-testing study and limit costs, it would be desirable if it could be performed using existing data. Prescription Event Monitoring and case–control surveillance would be excellent ways of addressing this, but only if the drug or disease in question, respectively, had been the subject of a prior study. Other methods of conducting case–control studies require gathering exposure data de novo.

As a last example, one might want to follow-up on a signal generated by a spontaneous reporting system, designing a study to investigate whether a drug, which has been on the market for, say, three years, is a cause of an extremely rare but serious illness, such as aplastic anemia. One's considerations would be similar to those above, but even Medicare or Medicaid databases would not be sufficiently large to include enough cases, given the delay in the availability of their data. One would have to gather data de novo. Assuming the drug in question is used mostly by outpatients, one could consider using Prescription Event Monitoring or a case–control study.

## Conclusion

Once one has decided to perform a pharmacoepidemiologic study, one needs to decide which of the resources described in the earlier chapters of this book should be used. By considering the characteristics of the pharmacoepidemiologic resources available as well as the characteristics of the question to be addressed, one should be able to choose those resources that are best suited to addressing the question at hand.

## Key Points

- There are many different approaches to performing pharmacoepidemiologic studies, each of which has its advantages and disadvantages.
- The choice of pharmacoepidemiologic resource must be tailored to the question to be addressed.
- One may want to use more than one data collection strategy or resource, in parallel or in combination.
- By considering the characteristics of the pharmacoepidemiologic resources available and the characteristics of the question to be addressed, one should be able to choose those resources that are best suited to address the question at hand.

## Further Reading

Anonymous (1986). Risks of agranulocytosis and aplastic anemia. A first report of their relation to drug use with special reference to analgesics. The international agranulocytosis and aplastic Anemia study. *JAMA* 256: 1749–1757.

Coulter, A., Vessey, M., and McPherson, K. (1986). The ability of women to recall their oral contraceptive histories. *Contraception* 33: 127–139.

Glass, R., Johnson, B., and Vessey, M. (1974). Accuracy of recall of histories of oral contraceptive use. *Br. J. Prev. Soc. Med.* 28: 273–275.

Klemetti, A. and Saxen, L. (1967). Prospective versus retrospective approach in the search for environmental causes of malformations. *Am. J. Public Health* 57: 2071–2075.

Mitchell, A.A., Cottler, L.B., and Shapiro, S. (1986). Effect of questionnaire design on recall of drug exposure in pregnancy. *Am. J. Epidemiol.* 123: 670–676.

Paganini-Hill, A. and Ross, R.K. (1982). Reliability of recall of drug usage and other health-related information. *Am. J. Epidemiol.* 116: 114–122.

Persson, I., Bergkvist, L., and Adami, H.O. (1987). Reliability of women's histories of climacteric oestrogen treatment assessed by prescription forms. *Int. J. Epidemiol.* 16: 222–228.

Rosenberg, M.J., Layde, P.M., Ory, H.W. et al. (1983). Agreement between women's histories of oral contraceptive use and physician records. *Int. J. Epidemiol.* 12: 84–87.

Schwarz, A., Faber, U., Borner, K. et al. (1984). Reliability of drug history in analgesic users. *Lancet* 2: 1163–1164.

Stolley, P.D., Tonascia, J.A., Sartwell, P.E. et al. (1978). Agreement rates between oral contraceptive users and prescribers in relation to drug use histories. *Am. J. Epidemiol.* 107: 226–235.

Strom, B.L., West, S.L., Sim, E., and Carson, J.L. (1989). Epidemiology of the acute flank pain syndrome from suprofen. *Clin. Pharmacol. Ther.* 46: 693–699.

**Part III**

**Special Issues in Pharmacoepidemiology Methodology**

# 13

# Validity of Drug and Diagnosis Data in Pharmacoepidemiology

*Mary Elizabeth Ritchey[1,2], Suzanne L. West[3], and George Maldonado[4]*

[1] Med Tech Epi, LLC, Philadelphia, PA, USA
[2] Center for Pharmacoepidemiology and Treatment Science, Rutgers University, New Brunswick, NJ, USA
[3] Gillings School of Global Public Health, University of North Carolina, Chapel Hill, NC, USA
[4] Division of Environmental Health Sciences, School of Public Health, University of Minnesota, Minneapolis, MN, USA

## Introduction

Accurate pharmacoepidemiologic study conclusions require assessment of valid data, regardless of whether the data originate from questionnaires, administrative claims, or electronic health records (EHRs). This chapter begins by discussing the validity of the drug and diagnostic information used by clinicians in patients' care. Next, we discuss measurement error, describing the different types of error and error detection methods, exploring how errors may affect the point estimate, and describing current techniques for mitigation. In the remainder of the chapter, we illustrate validity concerns when data from administrative claims, EHRs, or questionnaire responses are used, using as examples studies of the associations between nonsteroidal anti-inflammatory drugs (NSAIDs) and myocardial infarction (MI), and between NSAIDs and gastrointestinal (GI) bleeding.

## Clinical Problems to be Addressed by Pharmacoepidemiologic Research

Of particular concern to the subject of this book is the validity of data on drug exposure and disease occurrence, because the typical focus of pharmacoepidemiologic research is often the association between a medication and an adverse drug event. Further, many potential confounders of importance in pharmacoepidemiologic research (although certainly not all) are either drugs or diseases. Clinicians recognize that patients very often do not know the names of the drugs they are taking. Thus, it is a given that patients have difficulty recalling past drug use accurately, at least absent any aids to this recall. Superficially at least, patients cannot be considered reliable sources of diagnosis information either; in some instances, they may not even have been told the correct diagnosis, let alone recall it. Yet, these data elements are crucial to pharmacoepidemiology studies that ascertain data using questionnaires. Special approaches have been developed by pharmacoepidemiologists to obtain such data more accurately, from patients and other sources, but the success of these approaches needs to be considered in detail.

Besides self-reported data, pharmacoepidemiologists have been using administrative claims data for more than 30 years to evaluate drug safety. We discuss validity issues with using these data for research. However, the changing landscape of health care requires reassessing the validity of the data pharmacoepidemiologists are now using for their research and how these data impact clinical practice.

More and more, pharmacoepidemiologists are turning to EHR data for their research. Whereas the increased granularity of EHR data is a benefit for their use in pharmacoepidemiology, important limitations of these data include their potential incompleteness and lack of interoperability across health systems. Unless EHR data arise from "closed" health care systems where patients receive all their outpatient and inpatient care, the EHR data may represent only a portion of the patients' health problems and care received. If EHR data from multiple health systems are used, even if the health systems use the same EHR vendor, the data may need to be restructured so that they are consistent across all data arising from all health systems. The clinician reviewing evidence for patient care that arises from studies using EHR data trusts that these data have been curated sufficiently to produce robust and valid study findings.

## Methodological Problems to be Solved by Pharmacoepidemiologic Research

There are five major methodologic problems associated with validity of data for pharmacoepidemiologic research: indices of measurement error, quantitative measurement of

validity, quantitative measurement of reliability, measurement error in pharmacoepidemiologic research, and adjusting measures of association for measurement error.

### Indices of Measurement Error Relevant to Pharmacoepidemiologic Research

Two main comparisons may be drawn between two (or more) methods of data collection or sources of information on exposure or outcome: *validity* and *reliability*. Many different terms have been used to describe each, resulting in some confusion. Although the literature uses the term *validation* or *verification* to describe the agreement between two sources of information, *concordance* or *agreement* may more appropriately indicate comparison between data sources because *validation* requires a "gold standard." Though, in recognition that a method or source can be superior to another method or source without being perfect, the term "alloyed gold standard" is used.

### Quantitative Measurement of Validity

For a binary exposure or outcome measure, such as "ever" versus "never" using a particular drug, two measures of validity are used. *Sensitivity* measures the degree to which the inferior source or method correctly identifies individuals who, according to the superior method or source, possess the characteristic of interest (i.e. ever used the drug). *Specificity* measures the degree to which the inferior source or method correctly identifies individuals who, according to the superior method or source, lack the characteristic of interest (i.e. never used the drug). Figure 13.1 illustrates the calculation of sensitivity and specificity.

Sensitivity and specificity are the two sides of the validity "coin" for a dichotomous exposure or outcome variable. In general, sources or methods with higher sensitivity tend to have lower specificity, and methods with higher

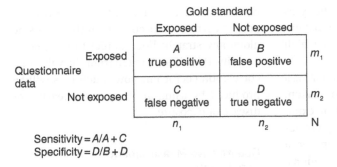

Sensitivity = $A/A + C$
Specificity = $D/B + D$

**Figure 13.1** Formulas for calculating sensitivity and specificity.

specificity tend to have lower sensitivity. In these very common situations, neither of the two sources or methods compared can be said to have superior overall validity. Depending on the study setting, either sensitivity or specificity may be the more important validity measure. Moreover, absolute values of these measures can be deceiving. For example, if the true prevalence of ever using a drug is 5%, then an exposure classification method or information source with 95% specificity (and perfect sensitivity) will almost double the measured prevalence to about 10%. The ultimate criterion of importance of a given combination of sensitivity and specificity is the degree of bias exerted on a measure of effect, such as an estimated relative risk due to measurement error.

As measures of validity, sensitivity and specificity have "truth" (i.e. the classification according to a gold standard or an alloyed gold standard) in their denominators. Investigators should take care not to confuse these measures with positive and negative predictive values (NPV), which include the inferior measure in their denominators. We distinguish here between the persons who *actually* do or do not have an exposure or outcome, and those who are *classified* as having it or not having it. The *positive predictive value* (PPV) is the proportion of persons classified as having the exposure or outcome who are correctly classified. The *negative predictive value* is the proportion of persons classified as lacking the exposure or outcome who are correctly classified. Predictive values are measures of performance of a

classification method or information source, not measures of validity. Predictive values depend not only on the sensitivity and specificity (i.e. on validity), but also on the true prevalence of the exposure or outcome. Thus, if a method or information source for classifying persons with respect to outcome or exposure has the same validity (i.e. the same sensitivity and specificity) in two populations, but those populations differ in their outcome or exposure prevalence, the source or method will have different predictive values in the two populations.

In some validation studies, one method or source may be used as a gold standard or as an alloyed gold standard to assess another method or source with respect to only one side of the validity "coin." Studies that focus on the completeness of one source, such as studies in which interview responses are compared with prescription dispensing records to identify drug exposures forgotten or otherwise unreported by the respondents, may measure (more or less accurately) the sensitivity of the interview data. However, such studies are silent on the specificity unless strong assumptions are made (e.g. that the respondent could not have obtained the drug in a way that would not be recorded in the prescription dispensing records). Similarly, validation of cases in a case–control study using self-report or administrative claims data often provides only the PPV that the cases are true cases and does not evaluate the NPV that the controls are truly controls. Ideally, one would design a validation study to calculate sensitivity and specificity, as well as positive and NPV and the key patient characteristics and other variables on which they depend.

For a drug exposure, a true gold standard is a list of all drugs the study participant has taken, including dose, duration, and dates of exposure. This drug list might be a diary of prescriptions that the study participants kept or a computerized database of filled prescriptions. However, neither of these data sources is a genuine gold standard. Prescription diaries cannot be assumed to be kept in perfect accuracy. For example, participants may tend to record drug use as more regular and complete than it actually was, or as more closely adhering to the typically prescribed regimen. Similarly, substantial gaps may exist between the point at which a prescription is filled and the time that it is ingested, if it is ingested at all (see Chapter 21 for discussion of adherence).

Two methods are used to quantify the validity of continuously distributed variables, such as duration of drug usage. The mean and standard error of the differences between the data in question and the valid reference measurement are typically used when the measurement error is constant across the range of true values (i.e. when measurement error is independent of where an individual's true exposure falls on the exposure distribution in the study population). With the caveat that it is generalizable only to populations with similar exposure distributions, the product–moment correlation coefficient may also be used.

High correlation between two measures does not necessarily mean high agreement. For instance, the correlation coefficient could be very high (i.e. close to 1), even though one of the variables systematically overestimates or underestimates values of the other variable. The high correlation means that the over- or underestimation is systematic and very consistent. When the two measures being compared are plotted against each other and they have the same scale, full agreement occurs only when the points fall on the line of equality, which is 45° from either axis. However, perfect correlation occurs when the points lie along any straight line parallel to the line of equality. It is difficult to tell from the value of a correlation coefficient how much bias will be produced by using an inaccurate measure of disease or exposure.

## Quantitative Measurement of Reliability

When the same data collection method or source of information is used more than once for the same information on the same individual, comparisons of the results measure the reliability of the method or information source. An example of a reliability study is a comparison of responses in repeat interviews using the same interview instrument. Reliability is not validity, although the term is sometimes used, inaccurately, as such. The term *reliability* tends to be used far too broadly to refer variously not only to reliability itself, but to agreement or validity as well. Researchers and others should take greater care with the way they use such terms.

When different data collection methods or different sources of information are compared (e.g. comparison of prescription dispensing records with interview responses), and neither of them can be considered distinctly superior to the other, the comparisons measure mere agreement. Agreement between two sources or methods does not imply that either is valid.

To evaluate reliability or agreement for categorical variables, the percentage agreement between two or more sources and the related (*kappa*, κ) coefficient are used. They are used only when two imperfect classification schemes are being compared, not when one classification method may be considered a priori superior to the other. The κ statistic is the percentage agreement corrected for chance. Agreement is conventionally considered poor for a κ statistic less than zero, slight for κ between zero and 0.20, fair for a κ of 0.21–0.40, moderate for a κ of 0.41–0.60, substantial for a κ of 0.61–0.80, and almost perfect for a κ of 0.81–1.00. Figure 13.2 illustrates the percentage agreement and κ calculations for a reliability assessment between questionnaire data and medical record information.

The intraclass correlation coefficient is used to evaluate the reliability of continuous variables. It reflects both the average differences in mean values and the correlation between measurements. The intraclass correlation coefficient indicates the degree to which the total measurement variation is due to the differences between the subjects being evaluated and to differences in measurement for one individual. When the data from two sets of measurements are identical, the intraclass correlation coefficient equals 1.0. Under certain conditions, the intraclass correlation coefficient is exactly equivalent to Cohen's weighted κ.

It is impossible to translate values of measures of agreement, such as κ, into expected degrees of bias in exposure or disease associations.

## Measurement Error in Pharmacoepidemiologic Research

Epidemiologic assessments of the effects of a drug on disease incidence depend on an accurate assessment of the study exposure, disease occurrence, and variables to be adjusted in the statistical analysis. Measurement error for any

of these factors may incorrectly identify a risk factor in the study that does not exist in the population or, conversely, may fail to detect a risk factor when one truly exists.

For example, when questionnaire data are used to study the association between drug A and disease B, study participants who forgot their past exposure to drug A would be incorrectly classified as nonexposed. Similarly, if a provider uses a diagnosis code to document the process of testing and ruling out a disease and then a researcher uses the diagnosis code as a study outcome, then the person would be incorrectly classified as having the outcome. This misclassification is a measurement error. Although the measurement process often involves some error, if this measurement error is of sufficient magnitude, the validity of the study's findings is diminished.

Surprisingly, measurement error is often ignored in epidemiologic studies. Jurek et al. reported the results of a random survey of studies published in three major epidemiology journals; they concluded the following for exposure-measurement error (EME): "Overall, the potential impact of EME on error in epidemiologic study results appears to be ignored frequently in practice (page 871)."

Measurement error is a potentially serious cause for concern in epidemiologic studies, and therefore, for several reasons, should not be ignored when analyzing and interpreting pharmacoepidemiologic study results. First,

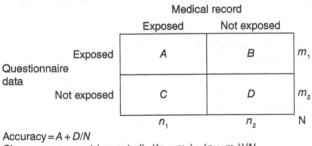

Accuracy $= A + D/N$

Chance agreement (expected) $= ((n_1 \times m_1) + (n_2 \times m_2))/N_2$

$$\kappa = \frac{\text{accuracy} - \text{chance agreement}}{1 - \text{chance agreement}}$$

**Figure 13.2** Formulas for calculating the percent agreement and κ.

small amounts of measurement error can cause large amounts of error in study results. For example, consider a pharmacoepidemiologic study of NSAID A versus NSAID B on GI bleed (Figure 13.3). In a study with a total number of study subjects equal to more than 22 000, if only 10 subjects are misclassified with respect to their exposure or disease (five with GI bleed who actually took NSAID B are incorrectly classified as having taken NSAID A, and five users of NSAID A without GI bleed are incorrectly classified as having GI bleed), the observed odds ratio (OR) would be 2.1 when the correct OR is in fact 1.0.

Second, measurement error can cause study results to overestimate or underestimate true effect sizes, and there is no simple rule for predicting the direction of the error in real-life situations. We now understand that these old and often-cited heuristics are not necessarily true, except under special conditions that are not likely to occur in practice: (i) "nondifferential misclassification always produces bias toward the null," and (ii) "bias toward the null always produces an observed relative risk that is an underestimate of the true relative risk." These heuristics are unlikely to be true in practice for the following reasons:

- Conditions beyond nondifferentiality are required to guarantee bias is toward the null (e.g. when the degree of exposure measurement error systematically differs across levels of a polychotomous or continuous exposure variable, or when errors in measuring the exposure and outcome are not independent).
- Even when the above conditions beyond nondifferentiality are met, exact nondifferentiality is required to guarantee bias is toward the null.
- Also required to guarantee bias is toward the null is either (i) the absence of other study biases (e.g. absence of confounding, absence of bias due to nonrandom subject selection/participation), or (ii) the combined effect of all other biases is also toward the null.
- Bias is a statistical term that is defined as the difference between the true value and the expected value of an estimator (i.e. the average of study results over hypothetical repetitions of the study). Bias is not the difference between the observed estimate for one repetition of the study and the true value. This important distinction was not appreciated in earlier writings on this topic, and even today we epidemiologists are not careful in our use of the term bias. Therefore, when bias is toward the null, the expected value of the estimator is shifted toward the null, but an observed estimate can be an overestimate of the true relative risk due to the influence of random error. (Similarly, when there is no bias of any kind, one observed estimate can be an overestimate or an underestimate of the true relative risk simply due to random error.)

Third, error in measuring variables to be adjusted in the analysis can result in only partial adjustment for the mismeasured variables.

Observed data (with 5 NSAID B cases misclassified as having taken NSAID A, and 5 without GI bleed misclassified as GI bleed)

|  | NSAID A | NSAID B |  |
| --- | --- | --- | --- |
| GI Bleed | 20 | 95 |  |
| Not GI Bleed | 1,995 | 20,000 | Observed OR = 2.1 |

Data after correcting for measurement error

|  | NSAID A | NSAID B |  |
| --- | --- | --- | --- |
| GI Bleed | 10 | 100 |  |
| Not GI Bleed | 2,000 | 20,000 | True OR = 1.0 |

**Figure 13.3** Small amount of measurement error can cause large error in study results.

## Adjusting Measures of Association for Measurement Error

One can use sensitivity analysis methods (also known as uncertainty analysis and bias analysis) to adjust measures of association for measurement error as well as for other study biases. (As used in this context, the meaning of the term *sensitivity* differs from its other epidemiologic meaning as the counterpart to specificity as a measure of classification validity.) Sensitivity analysis is the last line of defense against biases after every effort has been made to eliminate, reduce, or control them in study design, data collection, and data analysis. In a sensitivity analysis, one varies key assumptions or methods reasonably to see how sensitive the results of a study are to those variations.

One key assumption, usually implicit, in any study that does not quantitatively account for the possibility of error in measuring the study exposure or study outcome, is that the exposure and the outcome in a study have been measured accurately. With estimates of sensitivity and specificity from validation studies (from previous research or from a subsample within the study analyzed) or "guesstimates" from expert experience and judgment, one can modify this assumption and use sensitivity analysis methods to "back calculate" what the results might have looked like if more accurate methods had been used to classify participants with respect to outcome, exposure, or both.

For many years, a qualitative and informal version of this kind of assessment has been conducted. However, the net result is controversy, with investigators judging the bias small and critics judging it large. Further, in the absence of a formal sensitivity analysis, intuitive judgments, even those of the most highly trained and widely experienced investigators, can be poorly calibrated in such matters. Formal sensitivity analysis makes the assessment of residual bias transparent and quantitative, and forces the investigator (and other critics) to defend criticisms that in earlier times

would have remained qualitative and unsubstantiated. An important and well-known historical example is the bias from nondifferential misclassification of disease proposed by Horwitz and Feinstein to explain associations between early exogenous estrogen preparations and endometrial cancer. When proper sensitivity analyses were conducted, only a negligible proportion of those associations were explained by bias.

Epidemiologic applications of quantitative methods with a long history in the decision sciences have become accessible for quantifying uncertainties about multiple sources of systematic error in a probabilistic manner. These methods permit incorporation of available validation data, expert judgment about measurement error, uncontrolled confounding (see Chapter 22), and selection bias, along with conventional sampling error and prior probability distributions for effect measures themselves, to form uncertainty distributions. These approaches have been used practically in pharmacoepidemiology studies such as in assessing selection bias in a study of topical coal tar therapy and skin cancer among severe psoriasis patients; exposure misclassification and selection bias in a study of phenylpropanolamine use and stroke; selection bias, confounder misclassification, unmeasured confounding in a study of less than definitive therapy and breast cancer mortality; and other clinical and nonclinical applications.

Sometimes biases can be shown to be of more concern and sometimes of less concern than intuition or simple sensitivity analysis might suggest. Using these methods, assessment of systematic error can move from a qualitative discussion of "study limitations," beyond sensitivity analyses of one scenario at a time for one source of error at a time, to a comprehensive analysis of all sources of error simultaneously. The resulting uncertainty distributions can not only supplement but also supplant conventional likelihood and $p$-value functions, which reflect only random sampling error. As a result, much more realistic, probabilistic assessments of total uncertainty attending to effect measure estimates are available.

## Self-Reported Drug Data from Ad hoc Survey Studies: Recall Accuracy

The methodological literature on recall accuracy discussed above indicates that study participants have difficulty remembering drug use from the distant past, which contributes to misclassification of exposure in de novo studies. Researchers are using best practices in questionnaire design, including medication-specific and indication-specific questions, along with recall enhancements, which have been shown to produce better data. Calendars and photos of drugs augment recall to a greater degree than listing only the brand names of the drugs in question. These techniques – namely, photos, calendars, and the two different types of drug questions – have become the state of the art for collecting self-reported drug data by personal or telephone interview.

The literature to date suggests that recall accuracy of self-reported medication exposures is sometimes, but not always, influenced by type of medication, drug-use patterns, design of the data collection materials, and respondent characteristics. Given the current state of the literature, epidemiologists who plan to use questionnaire data to investigate drug–disease associations will need to consider which factors may influence recall accuracy in the design of their research protocols. Case example 13.1 summarizes the published literature on studies that have validated drug exposure information (NSAIDs) on health outcomes (MI and GI bleeding) from questionnaire data.

## The Influence of Medication Class

Several studies have compared self-reported recall accuracy for current or past medication use with prospectively collected cohort data or pharmacy, hospital, and outpatient medical record documentation. Overall, published studies indicate that people accurately remember ever having used a medication and when they first began using it, for some medications, although they do not remember brand names and duration of use as well. In general, inaccuracies correlated with more time elapsed between occurrence of exposure and its subsequent reporting. Accuracy of self-reporting varies by medication. For example:

- Chronically used medications (especially those with more refills) being recalled more often than acute exposures.
- First and most recent brands in a class are recalled more frequently than other medications in the class.
- Multiple medications in one class are recalled more frequently than single medication exposure.
- Salient exposures (those that prompted study initiation) are more accurately recalled than common and less disconcerting medications.

For prescription drugs, recall between self-reported use and medical records was moderately accurate, but over-the-counter medications and vitamin supplements had poorer recall. Discrepancies were due to both underreporting (e.g. respondent forgot that the medication was taken) and overreporting (e.g. physician record patient's use in chart from previous visit, even though patient stopped medication) and differed by therapeutic class. When self-reported data were compared with multiple sources, such as medical records and pharmacy dispensing, verification of self-reported use was higher than for a single source.

## The Influence of Questionnaire Design

As reported in a recent systematic review, several factors affect the accuracy of medication exposure reported via questionnaire. Researchers can facilitate recall and reporting of medication use by indication-specific questions, memory prompts (such as drug photo), a list of drug names, or a calendar to record life events. Medication-specific or indication-specific questions can identify most medications in current use, but a general medication question, such as "Have you taken any other medications?" failed to identify all medications respondents were currently taking. Similarly, open-ended questions such as "Have you ever used any medications?" yielded less than half of the affirmative responses for actual use of three different medications. Using the filter question ("Did you use any medications in the three months before or during your pregnancy?"), van Gelder and colleagues noted that many women failed to report medications that they had been dispensed for pain or infections. These findings could be attributed to poor recall, but they may be also due to women having chosen not to take the dispensed medications. If researchers choose to use open-ended medication questions, adding indication-specific questions that facilitate recall of medication exposures may be useful. Finally, 20–35% of respondents reported drug exposure only when asked medication-name-specific questions.

Response order may affect recall, as noted with malaria medications when respondents had more than one episode of malaria. Medications listed earlier tended to be selected more frequently than those listed later – a finding that may be related to "satisficing," which occurs when respondents expend the least psychological and emotional effort possible to provide an acceptable answer to a survey question rather than an optimal answer.

A comparison of self-report for current and recent medication use (within the past two years) with pharmacy records of dispensed prescriptions for multiple drug classes found that recall of the number of drug dispensingswas highest for cardiovascular medications (66%) and poorest for alimentary tract medications (48%). Recall was influenced by the number of regularly used medications: 71% for one drug, 64% for two

drugs, and 59% for three or more drugs, although duration of use was not related to recall. However, the questionnaire did not allow sufficient space to record all medications used in the time period for this study. Thus, if respondents were unable to record all medications due to space limitations, a misleading validation might have occurred: it appeared that respondents were unable to recall all their medications dispensed, according to the database.

Another methodological study evaluated whether question structure influenced the recall of currently used medications in 372 subjects with hypertension who had at least 90 days of dispensing in the PHARMO database. The questionnaire asked indication-specific questions first (e.g. medications used for hypertension, medications used for diabetes), followed by an open-ended question that asked whether the participants used any *other* medications not already mentioned. For hypertension, the sensitivity was 91% for indication-specific questions and 16.7% for open-ended questions. About 20% of participants listed medications on the questionnaire that were not in the database; a similar proportion failed to list medications on the questionnaire that were in use according to the pharmacy database. Based on these recall sensitivity results, indication-specific questions invoke better recall accuracy. However, to adequately assess question structure, a questionnaire could be designed to ask open-ended questions before indication-specific questions. This sequencing would allow a comparison of the number of medications recalled by each question structure.

## The Influence of Patient Population

Few studies have evaluated whether demographic and behavioral characteristics influence the recall of past medication use. Research suggests that education attainment and race/ethnicity may affect recall accuracy.

Studies are inconsistent for age, socioeconomic status, and smoking as predictors of recall accuracy, and no study found that recall accuracy varies by gender. The inconsistencies on the effect of age on recall accuracy might arise from differing study designs. The two studies that reported an age effect were methodological studies evaluating recall accuracy, whereas the two that reported no age effects were etiologic studies that reported verification of drug use as a measure of exposure misclassification for the association under study. Because of the paucity of information on predictors of recall, further research in this area is warranted.

## Self-Reported Diagnosis and Hospitalization Data from Ad hoc Studies: Recall Accuracy

Just as recall accuracy of past medication use varies by drug class, the recall accuracy of disease conditions varies by disease, particularly when it is chronic, like hypertension, or is viewed as threatening, such as sexual transmitted infections.

## The Influences of Medical Condition Type

Comparing patient self-report with data from a provider questionnaire (gold standard) on previous history of cardiovascular disease or GI events, researchers found better agreement for previous acute MI than for upper GI bleeding (see Case Example 13.1).

- The best reporting has been noted with conditions that are specific and familiar, such as diabetes mellitus, hypertension, asthma, and cancers such as breast, lung, large bowel, and prostate. However, assessing reporting accuracy is more difficult for common, symptom-based conditions such as sinusitis, arthritis, low back pain, and migraine headaches, which many people may have, or believe they have, without having been diagnosed by a clinician.

Both overreporting and underreporting was noted for cardiovascular conditions, depending on the data source used for comparison. In most instances of recall error, respondents who had incorrectly reported MIs and stroke had other conditions that they may have mistakenly understood as coronary heart disease, MI, or stroke. Underreporting was the primary reason for poor agreement comparing interview data to clinical evaluation, although it is unclear whether this is due to the respondent's unwillingness to admit to mental illness or underdiagnosis of the conditions.

## The Influences of Timing of Diagnosis and Its Emotional Effects on the Patient

Factors influencing accuracy of past diagnoses and hospitalizations also include the number of physician services for that condition and the recency of services. For reporting of diagnoses, the longer the interval between the date of the last medical visit for the condition and the date of interview, the poorer the recall for that condition. These differences in recall may be explained in part by recall interval, patient age, a cohort (generational) effect, or some intertwining of all three factors. Diagnoses considered sensitive by one generation may not be considered as such by subsequent generations. Further, terminology changes over time, with prior generations using different nomenclature compared with recent generations.

Conditions with substantial impact on a person's life are more accurately reported than those with little or no impact on lifestyle. More patients with current restrictions on food or beverage due to medical problems reported chronic conditions that were confirmed in medical records than did those without these restrictions. Similarly, those who had restrictions on work or housework reported their chronic conditions more often than those who did not have these restrictions. The major determinant of recall for spontaneous abortions was the length of the pregnancy at the time the

---

**Case Example 13.1    Fourrier-Reglat et al. (2010)**

---

*Background*

- Researchers may have to query the subject to assess medication exposure and outcome diagnoses. Accuracy of ad hoc questionnaire studies has been determined via comparison with pharmacy, practitioner, and hospital records.
- In some cases, pharmacy or medical records may not be available or there may be reason to question both the patient and practitioner rather than conducting medical record review. In addition, questionnaires can provide concurrence regarding patient history and indication for use, which are not available from claims data or easily found in many medical records.

*Question*

When questionnaires are self-administrated, is there concordance of patient-derived and physician-derived data on medical information such as previous medical history and initial indication for NSAID prescriptions?

*Approach*

- The Kappa statistic ($\kappa$) was used to measure concordance in self-administered questionnaires completed by 18 530 pairs of NSAID patients and their prescribers for the French national cohort study of NSAID and Cox-2 inhibitor users.
- Both patients and prescribers were asked about patients' previous history of cardiovascular events, including MI, and GI events, including upper digestive hemorrhage. Patients and prescribers were asked to identify which of the following was the initial indication for NSAID use: rheumatoid arthritis, psoriatic rheumatism, spondylarthritis, osteoarthritis, back pain, muscle pain/sprain/tendonitis, migraine/headache, flu-like symptoms, dysmenorrhea, or other indication.

*Results*

- Agreement between patients and prescribers was substantial for MI ($\kappa = 0.75$, 95% CI: 0.71–0.80), and minimal for upper GI bleeding ($\kappa = 0.16$, 95% CI: 0.11–0.22).
- With prescriber data as the gold standard, patient reports of MI provided moderately complete data (sensitivity: 77.7%; specificity: 99.6%, PPV: 74.1%, NPV: 99.6%), but reports of upper GI bleeding by patients were less well documented in the prescriber reports (sensitivity: 44.6%; specificity: 98.5%, PPV: 10.4%, NPV: 99.8%).
- For the index NSAID indication, the proportion of agreement ranged from 84.3% to 99.4%, and concordance was almost perfect ($k = 0.81$–1.00).

*Strengths*

- Concurrent evaluation of patients and prescribers allows corroboration of patient history and indication for medication usage, which are difficult to assess in claims and electronic health care records.
- Self-administered questionnaires provide data on a list of potential confounders that are often missing from electronic records.

*Limitations*

- Study was carried out in an established cohort in a single country. Results may not be generalizable to other data in other locations.
- Neither the patient nor the prescriber reports "truth"; accuracy of recall was not assessed in this study.

*Key Points*

- Prior history and indication for prescriptions are often missing from claims and electronic health care record databases. Questionnaires from both patients and prescribers may collect data on these potential confounders, as well as determine the reliability of the collected variables.

---

*(Continued)*

---

**Case Example 13.1    (Continued)**

- Patients and prescribers may have differing recall of patient history, especially as related to nonspecific diagnoses.
- Relying on patient-reported data may be necessary but inaccurate, especially for

over-the-counter medication use. However, corroboration with another information source, such as data from the prescriber, may provide an estimate of the reliability of patient-reported data.

---

event occurred: nearly all respondents who experienced spontaneous abortions occurring more than 13 weeks into the pregnancy remembered them, compared with just over half of respondents who experience such abortions occurring in the first six weeks of pregnancy.

Perhaps as a result of the emotional stress, lifestyle changes, and potential financial strain, hospitalizations tend to be reported accurately. Further, underreporting of hospitalizations occurred in 9% of patients when surgery was performed, compared with 16% of patients without a surgical procedure. Underreporting in those with only a one-day hospital stay was 28% compared with 11% for two to four day stays and approximately 6% for stays lasting five or more days.

Researchers also agree that respondents remember the type of surgery accurately. Recall accuracy was very good for hysterectomy and appendectomy, most likely because these surgeries are both salient and familiar to respondents. For induced abortions, marginal agreement occurred, as noted by records from a managed care organization: 19% of women underreported their abortion history, 35% overreported abortions, and 46% reported accurately, according to their medical records. Cholecystectomy and oophorectomy were not as well recalled and were subject to some overreporting. However, apparent overreporting may have been due to possible incompleteness of the medical records used for comparison.

### The Influence of Patient Population

The influence of demographic characteristics on reporting of chronic illness has been

thoroughly evaluated, although the results are conflicting. The most consistent finding is that recall accuracy decreases with age, although this may be confounded by recall interval, or cohort (generational) effects. Whether gender influences recall accuracy is uncertain. Men have been found to report better than women, independent of age, whereas conflicting evidence found that women reported better than men, especially in older age groups. Further studies indicate that gender and age differences depended on the disease under investigation, with women overreporting malignancies and men overreporting stroke. No differences were found for reporting of hospitalizations by age or gender.

Reporting of illnesses, procedures, and hospitalizations tends to differ by race/ethnicity, but most studies had much larger proportions of whites than nonwhites. Reporting by educational level was equivocal and was more complete for self-respondents than for proxy respondents. Those with a poor or fair current health status reported conditions more completely than those with good to excellent health status.

### The Influence of Questionnaire Design

Questionnaire design also influences the validity of disease and hospitalization data obtained by self report. Providing respondents with a checklist of reasons for visiting the doctor improves recall of all medical visits. Simpler questions yield better responses than more complex questions, presumably because complex questions require the respondent to first comprehend what is being asked and then provide an answer. Inherent redundancy in longer questions and greater time allowances to develop an answer may increase recall; however, longer questions may tire the respondents, leading to satisficing, as well as increase the cost of the research.

# Currently Available Solutions

## Following Best Practices for Questionnaire Design

Designing a questionnaire to collect epidemiologic data requires careful planning and pretesting. We suggest the following steps be considered during the design and initial analysis stages of a study requiring data collection via questionnaire:

1) Use validated instruments or validated questions whenever possible.
2) Consider question banks if new questions are required, such as World Bank's Living Standards Measurement Study and Q-Bank.
3) Use question assessment tools to determine the likelihood of response error. These tools include the Question Appraisal System, the Survey Quality Predictor (SQP), and the Question Understanding Aid (QUAID).
4) Strive for a fifth-grade literacy level if you must develop new survey questions to be used for a general population.
5) Pretest questions using cognitive testing to assess respondent comprehension of new questions.

## Developing a De novo Questionnaire

Although specific guidance on best practices for improving the ascertainment of diagnoses and hospitalizations is lacking, researchers developing questionnaires should be mindful of question wording and sequencing and response formats. Questionnaire designers should attend to the cognitive processes involved in developing a response, especially those related to saliency for the respondent. The typical rule of thumb for question sequencing is to ask general questions before delving into specific topics and to group questions according to topic. Response categories should be unambiguous, nonoverlapping, and exhaustive. When there is a possibility of biased response due to response ordering, it is best to randomize the response options to minimize the bias. Finally, satisficing is also possible when respondents are asked to identify the diagnoses they have been given previously.

With the increasing availability of broadband and the population's access to the Internet, more surveys are moving away from face-to-face and telephone interviewer administration to web-based surveys. This modality requires the same considerations for question design as described above, but because no interviewer is available, usability and how efficiently and effectively respondents can answer the web-based questions, should be tested as well.

To appreciate the accuracy of data derived by respondent recall, it is important to understand the how people process, organize, and recall autobiographical information, which is key to the response process. Creating and retrieving information from autobiographical memories is a three-step process. Information that comes in via sensory or emotional input (e.g. visual, hearing, semantic) is *encoded* into a construct that can be stored within the brain. The next step is *storage*, which refers to how the brain retains the information, typically in either short- or long-term memory. *Retrieval or recall* of memories requires re-accessing information that was previously encoded and stored. The recall of encoded or cataloged information from memory is thought to be facilitated by using important personal milestones. Thus, when respondents are asked to recall a visit to a doctor that may have occurred at a particular point in time, researchers believe that the respondents use scripts (a generic mental representation of the event) to help retrieval. In general, underreporting of medical conditions and health visits is more widespread as the interval since the event increases. Applying what we know about how autobiographical memory is organized and the recall process in general helps us to understand survey response. A respondent undergoes four key tasks when asked to answer a questionnaire:

- Question comprehension and interpretation.
- Search for and retrieval of information to construct an answer to the question.
- Judgment to discern the completeness and relevance of memory for formulating a response.
- development of the response based on retrieved memories.

If survey instrument developers pay too little attention to the first two key tasks, their questions may be too vague or complex for respondents to marshal retrieval processes appropriately. For discussion of the theory of survey response and the cognitive process underlying retrieval, see Tourangeau et al. (2000).

The following example illustrates the response process for recalling the date on which a respondent's depression was diagnosed (January 2015). The recall process begins with the respondent being uncertain whether the depression was diagnosed in 2014 or 2015. To work toward identifying the correct year, the respondent recalls that the depression occurred after he lost his job. The job loss was particularly traumatic because he and his wife just purchased their first home a few months previously, and now, with the loss of his income, they were at risk of losing the house. The home purchase was a landmark event for this respondent, and he remembers that it occurred in mid-2014, just as their children finished the school year. So, in 2014 he lost his job, near the end of the year because the holiday season was particularly grim. He remembers that his depression was diagnosed after the holidays, but was it January or February of 2015? It was January 2015 because he was already taking antidepressants by Valentine's Day, when he went out to dinner with his wife and he could not drink wine with his meal. This chronology is diagrammed in Figure 13.4. We describe below, how to use the response process to design

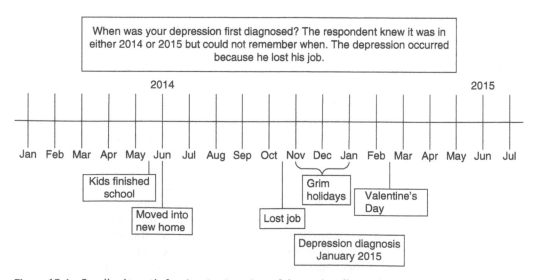

**Figure 13.4** Recall schematic for showing how date of depression diagnosis was determined.

questions to elicit the self-reported information requested.

As illustrated in Figure 13.4, landmark events probably serve as the primary organizational units of autobiographical knowledge and anchor information retrieval. In particular, the example shows how the respondent used landmark and other notable events, relationships among datable events, and general knowledge (holiday period and children finishing the school year) to reconstruct when his major depression was first diagnosed. An important caveat is that this respondent described above was willing to expend considerable effort searching his memory to determine when his depression was diagnosed, which may not be true for all respondents.

The process of *satisficing* occurs when respondents expend the least psychological and emotional effort possible to provide an acceptable answer to a survey question rather than an optimal answer. To minimize satisficing, questionnaire developers should consider the length of the instrument and the number of response categories. When faced with a long list of choices and depending on the mode of questionnaire administration (i.e. telephone versus self-administered), respondents may choose answers at the top or bottom of the list to minimize effort. Respondents with lower cognitive skills and less education, when challenged with discerning the best possible response, are more apt to settle for a satisfactory rather than an optimal response. Because accuracy of response is critical for pharmacoepidemiologic research, questionnaire developers must consider methods to minimize response burden leading to satisficing.

In addition to survey design and respondent motivation, measurement error can be attributed to improper training of interviewers and poor data entry quality. The degree to which one understands the measurement error associated with key variables is critical to the analysis can be assessed using several different modeling approaches, which Biemer, 2009 discusses in more detail.

## Conducting Validation Studies to Assess Self-Reported Data

Methodological studies that use alternative data sources such as prospectively collected data or databases of dispensed drugs can measure both sensitivity and specificity, if one assumes that the prescription database is a gold standard. In pharmacoepidemiology, lower sensitivity is often more of a concern than lower specificity. Questionnaires that underreport diseases or miss drug exposures because the medication was filled without using the pharmacy plan (e.g. when the co-pay is higher than the cost of the medication) – that is, data sources with low sensitivity – cannot be used to rigorously evaluate drug-disease associations. Alternatively, low specificity is often less of a problem in pharmacoepidemiology unless the characteristic with low specificity also has very low prevalence in the population being studied. For example, because the incidence of Stevens–Johnson syndrome is rare, a small degree of misclassification when using administrative claims data in which the case definition uses the ICD-9-CM code 695.1 will include several skin problems other than Stevens–Johnson (i.e. the false-positive rate will be high).

Besides the need for completeness on the individual level, the comparator database must have information for all persons whose information is to be assessed for accuracy. Systematic omissions of specific population groups, such as certain ethnic or racial groups, diminish the quality of the database.

## Considering the Influence of Comparator Selection on Validation Studies

Regardless of whether the medical record is paper or electronic, one needs to understand its availability, completeness, and accuracy to determine whether it is adequate for evaluating the accuracy of self-reported information. Retrieval of medical records depends not only on a person's ability to remember and report who prescribed the drug or diagnosed the condition in question, but on whether the health care provider recorded the information (and recorded it accurately) and on the availability of the medical record for review. If the medical record cannot be retrieved because the health care provider could not be identified, the provider had retired, or their record was destroyed or lost, the events cannot be verified.

In the US, health care is fragmented. Patients see multiple providers, are treated in several different health settings (e.g. chiropractors, podiatrists), and may become inpatients at several different hospitals. Thus, accessing patients' outpatient and inpatient medical records does not guarantee that a researcher will have all medical care provided and drugs prescribed to the patient. For example, if a researcher is able to access only the patients' primary care records, it is possible that the results of cardiology tests to confirm a diagnosis or medications for that diagnosis are not available. However, within integrated delivery systems that include primary care, multiple specialties, and inpatient care, there is a greater likelihood that the EHR will contain most of the care provided and medications prescribed to the patient.

In addition, exposure information about medications or important confounders (e.g. smoking) may be incomplete if clinicians do not ascertain this information and correctly enter it into the EHR. Another problem introduced by EHRs is the potential for errors inherent to electronic data entry, such as copying and pasting of incorrect data from other parts of the record, of expired or irrelevant clinical information, or of incorrect or unverified medication lists.

## Validation of Pharmacoepidemiologic Drug and Diagnosis Data from Electronic Encounter Databases

In addition to conducting de novo studies to evaluate drug–disease associations, a variety of computerized, administrative claims and EHR databases are available for pharmacoepidemiologic research, the structure, strengths, and limitations of which were reviewed in Chapters 8–10. One major advantage of using such databases for pharmacoepidemiologic research is the comparative validity of the drug data in lieu of questionnaire data, where recall bias is of concern, as previously described.

The drawbacks and limitations of these data systems are important. Their most critical limitation for pharmacoepidemiologic research is the manner in which health insurance is currently covered in the United States, typically through the employer. If the employer changes plans, which may occur annually, the employee changes among the plans offered by the employer, or the employee changes jobs, then the plan no longer covers that employee or his or her family. Thus, the continual enrollment and disenrollment of plan members hinders the opportunity for extended longitudinal analyses in both administrative claims and EHRs.

Diagnoses, procedures, medications, and other therapeutics are included in administrative claims and EHR data through structured coding systems. Each coding system has its own ontology and is separated into specific codes, based on an established hierarchy. Further, the coding systems are updated periodically to reflect changes in the practice of health care as well as to incorporate new therapies and processes. Both codes and the general structure and hierarchy differ between coding systems. In many cases, a single code is insufficient to define a variable and an *algorithm*, with required timing of codes or a sequential process for determining the level(s) of the variable, is needed. Algorithms developed in one coding system likely require translation to be useful in another coding system.

In addition to the structured data, many aspects of health care are captured within clinician notes, images and descriptions of procedure results, and other unstructured data. Performance of an algorithm can be enhanced through use of this unstructured information, by converting it into structured information (e.g. manually) for a specific project, or to modify and improve algorithm performance as cases are identified over time (e.g. machine learning). Previously developed algorithms are sometimes used for comparison, however patient charts (electronic or paper) are still often used as the reference standard for assessing validation.

Completeness and validity of data are the most critical elements in the selection of a database for research. *Completeness* is defined as the proportion of all exposures, events of interest, or both that occurred in the population covered by the database that appear in the computerized data. Missing subjects, exposures, or events could introduce bias in the study results. For example, completeness of the drug data may vary by income level if persons with higher incomes and drug copayments choose to obtain their medications at pharmacies not participating in a prescription plan, which is how pharmacy data are collected. Similarly, bias may be introduced in the association between a drug and a serious adverse drug reaction if hospitalizations for that adverse reaction are missing, e.g. if the researcher only has access to outpatient clinic data in the EHR.

## Special Considerations with Drug Data

A handful of studies to date have assessed dispensing associated with prescriptions via linked administrative claims and EHR data. These studies indicated that 70–77% of initial prescriptions are dispensed. Prescribed analgesics (i.e. pain medications, including NSAIDS) and lifestyle drugs (e.g. phosphodiesterase type 5 inhibitors) are least likely to be dispensed, while antimicrobials are most likely to be dispensed for an initial prescription. Substantial variation in dispensing was seen across medications within a class. In addition, results from Rowan suggests that <20% of patients taking analgesics and NSAIDS possessed adequate medication to be adherent throughout a 12 month period; this finding may be consistent with intermittent or "as needed" utilization.

In summary, drug and medical intervention data are often considered to be correct when using administrative claims data and EHRs for research. Although this is generally the case, researchers should be aware of whether and how prescribing, dispensing, and administration of drugs are captured within each database they are contemplating using. We will likely see greater emphasis on data linkage and incorporation of more unstructured data from clinical notes into pharmacoepidemiologic research, which may lead to increased need for validation of drug and medical intervention exposures in the future.

## Special Considerations with Diagnosis and Hospitalization Data

Unlike drug data where many researchers are comfortable with accuracy and completeness, inpatient and outpatient diagnoses in these databases raise considerable concern for investigators. The accuracy of outpatient diagnoses is more uncertain than inpatient diagnoses for several reasons. Hospitals employ experienced people to code diagnoses for reimbursement, which may not occur in physicians' offices where outpatient diagnoses are determined. Moreover, hospital personnel scrutinize inpatient diagnoses for errors, monitoring which does not typically occur in the outpatient setting.

Systematic errors as a result of diagnostic coding may influence the validity of both inpatient and outpatient diagnostic data. For example, diseases listed in administrative claims databases are often coded using the International Classification of Disease (ICD) system. Poorly defined diseases are difficult to code using the ICD system, and no way exists to indicate that an ICD code is coded for "rule-out" purposes. How health care plans address "rule-out" diagnoses is unclear; they likely do

---

**Case Example 13.2   Bustamante et al. (2019)**

*Background*
- A variety of electronic administrative databases are available for pharmacoepidemiologic research. One major advantage of using such databases for pharmacoepidemiologic research is the comparative validity of the drug data in lieu of questionnaire data, for which recall bias is always a concern.
- Algorithms using structured and unstructured data may have differing validity. Unstructured data may provide useful information for identifying an over-the-counter medication.

*Question*
Within the Veteran's Affairs (VA) administrative data, what is the reliability and validity of various measures of dispensing for aspirin?

*Approach*
- A retrospective cohort database study was conducted of 1 869 439 veterans who underwent colonoscopy within the VA in 1999–2014 to develop and evaluate three algorithms for identifying which patients received aspirin (over-the-counter or prescription). Charts reviewed to develop algorithms (number not stated); tested algorithms in 100 charts categorized as having aspirin use and 100 charts categorized with non-use.
  - Structured data from VA Meds: use of aspirin documented as *medicine* taken and *allergy* to aspirin assumed to confirm non-use of aspirin
  - Identified common terms from progress notes, included character distance between "aspirin" and dose indicators – identified terms consistent with aspirin use and non-use
  - Combined structured and unstructured data
- Assessed sensitivity, specificity PPV, and NPV of charts compared to manual chart review of free-text progress notes and pharmacy data

*Results*
Table 13.1 presents the sensitivity, specificity, PPV, and NPV for the three algorithms. The sensitivity dropped (minimally) as a wider array of data was incorporated into the algorithm, while the specificity, PPV, and NPV increased. Using both structured and unstructured data led to the highest specificity, PPV, and NPV.

*Strengths*
- Evaluation of sensitivity, specificity, PPV, and NPV provides the full picture of reliability and validity for algorithms assessing both prescription and over-the-counter medication use.
- Multiple predictive algorithms were assessed, showing the improvement in validity with the use of unstructured data (i.e. progress notes).
- Data were from routine clinical and billing processes, so no additional burden of data collection for research purposes was necessary.

**Table 13.1**   Sensitivity, specificity, PPV and NPV for three algorithms.

|  | Sensitivity (%) | Specificity (%) | PPV (%) | NPV (%) |
| --- | --- | --- | --- | --- |
| Structured data | 98 | 61 | 94 | 80 |
| Unstructured data | 98 | 95 | 95 | 98 |
| Both structured and unstructured data | 96 | 100 | 99 | 98 |

---

**Case Example 13.2    (Continued)**

*Limitations*

- The study was conducted in one database (VA) only; validation results for the algorithm may not be applicable to different databases or patient populations.
- Algorithms did not include other measures of patient condition, severity or treatment. Additional factors (e.g. age, diagnoses) may improve the reliability and validity of algorithms.

*Key Points*

- Validation of the specific codes or algorithm used to assess a medication or treatment can improve capture of over-the-counter medication use.
- Inclusion of unstructured data may substantially increase specificity, but it does so at the expense of sensitivity – this may be warranted with specificity increases substantially with only a small decrease in sensitivity, especially when PPV and NPV also increase.

---

become part of administrative claims data. In addition, reimbursement standards and patient insurance coverage limitations may influence the selection of ICD codes for billing purposes. The potential for abuse of diagnostic codes, especially outpatient codes, may occur when physicians apply to either an insurance carrier or the government for reimbursement and may be less likely in group model health maintenance organizations (HMOs), such as Kaiser Permanente.

Continuing with the NSAID example, we conducted a literature scan of published studies validating, MI or GI bleeding outcomes with use of NSAIDs in administrative claims databases. Administrative claims data are often compared with medical records in a validation study. Most of these studies provide only a PPV that indicates whether the coding scheme is accurately classifying observed measures as compared with another source. Case Example 13.3 summarizes the findings from a study using the data from the Veteran's Administration to identify upper GI events with an algorithm consisting of ICD-9 and Current Procedural Terminology (CPT) codes. The measurement characteristics of the diagnosis codes 'selected for the algorithm depended on which codes were used.

## Special Considerations with Distributed Data Systems

Multiple health data sources may be included within a single study or for ongoing surveillance. Simultaneous assessment of multiple data sources allows for better understanding of a larger population while also observing a diverse set of patients. These multidatabase studies or distributed data systems may have differences in information collected, coding systems, language (e.g. across different countries), and even the underlying practice of medicine and overarching system of health care. Thus, even in the situation where distributed data systems use a common data model, careful consideration is warranted regarding how to assess validity of drugs, other therapeutics, diagnoses, procedures, and health-related events within each administrative claims data source contributing to the distributed data system. Whenever EHR data are utilized, differences across sites warrant assessment of validity within each health system to improve overall accuracy.

## Best Practices

For the data in an administrative database to be considered valid, subjects who appear in the

---

**Case Example 13.3    Abraham et al. (2006)**

*Background*
- Databases differ in terms of demographic, clinical, diagnosis, and procedure data capture.
- New algorithms for identifying an outcome may have different reliability and validity than previously used algorithms, even in the same database. It is important to validate claims within each new database and to validate new algorithms upon development.

*Question*
Within the Veteran's Affairs (VA) administrative data, what is the reliability and validity of various measures of diagnosis for NSAID–related upper gastrointestinal events (UGIE)?

*Approach*
- A retrospective cohort database and medical record abstraction study was conducted of 906 veterans to determine the reliability and validity of ICD-9 and CPT codes to determine UGIE and to develop an algorithm to predict events among NSAID users.
- The ICD-9 codes used for UGIE were 531.x-534.x, and 578.x. CPT procedural codes were 432xx, 443xx, 435xx, 436xx, 440xx, 446xx, 44120, 78278, 7424x, 7425x, and 74260.

- Multivariable logistic regression analysis was used to derive a predictive algorithm using ICD-9 codes, CPT codes, source of code (outpatient/inpatient), and patient age. The algorithm was developed and tested in separate cohorts from VA data.

*Results*
Table 13.2 presents the sensitivity, specificity, PPV, and NPV for the three claims-based diagnoses of UGIE evaluated and the algorithm PPV among NSAID users. The sensitivity dropped as diagnosis included broader parameters, while the PPV increased. Using both ICD-9 and CPT codes led to the highest specificity and NPV.

*Strengths*
- Evaluation of sensitivity, specificity, PPV, and NPV provides the full picture of reliability and validity of claims for both patients diagnosed with UGIE and those without the diagnosis.
- Multiple diagnoses codes and a predictive algorithm were assessed, providing a robust evaluation for this data set, one that is suitable for future study and clinical decision-making.
- Data were from routine clinical and billing processes, so no additional burden of data

**Table 13.2**    Sensitivity, specificity, PPV and NPV for claims-based diagnoses of UGIE.

| Claims-based diagnosis of UGIE | Sensitivity (%) | Specificity (%) | Positive predictive value (%) | Negative predictive value (%) |
|---|---|---|---|---|
| Only ICD-9 codes for UGIE | 100 | 96 | 27 | 100 |
| ICD-9 and CPT codes for UGIE | 82 | 100 | 51 | 99 |
| ICD-9 and CPT algorithm for UGIE | 66 | 88 | 67 | 88 |
| Algorithm in only NSAID users | NA | NA | 80 | NA |

*Source:* Adapted from Abraham et al. (2006) with permission from John Wiley and Sons.
NA = not applicable. UGIE = upper gastrointestinal events.

---

**Case Example 13.3 (Continued)**

collection for research purposes was necessary.

*Limitations*

- The study was conducted in one database (VA) only; validation results for the algorithm may not be applicable to different databases or patient populations.
- Multivariable logistic regression did not include multiple demographic or clinical factors that may affect occurrence of outcome. Additional factors may improve the reliability and validity of algorithm.

*Key Points*

- Within the same database, different algorithms or codes used to assess a diagnosis may substantially affect the number of

diagnoses captured. For instance, use of both ICD-9 and CPT codes for UGIE substantially decreased the sensitivity and increased the PPV for UGIE within claims data. Thus, validation of the specific codes or algorithm used to assess a diagnosis is key to understanding the findings from pharmacoepidemiologic research.

- Inclusion of a broader base of diagnoses, procedures, or other factors forming an algorithm to provide a diagnosis may increase specificity, but it does so at the expense of sensitivity. Sensitivity, specificity, PPV, and NPV are *all* necessary to provide a complete picture of the agreement between claims data and medical records.

---

computerized files as having a drug exposure or disease should truly have that attribute, and those without the exposure or disease should truly not have the attribute. Validating the case definition for observational studies by comparing administrative databases with original documents, such as inpatient or outpatient medical records, is an important step to enhance research quality and credibility. Although many studies have reviewed original documents to validate the diagnoses under study or have referenced validation studies, a need still exists for validation of drug exposures and disease diagnoses in databases in which no previous validation has been performed. As medical practice changes, further validation of previously validated claims will be warranted.

Evaluating the completeness of the databases is much more difficult because it requires an external data source known to be complete. Although administrative claims and EHR databases have greatly expanded our ability to do pharmacoepidemiologic research, we need to ensure that tools, including the databases used for analyses, are complete and of the highest quality.

The investigator must be aware of the limitations of both the administrative database and the chosen comparison data set. The chosen comparator should provide sufficient data to validate both the exposure and outcome used for the study. A variable that provides linkage between the files in a data source, such as a medical record number, should be available so that accuracy can be evaluated within a subset of known study patients. For example, if a single claim contains six diagnosis codes and six months of claims were used to determine outcomes in patients, then all six diagnosis codes for all claims across the six-month study time must be available in a comparison data set to establish the validity of the outcome. A validation assessment should include evaluation of patients with and without the exposure or outcome. PPV, NPV, sensitivity, and specificity combined provide a complete understanding of the agreement between the two data sources.

The following is a broad overview of how to conduct a validation study in administrative claims or EHR data. First, choose a meaningful number of patients for validation. This sample size should be statistically grounded; however, considerations of data availability, cost, and labor are understandable. Next, extract the variables needed to determine cohort selection, exposure, outcome, and other variables for validation. Calculate measures of agreement and error rates (e.g. standard deviations) between the two data sets. Finally, consider strengths and limitations of the two data sets to ascertain validity and completeness of the data source to answer the study question.

## The Future

Methods for conducting pharmacoepidemiologic studies have shifted over the past several decades from reliance on studies requiring de novo data collection from individuals, to extensive use of electronic data from either administrative claims or EHRs to linked data sources and distributed data networks. Yet, de novo data collection will continue to be required to ascertain information on quality of life, patient reported outcomes, and medications either not included in pharmacy dispensing files or not reliably entered into EHRs, such as herbal and over-the-counter medications. In fact, with the advent of wearables and the Internet of Things, we anticipate that de novo collection of health data may increase in the coming years.

The improved computer technology that resulted in faster processor speeds and increased storage capacity facilitated storage of health care data in an electronic format, i.e. EHRs, and allowed development of distributed data networks, using data from multiple health plans. The availability of these data for research has improved researchers' ability to conduct studies, and increasing uptake of EHRs is leading to increased availability of more granular clinical data for pharmacoepidemiologic research (e.g. lab results and clinical notes). Initial evaluation of EHR data suggest great promise, and increased data quality and standardization of terminology and codes will be required to make these data, collected for clinical care, useful for research. Similar processes will be warranted for use of data from wearables and prior to integration of new data from biobanks, mobile apps, social media, or other sources into a rigorous research framework.

As part of the standardization process, data holders will have to document that their data are valid for conducting research and surveillance activities. This will require investigators to apply their knowledge and practices from use of administrative claims and EHR data to linked data from these novel sources. Both medication exposure and outcome diagnosis data from these novel sources do not carry the same level of comfort regarding validity as claims and EHR data. As these data are considered for research, we hope and expect to see studies validating their use.

## Key Points

- The validity of self-reported diagnosis and drug use data is a function of two properties: how accurately persons who have medical conditions or use drugs of interest are ascertained (sensitivity), and the accuracy with which those who do not have the conditions or do not use the drugs are identified (specificity).
- Misclassification of drug and diagnosis information obtained from study participants by questionnaires or interviews depends on factors such as the training and experience of interviewers, the elapsed time since the events of interest took place, and characteristics of the participants, such as their medical status and age.
- Misclassification can lead to over- or underestimation of the true association between the drug exposure and the outcome of interest.
- The medical record is typically used as the gold standard for verifying drug and diagnosis information, but it may be incomplete and, with the increasing focus on privacy, may be difficult to obtain.

# Further Reading

Abraham, N.S., Cohen, D.C., Rivers, B., and Richardson, P. (2006). Validation of administrative data used for the diagnosis of upper gastrointestinal events following nonsteroidal anti-inflammatory drug prescription. *Alimentary Pharmacology & Therapeutics* 24 (2): 299–306.

Bank, T.W. (2018). *Living Standards Measurement Survey - Questionnaires*. [cited 27 January 2018] Available from: http://go.worldbank.org/HZVSQMD5S0.

Biemer, P. Measurement errors in sample surveys. In: *Handbook of Statistics – Sample Surveys: Design, Methods and Applications* (eds. D. Pfeffermann and C.R. Rao), 281–316. The Netherlands: North-Holland.

Bland, J.M. and Altman, D.G. (1986). Statistical methods for assessing agreement between two methods of clinical measurement. *Lancet* 1 (8476): 307–310.

Bustamante, R., Earles, A., Murphy, J.D. et al. (2019). Ascertainment of aspirin exposure using structured and unstructured large-scale electronic health record data. *Medical Care* 57 (10): e60–e64.

Copeland, K.T., Checkoway, H., McMichael, A.J., and Holbrook, R.H. (1977). Bias due to misclassification in the estimation of relative risk. *American Journal of Epidemiology* 105 (5): 488–495.

Dean, E., Caspar, R., McAvinchey, G. et al. (2007). Developing a low-cost technique for parallel cross-cultural instrument development: the Question Appraisal System (QAS-04). *International Journal of Social Research Methodology* 10 (3): 227–241.

Dosemeci, M., Wacholder, S., and Lubin, J.H. (1990). Does nondifferential misclassification of exposure always bias a true effect toward the null value? *American Journal of Epidemiology* 132 (4): 746–748.

Fischer, M.A., Stedman, M.R., Lii, J. et al. (2010). Primary medication non-adherence: analysis of 195,930 electronic prescriptions. *Journal of General Internal Medicine* 25 (4): 284–290.

Flegal, K.M., Keyl, P.M., and Nieto, F.J. (1991). Differential misclassification arising from nondifferential errors in exposure measurement. *American Journal of Epidemiology* 134 (10): 1233–1244.

Fourrier-Reglat, A., Cuong, H.M., Lassalle, R. et al. (2010). Concordance between prescriber- and patient-reported previous medical history and NSAID indication in the CADEUS cohort. *Pharmacoepidemiology and Drug Safety* 19 (5): 474–481.

Gama, H., Correia, S., and Lunet, N. (2009). Questionnaire design and the recall of pharmacological treatments: a systematic review. *Pharmacoepidemiology and Drug Safety* 18 (3): 175–187.

Geisen, E. and Bergstrom, J.R. (2017). *Respondent-survey interaction*. In: *Usability Testing for Survey Research* (ed. M. Kaufmann), 21–49. Cambridge, MA: Elsevier.

Graesser, A.C., Wiemer-hastings, K., Kreuz, R. et al. (2000). QUAID: a questionnaire evaluation aid for survey methodologists. *Behavior Research Methods, Instruments, and Computers* 32: 254–262.

Greenland, S. (2005). Multiple-bias modelling for analysis of observational data [with discussion]. *Journal of the Royal Statistical Society: Series A (Statistics in Society)* 168 (2): 267–306.

Greenland, S., Lash, T.L., and Rothman, K.J. (2008). Bias analysis. In: *Modern Epidemiology* (eds. K.J. Rothman, S. Greenland and T.L. Lash), 345–380. Philadelphia, PA: Wolters Kluwer Health/Lippincott Williams & Wilkins.

Greenland, S. (2001). Sensitivity analysis, Monte Carlo risk analysis, and Bayesian uncertainty assessment. *Risk Analysis: An Official Publication of the Society for Risk Analysis* 21 (4): 579–583.

Horwitz, R.I. and Feinstein, A.R. (1978). Alternative analytic methods for case–control studies of estrogens and endometrial cancer. *The New England Journal of Medicine* 299 (20): 1089–1094.

Jurek, A.M., Maldonado, G., Greenland, S., and Church, T.R. (2006). Exposure-measurement error is frequently ignored when interpreting epidemiologic study results. *European Journal of Epidemiology* 21 (12): 871–876.

Jurek, A.M., Greenland, S., Maldonado, G., and Church, T.R. (2005). Proper interpretation of non-differential misclassification effects: expectations vs observations. *International Journal of Epidemiology* 34 (3): 680–687.

Jurek, A.M., Maldonado, G., and Greenland, S. (2013). Adjusting for outcome misclassification: the importance of accounting for case–control sampling and other forms of outcome-related selection. *Annals of Epidemiology* 23 (3): 129–135.

Krosnick, J. (2000). The threat of satisficing in surveys: the shortcuts respondents take in answering questions. *Survey Methods Newsletter* 20: 4–8.

Lash, T.L., Fox, M.P., and Fink, A.K. (2009). *Applying Quantitative Bias Analysis to Epidemiologic Data*. New York: Springer.

Lash, T.L., Fox, M.P., MacLehose, R.F. et al. (2014). Good practices for quantitative bias analysis. *International Journal of Epidemiology* 43 (6): 1969–1985.

Lash, T.L. and Fink, A.K. (2003). Semi-automated sensitivity analysis to assess systematic errors in observational data. *Epidemiology (Cambridge, Massachusetts)* 14 (4): 451–458.

Lessler, J.T. and Harris, B.S.H. (1984). *Medicaid Data as a Source for Postmarketing Surveillance Information*. Research Triangle Park, NC: Research Triangle Institute.

Maclure, M. and Willett, W.C. (1987). Misinterpretation and misuse of the kappa statistic. *American Journal of Epidemiology* 126 (2): 161–169.

Madow, W.G. (1967). Interview data on chronic conditions compared with information derived from medical records. Vital and health statistics. Series 2. *Data Evaluation and Methods Research* 23: 1–84.

Maldonado, G. (2008). Adjusting a relative-risk estimate for study imperfections. *Journal of Epidemiology and Community Health* 62 (7): 655–663.

Maldonado, G., Greenland, S., and Phillips, C. (2000). Approximately nondifferential exposure misclassification does not ensure bias toward the null. *American Journal of Epidemiology* 151: S39.

Mitchell, A.A., Cottler, L.B., and Shapiro, S. (1986). Effect of questionnaire design on recall of drug exposure in pregnancy. *American Journal of Epidemiology* 123 (4): 670–676.

Naleway, A.L., Belongia, E.A., Greenlee, R.T. et al. (2003). Eczematous skin disease and recall of past diagnoses: implications for smallpox vaccination. *Annals of Internal Medicine* 139 (1): 1–7.

Newton, K.M., Peissig, P.L., Kho, A.N. et al. (2013). Validation of electronic medical record-based phenotyping algorithms: results and lessons learned from the eMERGE network. *Journal of the American Medical Informmatics Association* 20 (e1): e147–e154.

Nichols, E., Olmsted-Hawala, E., Holland, T., and Riemer, A.A. (2016). Best Practices of Usability Testing Online Questionnaires at the Census Bureau: How rigorous and repeatable testing can improve online questionnaire design. In: *International Conference on Questionnaire Design, Development, Evaluation, and Testing* (QDET2). Miami, FL.

Phillips, C.V. (2003). Quantifying and reporting uncertainty from systematic errors. *Epidemiology (Cambridge, Massachusetts)* 14 (4): 459–466.

Phillips, C.V. and LaPole, L.M. (2003). Quantifying errors without random sampling. *BMC Medical Research Methodology* 3: 9.

Poole, C. (1985). Exceptions to the rule about nondifferential misclassification. *American Journal of Epidemiology* 122: 508.

C.f.D.C.a. Q-Bank. Prevention [cited 27 January 2018]. https://wwwn.cdc.gov/qbank

Ray, W. (2003). Evaluating medication effects outside of clinical trials: new-user designs. *American Journal of Epidemiology* 158: 915–920.

Ritchey, M.E., West, S.L., and Maldonado, G. (2019). Validity of pharmacoepidemiology drug and diagnosis data. In: *Pharmacoepidemiology*, 6e (eds. B.L. Strom, S. Hennessy and S.E. Kimmel), 948–990. Sussex: Wiley.

Rodgers, A. and MacMahon, S. (1995). Systematic underestimation of treatment effects as a result of diagnostic test inaccuracy: implications for the interpretation and design of thromboprophylaxis trials. *Thrombosis and Haemostasis* 73 (2): 167–171.

Rothman, K.J., Greenland, S., and Lash, T.L. (2008). Precision and statistics in epidemiologic studies. In: *Modern Epidemiology*, 3e (eds. K.J. Rothman, S. Greenland and T.L. Lash), 148–167. Philadelphia, PA: Lippincott, Williams & Wilkins.

Rothman, K.J., Greenland, S., and Lash, T.L. (2008). Validity in epidemiologic studies. In: *Modern Epidemiology* (eds. K.J. Rothman, S. Greenland and T.L. Lash), 128–147. Philadelphia, PA: Wolters Kluwer Health/ Lippincott Williams & Wilkins.

Rowan, C.G., Flory, J., Gerhard, T. et al. (2017). Agreement and validity of electronic health record prescribing data relative to pharmacy claims data: a validation study from a US electronic health record database. *Pharmacoepidemiology and Drug Safety* 26 (8): 963–972.

Smith, T.W. (2016). Optimizing Questionnaire Design in Cross-National and Cross-Cultural Surveys. In: *International Conference on Questionnaire Design, Development, Evaluation, and Testing* (QDET2). Miami, FL. Survey Quality Predictor (SQP) 2.1. [cited 27 January 2018]. http://sqp.upf.edu

Stange, K.C. (2009). The problem of fragmentation and the need for integrative solutions. *The Annals of Family Medicine* 7 (2): 100–103.

Tourangeau, R., Rips, L.J., and Rasinski, K. (2000). *The Psychology of Survey Response.* Cambridge, MA: Cambridge University Press.

Trifiro, G., Coloma, P.M., Rijnbeek, P.R. et al. (2014). Combining multiple healthcare databases for postmarketing drug and vaccine safety surveillance: why and how? *Journal of Internal Medicine* 275 (6): 551–561.

Tsou, A.Y., Lehmann, C.U., Michel, J. et al. (2017). Safe practices for copy and paste in the EHR. Systematic review, recommendations, and novel model for health IT collaboration. *Applied Clinical Informatics* 8 (1): 12–34.

Upadhyaya, S.G., Murphree, D.H., Ngufor, C.G. et al. (2017). Automated diabetes case identification using electronic health record data at a tertiary care facility. *Mayo Clinic Proceedings. Innovations, Quality & Outcomes* 1 (1): 100–110.

van Gelder, M.M., van Rooij, I.A., de Walle, H.E. et al. (2013). Maternal recall of prescription medication use during pregnancy using a paper-based questionnaire: a validation study in the Netherlands. *Drug Safety* 36 (1): 43–54.

Wacholder, S., Armstrong, B., and Hartge, P. (1993). Validation studies using an alloyed gold standard. *American Journal of Epidemiology* 137 (11): 1251–1258.

Watson, D.L. (1965). Health interview responses compared with medical records. *Vital and Health Statistics* 1 (46): 1–74.

West, S.L., Blake, C., Zhiwen, L. et al. (2009). Reflections on the use of electronic health record data for clinical research. *Health Informatics Journal* 15 (2): 108–121.

West, S.L., Savitz, D.A., Koch, G. et al. (1995). Recall accuracy for prescription medications: self-report compared with database information. *American Journal of Epidemiology* 142 (10): 1103–1112.

## 14

# Assessing Causality from Case Reports

*Bernard Bégaud[1] and Judith K. Jones[†]*

[1] *Clinical Pharmacology and Pharmacoepidemiology, Medical School, University of Bordeaux, Bordeaux, France*
[†] *Formerly Principal Consultant PharmaLex, Inc. 9302 Lee Highway. Suite 700, Fairfax, VA 220131, and Adjunct Faculty: The University of Michigan School of Public Health Summer Program, 1415 Washington Heights, 1700 SPH I, Ann Arbor, MI 48109-2029, USA*

## Introduction

An important component in clinical and epidemiological research is the assessment of the degree to which an observed or reported event is causally associated with a drug treatment. Several approaches to assessing this probability of a causal connection have been developed. This chapter reviews the basic principles, current approaches, and discusses their regulatory context and application.

## Clinical Problems to be Addressed by Pharmacoepidemiologic Research

The basic clinical problem is that adverse events may be associated with multiple causal factors. The task is to make a differential diagnosis and evaluate the degree to which the occurrence of an event is linked to a particular suspected causal agent: a drug or other pathophysiological mechanism.

In case reports of suspected adverse reactions to a medicinal product, data are often incomplete so causal assessment is challenging.

Moreover, adverse reactions to drugs can be acute, subacute, or chronic, can be reversible or not (e.g. birth defects and death), and can be quite rare or common. They can be pathologically unique or mimic almost the entire range of human pathology. Thus, defining general data parameters and criteria for assessing causality that will apply to most types of suspected adverse reactions is tricky.

Finally, in some instances, the assessment will have little public health or economic impact. Conversely, if continuation of a development program depends upon this assessment, the rigor of the approach used becomes critical.

## The Two Paradigms of Causality Assessment

For a clinical pharmacologist, causal inference, i.e. stating that a drug can cause a given event, can only ensue from an experimental design such as a randomized clinical trial. In this case, owing to the random allocation of exposure, the compared groups can be considered as identical with respect to all variables that could influence the probability of occurrence of the considered event. Therefore, a

*Textbook of Pharmacoepidemiology*, Third Edition. Edited by Brian L. Strom, Stephen E. Kimmel, and Sean Hennessy.
© 2022 John Wiley & Sons Ltd. Published 2022 by John Wiley & Sons Ltd.

statistically significant excess of cases in the exposed group, absent any other biases or the play of chance, signifies drug causation.

Pharmacoepidemiology deals with the real world where exposure is not allocated by chance but by human behavior. For this reason, compared groups never can be considered as identical in risk, and an excess risk observed in the exposed can also be explained by other factors or characteristics over- or under-represented in the treated population. Drug causation for a significant risk increase among the exposed can be established only after these confounders and putative other biases have been properly accounted for.

For both the clinical and epidemiological approaches, statistical inference relies on the same $2 \times 2$ contingency table:

|  | Event | No event |
|---|---|---|
| Exposed | $a$ | $b$ |
| Unexposed | $c$ | $d$ |
|  |  | $n$ |

If we leave the populational level, a quite different question is: *Did this drug cause this event in this particular person?* This is the scope of this chapter.

Assessing drug causation from individual case reports may seem incongruous for a statistician. Indeed, here we are dealing only with exposed cases, without the help of figures and data from the non-exposed or from exposed but non-diseased persons:

|  | Event | No event |
|---|---|---|
| Exposed | $a$ | ? |
| Unexposed | ? | ? |
|  |  | ? |

The situation is even worse since in many instances, such as passive safety surveillance schemes like spontaneous reporting, $a$ is only the reported fraction of the cases which have occurred in the exposed population. Because

of massive under-reporting, worsened by a probable subjective selection bias, this sample has a good chance to differ, in terms of its characteristics, from the whole population of exposed cases, the number of which remains unknown.

Answering the *"Did it"* question requires working only from what we know about this case, and then extracting what can be considered as relevant for assessing causation. This assessment will be based on common sense, medical knowledge, and/or probability theory.

# When is Assessing Causation from Cases Reports Useful?

Here are some examples where case-by-case causal assessment can offer real added value:

## Spontaneous Reporting

Historically, assessing causation at the individual level was the trademark of pharmacovigilance. For the most relevant adverse drug reactions reported by health professionals or patients, e.g. those which were serious or not previously reported, it was crucial to know whether the drug-event association had a good chance of being causal or simply coincidental. During the last 30 years of the twentieth century, dozens of drugs were withdrawn from the market owing to a safety profile judged "unacceptable" on the basis of case reports assessed as causal by the manufacturer or a regulatory agency. From a methodological point of view, this indisputably was the golden era of case-by-case causality assessment and more than 30 different methods and approaches were proposed during this fruitful period.

In several countries, assessment methods and algorithms were or still are widely used to discard spurious drug-event associations in order to decrease the background noise and the generation of false-positives.

As big health databases have been made accessible and allow large pharmacoepidemiologic studies to be designed, regulatory decisions have become more and more based on a causation assessed at the populational level. However, the case-by-case approach remains essential for associations difficult to appraise by epidemiological approaches, such as serious cases reported during the early phase of marketing or of a suspected very rare occurrence, when the constitution of an appropriate control group is difficult if not impossible or when a conservative decision could be made on the basis of a series of serious case reports.

### Clinical Trials and Pharmacoepidemiology

It is obvious that the clinical development of a novel drug may be hampered by the occurrence of a single case of an adverse reaction if this event is serious and drug causation is the more probable option. For example, for one case of death identified during clinical development totaling 900 exposed subjects, the risk estimate derived from Poisson probabilities would range from 3.3/100 000 to 6.2/1000. This emphasizes the strategic importance of a precise and reliable assessment of the causal nature of the link in this particular case.

A more common practice is to classify adverse events observed in the study groups according to the likelihood of drug causation, e.g. *not related*, *possible*, *probable*, etc. The same applies to pharmacoepidemiologic approaches like large post-marketing cohort studies, mainly when a dedicated control group is not available.

### Clinical Practice and Prescription

Appraising whether a drug treatment is responsible or not for the occurrence of an adverse event or of the worsening of a patient's state is a daily challenge in medical practice. In some instances, (e.g. oncology, cardiology), the decision of pursuing or not pursuing the treatment is vital and the help provided by a reliable diagnostic method is particularly valuable.

### Reports of Adverse Drug Reactions to Medical Journals

Cases published in the literature are one of the most respected and influential sources of data for drug safety surveillance. Owing to the impact of such publications, arguments for and against drug causation should be extensively listed and discussed. Sadly, many reports do not provide information on confounding therapies, medical conditions or data deemed essential for considering causality. Here too, operational guidelines or algorithms can have some added value, and some journals like *Therapies* or *Annals of Pharmacotherapy* have made the use of an operational algorithm mandatory.

### Hypothesis Generation and Research

The scope of causal assessment goes far beyond the issue of adverse drug reactions and pharmacovigilance. Its basic principles and structured approaches can apply to the broader question of the link between a factor, trait or exposure and an event, whatever its nature.

## Methodological Problems to be Addressed by Pharmacoepidemiologic Research

Adverse drug reactions are a major cause of mortality and morbidity, both in developed and developing countries. Decisions to minimize their public health and economic impact must be based on reliable conclusions as to the nature – causal or not – of the association between a drug exposure and a harmful event.

Two divergent philosophies have developed. Some discount the value of causality assessment of individual reactions, deferring judgment to the results of formal epidemiologic studies or clinical trials. In contrast, others contend that the information in single reports can be evaluated to determine some degree of association, and that this can be useful – sometimes critical – when considering discontinuation of a clinical trial or development or market withdrawal of a drug. The latter view has spurred the evolution of causal assessment from expert consensual opinion (global introspection) to structured algorithms and elaborate probabilistic approaches.

## Approaches for Assessing Causation from Individual Cases

For the sake of simplicity, three approaches for assessing causation from individual cases can be contrasted:

- Expert judgment/Global introspection.
- Structured guidelines and algorithms.
- Probabilistic approaches.

In practice, the differences among these approaches is not totally watertight: expert judgment can be used as a gold standard for weighting the decision criteria of an operational algorithm and probability concepts may be used when designing an algorithm.

### Expert Judgment/Global Introspection

Since case-by-case causality assessment tends to reproduce the medical diagnosis process, e.g. to determine the most probable cause of a disease, the most natural and common approach for assessing drug causation is indisputably global introspection. One or more experts review available information on the case, refer to current medical knowledge, and judge the likelihood that the adverse event resulted from drug exposure. However, if not structured, global introspection is known to suffer severe limitations, notably judgment errors and poor reproducibility.

It has been repeatedly shown that several experts working separately on the same set of case reports may express marked disagreements in their judgments. Moreover, the process is uncalibrated; for example, one assessor's "possible" might be another's "probable" or "doubtful." Worse, as for any subjective judgment, the same expert repeating the process after some weeks or months has a good chance of not duplicating his/her previous opinions.

Despite these weaknesses, global introspection continues to be used, notably by regulatory agencies and manufacturers, for assessing spontaneous reports whose serious events may call for a decision to be made. The same is true for severe or serious cases identified during the clinical development of a novel drug in the framework of "safety advisory boards."

Here, we are touching on the paradox of global introspection, which is not a reliable instrument per se, but can be considered as the gold standard in some circumstances. Such may be the case when a multidisciplinary group of senior experts is called upon in a systematic, structured, and interactive process such as the Delphi Method. For example, drug causation may be assessed by several experts working separately. They are required to express their final judgment for each case and to provide detailed arguments to substantiate it. Next, all disagreements are listed and then interactively discussed until a consensus is reached on each case. Even if time-consuming, and therefore not applicable to large case series, this approach can be considered as a sort of gold standard and has been used as such to calibrate various algorithmic or probabilistic methods.

## Structured Guidelines and Algorithms

Because expert judgment/global introspection, which is often plagued by subjectivity, haspoor reliability and reproducibility, an obvious improvement has been to force experts to follow a structured common thread, e.g. by obliging them to make their final judgment on the successive assessment of relevant criteria. These criteria can make reference to formal logic or common sense, to medical knowledge, or to literature data.

A good example of *formal logic* is the temporal association between the drug treatment and the event. The "cause" should always precede the first symptoms of the event ("*challenge*"); the suppression of the cause, i.e. stopping the treatment is expected to improve or to cure the situation ("*dechallenge*"), while the re-introduction of the cause, if any, is expected to make the event reappear ("*rechallenge*"). This should be interpreted in the light of the characteristics of the molecule (pharmacokinetic parameters) and of the event. For instance, for some of them, such as with death or irreversible lesions, no relapse can be expected. Similarly, as for the Bradford Hill criteria, a clear relationship between the dose and the intensity/severity of the event can be supportive of drug causation.

For criteria calling upon *medical knowledge*, there are arguments that allow alternative causes for the event to be ruled out or the biological or pharmacological plausibility: does the pharmacological properties of this drug allow such a manifestation to be expected? For *literature data*, one is obviously more inclined to draw a conclusion of drug causation if this type of reaction has been repeatedly reported with the suspected drug.

The first attempt at structuring the assessment of drug causation in individual cases was proposed in 1976 by Nelson Irey, a pathologist at the US Armed Forces Institute of Pathology. One year later, in 1977, two clinical pharmacologists, Fred Karch and Louis Lasagna, proposed the first structured algorithm for assessing case reports. The two approaches shared similar basic data elements:

- Timing relative to drug exposure,
- "Dechallenge",
- "Rechallenge",
- Presence/absence of other potential causal factors or alternative causes,
- Other supportive data, e.g. if previous cases were reported.

During the following two decades, no less than 30 methods, algorithms and others were designed and, for the most part, published. Although their functional architecture can be quite diverse, they generally consist in successively answering a certain number of questions in order to end up with an assessment of the probability of drug causation that is generally expressed in the form of qualifiers (e.g. "Not-related,""doubtful,""possible,""prob able,""certain") or, for some algorithms, of figures (e.g. 1, 2, 3, 4) or of a probability scale. Although, the number (from less than 10 up to 84) and the wording of questions may differ greatly, they roughly include five basic criteria: timing, dechallenge, rechallenge, confounding, and prior history of the event. Information relevant to each criterion is elicited by questions. The answers are restricted to "yes/no" (and for some methods "don't know") and then aggregated to derive the final causality score. This aggregation process can be discrete (the various questions being interdependent) relying on an algorithm, a decisiontree or a combination table, or continuous by summing notes or scores as in Figure 14.1 below.

The core issue that remains is the weight attributed to each question in the final score. On this point, each method has its own "personality" and it comes as no surprise that when used on the same set of case reports, several methods can provide discrepant estimates of the probability of drug causation. In fact, the two dozen methods proposed so far do not purport to have the same goals. Some are very basic algorithms aiming at roughly

**CAUSALITY ASSESSMENT**
**NARANJO SCORED ALGORITHM**

| QUESTION | ANSWER | | | SCORE |
|---|---|---|---|---|
| | Yes | No | Unk | |
| Previous reports? | +1 | 0 | 0 | _____ |
| Event after drug? | +2 | −1 | 0 | _____ |
| Event abate on drug removal? | +1 | 0 | 0 | _____ |
| + Rechallenge? | +2 | −1 | 0 | _____ |
| Alternative causes? | −1 | +2 | 0 | _____ |
| Reaction with placebo? | −1 | +1 | 0 | _____ |
| Drug blood level toxic? | +1 | 0 | 0 | _____ |
| Reaction dose-related? | +1 | 0 | 0 | _____ |
| Past history of similar event? | +1 | 0 | 0 | _____ |
| ADR confirmed objectively? | +1 | 0 | 0 | _____ |
| **Total Score** | | | | _____ |

**Figure 14.1** Simplified presentation of method proposed by Naranjo et al. Likelihood of drug causation is qualified by score (*Total Score*) obtained by summing individual scores from each of 10 questions.

classifying case reports in order to reject those for which drug causation is quite improbable. In other cases, the method was designed for a specific application like signal detection in routine safety surveillance where sensitivity is preferred, often at the cost of specificity, for a specific type of event such as liver injury, or for a given type of drug (vaccines, anticancer drugs, etc.). The most ambitious ones aim to provide "exact" appreciations of the probability of drug causation by means of meticulously tuning the respective weight of each question.

Fewer than one third of these methods have actually been used in routine practice: some because their use was recommended or made mandatory by some regulatory agencies (as it was the case for Australia and the Food and Drug Administration and still is in practice for France); others because they were developed by a pharmaceutical company for their own pharmacovigilance, and others because they were adopted by medical journals for the reporting of adverse drug reactions.

Despite their obvious weaknesses, algorithms offer a compromise between simplicity and added value for whomever intends to deal with drug causation. They dramatically decrease discrepancies between experts, markedly increase the reproducibility of estimates, and overall, provide a structured approach that makes the observer aware of the questions to be explored before concluding in terms of drug causation.

## Probabilistic Approaches

### Bayesian Approaches

In essence, the issue of drug causation belongs to the domain of probability, the aim being to quantify (from 0 to 1 or 0% to 100%) the probability that drug A caused the adverse event presented by a given person. In the absence of any relevant information for judging the nature of the link, the probability of drug causation is 50% (i.e. in the middle of a probability scale ranging from 0 to 1). In this case, the chances for drug causation and non-drug causation are equal (i.e. 50% each). Any evidence in favor of drug causation will move the estimate to the right (probability $>0.5$), while an argument against it will shift it left (probability $<0.5$). These basic probability rules have led some researchers to propose the Bayes' Theorem as the most satisfactory approach to the issue of drug causation.

Indeed, conditional probabilities allow the calculation of the probability that an event will occur or that an affirmation will be correct under certain conditions, e.g. that a test is positive or negative or a symptom is present or absent. The approach developed by Thomas Bayes (1702–1761) was to start from ana priori estimate of this probability (*prior probability*) that is then altered (increased or decreased) by what we learn about this particular case in order to obtain a final estimate called *posterior probability*.

For the sake of simplicity, it is easier to use odds rather than probabilities, the original Bayes' formulae being rather troublesome to use. In this case, the formulation is:

$$\text{Posterior Odds} = \text{Prior Odds} \times \text{LR}_1 \times \text{LR}_2 \times \text{LR}_3 \times \ldots \times \text{LR}_j$$

The odds (*Posterior* or *Prior*) are simply the probability that the drug was the cause of the event divided by the probability that it was not. The odds obviously being 1 when these probabilities are equal (50% or 0.5 each). Indeed:

$$\text{Odds} = \text{Probability} / \left(1 - \text{Probability}\right)$$

LRs are the *Likelihood Ratios* corresponding to each information component judged to be relevant for assessing the probability of drug causation in this particular case. For example, they may refer to the delay between the start of treatment and the occurrence of the event, to a particular clinical or biological sign, to the past medical history of the person, or to whatever appears relevant in this particular context. The value of each LR (which is simply an odds) is obtained by dividing the probability of the sign being present if the drug was the cause by the probability of the sign being present if it was not the cause. For example, if we learned from literature that, on average, 67% of persons presenting with the considered adverse event are female while the proportion of females among users is 42% in the source population, the LR for gender would be: 0.67/0.42 = 1.6 if the person was female and 0.33/0.58 = 0.57 if this person was male.

David Lane and colleagues have made this approach more operational by superposing the various LRs to be computed with the criteria universally used in algorithmic approaches: *challenge, dechallenge, rechallenge*, etc. An automated computerized version of the method has even been developed.

One can see from the Bayes' formula that the value used for the prior odds is the starting point and has a notable influence on the final result. In the absence of any pre-analysis information, the prior odds can be set arbitrarily to 1, i.e. one assumes that the chances that the drug under study was or was not the cause of the event are equal. In more favorable cases, it is possible to set the value of the prior odds more satisfactorily. This is for example the case when the drug is already known or suspected to cause the disease and a literature search provides reliable data on the strength of association between exposure to this drug and the probability of occurrence of the event in question. For example, if a pharmacoepidemiologic study has shown that such a drug treatment increased the probability of the disease by a factor (hazard ratio) of 4.5, one can deduce that the etiologic fraction of the risk among the exposed is:

$$\text{AFR}_E = \left(\text{HR} - 1\right) / \text{HR or} \left(4.5\ 1\right) / 4.5 = 0.78$$

In other words, on average, the probability for drug causation is 78% for each exposed individual in this study. Therefore, the prior odds (probability of drug causation divided by the probability of non-drug causation) is: 0.78/ (1 – 0.78) = 3.5. Or, more simply:

$$\text{Prior Odds} = \text{HR} - 1$$

Starting from the two examples above, the probability estimate would be (if the case was a male):

$$\text{Posterior Odds} = 3.5 \times 0.57 = 1.99$$

At this stage, and before pursuing the computation with other, and probably more relevant LRs (timing, clinical and/or biological feature, medical history, alternative causes, etc.), the drug is twice as likely to be responsible than it is not. To that end, odds can easily be, if wished, converted into a probability for drug causation:

$$\text{Probability} = \text{Odds} / (\text{Odds} + 1) \text{ or, for our interim result}: 1.99 / 2.99 = 66\%.$$

Although rather complex to handle, a major advantage of the Bayesian approach is that it relies on healthy probabilistic concepts, respects the basic rules of probability and provides a scientifically valid estimate of probability.

### Other Probabilistic Approaches

The logistic function was proposed by Arimone et al. to convert the individual estimates of seven criteria (roughly those commonly used by algorithmic and Bayesian approaches) into a probability of drug causation varying from 0 to 1:

$$p = \frac{1}{1 + \exp\left[-\left(\alpha + \sum_{i=1}^{7} \beta_i X_i\right)\right]}$$

$\alpha$ is similar to the Bayesian prior odds, $X_1$ to $X_7$ are the results of the individual assessments of the seven criteria, and $\beta_1$ to $\beta_7$ are the relative weights attributed to each criterion after the validation against a gold standard. Assessments were made simple owing to an automated computerized process.

## Calibration

When designing a method for assessing drug causation, the main challenge is to make sure that the estimates it provides are valid. As no indisputable gold standard exists, several workarounds have been proposed:

- The most satisfactory ones may arguably, be Bayesian approaches and multidisciplinary experts' judgment optimized by the Delphi process.
- It would be tempting to use cases for which one can be almost certain that the drug was or was not the cause of an event. For example, this might involve a well-documented reaction with this drug that occurs after an expected delay, which relapses after treatment cessation, reappears after its reintroduction and for which no other cause has been found. However, following such a caricatural logic gives no guarantee that the method will provide consistent results in the situations where uncertainty is the main reason for using it such as in the vast majority of cases.
- A more sensible approach would be to use, when available, the data from a cohort study or a large-scale trial using a non-exposed control group. The value of the hazard ratio makes it possible to calculate the etiologic fraction of the risk in exposed and, therefore, the proportion and the number of cases of the event attributable to exposure. In an ideal world, this proportion and number should be confirmed by the individual assessment of all exposed cases with the method under study.

## Choosing the Appropriate Approach

To date, it is obvious that there is no unique method for assessing drug causation that can be adopted by all stakeholders in the domain of drug safety. Moreover, if used on the same set of cases, one could expect the results to be discrepant. Nevertheless, one should bear in mind the following:

- A structured approach is always preferable to a non-structured assessment, which intrinsically has poor reliability and poor reproducibility.

- Beyond the Holy Grail quest for the "universal" method, the choice should first be guided by the context:
  - *How will the evaluation be used and who will perform the evaluation?*
  - *The importance of the accuracy of the judgment.* If the evaluation will determine either the continuation of a clinical trial or the continued marketing of a drug, then its accuracy may be critical, so a probabilistic approach would be more appropriate. Conversely, if little hinges upon the judgment, unrefined estimates and methods may suffice.
  - *The number of causality evaluations to be made* must also be weighed against the time required to make judgments on large numbers of reports, a dilemma for regulatory agencies and sponsors. Here, the need for accurate judgments is pitted against the volume of evaluations to be considered.

## The Future

The field of adverse reaction causality assessment has many unresolved issues, both methodological and practical. Originally there was hope a consensus method would be found, but the current state of the field suggests that this is unlikely for several reasons.

First, some individuals and institutions have adopted one or a few methods and have committed to their use, often through their choice of data collecting systems or software. Second, practical aspects in using them appear to play a very real role. Although discussed with excitement as the possible "gold standard" for adverse reaction causality, the Bayesian method has not been widely embraced, partly because it is difficult to use without automation. With the lifting of that barrier, and with further practical applications, its potential may be realized. Third, the misuse of judgment terms or scores within the legal arena has generated concern, particularly

given the fact that there is no reliable standard terminology.

All of these factors suggest the need for further work in several areas:

- Determining the *applications* of causality assessment, i.e. the "output" of the process, to better define the desired rigor, accuracy, and usability of the methods. There will probably always be the need for simpler and rougher methods, as well as more complete and rigorous methods when the determination has considerable impact.
- Further defining the *critical elements needed* for evaluation of causality for different types of adverse reactions (e.g. hepatic, hematological, skin, etc.) so that this information may be collected at the time of reporting or publishing a spontaneous event.
- Gathering of data on *critical elements* of the specific adverse events in the course of both clinical trials and epidemiologic studies. Risk factor, history, timing, characteristics, and resolution patterns of adverse events should be described in these studies and incorporated into general data resources on the characteristics of medical events and diseases.
- Further work on *automation* of the causality evaluation process. Global introspection is still widely used because of the cumbersome nature of many of the more complete methods. Convenient access to the proper questions, set out in logical order, as well as background data meeting quality criteria on the state of information to date, has potential for considerably improving the state of adverse reaction causality evaluation.
- Consideration of *new and different* approaches. Although it is likely that further work will be based on one or more of the many available methods, other interesting approaches have emerged. For example, as part of work on patient safety in the US, "root cause analysis" is used to identify important contributors to adverse events in clinical settings. This approach creates

functional maps of possible contributing factors to identify not only a cause but also preventative measures. Another approach is the *N*-of-1 trial, which can evaluate the causality of adverse events in individuals, particularly those who have experienced multiple reactions to drugs. Other potentially promising approaches include expert systems, machine learning, neural networks and other sophisticated approaches.

## Key Points

- Applications of a structured causality method can standardize and help reduce biases in assessing the possible cause-effect relationship of an event to a drug exposure.
- The use of a clinical non-structured approach ("global introspection") to assess adverse events believed to be associated with a drug has been shown to yield inconsistent results between raters; its lack of structure does not further the development of the hypothesis raised in the report of the event.
- The choice of a method is based upon the use of judgment; if pivotal to the continued development of a drug, the most rigorous methods such as the Bayesian approach may help; if used to sort out well-documented cases that may probably be associated with a drug, then simple algorithms or scoring algorithms usually suffice.
- The components of causality assessment methods can help structure data collection on individual and groups of cases; ultimately, these aggregate data can improve the description of the event of interest, and possibly its relationship to a drug, or the disease of indication.
- The detailed probabilistic and explicit approach in the Bayesian method can, if data are available, provide a basis for developing more precise statements of the hypothesis that is posed in a spontaneous report of a suspected adverse drug reaction.

## Further Reading

Agbabiaka, T.B., Savović, J., and Ernst, E. (2008). Methods for causality assessment of adverse drug reactions: a systematic review. *Drug Saf.* 31 (1): 21–37.

Arimone, Y., Bégaud, B., Miremont-Salamé, G. et al. (2006). A new method for assessing drug causation provided agreement with experts' judgment. *J. Clin. Epidemiol.* 59 (3): 308–314.

Benahmed, S., Picot, M.C., Hillaire-Buys, D. et al. (2005). Comparison of pharmacovigilance algorithms in drug hypersensitivity reactions. *Eur. J. Clin. Pharmacol.* 61 (7): 537–541.

Bénichou, C. and Danan, G. (1994). A new method for drug causality assessment: RUCAM. In: *Adverse Drug Reactions. A Practical Guide to Diagnosis and Management*, 277–284. New York: Wiley.

Collet, J.-P., MacDonald, N., Cashman, N., and Pless, R. (2000). The advisory committee on causality assessment. Monitoring signals for vaccine safety: the assessment of individual adverse event reports by an expert advisory committee. *Bull. World Health Organ.* 78: 178–185.

Drug Information Association (1986). Proceedings of the Drug Information Association Workshop, Arlington, Virginia, February. *Drug Inf. J.* **20**: 383–533.

Irey, N.S. (1976). Adverse drug reactions and death: a review of 827 cases. *JAMA* 236: 575–578.

Jones, J.K. (2020). Assessing causation from case reports. In: *Pharmacoepidemiology*, 6e (eds. B.L. Strom, S.E. Kimmel and S. Hennessy), 725–745. Wiley.

Karch, F.E. and Lasagna, L. (1977). Toward the operational identification of adverse drug reactions. *Clin. Pharmacol. Ther.* 21: 247–254.

Kelly, W.N., Arellano, F.M., Barnes, J. et al. (2007). Guidelines for submitting adverse event reports for publication. *Pharmacoepidemiol. Drug Saf.* 16: 581–587.

Kramer, M.S., Leventhal, J.M., Hutchinson, T.A., and Feinstein, A.R. (1979). An algorithm for the operational assessment of adverse drug reactions. I background, description, and instructions for use. *JAMA* 242: 623–632.

Lane, D.A., Kramer, M.S., Hutchinson, T.A. et al. (1987). The causality assessment of adverse drug reactions using a Bayesian approach. *Pharm. Med.* 2: 265–283.

Macedo, A.F., Marques, F.B., and Ribeiro, C.F. (2006). Can decisional algorithms replace global introspection in the individual causality assessment of spontaneously reported ADRs? *Drug Saf.* 29 (8): 697–702.

Miremont-Salamé, G., Théophile, H., Haramburu, F., and Bégaud, B. (2016). Causality assessment in pharmacovigilance: the French method and its successive updates. *Therapie* 71: 179–186.

Naranjo, C.A., Busto, U., Selers, E.M. et al. (1981). A method for estimating the probability of adverse drug reactions. *Clin. Pharmacol. Ther.* 30: 239–245.

Péré, J.C., Bégaud, B., Harambaru, F., and Albin, H. (1986). Computerized comparison of six adverse drug reaction assessment procedures. *Clin. Pharmacol. Ther.* 40: 451–461.

Stephens, M.D. (1987). The diagnosis of adverse medical events associated with drug treatment. *Adverse Drug React. Acute Poisoning Rev.* 6: 1–35.

Venulet, J., Ciucci, A.G., and Berneker, G.C. (1986). Updating of a method for causality assessment of adverse drug reactions. *Int. J. Clin. Pharmacol. Ther. Toxicol.* 24: 559–568.

Yerushalmy, J. and Palmer, C.E. (1959). On the methodology of investigations of etiologic factors in chronic diseases. *J. Chronic Dis.* 10 (1): 27–40.

Zapater, P., Such, J., Perez-Mateo, M., and Horga, J.F. (2002). A new Poisson and Bayesian-based method to assign risk and causality in patients with suspected hepatic adverse drug reactions: a report of two new cases of Ticlopidine-induced hepatotoxicity. *Drug Saf.* 25: 735–750.

# 15

# Molecular Pharmacoepidemiology

*Christine Y. Lu[1] and Stephen E. Kimmel[2]*

[1] *Harvard Medical School & Harvard Pilgrim Health Care Institute, Boston, MA, USA*
[2] *University of Florida, Gainesville, FL, USA*

## Introduction

Precision medicine has been defined by the National Institutes of Health (NIH) in the United States as an "approach to disease prevention and treatment based on people's individual differences in environment, genes and lifestyle." Genomic technologies are increasingly available, and their use in clinical care has grown substantially over the last decade. There are different types and applications of genomic technologies, including disease screening, diagnosis, prognosis, risk assessment or susceptibility, informed reproductive choices, and pharmacogenetics.

One of the most challenging aspects of clinical pharmacology and pharmacoepidemiology is to understand why individuals and groups of individuals respond differently to a specific drug therapy, both in terms of beneficial and adverse effects. Reidenberg observed that, while the prescriber has basically two decisions to make while treating patients (i.e. choosing the right drug and choosing the right dose), interpreting the inter-individual variability in outcomes of drug therapy includes a wider spectrum of variables, including the patient's health profile, prognosis, disease severity, quality of drug prescribing and dispensing, adherence with prescribed drug regimen (see Chapter 21), and last, but not least, the genetic profile of the patient.

The effects of genes and other biomarkers on drug response can be studied using molecular pharmacoepidemiology. Molecular pharmacoepidemiology is the study of the manner in which molecular biomarkers alter the clinical effects of medications in populations. Just as the basic science of pharmacoepidemiology is epidemiology, applied to the content area of clinical pharmacology, the basic science of molecular pharmacoepidemiology is epidemiology in general and molecular epidemiology specifically, also applied to the content area of clinical pharmacology. Thus, many of the methods and techniques of epidemiology apply to molecular pharmacoepidemiologic studies. However, there are features of molecular pharmacoepidemiology that are unique, as discussed later in this chapter. Most of the discussion will focus on studies related to genes, but the methodological considerations apply equally to studies of proteins (e.g. proteomics) and other biomarkers, such as the microbiome (the genes within the microbial cells, primarily bacteria in the gut, harbored within each person) and mRNA (messenger RNA that results from DNA transcription.

On average for each medication, it has been estimated that about one out of three treated patients experience beneficial effects, one out of three do not show the intended beneficial effects, 10% experience only side effects, and the rest of the patient population is nonadherent so that the response to the drug is difficult to assess. This highlights the challenge of individualizing therapy to produce a maximal beneficial response and minimize adverse effects. Although many factors can influence medication efficacy and adverse effects, including age, drug interactions, and medication adherence (see Chapter 21), genetics is an important contributor in the response of an individual to a medication. Genetic variability can account for a large proportion (e.g. some estimates range from 20% to 95%) of variability in drug disposition and medication effects.

In addition to altering dosing requirements, genetics can influence response to therapy by altering drug targets or the pathophysiology of the disease states that drugs are used to treat.

## Definitions and Concepts

### Genetic Variability

Building on the success of the various human genome initiatives, it is now estimated that there are approximately 25 000 regions of the human genome that are recognized as genes because they contain *deoxyribonucleic acid (DNA)* sequence elements including exons (sequences that encode proteins), introns (sequences between exons that do not directly encode amino acids), and regulatory regions (sequences that determine gene expression by regulating the transcription of DNA to RNA, and then the translation of RNA to protein). Some of these sequences have the ability to encode *RNA* (*ribonucleic acid*, the encoded messenger of a DNA sequence that mediates protein translation) and proteins (the amino acid sequence produced by the translation of RNA). In addition, we are learning a great deal

about genomic regions that do not encode RNA or protein, but play important roles in gene expression and regulation such as epigenetics (changes in DNA expression that occur but are not related to the base order, such as DNA-methylation). In addition, changes in the DNA of microbial cells (the microbiome) can influence human response to medications.

Thanks to numerous human genome initiatives, we also have substantial information about inter-individual variability in the human genome. The most common form of genomic variability is a *single nucleotide polymorphism (SNP)*, which represents a substitution of one nucleotide (i.e. the basic building block of DNA, also referred to as a "base") for another, which is present in at least 1% of the population. Each person has inherited two copies of each allele (one from the paternal chromosome and one from the maternal chromosome). The term allele refers to the specific nucleotide at one point in the genome inherited either from the father or mother, and the combination of alleles in an individual is denoted a *genotype*. When the two alleles are identical (i.e. the same nucleotide sequence on both chromosomes), the genotype is referred to as "homozygous;" when the two alleles are different (i.e. different nucleotide sequences on each chromosome), the genotype is referred to as "heterozygous." Approximately 10 million SNPs are thought to exist in the human genome, with an estimated two common missense (i.e. amino acid changing) variants per gene.

However, SNPs are not the only form of genetic variation that may be relevant to human traits and diseases. For example, copy number variants (CNV), sections of the genome that have repeats of base pairs, have also been recently identified as another common form of genomic variation that may have a role in disease etiology. DNA methylation, where methyl groups are added to DNA, thus changing the activity of DNA (which itself is regulated by genetics), and variability in the gut microbiome can also alter drug response.

Finally, we also recognize that the genome is not simply a linear nucleotide sequence, but that population genomic structure exists in which regions as large as 100 kilobases (a kilobase being a thousand nucleotides, or bases) in length define units that remain intact over evolutionary time. These regions define genomic block structure that may define *haplotypes*, which are sets of genetic variants that are transmitted as a unit across generations.

Thus, the complexity of genome structure and genetic variability that influences response to medications provides unique challenges to molecular pharmacoepidemiology.

## Pharmacogenetics and Pharmacogenomics

While the term *pharmacogenetics* is predominantly applied to the study of how genetic variability is responsible for differences in patients' responses to drug exposure, the term *pharmacogenomics* also encompasses approaches simultaneously considering data about thousands of genotypes, as well as responses in gene expression to existing medications. Although the term "pharmacogenetics" is sometimes used synonymously with pharmacogenomics, the former usually refers to a candidate-gene approach as opposed to a genome-wide approach in pharmacogenomics (both discussed later in this chapter).

## The Interface of Pharmacogenetics and Pharmacogenomics with Molecular Pharmacoepidemiology

Pharmacogenetic and pharmacogenomic studies are usually designed to examine intermediate endpoints between drugs and outcomes (such as drug levels, pharmacodynamic properties, or surrogate markers of drug effects) and often rely on detailed measurements of these surrogates in small groups of patients in highly controlled settings. Molecular pharmacoepidemiology focuses on the effects of genetics on clinical outcomes and uses larger observational and experimental methods to evaluate the effectiveness and safety of drug treatment in the population. Molecular pharmacoepidemiology uses similar methods as pharmacoepidemiology to answer questions related to the effects of genes on drug response. Thus, molecular pharmacoepidemiology answers questions related to:

1) The population prevalence of SNPs and other genetic variants,
2) Evaluating how these genetic variants alter disease outcomes,
3) Assessing the impact of gene–drug and gene– gene interactions on drug response and disease risk, and
4) Evaluating the usefulness and impact of genetic tests in populations exposed, or to be exposed, to drugs.

There are, however, some aspects of molecular pharmacoepidemiology that differ from the rest of pharmacoepidemiology. These include the need to understand the complex relationship between medication response and the vast number of potential molecular and genetic influences on this response; a focus on interactions among these factors and interactions between genes and environment (including other medications) that raise issues of sample size and has led to interest in novel designs; and the need to parse out the most likely associations between genes and drug response from among the massive number of potentially important genes identified through bioinformatics (the science of developing and utilizing computer databases and algorithms to accelerate and enhance biological research). As stated previously, the basic science of epidemiology underlies molecular pharmacoepidemiology just as it underlies all pharmacoepidemiology. What is different is the need for approaches that can deal with the vast number of potential genetic influences on outcomes; the possibility that "putative" genes associated with drug response may not be the actual causal genes, but rather a gene near or otherwise associated with the causal gene on the chromosome in the population studied (and that may not be similarly linked in other populations); the potential that multiple genes, each with a relatively small effect, work together to alter drug response; and the focus on complex interactions between and among genes, drugs, and environment. By discussing the potential approaches to these challenges in this chapter, it is hoped that both the similarities and differences between pharmacoepidemiology and molecular pharmacoepidemiology will be made clear.

## Clinical Problems to be Addressed by Pharmacoepidemiologic Research

It is useful to conceptualize clinical problems in molecular pharmacoepidemiology by thinking about the mechanism by which genes can affect drug response.

### Three Ways That Genes Can Affect Drug Response

The effect that a medication has on an individual can be affected at many points along the pathway of drug distribution and action. This includes absorption and distribution of medications to the site of action, interaction of the medication with its targets, metabolism of the drug, and drug excretion (see Chapter 4). These mechanisms can be categorized into three general routes by which genes can affect a drug response: pharmacokinetic, pharmacodynamic, and gene–drug interactions in the causal pathway of disease. These will be discussed in turn below.

### Pharmacokinetic Gene–Drug Interactions

Genes may influence the pharmacokinetics of a drug by altering its metabolism, absorption, or distribution. Metabolism of medications can either inactivate their effect or convert an inactive prodrug into a pharmacologically active compound. The genes that are responsible for variable metabolism of medications are those that code for various enzyme systems, especially the cytochrome P450 enzymes.

The gene encoding CYP2D6 represents a good example of the various ways in which polymorphisms can alter drug response. Many drug-CYP2D6 genetic variant interactions have been reported based on experimental or epidemiologic associations. CYP2D6 is one of the most common pharmacogenomic markers included in drug labeling by the US Food and Drug Administration (FDA) and the European Medicines Agency (EMA). Some of the genetic variants lead to low or no activity of the CYP2D6 enzyme whereas some individuals have multiple copies of the gene, leading to increased metabolism of drugs. Thus, patients using CYP2D6-dependent antipsychotic drugs (e.g. haloperidol) who are poor metabolizers (low CYP2D6 activity) are more than four times more likely to need anti-Parkinsonian medication to treat side effects of the antipsychotic drugs than high metabolizers. The decreased metabolic activity of CYP2D6 may also lead to lower drug efficacy, as illustrated for codeine, which is a prodrug that is metabolized to the active metabolite, morphine, by CYP2D6. It has been estimated that approximately 6–10% of Caucasians have variants that result in CYP2D6 genotypes that encode dysfunctional or inactive CYP2D6 enzyme, in whom codeine is an ineffective analgesic. There also is important interethnic variability of CYP2D6 alleles and phenotypes. An analysis of CYP2D6 allele-frequency data from >60 000 individuals suggests that diplotype frequencies predicting poor metabolism are highest among Europeans and the Ashkenazi Jewish population (about 5–6%) and lowest among East and South Central Asians,

Oceanians, and Middle Easterns (<1% in each of these populations). In contrast, diplotype frequencies predicting ultrarapid metabolism were highest in Oceanian (21.2%), followed by Ashkenazi Jews and Middle Easterns (about 11% in each of these populations) and lowest in East Asians (1.4%).

However, predicting clinical outcomes in daily practice based on such CYP2D6 genetic data in a valid fashion remains complex. Drug–gene associations shown in one study cannot always be replicated in another one. Obviously, variance in drug response has many determinants and singling out only one genetic factor fails to account for the co-occurrence, interplay, and interactions of several other factors (e.g. disease severity, exposure variability over time, physiological feedback mechanisms, and testing bias), all also important for molecular pharmacoepidemiology.

In addition to metabolism, genes that alter the absorption and distribution of medications may also alter drug levels at tissue targets. These include, for example, genes that code for transporter proteins such as the ATP-binding cassette transporter proteins (ABCB, also known as the multidrug-resistance [MDR]-1 gene), which has polymorphisms that have been associated with, for example, resistance to antiepileptic drugs. Patients with drug-resistant epilepsy (approximately one of three patients with epilepsy is a nonresponder) are more likely to have the CC polymorphism of ABCB1, which is associated with increased expression of this transporter drug-efflux protein. Of note, the ABCB1 polymorphism falls within an extensive block of linkage disequilibrium (LD). LD is defined by a region in which multiple genetic variants (e.g. SNPs) are correlated with one another due to population and evolutionary genetic history. As a result, a SNP may be statistically associated with disease risk, but is also in LD with the true causative SNP. Therefore, the SNP under study may not itself be causal but simply linked to a true causal variant. One of the major challenges in genetics research at this time is developing methods that can identify the true causal variant(s) that may reside in an LD block.

## Pharmacodynamic Gene–Drug Interactions

Once a drug is absorbed and transported to its target site, its effect may be altered by differences in the response of drug targets. Therefore, polymorphisms in genes that code for drug targets may alter the response of an individual to a medication.

For example, polymorphisms of the β(2)-adrenergic receptor (β(2)-AR) might affect response to β-agonists (e.g. albuterol) in asthma patients. In particular, the coding variants at position 16 within the β(2)-AR gene (β(2)-AR-16) have been suggested to determine patient response to albuterol treatment (see Case Example 15.1).

Pharmacodynamic gene–drug interactions may also affect the risk of adverse reactions. One example is a polymorphism in the gene coding for the bradykinin B2 receptor that has been associated with an increased risk of angiotensin converting enzyme (ACE) inhibitor-induced cough. Cough is one of the most frequently seen adverse drug reactions (ADRs) in ACE therapy and very often a reason for discontinuation of therapy. The TT genotype and T allele of the human bradykinin B(2) receptor gene were found to be significantly higher in patients with cough. However, similar to many other studies, replication of these findings has been limited. Further research using genome-wide association studies (GWAS) has suggested that other SNPs are related to intolerance to ACE inhibitors, but again requires replication.

## Gene–Drug Interactions and the Causal Pathway of Disease

Along with altering the pharmacokinetic and pharmacodynamic properties of medications, genetic polymorphisms may also alter the disease state that is the target of drug therapy. For example, antihypertensive medications that work by a particular mechanism, such as the

---

**Case Example 15.1**

*Background*
*Regular use* of inhaled B-agonists for asthma may produce adverse effects and be no more effective than *as-needed* use of these drugs.

*Question*
Can genetic polymorphisms in the B2-agonist receptor alter responsiveness to inhaled B-agonists?

*Approach*
- Perform genetic analysis within a randomized clinical trial of regular versus as-needed use of inhaled B-agonists, and
- Compare the effects of multiple genetic polymorphisms on drug-response.

*Results*
- Regular use of inhaled B-agonist is associated with decline in efficacy among those with B(2)-AR-16 variants but not among those with other variants tested.
- No effect of genotype in those using inhaled B-agonists in an as-needed manner.

*Strengths*
- Randomized trial design eliminates confounding by indication for frequency of medication use.

- Candidate genes enhances biological plausibility.

*Limitations*
- Multiple polymorphisms tested on multiple outcomes leads to concern of false positives.
- LD: polymorphisms identified could be "innocent bystanders" by being linked to the true causative mutations.

*Key Points*
- Genetic polymorphisms of drug targets may alter drug response.
- Because of the concern of false positives and/or LD, replication studies and mechanistic studies remain critical to identifying true putative mutations that alter drug response.
- Effects of a gene may vary by the pattern of drug use, making it important to consider all aspects of drug use (dose, duration, frequency, regularity, etc.) in molecular pharmacoepidemiology studies.

---

increasing sodium excretion of some antihypertensive medications, may have different effects depending on the susceptibility of the patient to the effects of the drug. Patients with a polymorphism in the α-adducin gene may have greater sensitivity to changes in sodium balance. A case–control study has suggested that those with the α-adducin polymorphism may be more likely to benefit from diuretic treatment than those without the polymorphism.

Genetic variability in disease states also can be critical for tailoring drug therapy to patients with a specific genotype related both to the disease and drug response. One example is the humanized monoclonal antibody trastuzumab

(Herceptin®), which is used for the treatment of metastatic breast cancer patients with overexpression of the HER2 oncogene. The HER2 protein is thought to be a unique target for trastuzumab therapy in patients with this genetically associated overexpression, occurring in 10–34% of females with breast cancer. The case of trastuzumab, together with another anticancer drug, imatinib, which is especially effective in patients with Philadelphia chromosome-positive leukemias, has pioneered successful genetically targeted therapy. The association of somatic mutations to drug response has received substantial interest. There are many targeted therapies now available that block the growth and spread of cancer by interfering with specific molecules that are involved in the growth, progression, and spread of cancer.

Genetic polymorphisms that alter disease states can also play a role in drug safety. For example, factor V Leiden mutation, present in about 1 out of 20 Caucasians, is considered an important genetic risk factor for deep vein thrombosis and embolism. A relative risk of about 30 in factor V carriers and users of oral contraceptives compared to noncarriers and non-oral-contraceptive users has been reported. This gene–drug interaction has also been linked to the differential thrombotic risk associated with third-generation oral contraceptives compared with second-generation oral contraceptives. Despite this strong association, Vandenbroucke et al. have calculated that mass screening for factor V would result in denial of oral contraceptives for about 20000 women positive for this mutation in order to prevent 1 death. Therefore, these authors concluded that reviewing personal and family thrombosis history, and only if suitable, factor V testing before prescribing oral contraceptives, is the recommended approach to avoid this adverse gene–drug interaction. This highlights another important role of molecular pharmacoepidemiology: determining the utility and cost-effectiveness (see also Chapter 18) of genetic screening to guide drug therapy.

## The Interplay of Various Mechanisms

It is useful to conceptualize how the effects of genetic polymorphisms at different stages of drug disposition and response might influence an individual's response to a medication. As an example, an individual may have a genotype that alters the metabolism of the drug, the receptor for the drug, or both. Depending on the combination of these genotypes, the individual might have a different response in terms of both efficacy and toxicity (see Table 15.1). In the simplified example in Table 15.1, there is one genetic variant that alters drug metabolism and one genetic variant that alters receptor response to a medication of interest. In this example, among those who are homozygous for the alleles that encode normal drug metabolism and normal receptor response, there is relatively high efficacy and low toxicity. However, among those who have a variant that reduces drug metabolism, efficacy at a standard dose could actually be greater (assuming a linear dose–response relationship within the possible drug levels of the medication) but toxicity could be increased (if dose-related). Among those who have a variant that reduces receptor response, drug efficacy will be reduced while toxicity may not be different from those who carry genotypes that are not associated with impaired receptor response (assuming

**Table 15.1** Hypothetical response to medications by genetic variants in metabolism and receptor genes.

| | Drug response | | |
| --- | --- | --- | --- |
| Gene affecting metabolism[a] | Gene affecting receptor response[a] | Efficacy | Toxicity |
| Wild-type | Wild-type | 70% | 2% |
| Variant | Wild-type | 85% | 20% |
| Wild-type | Variant | 20% | 2% |
| Variant | Variant | 35% | 20% |

*Source:* Data from Evans and McLeod (2003).
[a] Wild-type associated with normal metabolism or receptor response and variants associated with reduced metabolism or receptor response.

that toxicity is not related to the receptor responsible for efficacy). Among those who have variants for both genes, efficacy could be reduced because of the receptor variant (perhaps not as substantially as those with an isolated variant of the receptor gene because of the higher effective dose resulting from the metabolism gene variant), while toxicity could be increased because of the metabolism variant.

## The Progression and Clinical Application of Molecular Pharmacoepidemiology

Medications with a narrow therapeutic index are good targets for the use of molecular pharmacoepidemiology to improve the use and application of medications. One example is warfarin. This example illustrates both the logical progression of pharmacogenetics through molecular pharmacoepidemiology and the complexity of moving pharmacogenetic data into practice. The enzyme primarily responsible for the metabolism of warfarin to its inactive form is the cytochrome P450 2C9 variant (CYP2C9). Case Example 15.2 illustrates both the logical progression of pharmacogenetics through molecular pharmacoepidemiology and the complexity of moving pharmacogenetic data into practice.

Another pertinent example is in oncology. Markers predicting response to anti-cancer drugs are mostly related to the fact that drug efficacy can be greatly influenced by alterations in drug targets and in related proteins present in tumor cells. Therefore, cancer targeted therapies, directed to a specific cancer alteration, may only be indicated for the subgroup of patients with tumors carrying that molecular target. Examples include trastuzumab and imatinib mentioned earlier in the chapter.

It is important to note that novel treatment strategies can be based on a specific genetic characteristic regardless of the type or subtype of cancer. For instance, in 2017 the US FDA approved pembrolizumab for treatment of unresectable or metastatic solid tumors that have a biomarker, microsatellite instability-high (MSI-H) or mismatch repair deficient (dMMR), in adult and pediatric patients. This is the first drug approval based on a tumor's biomarker without regard to the tumor's original location.

## Methodological Problems to be Addressed by Pharmacoepidemiologic Research

The same methodological problems of pharmacoepidemiology must be addressed in molecular pharmacoepidemiology. These problems include those of chance and statistical power, confounding, bias, and generalizability (see Chapters 2, 3, and 22).

However, the complex relationship between medication response and molecular and genetic factors generates some unique challenges in molecular pharmacoepidemiology. These challenges derive from the large number of potential genetic variants that can modify the response to a single drug, the possibility that there is a small individual effect of any one of these genes, the low prevalence of many genetic variants, and the possibility that a presumptive gene–drug response relationship may be confounded by the racial and ethnic mixture of the population studied. Thus, the methodological challenges of molecular pharmacoepidemiology are closely related to issues of statistical interactions, type I and type II errors, and confounding. First and foremost, however, molecular pharmacoepidemiologic studies rely on proper identification of putative genotypes. In addition, in all research of this type, use of appropriate laboratory methods, such as high-throughput genotyping technologies, is necessary. Similarly, appropriate quality control procedures must be considered to

**Case Example 15.2**

The complexity of the progression and clinical application of molecular pharmacoepidemiology

*Background*
Warfarin is a narrow therapeutic index drug. Underdosing or overdosing, even to a minimal degree, can lead to significant morbidity (thromboembolism and/or bleeding).

*Question*
Can genetic variants be identified and used to alter the dosing of warfarin and thus improve safety and effectiveness?

*Approach and Results*
- Multiple study designs have been used to address this question.
- Pharmacogenetic studies identified the effect of CYP2C9 polymorphisms on warfarin metabolism. Additional research clearly demonstrated that the vitamin K epoxide reductase complex 1 (VKORC-1) gene is responsible for coding the target for warfarin.
- Numerous observational studies then demonstrated differential response to warfarin in patients with CYP2C9 and VKORC1 variants, particularly for the outcome of the required maintenance dose of warfarin.
- The development of algorithms to predict a maintenance warfarin dose that combines clinical and genetic data then suggested that improvements may be made by incorporating genetic data into dosing algorithms. However, small clinical trials did not demonstrate the utility of genotyping.
- Large-scale trials were performed to answer the important question of clinical utility. The Clarification of Optimal Anticoagulation through Genetics (COAG) trial demonstrated no benefit of pharmacogenetic dosing on anticoagulation control overall, and worsening of anticoagulation control with pharmacogenetic

dosing in African Americans. The EU-PACT UK trial demonstrated improvement in anticoagulation control. A third trial, the GIFT trial, examined pharmacogenetic dosing in orthopedic patients, compared with a clinical algorithm dosing arm. This trial demonstrated benefit from pharmacogenetic dosing, but could not address the question of the effects of pharmacogenetics in African Americans due to the enrolment of very few African American patients. Together, these trials demonstrate the need for, and benefit of, pharmacogenetic clinical trials testing different strategies in different patient populations.

*Strengths*
A logical series of studies, each with its own strengths and limitations, has improved our understanding of genetic variability in response to warfarin.

*Limitations*
- No randomized trials have yet shown that one can reduce adverse events and enhance effectiveness of warfarin by knowing a patient's genetic make-up.
- Only about 50% of variability in warfarin response can be explained by existing algorithms–other polymorphisms or clinical factors (e.g. adherence) may be important.

*Key Points*
- The process of fully understanding the effects of polymorphisms on drug response requires multiple studies and often substantial resources.
- Our understanding of genetic variants has progressed so rapidly that new questions are often raised that have implications for clinical practice even as old ones are answered.
- Before using genetic data to alter drug prescribing, prospective evaluation is needed.

obtain meaningful data for research and clinical applications. Recent next-generation sequencing (NGS) techniques have only highlighted further the need for, and complexity of, obtaining valid genotyping results. This section will focus on the methodological challenges of studying interactions, minimizing type I and type II errors, and accounting for confounding, particularly by population admixture (defined below).

## Interactions

Along with examining the direct effect of genes and other biomarkers on outcomes, molecular pharmacoepidemiologic studies must often be designed to examine effect modification between medication use and the genes or biomarkers of interest. That is, the primary measure of interest is often the role of biomarker information on the effect of a medication. For purposes of simplicity, this discussion will use genetic variability as the measure of interest.

Effect modification is present if there is a difference in the effect of the medication depending on the presence or absence of the genetic variant. This difference can be either on the multiplicative or additive scale. On the multiplicative scale, interaction is present if the effect of the combination of the genotype and medication exposure relative to neither is greater than the product of the measure of effect of each (genotype alone or medication alone) relative to neither. On the additive scale, interaction is present if the effect of the combination of the genotype and medication exposure is greater than the sum of the measures of effect of each alone, again all relative to neither.

For studies examining a dichotomous medication exposure (e.g. medication use versus nonuse), a dichotomous genetic exposure (e.g. presence versus absence of a genetic variant), and a dichotomous outcome (e.g. myocardial infarction occurrence versus none), there are two ways to consider presenting and analyzing interactions. The first is as a stratified analysis, comparing the effect of medication exposure versus non-exposure on the outcome in two strata: those with the genetic variant and those

**Table 15.2** Two ways to present effect modification in molecular pharmacoepidemiologic studies using case–control study as a model.

| Stratified analysis | | | | | |
|---|---|---|---|---|---|
| Genotype | Medication | Cases | Controls | Odds ratio | Information provided |
| + | + | a | b | ad/bc | Effect of medication vs. no medication among those with the genotype |
| | − | c | d | | |
| − | + | e | f | eh/fg | Effect of medication vs. no medication among those without the genotype |
| | − | g | h | | |

| 2 × 4 Table | | | | | |
|---|---|---|---|---|---|
| Genotype | Medication | Cases | Controls | Odds ratio | Information provided |
| + | + | a | b | ah/bg = A | Joint genotype and medication vs. neither |
| + | − | c | d | ch/dg = B | Genotype alone vs. neither |
| − | + | e | f | eh/fg = C | Medication alone vs. neither |
| − | − | g | h | Reference | Reference Group |

without (e.g. see Table 15.2). The second is to present a 2×4 table (also shown in Table 15.2). In the first example (stratified analysis), one compares the effect of the medication among those with the genetic variant to the effect of the medication among those without the genetic variant. In the second example (the 2×4 table), the effect of each combination of exposure (i.e. with both genetic variant and medication; with genetic variant but without medication; with medication but without genetic variant) is determined relative to the lack of exposure to either. The advantage of the 2×4 table is that it presents separately the effect of the drug, the gene, and both relative to those without the genetic variant and without medication exposure. In addition, presentation of the data as a 2×4 table allows one to directly compute both multiplicative and additive interactions. In the example given in Table 15.2, multiplicative interaction would be assessed by comparing the odds ratio for the combination of genotype and medication exposure to the product of the odds ratios for medication alone and genotype alone. Multiplicative interaction would be considered present if the odds ratios for the combination of medication and genotype (A in Table 15.2) was greater than the product of the odds ratios for either alone (B×C). Additive interaction would be considered present if the odds ratio for the combination of genotype and medication use (A) was greater than the sum of the odds ratios for medication use alone and genotype alone (B+C). The 2×4 table also allows the direct assessment of the number of subjects in each group along with the respective confidence interval for the measured effect in each of the groups, making it possible to directly observe the precision of the estimates in each of the groups and therefore better understand the power of the study. Furthermore, attributable fractions can be computed separately for each of the exposures alone and for the combination of exposures. In general, presenting the data in both manners is optimal because it allows the reader to understand the effect of each of the

exposures (2×4 table) as well as the effect of the medication in the presence or absence of the genotypic variant (stratified table).

## Type I Error

The chance of type I error (concluding there is an association when in fact one does not exist) increases with the number of statistical tests performed on any one data set (see also Chapter 3). It is easy to appreciate the potential for type I error in a molecular pharmacoepidemiologic study that examines, simultaneously, the effects of multiple genetic factors, the effects of multiple nongenetic factors, and the interaction between and among these factors. One of the reasons cited for nonreplication of study findings in molecular pharmacoepidemiology is type I error. Limiting the number of associations examined to those of specific candidate genetic variants that are suspected of being associated with the outcome is one method to limit type I error in pharmacoepidemiology. However, with increasing emphasis in molecular pharmacoepidemiologic studies on identifying all variants within a gene (and all variants within the genome) and examining multiple interactions, this method of limiting type I error is often not tenable. Some other currently available solutions are discussed in the next section.

## Type II Error

Because it has been hypothesized that much of the genetic variability leading to phenotypic expression of complex diseases results from the relatively small effects of many relatively low prevalence genetic variants, the ability to detect a gene–response relationship is likely to require relatively large sample sizes to avoid type II error (concluding there is no association when in fact one does exist). The sample size requirements for studies that examine the direct effect of genes on medication response will be the same as the requirements for examining direct effects of individual risk factors on outcomes. With relatively low prevalences of polymorphisms and often low incidence of outcomes (particularly in studies of ADRs), large sample sizes are typically required to detect even modest associations. For such studies, the case–control design (see Chapter 2) has become a particularly favored approach for molecular pharmacoepidemiologic studies because of its ability to select participants based on the outcome of interest, and its ability to study the effects of multiple potential genotypes in the same study.

Studies that are designed to examine the interaction between a genetic polymorphism and a medication will require even larger sample sizes. This is because such studies need to be powered to compare those with both the genetic polymorphism and the medication exposure with those who have neither. As an example, the previously mentioned case–control study of the α-adducin gene and diuretic therapy in patients with treated hypertension examined the effects of the genetic polymorphism, the diuretic therapy, and both in combination. There were 1038 participants in the study. When comparing the effect of diuretic use with no use and comparing the effect of the genetic variant with the nonvariant allele, all 1038 participants were available for comparison (Table 15.3). However, when examining the effect of diuretic therapy versus nonuse

among those with the genetic variant, only 385 participants contributed to the analyses.

In order to minimize false negative findings, further efforts must be made to ensure adequate sample sizes for molecular pharmacoepidemiologic studies. Because of the complex nature of medication response, and the likelihood that at least several genes are responsible for the variability in drug response, studies designed to test for multiple gene–gene and gene–environment interactions (including other medications, environmental factors, adherence to medications, and clinical factors) will, similarly, require large sample sizes.

## Confounding by Population Admixture

When there is evidence that baseline disease risks and genotype frequencies differ among ethnicities, the conditions for population stratification (i.e. population admixture or confounding by ethnicity) may be met. Population admixture is simply a manifestation of confounding by ethnicity, which can occur if both baseline disease risk and genotype frequency vary across ethnicity. For example, the African–American population represent admixture of at least three major continental ancestries (African, European, and Native American). The larger the number of ethnicities involved

**Table 15.3** Gene-exposure interaction analysis in a case–control study.

| Diuretic Use | Adducin Variant | Cases | Controls | Odds Ratio (OR) for Stroke Myocardial Infarction |
|---|---|---|---|---|
| 0 | 0 | $A_{00}$ 103 | $B_{00}$ 248 | 1.0 |
| 0 | 1 | $A_{01}$ 85 | $B_{01}$ 131 | 1.56 |
| 1 | 0 | $A_{10}$ 94 | $B_{10}$ 208 | 1.09 |
| 1 | 1 | $A_{11}$ 41 | $B_{11}$ 128 | 0.77 |

*Source:* Data from Psaty et al. (2002).

in an admixed population, the less likely that population stratification can be the explanation for biased associations. Empirical data show that carefully matched, moderate-sized case–control samples in African–American populations are unlikely to contain levels of population admixture that would result in significantly inflated numbers of false-positive associations. There is the potential for population structure to exist in African–American populations, but this structure can be eliminated by removing recent African or Caribbean immigrants, and limiting study samples to resident African–Americans. Based on the literature that has evaluated the effects of confounding by ethnicity overall, and specifically in African–Americans, there is little empirical evidence that population stratification is a likely explanation for bias in point estimates or incorrect inferences. Nonetheless, population admixture must be considered in designing and analyzing molecular pharmacoepidemiologic studies to ensure that adequate adjustment can be made for this potential confounder. It is important to note that poor study design may be more important than population stratification in conferring bias to association studies.

## Currently Available Solutions

### Identifying Additional Genetic Contributions to Drug Response

A great concern of the identification of low penetrance alleles (those in which few of the individuals who have the allele exhibit the clinical symptoms associated with that allele) is that they have not yet been able to explain the majority of the estimated genetic contribution to disease etiology. Based on studies of families or phenotypic variability, most loci have been found to explain less than half (and at times as little as 1%) of the predicted heritability of many common traits. This "missing

heritability" of complex disease suggests that other classes of genetic variation may explain much of the genetic contribution to common disease.

There are two primary approaches for gene discovery: candidate gene association studies and genome-wide studies. In the former, genes are selected for study on the basis of their plausible biological relevance to drug response. While this allows for identification of variants with a priori biological plausibility, it is limited by our partial knowledge of which genetic variants may actually be responsible for variable drug effects. In the latter, DNA sequences are examined for associations with outcomes, initially irrespective of biological plausibility. The benefit of this approach is that it does not rely on our limited knowledge of genetics; the disadvantage is that the biological plausibility of the findings may then need to be confirmed.

One example of the genome-wide approach are GWAS. GWAS rely on LD, defined above as the correlation between alleles at two loci. The GWAS approach uses DNA sequence variation (e.g. SNPs) found throughout the genome, and does not rely on a priori functional knowledge of gene function. A number of factors influence the success of these studies. Appropriate epidemiologic study designs and adequate statistical power remain essential. Thorough characterization of LD is essential for replication of GWAS: the haplotype mapping (HapMap) consortium and other groups have shown that the extent of LD varies by ethnicity, which may affect the ability to replicate findings in subsequent studies. Particularly informative SNPs that best characterize a genomic region can be used to limit the amount of laboratory and analytical work in haplotype-based studies. It has been hypothesized that studies that consider LD involving multiple SNPs in a genomic region (i.e. a haplotype) can increase power to detect associations by 15–50% compared with analyses involving only individual SNPs. Finally, even if genome-wide scans may identify markers associated with the trait of interest, a challenge will be to identify the causative SNPs.

Newer, sequencing technologies have made it possible to study rarer genetic variants. While Sanger sequencing is still considered the gold standard in clinical testing, its limitations include low throughput and high cost. Broadly, NGS describes technologies that utilize clonally amplified or single-molecular templates that are then sequenced in a massively parallel fashion. The advance of NGS technologies has been enabled by innovation in sequencing chemistries, better imaging, microfabrication, and information technology. In addition, bioinformatics tools for data analysis and management and sample preparation methods have rapidly evolved along with the sequencing technologies, translating to reductions in the amount of input materials required. In 2013, the US FDA approved marketing for the first time for a next-generation sequencer, Illumina's MiSeqDx, which allows the development and use of innumerable new genome-based tests.

Clearly, candidate gene and genome-wide approaches are not mutually exclusive. Both have the potential to identify important variants that may be clinically useful.

## Interactions

Along with traditional case–control and cohort studies, the case-only study can be used for molecular pharmacoepidemiologic studies designed to examine interactions between genes and medications. In this design, cases, representing those with the outcome or phenotype of interest, are selected for study, and the association between genetic variants and medication use is determined among these cases. Assuming that the use of the medication is unrelated to the genotype, the case-only study provides a valid measure of the interaction of the genotype and the medication on the risk of the outcome.

One strength of the case-only study design is that it eliminates the need to identify controls,

often a major methodological and logistical challenge in case–control studies. One limitation of the case-only design is that it relies on the assumption of independence between exposure (medication use) and genotype. Although this assumption may be valid (in the absence of knowing genotype clinically, it may be reasonable to assume that the use of the medication is not related to patients' genotypes), it is certainly possible that, within observational studies, the genotype, by altering response to medications targeted at a specific disease, could affect the medications being prescribed to patients. Another method is to perform the case-only study within a randomized trial, where drug use is randomly assigned.

## Type I Error and Replication

Given concerns of type I error (along with other methodologic concerns such as uncontrolled confounding, publication bias, and LD), a key issue in molecular epidemiology is the ability to replicate association study findings. Replication of association studies is required not only to identify biologically plausible causative associations, but also to conclude that a candidate gene has a meaningful etiological effect.

The lack of replication can be explained by false positive reports (e.g. spurious associations), by false negative reports (e.g. studies that are insufficiently powerful to identify the association), or by actual population differences (e.g. the true associations are different because of differences in genetic background, exposures, etc.).

In order to achieve believable, replicable association results, investigators must consider factors that influence the design, analysis, and interpretation of these studies. These include adequate sample size, proper study design, and characterization of the study population, particularly when replication studies themselves are not comparable in terms of participant characteristics or other confounding factors.

Adequate reporting of genetic association studies is important to allow assessment of their strengths and weaknesses. The STREGA statement (Strengthening the Reporting of Genetic Association studies) is an extension of the STROBE statement (Strengthening the Reporting of Observational Studies in Epidemiology) that provides a checklist to help researchers and journals.

Data analytical methods can complement replication studies to address multiple testing and type I error. Bonferroni correction is the most basic approach for adjusting multiple testing. However, this method is considered too conservative for tightly linked SNPs and it may wipe out many small effects that one may actually expect (i.e. increase risk of type II errors). The false discovery rate (FDR) approach is less conservative for controlling for multiple analyses of the data. The FDR method estimates the expected proportion of false-positives among associations that are declared significant, which is expressed as a q-value. Under a Bayesian approach there is no penalty for multiple testing because the prior probability of an association should not be affected by the tests that the investigator chooses to conduct. However, without strict standards, one may choose an exaggerated prior plausibility of a model that is supported a posteriori.

### Type II Error

Reducing type II error (concluding that there is no association when one does exist in fact) essentially involves a logistical need to ensure adequate sample size (see also Chapter 3). One approach to increasing the sample size of molecular pharmacoepidemiologic studies is to perform large, multicenter collaborative studies. Another is to combine multiple, separately performed cohorts.

Another potential solution to minimizing type II error is through meta-analysis, whereby smaller studies, which are, individually, not powered to detect specific associations (such as interactions) are combined in order to improve the ability to detect such associations (see Chapter 20).

### Confounding by Population Admixture

Although population stratification is unlikely to be a significant source of bias in epidemiologic association studies, this assumes adequate adjustment for population genetic structure. A number of analytical approaches exist to either circumvent problems imposed by population genetic structure or that use this structure in gene identification. The "structured association" approach identifies a set of individuals who are drawing their alleles from different background populations or ethnicities. This approach uses information about genotypes at loci that lie in regions other than the location of the gene of interest (i.e. "unlinked markers") to infer their ancestry (often referred to as ancestry informative markers) and learn about population structure. It further uses the data derived from these unlinked markers to adjust the association test statistic. By adjusting for these ancestry informative markers, one can adjust for differences in ancestry.

## The Future

Scientific and clinical developments in biology and molecular biology, particularly in the field of genomics and other biomarkers, have and will continue to affect the field of pharmacoepidemiology in a significant way. Translating biomarkers from the lab and experimental studies to clinical practice has been a difficult path. Often, initial promising findings on drug-gene interactions to predict clinical drug responses could not be replicated in subsequent studies. For sure, the ability of genes and other biomarkers to improve patient care and outcomes will need to be tested in properly controlled studies, including randomized controlled trials in some circumstances. The positive and negative predictive value of carrying a genetic variant will be important determinants of the ability of the variant to improve outcomes. Those genetic variants with good test characteristics may still need to be evaluated in properly controlled trials. Such studies could examine several ways to incorporate genetic testing into clinical practice, including the use of genetic variants in dosing algorithms, in selection of a specific therapeutic class of drug to treat a disease, and in avoidance of using specific medications in those at high risk for ADRs. These scientific advances are also finding their way into drug discovery and development in order to rationalize drug innovation and to identify good and poor responders, both in terms of efficacy and safety, of drug therapy in an earlier phase. The cost-effectiveness of such approaches is also of great interest because the addition of genetic testing adds cost to clinical care (see also Chapter 18). Research will be needed to determine the cost-effectiveness of new biomarker and genetic tests as they are developed.

NGS will also require the development of novel approaches to data analyses. There are three levels of analysis that are conducted by NGS technologies: (i) targeted gene panels focus on a limited set of genes allowing for greater depth of coverage. The advantages include higher analytical sensitivity and specificity, and improved ability to interpret the results in a clinical context because only genes with an established role in the disease are sequenced, (ii) exome sequencing tests all coding regions of the human genome, and (iii) whole-genome sequencing analyzes the entire three billion bases of the genome. The targeted approach to genome sequencing is the more widespread clinical implementation of NGS technologies. This is because only some of the enormous amount of genetic information generated by exome or whole-genome sequencing can be interpreted and is actionable. Along with the bioinformatics challenges of managing and validating such large data sets, a significant amount of information will be novel and/or of unknown clinical importance.

A major area that requires further development is in establishing the clinical utility of the identified markers/strategies for patients and healthcare systems. The level of evidence required to establish that a marker is clinically useful and should be introduced for routine use has been discussed extensively but consensus has not been reached. Genetic and molecular studies are increasingly being incorporated in large clinical trials, which can lead to the identification of subgroups of patients with clear benefit from drugs, accelerating the discovery of effective therapies for selected populations. Another challenge to the implementation of genetic testing is the fact that pharmacogenetics knowledge is constantly being updated. Clinicians need to interpret the results of these tests in accordance with current understanding of the association between pharmacogenetic variation and drug effects.

What this all means for the future of pharmacoepidemiology is a challenging question. Genotype data will increasingly become available and will enrich pharmacoepidemiologic analysis. New methods (e.g. sequencing) will provide new opportunities but also new challenges to analyzing pharmacoepidemiologic data. Further, although it is useful to characterize the three different pathways of how drug-gene interactions may occur as was done in this chapter, this stratification is most likely an oversimplification of the large plethora of possible mechanisms of how drugs, genes, and patient outcomes are interrelated. All these may have consequences for how molecular pharmacoepidemiologic studies are designed, conducted, and analyzed. In addition, the more that genotype testing is applied in clinical practice, the more drug exposure will be influenced by such tests, making genotype and drug exposure non-independent factors.

Finally, just as for all research, the ethical, legal, and social implications of genetic testing must be considered and addressed (see also

Chapter 16). Pharmacogenetic testing raises issues of privacy concerns, access to health care services, and informed consent. For example, concern has been raised that the use of genetic testing could lead to targeting of therapies to only specific groups (ethnic or racial) of patients, ignoring others, and to loss of insurance coverage for certain groups of individuals. There is also a concern that medicines will be developed only for the most common, commercially attractive genotypes, leading to "orphan genotypes." Equally importantly, as more and more genetic data are collected on individuals as part of routine clinical care, the requirements and methods for returning unanticipated genetic results must be carefully determined and implemented.

All of these issues are challenges to overcome as we continue to reap the benefits of the tremendous strides made in determining the molecular basis of disease and drug response.

## Key Points

- Genes can affect a drug response via: alteration of drug pharmacokinetics, pharmacodynamic effects on drug targets, and gene–drug interactions in the causal pathway of disease.
- Molecular pharmacoepidemiology is the study of the manner in which molecular biomarkers (often, but not exclusively, genes) alter the clinical effects of medications in populations.
- Molecular pharmacoepidemiology answers questions related to: the population prevalence of SNPs and other genetic variants; evaluating how these SNPs alter disease outcomes; assessing the impact of gene–drug and gene–gene interactions on disease risk; and evaluating the usefulness and impact of genetic tests in populations exposed, or to be exposed, to drugs.
- Identifying genes that alter drug response for molecular pharmacoepidemiology studies can use a candidate gene approach or a genome-wide approach; these approaches are complementary, not mutually exclusive.
- The methodological challenges of molecular pharmacoepidemiology are closely related to issues of statistical interactions, type I and type II errors, and confounding.
- Case-only studies can be used to measure the interaction between genetic variants and medications and eliminate the difficulty and inefficiency of including a control group. However, they rely on the assumption of independence between medication use and genetic variants among those without disease, an assumption that may not be met.
- Given concerns of type I error (along with other methodological concerns such as uncontrolled confounding and LD), a key issue in molecular epidemiology is the ability to replicate association study findings.
- Because genetic variability leading to phenotypic expression of complex diseases results from the relatively small effects of many relatively low prevalence genetic variants, the ability to detect a gene–response relationship is likely to require relatively large sample sizes to avoid type II error. Methods to ensure adequate sample sizes include the use of large, multicenter collaborative studies; assembly and genotyping of large, relatively homogenous populations for multiple studies; and meta-analysis.
- Population stratification can distort the gene-medication response association. Although unlikely to be a significant source of bias in well-controlled epidemiological association studies, a number of analytical approaches exist to either circumvent problems imposed by population genetic structure or that use this structure in gene identification.
- The ability of genes and other biomarkers to improve patient care and outcomes needs to be tested in properly controlled studies, including randomized controlled trials in

some cases. Similarly, the cost-effectiveness of such approaches must be justifiable given the additional costs of genetic testing in clinical care.

- The ethical, legal, and social implications of genetic testing must be considered and addressed, just as they must be considered for all research.

## Further Reading

Botto, L.D. and Khoury, M.J. (2004). Facing the challenge of complex genotypes and gene–environment interaction: the basic epidemiologic units in case–control and case-only designs. In: *Human Genome Epidemiology* (eds. M.J. Khoury, J. Little and W. Burke), 111–126. New York: Oxford University Press.

Bournissen, F.G., Moretti, M.E., Juurlink, D.N. et al. (2009 Apr). Polymorphism of the MDR1/ABCB1 C3435T drug-transporter and resistance to anticonvulsant drugs: a meta-analysis. *Epilepsia* 50 (4): 898–903.

Caraco, Y., Blotnick, S., and Muszkat, M. (2008). CYP2C9 genotype-guided warfarin prescribing enhances the efficacy and safety of anticoagulation: a prospective randomized controlled study. *Clin. Pharmacol. Ther.* 83: 460–470.

Evans, W.E. and McLeod, L.J. (2003). Pharmacogenomics–drug disposition, drug targets, and side effects. *N. Engl. J. Med.* 348: 528–549.

Fleeman N, Dundar Y, Dickson R, et al. Cytochrome P450 testing for prescribing antipsychotics in adults with schizophrenia: systematic review and meta-analyses. *Pharm. J.* 2011 Feb;11(1):1–14.

Gaedigk, A., Sangkuhl, K., Whirl-Carrillo, M. et al. (2017). Prediction of CYP2D6 phenotype from genotype across world populations. *Genet. Med.* 19: 69–76. https://doi.org/10.1038/gim.2016.80. Epub 2016 Jul 7.

Kimmel, S.E., French, B., Kasner, S.E. et al. (2013). A pharmacogenetic versus a clinical algorithm for warfarin dosing. *N. Engl. J. Med.* 369: 2283–2293.

Klein, T.E., Altman, R.B., Eriksson, N. et al. (2009). Estimation of a warfarin dose with clinical and pharmacogenetic data. International Warfarin Pharmacogenetics Consortium. *N. Engl. J. Med.* 360: 753–764.

Lohmueller, K.E., Pearce, C.L., Pike, M. et al. (2003). Meta-analysis of genetic association studies supports a contribution of common variants to susceptibility to common disease. *Nat. Genet.* 33: 177–182.

Mallal, S., Phillips, E., Carosi, G. et al. (2008). HLA-B*5701 screening for hypersensitivity to abacavir. *N. Engl. J. Med.* 358: 568–579.

Manolio, T.A., Collins, F.S., Cox, N.J. et al. (2009). Finding the missing heritability of complex diseases. *Nature* 461: 747–753.

Psaty, B.M., Smith, N.L., Heckbert, S.R. et al. (2002). Diuretic therapy, the alpha-adducin gene variant, and the risk of myocardial infarction or stroke in persons with treated hypertension. *JAMA* 287: 1680–1689.

Roden, D.M., McLeod, H.L., Relling, M.V. et al. (2019 Aug 10). Pharmacogenomics. *Lancet* 394 (10197): 521–532.

Roses, A.D. (2008). Pharmacogenetics in drug discovery and development: a translational perspective. *Nat. Rev. Drug Discov.* 7 (10): 807–817.

Thomas, D. (2010 Apr). Gene-environment-wide association studies: emerging approaches. *Nat. Rev. Genet.* 11 (4): 259–272.

Tse, S.M., Tantisira, K., and Weiss, S.T. (2011). The pharmacogenetics and pharmacogenomics of asthma therapy. *Pharm. J.* 11: 383–392.

Veenstra, D.L. (2004). The interface between epidemiology and pharmacogenomics. In: *Human Genome Epidemiology* (eds. M.J. Khoury, J. Little and W. Burke), 234–246. New York: Oxford University Press.

Wang, Y., Localio, R., and Rebbeck, T.R. (2006). Evaluating bias due to population stratification in epidemiologic studies of gene–gene or gene–environment interactions. *Cancer Epidemiol. Biomark. Prev.* 15 (1): 124–132. https://doi.org/10.1158/1055-9965.EPI-05-0304. PMID: 16434597.

# 16

# Bioethical Issues in Pharmacoepidemiologic Research

*Laura E. Bothwell[1], Annika Richterich[2], and Jeremy Greene[3]*

[1] Yale School of Public Health, New Haven, Connecticut, USA
[2] Maastricht University, Maastricht, The Netherlands
[3] Johns Hopkins University, Baltimore, Maryland, USA

## Introduction

Because the bioethical issues involved in pharmacoepidemiologic research are closely related to changing patterns of drug usage and changing technologies of surveillance and data analysis, it is impossible to understand them without attention to historical and sociological perspectives. The field of pharmacoepidemiology emerged as a result of broader recent developments in medical therapeutics, concomitant to the expansion and refinement of the field of bioethics. Some key bioethical principles relevant to pharmacoepidemiologic research have remained significant over time, others have only gained attention in recent years. This chapter briefly introduces historical and sociological dimensions of pharmacoepidemiology from an international perspective, with an eye toward commonalities and differences in national variations in ethical approaches to the field.

It is widely believed that pharmacoepidemiologic studies should create data that benefit public health, improve drug safety, and ensure efficacy. The protection of research subjects' rights and safety, their wellbeing, dignity, autonomy and privacy, as well as the reliability and robustness of generated data are relatively

universal normative cornerstones of pharmacoepidemiology ethics. The same goes for the injunction that objectives and results of pharmacoepidemiologic research should be independent from economic and promotional interests of pharmaceutical companies or device manufacturers. Yet these principles are not simple to implement systematically at an international level. In this chapter, we explore the emergence and conduct of pharmacoepidemiologic research in three major global settings in which the field developed (North America, Europe, and East Asia) and some of the key challenges, tensions, and trends in historic and current international ethical policies toward pharmacoepidemiology.

## Clinical Problems to be Addressed by Pharmacoepidemiologic Research

### The Emergence, Changing Methods, and Moral Stakes of Pharmacoepidemiology in Twentieth Century North America

In 1962 a series of epidemiological reports initiated by the German physician Widukind Lenz connected a recent increase in phocomelia, a birth defect which resulted in grossly visible limb deformities, with maternal use of the popular new anti-nausea medicine Contergan (thalidomide). Images of thalidomide children became an international symbol of the ethical failure of the medical profession and the regulatory state to protect vulnerable populations from the harmful effects of widely marketed new drugs. Contergan had been extensively marketed to physicians and consumers alike, and its premarket testing and post-market promotion had emphasized its remarkably *nontoxic* safety profile by available standards of clinical pharmacology. As Lenz's work was read internationally, his careful use of the correlative techniques of infectious disease epidemiology within the terrain of prescription drug use documented not only the unseen dangers of newly marketed drugs but also the need for a new discipline of pharmaceutical epidemiology to scour observational data for therapeutic effects and adverse reactions that could clearly be associated with drug use in clinical practice.

The recognition that the risks of new drugs could be better understood when they were consumed by broad numbers of patients had been evident long before Lenz's epidemiology of thalidomide-associated phocomelia. Indeed, the history of federal drug regulation in the United States can be recounted as a succession of measures taken in response to dangers of drugs that became apparent after widespread consumption by the general public. However, until the 1960s the Food and Drug Administration (FDA) had very limited authority in the post-market regulation of drugs. The agency had neither direct means to control physician prescriptions nor resources to gather data on prescribing of newly marketed drugs. While the Committee on Pharmacy and Chemistry of the American Medical Association (AMA) nominally maintained more influence in both arenas, it depended entirely upon voluntary physician reports, and Committee members complained loudly that the system itself was doomed to failure; as one report noted, "physicians reported only a small fraction of all cases and the total number of patients receiving a drug was unknown."

The 1962 Kefauver-Harris Amendments – passed largely on the strength of popular moral outrage over thalidomide – demanded pharmaceutical manufacturers establish records and make reports to the FDA of "data relating to clinical experience and other data or information, received or otherwise obtained" for all new drugs. By 1967 the agency had developed a protocol requiring manufacturers to seek and report any reported or published case reports related to putative side effects of their marketed products. Any novel or unexpected adverse effect was to be reported to the agency within 15 days; other information "pertinent to the safety or effectiveness of the drug" was to be reported quarterly for the first year after approval, twice in the second year, and annually thereafter. Yet this kind of information could become actionable only after years of case reports, and then only if one of the relatively few FDA staffers took active interest in pursuit of a specific question of drug harm.

The hospital became the center of early programs of pharmacoepidemiologic surveillance. By 1964, the FDA and AMA had built a surveillance program involving more than 600 hospitals, which became the focus of early pharmacoepidemiologic research by Johns Hopkins University's Leighton Cluff, Harvard University's Thomas Chalmers, and Tufts University's Hershel Jick. Yet the data were still only as good as the reporting physicians' records. As Leighton Cluff noted, an early validation system of reporting efforts at the Johns Hopkins Hospital "proved completely unsatisfactory for detecting drug reactions. . .[d]uring recent daily intensive surveillance of one hospital service, four times as many reactions were detected than had been reported on the cards from the entire hospital." Would-be epidemiologists of adverse drug effects needed a way to circumvent the physician as reporting device – and the digitization of data provided an appealing solution. Cluff's attempts at computerized drug monitoring involved the creation of three linked datasets for every drug received by every patient in a dedicated hospital ward. D. J. Finney, another early theorist of computerized drug monitoring, expressed these data sets as a linked "P-D-E system," in which P(atient) population data would be systematically gathered within a set geographic or hospital catchment area, the D(rug) data would include records of all relevant prescriptions, and E(vent) collection would record all untoward reactions potentially attributable to the drugs prescribed.

Proponents of drug monitoring imagined a linked system of inpatient surveillance wards circling the globe, which could act as pharmacovigilance sensors, detecting early signals of possible drug harms and providing descriptive data regarding their frequency, severity, and relative strength of association. Finney predicted that surveillance would change pharmacoepidemiology from a reactive into a proactive field. Allowing that "much is due to Lenz for his discovery in 1961 [that thalidomide was associated with phocomelia]," he also boasted that "a *monitor* could have signaled a warning 1½–2 years earlier." Automated inpatient surveillance systems liberated pharmacoepidemiology from the "weak link" of the reporting physician. With public and private support from the United States Public Health Service and the Pharmaceutical Manufacturers Association, Dennis Slone, Hershel Jick, and Ivan Borda demonstrated the feasibility of implementing an automated hospital-based drug monitor system in 1966. Based at the Lemuel Shattuck Hospital, the Boston Collaborative Drug Surveillance Program bypassed the physician by hiring a drug surveillance nurse "whose primary role is the acquisition of accurate data." The Boston team became a model for an automated drug surveillance program that functioned "largely independent of clinical judgment in establishing a connection between a drug and an adverse event."

Early results showed that drug-related events were both more frequent and less severe than had previously been anticipated. More than one-third of patients on the Shattuck wards experienced at least one drug-associated adverse reaction during the first year of study. By 1967 the Boston group had established a numerator/denominator approach for comparing drug usage between long-term and acute hospitals through a network of five hospitals in Boston. By 1968, over 2500 patients had been entered and discharged from the surveillance system, with over 26 000 monitored drug exposures, representing more than 700 individual drugs. Commonly-prescribed drugs, such as digoxin and heparin, could be reported in detail, yielding novel information related to their clinical pharmacology and their interactions with other drugs. The system enabled the observation of not only obvious drug reactions (such as a rash) but also other clinical events (such as heart attacks or kidney failure) that could only be associated with drugs by careful epidemiologic surveillance.

As the Boston Collaborative Drug Surveillance Program escalated its activities and exported its methods to other sites, these new data provoked a series of drug scandals that emphasized both the utility and the limitations of the new forms of pharmacovigilance. Clioquinol, an anti-infective that had been in use since the 1930s, was found to be associated with subacute myelo-optic neuropathy in 1970, over three decades after its initial introduction. An association between the synthetic estrogen diethylstilbestrol (DES) and a rare form of cervical clear cell adenoma was reported in 1971, with evidence of a 20-year latency period between the use of the drug and detection of the cancer. The beta-blocker practolol became the focus of a broad scandal after it was associated with a potentially fatal inflammation of the skin and soft tissues (oculomucocutaneous syndrome) some five years after its broad release on the British market. These examples simultaneously elucidated the scientific and ethical necessity for drug surveillance units and underscored the impossibility of inpatient surveillance systems to capture drug-disease associations in which three decades or more might pass between drug exposure and adverse events. As Jick warned, in a systematic proposal for the theory and design of the emerging field of pharmacoepidemiology, the ability to study "drug-illness relations" required distinct methods depending on the time course and prevalence of prescription-related adverse events. High-frequency events in high-prevalence diseases could be detected swiftly by case report, low-frequency events in high-prevalence diseases required careful active ongoing surveillance, and low-frequency events in low-prevalence diseases might simply never be adequately described.

Many early pharmacoepidemiologic researchers viewed scientific quality and ethics as complementary: more rigorous data collection of drug-related events carried ethical benefits by enhancing medical practitioners' capacity to "do no harm" to patients. As early pharmacoepidemiologic work also coincided with the development of bioethics as a field, critical principles of informed consent, external review of research protocols, and protection of patient privacy began to influence pharmacoepidemiologic investigators' thinking in the US and internationally, as described below.

To address the growing problems of drug safety, prescription surveillance needed to extend outwards: spatially, from the monitored wards of the hospital to the messier universe of outpatient care; temporally, from links visible in days or weeks of measurable hospital time to the longer stretches of months and years required to understand the impacts of chronic medication use; and thematically, from the isolated connection of drug and disease to the study of all steps of diagnosis, prescription, adherence, consumption, and presentation that might extend in between. In the United States, this project would find its boldest form in the Joint Commission on Prescription Drug Use, formed in response to a press conference held by Senator Edward Kennedy on 30 November 1976, at which he announced that the new science of drug utilization studies

had provided irrefutable evidence that prescription drugs were ill-used in American society. Kennedy called for Congress to work with the medical profession and the pharmaceutical industry to sponsor a public-private body of expertise whose explicit purpose would be to establish a post-market surveillance system for prescription drugs. As the Commission would note in its final report, the purpose of systematic prescription surveillance was "not merely to learn 'something' about a drug but to glean information that is useful in improving the rational use of drugs."

Conceived as a public-private venture, the Commission ran from 1976 until 1979 and issued its final report in the first month of 1980. The Commission worked to integrate the social, epidemiological, marketing, and policy interests in prescriptions as a source of data. Initially, the prospects for a harmonization of these four perspectives seemed auspicious. At the first meeting, Howard L. Binkley, Vice President for Research and Planning of the Pharmaceutical Manufacturers Association, provided a description and critique of presently available sources of data on trends in the prescribing and dispensing of prescription drugs, with an emphasis on how market research data could be linked to broader systems of private and public claims and outcomes data. Yet as the Commission assessed its findings by 1979, it became clear that although several data sets existed, no individual data set contained enough information to deliver sufficient granularity to allow the full assessment of drug use in outpatient practice.

The Commission began to interview hybrid data sources that illustrated new links between the public and private nature of prescriber data sets. Fledgling health maintenance organizations such as Kaiser Permanente and the Group Health Cooperative of Puget Sound developed in-house proprietary databases that linked both prescription claims and outcomes data in the same place. Exploratory work by Hershel Jick following the use of the blockbuster anti-ulcer drug Tagamet (cimetidine) in Puget Sound pharmacies suggested that this approach could be quite promising indeed. Another hybrid form was introduced by Noel Munson, a spokesman from Prescription Card Services (PCS), a private prescription data company that acted as a "fiscal intermediary" for public payment groups like Medicare and Medicaid and other groups that paid for prescription drugs. But these individual companies (e.g. PCS) appeared to code their data according to their own proprietary software. Even within the Medicaid system, the promise of effortless data linkage remained a dream in the late 1970s, complicated by wide state-by-state discrepancies in patterns of coding, storing, and retrieving prescription data.

If the 1980 publication of the Joint Commission report represented a high point of collaboration between market researchers, epidemiologists, policy reformers, and sociologists in imagining an early "big data" universe for therapeutic surveillance, it also represented a dream of collaborative work that would soon dissipate. Like many other grand designs for federally-sponsored health programs conceived in the later 1970s and proposed in the early 1980s, its speculative structures would never materialize, its measures would be left unfunded, and subsequent calls for a center for post-marketing surveillance would be repeated, and unfunded, every few years for several decades. Only in the past decade, with the passage of the Food and Drug Administration Amendments Act of 2007 (FDAAA), would a substantial US public investment be made in the construction of a linked public prescription database for pharmacoepidemiologic research with the creation of the FDA's new automated pharmacovigilance program, the Sentinel Initiative, which officially launched in 2016.

## European Pharmacoepidemiologic Trends and Ethics

In Europe, several nations with centralized national health systems like England and Sweden created prescription surveillance systems by the second half of the twentieth century. Scandinavian countries in particular had long histories of centrally organized pharmacy records and more tightly controlled national formularies of allowable drugs. Moreover, the World Health Organization had set up a regional European Drug Utilization Group in Oslo which held a prominent conference on the overprescribing of prescription drugs in 1969 and then proceeded to develop methods of comparing utilization across drug classes and across national pharmacy standards. Ironically, even in countries such as Sweden, much of the prescription data came from the private sector. Still, pharmacoepidemiologic research in Europe continued to receive substantial public support throughout the 1970s, 1980s, and 1990s.

The founding of the European Medicines Agency (EMA) in 1995 was a crucial step toward a pan-European supervision of medicines. The decentralized agency is critical to the European Medicines Regulatory Network (EMRN), partnering with the European Commission (EC) and national authorities of European Economic Area (EEA) member states (the Heads of Medicines Agencies [HMA] network). The EMRN's main objective is to achieve a consistent approach to medicines regulation across the European Union (EU). In collaboration with the network partners, the EMA oversees the scientific evaluation, safety and efficacy monitoring of human (and veterinary) medicines in the EU. For most innovative medicines, including those for rare diseases, a central assessment and marketing authorization coordinated by the EMA is compulsory. In cases of human medicines, the EMA's Committee for Medicinal Products for Human Use (CHMP) carries out a scientific assessment, based on which the EC decides whether to grant marketing authorization. Once granted, such a centralized marketing authorization is valid across the EU. Predominantly though, medicines in the EU are authorized by member states' national authorities.

Shared, key ethical requirements in European pharmacoepidemiologic research came to include beneficence, transparency, scientific independence, and integrity. Yet, inconsistent application and authorization procedures for clinical studies in EU and EEA member states have long been criticized. This also applies to pharmacoepidemiology and pharmacovigilance. Especially for multinational, non-interventional studies (NIS), it has been lamented that "[. . .] a patchwork of regulations and codes of conduct have to be followed."

Partly in response to some of these issues, since the early 2000s new EU regulations, directives and guidelines have been introduced. These aim to facilitate ethical, effective pharmacoepidemiologic practices in and across different member states. Currently, crucial regulatory changes are underway that will affect pharmacoepidemiology and pharmacovigilance in the EU.

The EU pharmacovigilance legislation aims to minimize risks and harms posed by adverse drug reactions (ADRs). Its implementation is overseen by the EMA, EU member state authorities, and the EC. Key legal documents for the pharmacovigilance legislation and pharmacoepidemiologic studies are EU regulation No. 1235/2010 and directive 2010/84/EC. In effect since 2012, the regulation outlines measures for safeguarding patients' safety and rights and asserts the crucial role of healthcare professionals in reporting ADRs. It moreover acknowledges the necessity to develop EU/EEA wide "[. . .] harmonized guiding principles for, and regulatory supervision of, post-authorization safety studies that are requested by competent authorities and that are non-interventional, that are initiated, managed or financed by the marketing authorization holder." Among other deliverables, the regulation established the EudraVigilance database as a main platform for the obligatory reporting of ADRs by marketing authorization holders and respective national authorities.

In response to the benfluorex scandal, the legislation was amended in 2012. Servier pharmaceuticals' Mediator (benfluorex), marketed as an add-on for diabetes and hyperlipidemia, was under pharmacovigilance investigation in France since 1998. It was found in 2003 that the drug caused cardiovascular complications. In response, Servier did not re-apply for marketing authorization in Spain and Italy, effectively withdrawing the product from the market in those countries. However, benfluorex continued to be available and approved for diabetes treatment in France and other countries until 2009. Only then was the benfluorex authorization fully revoked; its efficacy was found to be limited and it risked causing cardiac valvulopathy. Subsequently, EU regulation No. 1027/2012 and Directive 2012/26/EC were published, amending the 2010 EU pharmacovigilance legislation. The amendments especially addressed the issue that safety measures for medicinal products need to be implemented consistently and in a timely fashion in all member states where respective products were authorized.

The benfluorex scandal points to broader challenges regarding pharmacovigilance and pharmacoepidemiologic research in the EU: regulations and guidelines need to be applied across multiple states and to different actors, including national marketing authorization holders and applicants. While the legislation outlines fairly broad objectives, responsibilities, and issues, these are specified in concrete deliverables. One of these deliverables was the founding of the EMA Pharmacovigilance Risk Assessment Committee (PRAC) which monitors and assesses drug safety in the EU. Moreover, it initiated the development of the EMA's Good Pharmacovigilance Practices (GVP) guideline, (described below).

The European Network of Centres for Pharmacoepidemiology and Pharmacovigilance (ENCePP) was established in 2006 and is coordinated by the EMA. It is an expertise and resource network focused on pharmacoepidemiology and pharmacovigilance in Europe. It consists of partners that are public and not-for-profit organizations, including research and pharmacovigilance centers, university hospitals, healthcare database hosts, and electronic registry sponsors. For-profit organizations, e.g. contract research institutions, may only participate if they conduct pharmacoepidemiologic and/or pharmacovigilance studies commissioned by third parties. While pharmaceutical companies are not eligible for becoming ENCePP partners, the network provides relevant resources and allows for these companies to be involved in public document reviews.

The ENCePP offers crucial guideline documents for pharmacoepidemiology and pharmacovigilance: a Code of Conduct; the ENCePP Checklist for Study Protocols; and the ENCePP Guide on Methodological Standards in Pharmacoepidemiology. The Code lays down rules and principles aimed at ensuring transparency and scientific independence. While adherence to the Code is voluntary, it is required to receive the ENCePP Seal. Conditions for receiving the Seal are, among others, that a study is entered in the EU post-authorization study (PAS) Register and that it is of scientific and public health relevance, rather than mainly pursuing results which may promote certain medicinal products. The Checklist is meant to ensure that studies adhere to epidemiological principles, while also considering methodological transparency and the need for public outreach.

## East Asian Pharmacoepidemiologic Trends and Ethics

East Asian investigators have made major contributions to the field of pharmacoepidemiology. Researchers in South Korea, Japan, and Taiwan have linked into comprehensive data systems on insurance claims created through universal insurance coverage of these entire national populations. To help protect patient privacy, these databases have been made available for drug safety research only to researchers in non-profit organizations who must apply and undergo ethical review.

The Korea Food and Drug Administration (KFDA) launched an ADR reporting system in 1988, although the reporting rate was initially very low. In 2004, the KFDA mandated that pharmacists and pharmaceutical companies report ADRs. The KFDA also established regional pharmacovigilance centers in university hospitals that now provide nearly complete coverage of the country. The KFDA funded a pharmacovigilance research network (PVNet) among these centers, and researchers in the network use their data for studying adverse events. The Korean national health insurance (NHI) database also contains all information on insurance claims made and prescriptions for approximately 50 million Koreans, and this has been used for pharmacovigilance.

In Japan, drug manufacturers are required to report ADRs to the Pharmaceuticals and Medical Devices Agency (PMDA). A partial ADR dataset is available to researchers through the PMDA website. Healthcare professionals report adverse drug events to the Ministry of Health, Labor and Welfare. Japan made its national insurance claims database available for drug safety researchers in 2011. The database covers the entire population of 128 million and includes basic patient characteristics, drug prescription and dispensing, medical procedures, hospital admission, and annual health check data (for some patients). To protect patient privacy, Japan's national database is usually not available for purchase and may only be shared in some cooperative research projects. The Japanese government has also created the Medical Information for Risk Assessment Initiative (MIHARI) to access data from different sources and create a central database with a common data format.

Taiwan requires mandatory reporting of serious adverse reactions by medical institutions, pharmacies, and drug and device companies, as well as obligatory safety reports for newly marketed drugs over a five-year surveillance period. In Taiwan, the National Adverse Drug Reactions Reporting System has been the primary source for post-marketing surveillance of adverse drug events. Taiwan's single-payer NHI program was created in 1995 and covers more than 99% of the population. The NHI Research Database is thus a highly comprehensive data set including basic patient data, care record and expenditure claims, and pharmaceutical reimbursements. There are also subject datasets available to researchers on topics such as traditional Chinese medicine, cancer, diabetes, dental, catastrophic illness, or psychiatric care. Patients and medical facilities are de-identified for pharmacoepidemiologic research use of the NHI Research Database. To protect patient privacy, researchers using Taiwan's NHI Research Database also receive data for 10% or less of the population. Ethical policies for data privacy stipulate that no individual-level data can be shared with researchers from other countries.

China and other East Asian countries also have been creating national healthcare claims databases. In China, the Shanghai Center for Adverse Drug Reaction Monitoring has operated a drug surveillance and evaluation system since 2001 that works with patient information from 10 Shanghai hospitals. The Asian Pharmacoepidemiology Network (AsPEN) was recently established as a multi-national research network for pharmacoepidemiological research that promotes international communication among academia, government, industry, and consumers. The network functions to promptly identify drug safety issues.

Pharmacoepidemiology ethics in East Asia are similar in many ways to those of Western countries, including features such as institutional ethical review and guiding principles such as beneficence, justice, autonomy, and data privacy. However, experts on East Asian bioethics have also recognized some distinctions. For example, scholars have contended that much East Asian bioethical thinking reflects value systems that emphasize the family and public interest ahead of the individual

rights of the liberal subject that characterize much of Western bioethics. The family is often depicted as responsible for taking care of members who become sick, and medical decision-making has often been family-based. Some have also noted a plurality of ethical perspectives within East Asia, contending that a simple Eastern and Western bioethical dichotomy of communitarian versus individualistic values would be overly simplistic. Others have viewed bioethics as a Western entity, promoting the development of Asian bioethics based more on the traditions, philosophies, religions, and perspectives of the region's cultures. Future policies should consider these issues as core principles for pharmacoepidemiologic research ethics are discussed.

## Methodologic Problems to be Solved by Pharmacoepidemiologic Research

More work remains to establish international ethical policy harmonization while also promoting practices that support cultural variation in ethical values. Yet, as pharmacoepidemiological practices developed in different national contexts that have been incorporated into increasingly globalized flows of pharmaceuticals and pharmaceutical-related information, a number of ethical principles and practices have been adopted widely across international settings in an effort to establish consistent pharmacoepidemiologic methodology. The expansion of the field of pharmacoepidemiology has coincided with the establishment and institutionalization of the discipline of bioethics. Numerous critical ethical concepts took hold early in pharmacoepidemiology and have remained significant over time. For example, privacy of medical data is a historically consistent value, guiding the ethics of global pharmacoepidemiologic research. Pharmacoepidemiologic research protocols and/or database designs have also often been subjected to evaluation by institutional review boards as external review has become increasingly widespread for biomedical research since the second half of the twentieth century, although there is variation in the nature of this review (for example, some pharmacoepidemiologic research has been reviewed by institutional or national ethics boards, as well as by privacy boards). Some countries also do not require ethical review for de-identified data sets.

## Informed Consent

Informed consent became increasingly valued as a critical standard of international research ethics following its establishment as a cornerstone of the 1964 Declaration of Helsinki, a groundbreaking statement of international human experimentation ethics. However, the role of informed consent has been perceived differently in interventional versus non-interventional research studies. Many ethicists of international human subject research have argued that since pharmacoepidemiologic research involves relatively low risks to participants, patient consent is necessary only for studies that involve contact with patients/research subjects, such as for direct intervention or prospective gathering of information. There has been a broad acceptance among ethicists allowing researcher access to identifiable medical records for pharmacoepidemiologic research without explicit individual subject authorization. Research has also found that public opinion has echoed the views of professional ethicists that pharmacoepidemiologists should be permitted to use identifiable patient records, without patient consent, to study drug safety as long as existing ethical guidelines and relevant laws are followed.

A number of nations, however, require explicit informed consent from each study participant, and there are also international variations in requirements for electronic consent versus hard copy written consent. Ethical regulatory disharmony causes differences in study

conduct between countries and increases the cost of assembling multinational data. This poses challenges for conducting large international studies capable of detecting rare events. Additionally, requirements of explicit individual informed consent are problematic in that they can corrupt data by preventing a post-marketing pharmacoepidemiologic study from detecting fatal or serious events since people who have died are unable to provide informed consent. Thus, it is unsurprising that ethicists weighing risks and benefits have tended to contend that individual consent is not essential for the use of patient records in pharmacoepidemiologic research.

However, over time it has become normative that pharmacoepidemiologists must also meet certain requirements when conducting research in which participant consent is waived. These requirements often include that the use of protected health information involves no more than minimal risk to patients, the research could not be effectively conducted without access to the protected health information and/or the waiver of individual consent, the privacy risks to individuals are reasonable in relation to any value to the individuals of the knowledge expected to result from the study, there is a sound plan to protect patients from the improper use or disclosure of their information, there is a plan to destroy identifiers at the earliest opportunity consistent with the research, and the data will not be shared with external parties to the research.

Recent attention has been given to the waiver of patient informed consent to use data on substances of abuse or drugs that carry social stigma. Patient privacy is essential in these areas of research; however, requiring informed consent for each patient or allowing retraction of sensitive drug information from patient records leads to partial data sets that impede the ability of researchers to study the impact of these substances on patient health outcomes. The negative consequences of failing to collect sound pharmacoepidemiologic data on the health effects of these substances are likely worse than the relatively minimal risk associated with waiver of patient consent. However, in such circumstances, the highest precautions should be taken to protect patient privacy, such as de-identifying data through secure codes or potentially having extra ethics training requirements for all researchers using data on stigmatized or abused substances.

## Ethics of Surveillance

Surveillance has long evoked public concern regarding privacy, confidentiality, and autonomy. This is relevant to post-marketing surveillance, since health information is seen as highly sensitive and personal. Thus, pharmacoepidemiologic researchers need to balance possible risks to a larger population against the harms concerning individuals, such as a possible infringement of privacy. While privacy is highly important to the ethics of pharmacoepidemiologic research, privacy is not an absolute value, nor does it seem to have been perceived as such in public health surveillance history. Rather, privacy is one of multiple values that are balanced in public health surveillance. It has been argued that ensuring privacy is part of the broader value of protecting autonomy. Yet other key principles to be balanced in pharmacoepidemiologic research include beneficence to promote research that adds to the existing knowledge base of medicine to improve patient health and prevent mortality; non-maleficence, or the prevention of patient harm; and justice, which manifests as the fair distribution of research burdens and benefits among people.

Risks of surveillance can be minimized through confidentiality and data anonymization. Such strategies are ethically imperative, since they safeguard individuals' rights, privacy, autonomy, and dignity. Applying the highest ethical standards and communicating with the public about potential criticism is also important for a positive public perception of pharmacoepidemiology.

While there have been some disagreements, international ethics policies have developed some common stances toward ethical review of drug surveillance. Certain pharmacoepidemiologic research tends to qualify as exempt from ethics board review or qualifies for expedited review by an ethics board chair or a designated member. For studies in which it is not possible for investigators to identify the individual patients, ethics board review is often not required. For example, the US 45 Code of Federal Regulations 46.101 exempts from institutional review "research involving the collection or study of existing data, documents, records, pathological specimens, or diagnostic specimens, if these sources are publicly available or if the information is recorded by the investigator in such a manner that subjects cannot be identified, directly or through identifiers linked to the subjects." In many countries, research is also often eligible for expedited review if it poses no more than minimal risk to patients and involves a retrospective analysis of existing records. Still, ethics review policies vary internationally and by institutional practice, depending inter alia on respective national/state regulations, posing challenges for global collaborative studies. This may lead to inconsistent risk–benefit assessments and variations in balancing subjects' protection (e.g. regarding safety and privacy) against public health interests.

## Ethical Benefits of Pharmacoepidemiologic Research for Data Integrity

From a broader ethical perspective, it is increasingly clear that the expansion of pharmacoepidemiological research can provide added benefits to drug research by detecting groups at risk for adverse events. Thus, the field can play an important role in reducing drug safety data inequalities. For example, expanding drug outcomes data for groups such as minorities or small/rare genetic subpopulations who may have treatment outcome variations that can only be identified and/or adequately quantified and measured through large post-marketing pharmacoepidemiologic studies may provide substantial benefits for members of these populations. There is also limited data on the efficacy and safety of drugs in children due to the fact that historically, children have often not been included in randomized controlled trials (RCTs). Pharmacoepidemiologic research helps to fill these research gaps. However, it would be ethically problematic for pharmacoepidemiology to be relied on solely to provide missing data on children, minorities, or other subgroups in lieu of RCTs, particularly in cases when RCTs could produce more robust data.

Further, pharmacoepidemiologic studies are usually conducted after drug approval, and there is high variability in the frequency and design of post-marketing pharmacoepidemiologic research. Such studies are not necessarily required, and so are not a consistently reliable source of information on drug outcomes among diverse demographic groups. Clinical trials are usually required for drug approval and are thus a mechanism for ensuring broader implementation of policies requiring the inclusion of diverse research subjects. Ultimately, consistent with recurring concerns over ethical practices in pharmacoepidemiologic research in general, ethicists have noted that pharmacoepidemiology related to subpopulations would benefit from a more explicit legal ethical framework, particularly to clarify ethical requirements for data sharing.

## Problems of Conflicts of Interest for Drug Industry Research

Academia-industry collaborations have become a critical area of concern for the ethics of pharmacoepidemiologic research, particularly in recent decades as pharmaceutical profits have soared and the stakes have been raised for the outcomes of research on drug safety and efficacy. There is an inherent conflict of interest in research that is funded by drug companies to assess their own products. Academic settings in which researcher success and

advancement depend on obtaining external funding also can exacerbate the ethical problems resulting from direct relationships between drug companies and the pharmacoepidemiologists evaluating their products. Investigators in such environments are under professional pressure to secure funding, and in a climate of heightened competition for public funding sources, an academician who establishes a positive working relationship with a pharmaceutical research sponsor may increase his/her chances of obtaining future funding from that sponsor. This can create an incentive, whether subconscious or acknowledged, for researchers to conduct studies that sponsoring drug companies will find favorable. Indeed, studies have shown a trend toward more favorable efficacy results and conclusions for industry-sponsored drug research than research sponsored by other sources, finding a bias in industry-funded research that cannot be otherwise explained by standard assessments of risk of bias. There are a number of feasible solutions to address the ethical conflicts of interest in industry-funded research, as described below.

## Currently Available Solutions

### Good Pharmacoepidemiology and Pharmacovigilance Practices

The International Society for Pharmacoepidemiology (ISPE) has created Guidelines for Good Pharmacoepidemiology Practice (GPP), which provide a model for key pharmacoepidemiologic research ethics policies. The guidelines recommend that researchers include a description of quality control procedures; plans for protecting human subjects; confidentiality provisions; ethical conditions under which a study would terminate; the use of Data Safety Monitoring Boards where appropriate; institutional review board and informed consent considerations in accordance with local laws; research study registration; and plans for disseminating study results. However, ISPE GPP policies are nonbinding and therefore do not resolve concerns regarding national variations in ethical oversight and requirements by regulatory agencies for post-marketing pharmacoepidemiologic work.

EU policies provide a useful example of transnational efforts at regulatory standardization of GVPs. EU documents concerning biomedical research in general and pharmacoepidemiologic research in particular commonly speak of two types of clinical studies, broadly speaking: interventional, i.e. experimental, and non-interventional, sometimes called observational research. On the one hand, pharmacoepidemiologic research relies on non-interventional study designs such as case–control or cohort studies. On the other hand, interventional, randomized clinical trials (RCTs) are an important element of post-marketing pharmacoepidemiology studies (see Chapter 17).

The EMA defines GVPs as "a set of measures drawn up to facilitate the performance of the safety monitoring of medicines in the European Union." It includes chapters on pharmacovigilance processes as well as product- and population-specific considerations. For EU pharmacoepidemiologic post-authorization safety studies (PASS), module VIII is particularly relevant. PASS may be interventional or non-interventional. Although the module touches upon interventional studies too, emphasis is put on non-interventional PASS.

In accordance with the EU pharmacovigilance legislation, the GVP stipulates that the EMA needs to ensure that protocols and abstracts of PASS results are published. While the primary/lead investigator is responsible for the information provided, the registration may be made by, for example, research center staff or representatives of pharmaceutical companies funding a study. Where possible, this should be done before the study commences. Practically, registration and publication are processed through the EU PAS register, hosted by the ENCePP. As the ethics review procedure and requirements for respective committees depend on national legislation, information on individual application procedures is not included in the GVP. While there is no EU regulation or directive for NIS, interventional studies are covered in the Clinical Trials Regulation (CTR).

In the EU, methodological, ethical, and legal requirements for pharmacoepidemiologic research hinge significantly on whether a study is categorized as a "clinical trial" or as "non-interventional/non-experimental." Both categories are defined as "clinical studies" aimed at discovering or confirming the (adverse) effects of medicinal products. For pharmacoepidemiologic studies involving clinical trials, the introduction of the EU CTR No. 536/2014 will soon be decisive. The CTR was adopted on 16 April 2014 and entered into force on 16 June 2014. For the regulation to become applicable, an EU-wide clinical trials portal and database is required. Both need to undergo an independent audit. According to the EMA, the Regulation was supposed to come into application in late 2019, starting a transition period of three years. However, due to technical difficulties concerning the platform and database, this has been postponed and EMA's Management Board agreed to proceed with the audit in December 2020 (see European Commission n.d.). The CTR is meant to harmonize research practices and to ensure the highest methodological and ethical standards across all EU as well as EEA EFTA (European Economic Area, European Free Trade Association) member states. To what extent it will deliver on these promises is under discussion. The regulation replaces the "Clinical Trials Directive" 2001/20/EC which is said to have "[. . .] failed to achieve its goal of simplifying the scientific and ethical review of clinical trials in the EU."

Moreover, the ENCePP had problematized the NIS definition given in the 2001 directive. The ENCePP raised the issue that the definition was not sufficiently specific and created uncertainty as to what counts as NIS or RCT. Pharmacoepidemiologic prospective case-control studies – like the International Primary Pulmonary Hypertension Study investigation of primary pulmonary hypertension (PPH) occurrence in association with anorectic agents – would classify as a clinical trial according to the 2001 directive. Its ambiguous NIS definition was thus criticized for impeding the conduct of pharmacoepidemiologic studies.

The ENCePP Guide on Methodological Standards in Pharmacoepidemiology (Revision 6, July 2017) lays down rules and principles for transparency and scientific independence. Chapter 9 of the Guide deals with ethical aspects of pharmacoepidemiology, focusing on patient and data protection and scientific integrity and ethical conduct. It identifies key values based on documents such as the ADVANCE Code of Conduct for Collaborative Vaccine Studies, the GPPs of the ISPE, and the Good Epidemiology Practice (GEP) guidelines of the International Epidemiological Association. The Guide highlights that "[p]rinciples of scientific integrity and ethical conduct are paramount in any medical research" and points out that the abovementioned ENCePP code of conduct "[. . .] offers standards for scientific independence and transparency of research in pharmacoepidemiology and pharmacovigilance." In addition, the Guide highlights core values, such as best science, strengthening public health, and improving transparency, as stressed by the ADVANCE Code of Conduct. It moreover emphasizes the need for ensuring scientific autonomy, beneficence, non-maleficence and justice, according to the four general ethical principles defined in the GEP guidelines.

## Protections against Conflicts of Interest for Drug Industry-Sponsored Research

While industry-sponsored research creates real challenges for conflicts of interest, industry also has an interest in maintaining public trust in product integrity, as well as an interest in compliance with regulatory ethical and methodological requirements to obtain drug approval. Thus, there is some incentive for industry to address concerns about conflicts of interest. The Board of Directors of the ISPE has published a set of principles for academia-industry collaboration that can be helpful in managing industry conflicts of interest. It includes the importance of transparent research agreements, open and complete disclosure of conflicts of interest, registration of research protocols in public sites such as the ENCePP registry or http://ClinicalTrials.gov, compliance with local laws, clarity on confidentiality of proprietary information while also ensuring reporting of all relevant and important information to regulators, the potential value of having a steering committee and/or an independent advisory committee to the research, and an obligation to disseminate and publish research findings of potential scientific or public health importance irrespective of results.

While all of these principles are helpful in managing financial conflicts of interest, they do not eliminate the inherent problem of drug companies having a stake in the outcomes of research that they sponsor or the ethical concerns associated with the power dynamics of industry directly funding investigators as described above. To eliminate these underlying ethical problems, the direct relationships in which companies fund individual investigators to assess specific products would need to be severed. Alternative models that eliminate these ethical conflicts can be easily envisaged. For example, the British Drug Safety Research Unit (DSRU), an independent charity supported by the National Health Service, conducts publicly funded pharmacoepidemiologic research. Still, the organization conducts a large amount of research funded by unconditional donations from pharmaceutical companies. Yet, the companies have no control on the conduct or the publication of the studies conducted by the DSRU. This helps to mitigate the pressure of inherent conflicts of interest in industry-funded research. Given that industry funding may lead to biased study results, a comprehensive solution could build from the DSRU model, for example by requiring sponsors of new drugs to contribute an unconditional fee to drug regulators that would fund pharmacoepidemiologic research. By making such contributions mandatory rather than voluntary, investigators could conduct studies without concern as to whether results may influence future industry donation decisions. In the US, for example, the expansion of the FDA's Prescription Drug User Fee could easily establish a fund for pharmacoepidemiologic research.

## The Future

The ethical conduct of pharmacoepidemiologic studies is of crucial importance for subjects' safety, health and wellbeing. Moreover, it is decisive for the public perception of pharmacoepidemiology. Research in this field is rooted in the moral obligation to preempt or at least minimize medicine-related harms and health hazards. Implementing highest ethical standards helps to avoid potential damage to the public image of the field and public trust in claims of pharmacoepidemiological research as a disinterested form of expert knowledge. Such damage may be related to research practices compromised by economic interests or misconduct of the pharmaceutical industry. Thus, scientific integrity, independence, and transparency will continue to be crucial for the ethics of pharmacoepidemiologic research.

Even in the recent past, regulatory amendments relevant to pharmacoepidemiology and pharmacovigilance were often triggered by scandals, although a dream to make pharmacoepidemiology a proactive, rather than a reactive, field can be traced back to the 1960s if not earlier. Adjusted, new, and emerging regulations and guidelines aim at promoting ethical pharmacoepidemiologic research that effectively identifies and reports ADRs, thus allowing for timely responses. New policies must also be more thoroughly transnational and attentive to global variations in ethical beliefs. A main challenge is and will be to translate inevitably general documents into practical instructions and relevant local practices.

In the future, national regulatory authorities, universities, and research centers will continue working to align requirements toward coherent pharmacoepidemiologic research ethics. It is to be expected that further regulatory efforts will be invested in streamlining requirements for ethics review boards and ethical guidelines for NIS, especially across the EU. Although recent regulations and directives in the EU hope to address several, pressing issues, many of these are complicated anew by the United Kingdom's announced withdrawal from the EU. This has already triggered practical changes, such as the relocation of the EMA from London to Amsterdam in March 2019. Moreover, legal uncertainties are underway, as it has been disclosed by the *UK Department for Exiting the European Union* that the post-Brexit guidelines for clinical studies in the UK may deviate from EU legislation.

Transparency has been stressed as a key element for ensuring ethical pharmacoepidemiologic practices. Moreover, data sharing is pivotal for effective pharmacoepidemiology and pharmacovigilance. At the same time, researchers are required to safeguard the subjects' privacy and dignity. Developments such as the open data movement on the one hand and regulations aimed at protecting individuals' privacy on the other hand put researchers in a difficult position. At an increasing rate, there is a tendency to require public accessibility of scientific results and even data. Simultaneously, privacy concerns and potential regulations may pose challenges for data (re-)use in pharmacoepidemiologic studies.

Heightened attention has already been paid to the environmental, polluting effects of pharmaceutical residues. Regulatory documents, such as the EU pharmacovigilance legislation, acknowledge that "[t]he pollution of waters and soils with pharmaceutical residues is an emerging environmental problem." Research examining the adverse effects of pharmaceuticals on the environment has been labeled as *pharmacoenvironmentology*. With its focus on the environmental impact of drugs given at therapeutic doses, it is considered part of pharmacovigilance. Assuming that environmental issues will continue to be high on the political and scientific agenda, pharmacoepidemiologic expertise will be increasingly needed to assess medicines as pollutants. In this context, pharmacoepidemiologists will need to employ and expand their methodological repertoire for studies investigating medicines' adverse effects on the environment. This development might also imply an amplified need for novel, interdisciplinary research collaboration involving pharmacoepidemiologists. Such collaboration is also characteristic for another emerging intersection, between pharmacoepidemiology, computer, and data science.

Research at the intersection of digital services, big data, and public health is a potentially promising, but precarious field. It has been demonstrated that emerging, digital data sources like social networking sites can function as complementary resources for pharmacoepidemiology. The use of such data sources, often referred to as a type of "big data," is atypical for pharmacoepidemiologic studies, but may become more common in the future. Research drawing on "big data" may take place outside of medical departments or hospitals, e.g. conducted by data scientists. Big data and emerging data science approaches have created new possibilities for pharmacoepidemiologic research. For example, Freifeld et al. used data from the social networking site and microblogging service Twitter to monitor ADRs.

The term "big data" has become associated with various leaks and scandals. The United Kingdom *Science and Technology Committee* concluded in a 2015 report that data misuses and leaks have led to public skepticism concerning the use of big data. Not only such negative connotations, but also scientific concerns regarding users' consent, autonomy, and privacy raise ethical questions about big data research. Pharmacoepidemiologic research involving big data requires careful ethical considerations for the individuals' generating such data, for example users of social networking sites. Moreover, pharmacoepidemiologists need to consider the biases inherent to digital data sources: such bias can be caused by big data retrieved from populations that do not allow for generalizations. For instance, since individuals included in a digital data sample may represent only those using an expensive/innovative technical device or service, these users could be on average younger or above average in access to health-promoting resources. In addition, the quality of such data may differ from other sources of data (e.g. medical records).

Research involving these alternative sources of data is subject to different laws and regulatory frameworks when conducted in different global settings. For the United States, access to health relevant information via social networking sites such as Facebook is at present legally possible, due to the lack of protection for health-relevant data retrieved outside of the traditional health care and research system. With regards to medical privacy, the Electronic Frontier Foundation (EFF) points out that social networking sites and other online services compromise US citizens' control over their health data: "The baseline law for health information is the Health Insurance Portability and Accountability Act (HIPAA). HIPAA offers some rights to patients, but it is severely limited because it only applies to an entity if it is what the law considers to be either a 'covered entity' — namely: a health care provider, health plan, or health care clearinghouse — or a relevant business associate (BA)." This also implies that content such as Facebook or Twitter data, despite their actual use as health indicators, are currently not protected under

HIPAA. Yet, although arguably unlikely, this may change in the future. In addition, scientists should not conflate legal with ethical requirements.

With regard to biomedical research, it has been pointed out that the ethical implications of big data research are, at least partly, uncharted territory. Additional ethical considerations for pharmacoepidemiologic research involving big data are thus needed. This applies to the autonomy of data subjects, but also to new corporate stakeholders and public-private partnerships. The latter may not merely involve pharmaceutical companies or device manufacturers. Internet and technology corporations may also play a role and require ethical as well as legal oversight, since they control access to digital data that could further complement pharmacoepidemiology in the future.

## Acknowledgement

The authors would like to thank Philip Phan for assistance with literature searches.

## Key Points

- From an ethical perspective, pharmacoepidemiologic research has helped to address the ethical problem of drug safety scandals that occurred as a result of the release of poorly understood and inadequately tested drugs onto the marketplace. More rigorous pharmacoepidemiologic data on drug outcomes enhanced medical practitioners' capacity to "do no harm" to patients.
- Pharmacoepidemiology has developed in varied international social contexts in recent history. Global researchers share common experiences and ethical challenges such as concerns over informed consent, external review of research protocols, protection of patient privacy, and questions of conflicts of interest. However, pharmacoepidemiologic work within different national or private data systems has created specific areas of ethical demands and emphases in different settings. This history is reflected in the varied global landscape of ethical discussions and policies.
- There is more work to be done to consider how pharmacoepidemiology ethics can be inclusive of diverse cultural approaches to bioethics while also streamlining global ethical regulatory standards where appropriate.
- In the future, as the field of pharmacoepidemiology continues to rely on changing technological and data platforms and evolves to address new areas of pharmacovigilance such as pharmacoenvironmentology, ethical reflections and policies should continue to evolve and develop, as well.

| Case Example 16.1 |
| --- |

| Evaluation of Facebook and Twitter monitoring to detect safety signals for medical products: an analysis of recent FDA safety alerts (Pierce et al. 2017)<br><br>*Background*<br>The use of "big data" retrieved from social networking sites is rather uncommon for pharmacoepidemiologic studies, at least for now. Due to the methodological novelty of approaches involving such data, ethical issues are to some extent still uncharted | territory. Also, their methodological effectiveness, that is whether they can indeed complement pharmacoepidemiologic approaches, and their reliability are still under investigation.<br><br>*Question*<br>The authors aimed to examine whether, post-approval, adverse effects were reported sooner on social media than via the *US Food and Drug Administration's Adverse Event Reporting System* (FAERS). |

*(Continued)*

---

**Case Example 16.1    (Continued)**

*Approach*

In a retrospective approach, the authors retrieved data from the social networking site Facebook and the microblogging service Twitter. These were scanned for signals correlating with 10 post-marketing safety signals reported in FAERS and flagged by the FDA. For example, the authors examined whether tweets indicated symptoms of vasculitis caused by Dronedarone or angioedema caused by Pradaxa. Potentially relevant posts were then compared with those reported in FAERS, assessing where symptoms were reported first.

*Results*

The study did not yield a clear outcome. While some relevant social media data indicated adverse effects for Multaq (Dronaderone) before these were reported by the FDA, this was not the case for others.

*Strengths*

Provided that approaches like these were to become effective and reliable, harvesting and analyzing data from social media could complement existing pharmacoepidemiologic methods. Data from social media might particularly serve as early warning signals.

*Limitations*

In a letter to the editor, Wiwanitkit (2017) raised concerns over this study, questioning the validity and reliability of social media data. The commentator criticized that "[. . .] the basic issue with these social media platforms is of confidentiality and privacy." This raises the issue of whether it is ethical to use social media data in the first place. In this context, one should also consider the complexity and challenge of fully anonymizing big data. Moreover, others have pointed out that when entering public-private collaborations, researchers need to go beyond questions concerning the quality of research or

privacy (Sharon 2016). Studies such as the one conducted by Pierce et al. need to be carefully examined with regard to power asymmetries in access to data and control over technology platforms. For example, while some of the authors were employed by the US FDA, others indicated that they were employees of a technology company intending to commercialize the software platform used in the research – a conflict of interest. Such public–private partnerships also lead to dependencies between partners and put involved companies in a powerful position: this concerns the corporate ownership of public health data on the one hand and researchers' reliance on commercial technologies on the other. Ethical issues aside, one should also not forget that the effectiveness of such novel approaches and their place in the methodological repertoire of pharmacoepidemiology are still under scrutiny.

*Key Points*

- Data, in this case user-generated content, retrieved from social networking sites such as Facebook and Twitter are being explored as complementary sources for pharmacovigilance.
- The methodological effectiveness and reliability of pharmacoepidemiologic studies involving data from online sources such as social media have not been confirmed.
- Ethical issues concerning such studies go beyond matters of privacy and confidentiality: they raise issues of power asymmetries, dependencies, and conflicts of interest.
- Ethics boards and comparable oversight committees must gain further expertise to review pharmacoepidemiologic research projects and approaches involving user-generated big data.

# Further Reading

Abou-El-Enein, M. and Schneider, C. (2016). Deciphering the EU clinical trials regulation. *Nature Biotechnology* 34: 231–233.

Carpenter, D.P. (2010). *Reputation and Power.* Princeton, NJ: Princeton University Press.

European Commission (n.d.). 'Clinical trials - Regulation EU No. 536/2014'. Retrieved from: https://ec.europa.eu/health/human-use/clinical-trials/regulation_en (accessed on 26 October 2020).

Freifeld, C.C., Brownstein, J.S., Menone, C.M. et al. (2014). Digital drug safety surveillance: monitoring pharmaceutical products in twitter. *Drug Safety* 37 (5): 343–350.

Hedgecoe, A. (2016). Scandals, ethics, and regulatory change in biomedical research. *Science, Technology, & Human Values* 42 (4): 577–599.

International Society of Pharmacoepidemiology Public Policy Committee (2016). Guidelines for Good Pharmacoepidemiology Practice (GPP). *Pharmacoepidemiology and Drug Safety* 25: 188–191.

Kimura, T., Matsushita, Y., Kao Yang, Y.-H. et al. (2011). Pharmacovigilance systems and databases in Korea, Japan, and Taiwan. *Pharmacoepidemiology and Drug Safety* 20: 1237–1245.

Merz, J.F. (2001). Introduction: a survey of international ethics practices in pharmacoepidemiology and drug safety. *Pharmacoepidemiology and Drug Safety* 10 (7): 579–581.

Pierce, C.E., Bouri, K., Pamer, C. et al. (2017). Evaluation of Facebook and Twitter monitoring to detect safety signals for medical products: an analysis of recent FDA safety alerts. *Drug Safety* 40 (4): 317–331.

Pratt, B., Van, C., Cong, Y. et al. (2014). Perspectives from South and East Asia on clinical and research ethics. *Journal of Empirical Research on Human Research Ethics* 9 (2): 52–67.

Ramirez, I. (2015). Navigating the maze of requirements for obtaining approval of non-interventional studies (NIS) in the European Union. *GMS German Medical Science* 13 https://doi.org/10.3205/000225.

Sethi, N. (2014). The promotion of data sharing in pharmacoepidemiology. *European Journal of Health Law* 21 (3): 271–296.

Sharon, T. (2016). The Googlization of health research: from disruptive innovation to disruptive ethics. *Personalized Medicine* 13 (6): 563–574.

Urushihara, H., Parmenter, L., Tashiro, S. et al. (2017). Bridge the gap: the need for harmonized regulatory and ethical standards for postmarketing observational studies. *Pharmacoepidemiology and Drug Safety* 26: 1299–1306.

Vayena, E., Salathé, M., Madoff, L.C., and Brownstein, J.S. (2015). Ethical challenges of big data in public health. *PLoS Computational Biology* 11 (2): e1003904.

Wiwanitkit, V. (2017). Comment on: "Evaluation of Facebook and Twitter monitoring to detect safety signals for medical products: an analysis of recent FDA safety alerts". *Drug Safety* 40 (8): 755–755.

Wettermark, B. (2013). The intriguing future of pharmacoepidemiology. *European Journal of Clinical Pharmacology* 69 (1): 43–51.

# 17

# The Use of Randomized Controlled Trials for Pharmacoepidemiology

*Samuel M. Lesko[1], Allen A. Mitchell[2], and Robert F. Reynolds[3]*

[1] *Northeast Regional Cancer Institute, and Geisinger Commonwealth School of Medicine, Scranton, PA, USA*
[2] *Slone Epidemiology Center at Boston University, Boston, MA, USA*
[3] *Epidemiology, Research and Development, GlaxoSmithKline, New York, NY, USA*

## Introduction

When properly conducted, randomized controlled trials (RCTs) are considered the gold standard for demonstrating the efficacy and safety of a medicine for regulatory approval. During the premarketing phases of drug development, RCTs typically involve highly selected subjects and in the aggregate include at most a few thousand patients. These studies are designed to be sufficiently large to provide evidence of a beneficial clinical effect and to exclude large increases in risk of common adverse clinical events. However, premarketing trials are rarely large enough to detect relatively small differences in the risk of common adverse events or to estimate reliably the risk of rare events. Identification and quantification of these potentially important risks require large studies, which typically are conducted after a drug has been marketed. Because of design complexity and costs, large controlled trials are not generally conducted in the postmarketing setting. Rather, observational designs are commonly used to evaluate the safety of medicines post-approval. The authors' search for the best method to minimize the potential for bias yet remain relevant to real world clinical practice led to selecting a large simple trial design to assess the risk of serious but rare adverse reactions. The resulting experience of studying risks associated with pediatric ibuprofen and atypical antipsychotic use serves as the basis for this chapter (see Case Example 17.1 and Further Reading) and may prompt others to consider randomized trials, including large simple and pragmatic trials, for the postmarketing assessment of drug safety.

## Clinical Problems to be Addressed by Pharmacoepidemiologic Research

Pharmacoepidemiologic methods are used to quantify risks and benefits of medications that could not be adequately evaluated in studies performed during the premarketing phase of drug testing. While this chapter considers only the assessment of the risks of medications, the principles involved also apply to the postmarketing evaluation of the benefits of medications.

As noted in Chapters 1 and 3, premarketing studies are typically too small to detect modest

---

**Case Example 17.1    (See Lesko et al.)**

*Background*
- The use of nonsteroidal anti-inflammatory drugs is associated with an increased risk of GI bleeding and renal failure in adults.
- In 1989, ibuprofen suspension (an NSAID) was approved for use in children by prescription only.
- The risk of rare but serious adverse events among children treated with ibuprofen suspension must be documented before this medication can be considered for a switch from prescription to over-the-counter use in children.
- Confounding by indication is likely in observational studies of prescription ibuprofen use in children.

*Question*
Is the use of ibuprofen suspension in children associated with an increased risk of rare but serious adverse events?

*Approach*
- Conduct a large simple randomized trial of ibuprofen use in children.
- A randomized trial involving nearly 84 000 children 12 years of age and younger with a febrile illness was conducted.

*Results*
The risk of rare but serious adverse events (hospitalization for GI bleeding, acute renal failure, anaphylaxis and Reye syndrome) was not significantly greater among children treated with ibuprofen compared to those treated with acetaminophen.

*Strengths*
- The large sample size allowed evaluation of rare events.
- Randomization effectively controlled for confounding, including confounding by indication.

*Limitations*
- The use of an active control treatment (acetaminophen) precludes using these data to compare the risk of ibuprofen to that of placebo in febrile children.
- Because medication exposure was limited to the duration of an acute illness, this study cannot be used to assess the risk of long-term ibuprofen use in children.

*Key Points*
- When confounding by indication is likely, a RCT may be the only study design that will provide a valid estimate of a medication's effect.
- Large, simple, RCTs can be successfully conducted to evaluate medication safety.
- By keeping the study simple, it is possible to conduct a large, practice-based study and collect data that reflects current ambulatory medical practice.

---

differences in the incidence rates (e.g. relative risks of 2.0 or less) for common adverse events or even large differences in the incidence rates for rare events, such as those that affect 1/1000 treated patients. Modest differences in risk of non-life-threatening adverse events can be of substantial public health importance, particularly if the medication is likely to be used by large numbers of patients. If there are post-licensing questions about the safety of a drug, large observational studies are typically used to satisfy the sample sizes needed to identify (or rule out) the relevant risks. However, findings from observational studies are often contested as the basis for regulatory and clinical decisions. Epidemiologic studies of medication exposures and their effects have difficulty measuring and controlling for confounding in general and confounding by indication for drug use (and/or severity of disease) specifically. Uncontrolled or incompletely controlled confounding can easily account for modest associations between a drug and an adverse clinical event (see Chapter 2 and Case Example 17.1).

In observational studies, weak associations deserve attention with respect to uncontrolled confounding. Although there are important exceptions, the general view is that the stronger the association, the more likely the observed relationship is causal. This is not to say that a weak association (e.g. a relative risk ≤1.5) can never be causal; rather, it is more difficult to infer causality because such an association, even if statistically significant, can more likely be an artifact of confounding. As an example, consider an analysis where socioeconomic status is a potential confounder and education is used as a surrogate for this factor. Because the relation between years of education completed (the surrogate) and socioeconomic status (the potential confounder) is, at best, imperfect, analyses controlling for years of education can only partially control for confounding. Thus, it is advisable to use extreme caution in making causal inferences from small relative risks derived from observational studies. When there is concern about residual confounding prior to embarking on an observational study, one may wish to consider using a non-observational study design.

# Methodological Problems to be Solved by Pharmacoepidemiologic Research

Confounding by indication (also referred to as indication bias, channeling, confounding by severity, or contraindication bias) may be a particular problem for postmarketing drug studies. According to Slone et al., confounding by indication exists when "patients who receive different treatments differ in their risk of adverse outcomes, independent of the treatment received." In general, confounding by indication occurs when an observed association between a drug and an outcome is due to the underlying illness (or its severity) and not to any effect of the drug (see also Chapter 22). As with any other form of confounding, one can, in theory, control for its effects if one can reliably measure and control for the underlying risk of illness. In practice, however, this often is not easily done.

When confronted with the task of assessing the safety of a marketed drug product, the pharmacoepidemiologist must evaluate the specific hypothesis to be tested, estimate the magnitude of the hypothesized association, and determine whether confounding by indication is possible. If incomplete control of confounding is likely, it is important to recognize the limitations of observational research designs and consider conducting a randomized study design. There is nothing inherent about a randomized design that precludes a pharmacoepidemiologist from designing and carrying it out. To the contrary, the special skills of a pharmacoepidemiologist can be very useful in performing large scale randomized trials that use epidemiologic follow-up methods.

## Overview of Classic RCTs

As noted above, RCTs are most commonly used during the premarketing phases of drug development to demonstrate a drug's efficacy (and to gather general information concerning safety). By randomization, one hopes to equalize the distributions of confounding factors, whether they are known or unknown. Therefore, the assigned treatment is the most likely explanation for any observed difference between treatment groups in the clinical outcomes (improvement in the illness or the occurrence of adverse clinical events). By definition, participants in observational studies are not assigned treatment at random. In clinical practice, the choice of treatment may be determined by the stage or severity of the illness, by the underlying risk of developing the outcome of interest, or by the patient's poor response to or adverse experience with alternative therapies, any of which can introduce bias.

## Sample Size

In homogeneous populations, balanced treatment groups in RCTs can be achieved with relatively small study sizes. In heterogeneous populations (e.g. children less than 12 years of age), a large sample size may be required to insure the equal distribution of uncommon confounders among study groups (e.g. infants versus toddlers versus school-age children). Study size is determined by the need to assure balance between treatment groups and the magnitude of the effect to be detected (see Chapter 3). Large randomized studies minimize the chance that the treatment groups are different with respect to potential confounders and permit the detection of small differences in common clinical outcomes or large differences in uncommon ones (see Chapter 3).

## Masking Treatment Assignment

Concealed (or masking) treatment assignment is used to minimize detection bias and is particularly important where the outcome is subjective. Reporting of subjective symptoms by study participants and the detection of even objectively defined outcome events may be influenced by knowledge of the medications used. For example, if a patient complains of abdominal pain, a physician may be more likely to perform a test for occult blood in the stool if that patient was being treated with an NSAID rather than acetaminophen. Thus, follow-up data collection will only be unbiased if both parties (patient and investigator) are unaware of the treatment assigned. Concealing may be difficult to achieve and maintain, particularly if either the study or control medication produces specific symptoms (i.e. side effects) or easily observable physiologic effects (e.g. nausea or change in pulse rate).

## Choice of Control Treatment

The hypothesis being tested determines the choice of control treatment. Placebo controls are most useful for making comparisons with untreated disease but may not represent standard of care and have been challenged as unethical in some circumstances. Further, it may be difficult to maintain masking in placebo-controlled studies, as noted above. Studies employing an active control typically utilize usual drug treatments, which frequently represent the standard of care. Although often considered more ethical and easier to keep concealed because the illness and symptoms are not left untreated, these studies do not permit comparison with the natural history of the illness.

## Data Collection

Data collection in a premarketing clinical trial is generally resource intensive. Detailed descriptive and clinical data are collected at enrollment, and extensive clinical and laboratory data are collected at regular and often frequent intervals during follow-up. In addition to the data needed to test the hypothesis of a clinical benefit, premarketing trials of medications must also assess general safety and therefore must collect extensive data on symptoms, physical signs, and laboratory evaluations.

## Data Analysis

In observational studies, data analyses may be quite complex because of the need to adjust for potential confounders. In contrast, analysis of the primary hypothesis in many clinical trials is straightforward and involves a comparison of the outcome event in different groups. Analyses involving repeated measures, subgroups of study subjects, or adjustment to control for incomplete or ineffective randomization may be performed, albeit adding complexity.

## Generalizability of Results

The usual clinical trial conducted during the pre-marketing evaluation of a drug almost always involves highly selected patients; as a consequence, the results of the trial may not be generalizable to the large numbers of patients who may use the medication after licensing. Observational studies offer an advantage in that they can reflect the real-world experience of medication use and clinical outcomes, and because their modest costs permit studies involving large numbers of patients.

### Limitations of RCTs

Methodological strengths notwithstanding, there are several features of the classic RCT that limit its use as a postmarketing study design. First, it may be unethical to conduct a study in which patients are randomly assigned a potentially harmful treatment. For example, an RCT to test the hypothesis that cigarette smoking increases the risk of heart disease would not be acceptable. Second, the complexity and cost of traditional premarket RCTs, with their detailed observations and resource-intensive follow-up, make very large studies of this type generally infeasible. However, if the study can be simplified and use the epidemiologist's tools to track patients and collect follow-up data, it may be possible to both control costs and make a large study feasible. Third, RCTs, by design, do not study the safety of a medicine as it is actually prescribed by physicians and used by patients once on the market. A simplified design, such as the large, simple trial (LST), merges the ideal characteristics of the RCT (randomization) with those of an observational epidemiology study (follow-up with minimal intervention). The adoption of as many pragmatic elements as possible to mimic usual care practice while protecting study validity in theory yields results that are more informative for regulatory decisions and public health policy.

## Currently Available Solutions

### Large Simple Trials

LSTs may be the best solution when it is not possible to completely control confounding by means other than randomization, and the volume and complexity of data collection can be kept to a minimum (see Table 17.1). The US Salk vaccine trial of the 1950s is an early example of a very large trial. More recently, large randomized trials have been used to test the efficacy of therapeutic interventions, especially in cardiology, or to evaluate dietary supplements or pharmaceuticals for primary prevention of cardiovascular disease and cancer. This approach has also been used successfully to evaluate the risk of adverse drug effects when the more common observational designs have been judged inadequate. LSTs are just very large randomized trials made simple by reducing data collection to the minimum needed to test only a single hypothesis (or at most a few hypotheses). Randomization of treatment assignment is the key feature of the design, which controls for confounding by both known and unknown factors, and the large study size provides the power needed to evaluate small risks of common events as well as large risks of rare events.

It is useful to note that while LSTs may appear to be similar to pragmatic trials, they can differ in important ways. Both are randomized studies; pragmatic trials are intended to provide widely generalizable results and while they may be large, that is not always the case; by definition, LSTs are large to assess rare events and small relative risks but may not be generalizable. The two designs share similarities when LSTs may have so few exclusion criteria as to make them "pragmatic" (generalizable).

### How Simple Is Simple?

Yusuf et al. (1984) suggest that very large randomized studies of treatment-related mortality collect only the participants' vital status at the conclusion of the study. Because the question of drug safety frequently concerns outcomes less severe than mortality, these ultra simple trials may not be sufficient. Hasford has suggested an alternative in which "large trials with lean protocols" include only *relevant* baseline, follow-up, and outcome data. Collecting far fewer data than is common in the usual RCT is the key feature

**Table 17.1** Typical design characteristics of a large simple trial (LST) compared to those of a randomized controlled trial (RCT).

| Design Characteristic | LST | RCT |
|---|---|---|
| Randomization | Yes | Yes |
| Medicine Assignment | Concealed if feasible, assignment may be known, dose adjustment permitted | Concealed |
| Sample size | Larger (thousands) | Smaller (hundreds) |
| Inclusion criteria | Broad (e.g. per approved medicine label) | Narrow (e.g. excludes patients with co-morbid conditions, using multiple medications, pregnant women, elderly) |
| Questionnaire/Case Report Form (CRF)/Interview | Minimal, brief | Complex, lengthy |
| Endpoints | Hard endpoints (mortality, hospitalization or life-threatening events) | Virtually Any |
| Required patient visits and procedures | Few, if any; Follows normal practice schedule and assessments | Yes, frequent; Visits and tests far greater than expected in clinical practice |
| Primary source of investigators or enrolling physicians | Primary care provider/Community-based | Clinical research/Academic centers |
| Site monitoring | Minimal | Frequent |
| Followed after randomized treatment discontinued | Yes | No, or for limited duration post-discontinuation (e.g. 30 days) |
| Primary analytic method | Intent to treat (ITT) | ITT |

of both approaches. With simplified protocols that take advantage of epidemiologic follow-up methods, very large trials can be conducted to test hypotheses of interest to pharmacoepidemiologists.

**Power/Sample Size**

Study power is a function of the number of events observed during the course of the study, which in turn is determined by the incidence rate for the event, the sample size, and the duration of observation or follow-up (see Chapter 3). Power requirements can be satisfied by studying a population at high risk, enrolling a large sample size, or conducting follow-up for a prolonged period. The appropriate approach will be determined by the goal of the study and the hypothesis to be tested. Allergic or idiosyncratic events may require a very large study population, and events with

long latency periods may be best studied with long duration follow-up. However, power is not the only factor to consider. For example, while an elderly population may be at high risk for gastrointestinal bleeding or cardiovascular events, a study limited to this group may lack generalizability and would not provide information on the risk of these events in younger adults or children.

**Data Elements**

The data collection process can be kept simple by examining primary endpoints that are objective, easily identified, and verifiable. Because confounding is controlled by randomization, data on potential confounders need not be collected. Rather, a few basic demographic variables can be collected at enrollment in order to characterize the population and to confirm that randomization was achieved.

### Data Collection

The data collection process itself can be simplified; follow-up data can be collected by mail or web-based questionnaires, or telephone interviews conducted with the study participants. Because the study will involve clear and objective outcomes (see below), which can be confirmed by medical record review or other means, self-report by the study participants can be an appropriate source of follow-up data. Other sources of follow-up data could include electronic medical records (e.g. for LSTs conducted among subscribers of a large health insurance plan) or vital status records for fatal outcomes (e.g. the US National Death Index).

The primary advantage of simplicity is that it allows very large groups of study participants to be followed at reasonable cost. However, a simple trial cannot answer all possible questions about the safety of a drug but must be limited to testing, at most, a few related hypotheses.

### When Is a Large Simple Randomized Trial Appropriate?

LSTs are appropriate when the conditions in Table 17.2 apply.

### Important Research Question

Although a simple trial will cost less per subject than a traditional clinical trial, the total cost of a large study (in money and human resources) will still be substantial. The cost will usually be justified only when there is a clear need for a reliable answer to a question concerning the risk of a serious outcome. A minor medication side effect such as headache or

**Table 17.2** Conditions appropriate for the conduct of a large simply randomized trial.

| |
|---|
| The research question is important. |
| Genuine uncertainty exists about the likely results. |
| Confounding by indication is likely. |
| The absolute risk is small, or the relative risk is small, regardless of the absolute risk. |

nausea may not be trivial for the individual patient but may not warrant the expense of a large study. On the other hand, if the question involves the risk of premature death, permanent disability, hospitalization, or other serious events, the cost may well be justified.

### Uncertainty Must Exist

An additional condition has been referred to as the "uncertainty principle." Originally described by Gray et al. as a simple criterion to assess subject eligibility in LSTs, it states that "both patient and doctor should be *substantially uncertain* about the appropriateness, for this particular patient, of each of the trial treatments. If the patient and doctor are *reasonably certain* that one or other treatment is inappropriate then it would not be ethical for the patient's treatment to be chosen at *random*." This principle (also known as equipoise) should be applied to determine the appropriateness of performing all RCTs, including an LST of an adverse clinical event. Very large randomized trials are justified only when there is true uncertainty about the risk of the treatment in the population. Apart from considerations of benefit, it would not be ethical to subject large numbers of patients to a treatment that was reasonably believed to place them at increased risk, however small, of a potentially serious or permanent adverse clinical event. The concept of uncertainty can thus be extended to include a global assessment of the combined risks and benefits of the treatments being compared. One treatment may be known to provide superior therapeutic benefits, but it may be unknown whether the risks of side effects outweigh this advantage. For example, the antiestrogen tamoxifen may improve breast cancer survival, but may do so only at the cost of an increased risk of endometrial cancer. Appropriately, a randomized trial was undertaken to resolve uncertainty in this situation.

### Power and Confounding

LSTs will only be needed if: (i) the *absolute* risk of the study outcome is small and there are concerns about confounding by indication, *or* (ii) the *relative* risk is small (in which case, there are inherent concerns about residual confounding from any source). By contrast, LSTs would not be necessary if the *absolute* risk were large, because premarket or other conventional RCTs should be adequate, or where uncontrollable confounding is not an issue, because observational studies would suffice. Also, if the *relative* risk were large (and confounding by indication and other potential biases inherent in observational studies are not concerns), observational studies would be appropriate.

### No Interaction Between Treatment and Outcome

An additional requirement for LSTs is that important interactions between the treatment and patient characteristics (effect modification) are unlikely. In other words, the available evidence should suggest that the association will be qualitatively similar in all patient subgroups. Variation in the strength of the association is acceptable among subgroups, but there should be no suggestion that the effect would be completely reversed in any subgroup. Because of the limited data available in a truly simple trial, it may not be possible to test whether an interaction has occurred, and the data collected may not be sufficient to identify relevant subgroups. Because randomization only controls confounding for comparisons made between the groups that were randomized, subsets of these groups may not be strictly comparable with respect to one or more confounding factors. Thus, if clinically important interaction is considered likely, additional steps must be taken to permit the appropriate analyses (e.g. stratified randomization). This added complexity may result in a study that is no longer a truly simple trial.

### When is an LST Feasible?

LSTs are feasible when the conditions in Table 17.3 are met.

**Table 17.3** Conditions which make a large, simple randomized trial feasible.

---

The study question can be expressed as a simple testable hypothesis.

The treatment to be tested is simple (uncomplicated).

The outcome is objectively defined (e.g. hospitalization, death).

Epidemiologic follow-up methods are appropriate.

The patient and physician population are motivated to participate by a meaningful research question.

---

### Simple Hypothesis

LSTs are best suited to answer focused and relatively uncomplicated questions. For example, an LST can be designed to test the hypothesis that the risk of hospitalization for any reason, or for acute gastrointestinal bleeding, is increased in children treated with ibuprofen. However, it may not be possible for a single LST to answer the much more general question, "Is ibuprofen safe with respect to all possible outcomes in children?"

### Simple Treatments

Simple therapies (e.g. a single drug at a fixed dose for a short duration) are most amenable to study with LSTs. They are likely to be commonly used, so that it will be feasible to enroll large numbers of patients, and the results will be applicable to a sizeable segment of the population. Complex therapeutic protocols are difficult to manage, can reduce patient adherence, and by their very nature may not be compatible with the simple trial design.

### Objective and Easily Measured Outcomes

The outcomes to be studied should be objective and easy to define, identify, and recall. An example might include hospitalization for acute gastrointestinal bleeding. Study participants may not correctly recall the details of a hospital admission, or even the specific reason for admission, but they likely will recall the fact that they were admitted, the name of the hospital, and at least the approximate date of admission. Medical records can be obtained to document the details of the clinical events that occurred. Events of this type can be reliably recorded using epidemiologic follow-up methods (e.g. questionnaires, telephone interviews, or linkage with public vital status records). On the other hand, clinical outcomes that can be reliably detected only by detailed in-person interviews, physical examinations, or extensive physiologic testing may not be amenable for study in simple trials.

### Cooperative Population

A study population motivated by the research question will greatly increase the probability of success. Striking examples are the large populations in the Physicians' and Women's Health Studies; the success of these studies is at least partly due to the willingness of large numbers of knowledgeable health professionals to participate. Because of the participants' knowledge of medical conditions and symptoms and participation in the US health care system, relatively sophisticated information was obtained using mailed questionnaires, and even biologic samples were collected.

### Logistics of Conducting an LST

An LST may be appropriate and feasible, but it will only succeed if all logistical aspects of the study are kept simple as well. In general, LSTs will involve an oversight body, sometimes organized as a Scientific Steering Committee comprised of epidemiologic, statistical and clinical experts who are responsible for the scientific conduct of the study, as well as a central data coordinating facility, and a network of enrollment sites (e.g. offices of collaborating physicians or other health care providers). Health care professionals (e.g. physicians, nurse practitioners, and pharmacists in private practice or members of large health care organizations) can participate by recruiting eligible patients. Alternative methods to identify and enroll eligible subjects (e.g. direct mailings to professional groups, print or online ads,

emails and mobile phone text messages) may be appropriate for some studies. Because success depends on the cooperation of multiple health care providers and a large number of patients, it is best to limit the demands placed on each practitioner (or his/her clinical practice). One approach is to have the practitioner identify eligible subjects, obtain permission to pass their names to a central study staff, and leave to the study staff the task of explaining study details, enrollment, and obtaining informed consent. Another approach is to provide comprehensive training prior to site initiation followed by support to local administrative staff throughout the course of the study, particularly for research-naïve and inexperienced sites. Obtaining informed consent, baseline data, and the medicine assignment are best handled during a single visit.

To facilitate patient recruitment and to maximize generalizability of the results, minimal restrictions should be placed on patient eligibility. Patients with a medical contraindication or known sensitivity to either the study or control drug should not, of course, be enrolled, but other restrictions should be kept to a minimum and should ideally reflect only restrictions that would apply in a typical clinical setting.

Substantial bias can be introduced if either physician or patient can choose not to participate after learning (or guessing) which treatment the patient has been assigned. Therefore, patients should be randomized only after eligibility has been confirmed and the enrollment process completed.

### Importance of Complete Follow-up

Because dropouts and losses to follow-up may not be random but may be related to adverse treatment effects, it is important to make every effort to obtain follow-up data on all subjects. A study with follow-up data on even tens of thousands of patients may not be able to provide a valid answer to the primary study question if this number represents only a modest proportion of those randomized. The duration of the follow-up period can affect the completeness of follow-up data collection. If it is too short, important outcomes may be missed (i.e. some conditions may not be diagnosed until after the end of the follow-up period). On the other hand, as the length of the follow-up period increases, the number lost to follow-up or exposed to the alternate treatment (contaminated exposure) increases. In the extreme, a randomized trial becomes an observational cohort study because of selective dropouts in either or both of the treatment arms. Beyond choosing a motivated and interested study population, the investigators can minimize losses to follow-up by maintaining contact with all study participants. Regular mailings of supplies of medication, a study newsletter, or email reminders can be helpful, and memory aids such as medication calendar packs or other devices may help maintain adherence with chronic treatment schedules.

### Follow-up Data Collection

An important element of a successful LST is that the burden to health care providers for follow-up data collection is minimized. Busy health care providers cannot be expected to commit the time required to obtain systematically even minimal follow-up data from large numbers of subjects. However, the clinician who originally enrolled the subject may be able to provide limited follow-up data (e.g. vital status) or a current address or telephone number for the occasional patient who would otherwise be lost to follow-up. A mailed or electronic questionnaire, supplemented by telephone follow-up when needed, is effective. The response rate will likely be greatest if the questions are both simple and direct and minimal time is required to complete the questionnaire. Medical records can be reviewed to verify important outcomes, such as rare adverse events, and the work needed to obtain and abstract the relevant records should be manageable. If there is a need to confirm a diagnosis or evaluate symptoms, a limited number of participants can be referred to their enrolling health care provider for examination or to have blood or other studies performed,

although as previously noted this can make the trial far more complex. In addition, a search of public records (e.g. the National Death Index in the US) can identify study subjects who have died during follow-up.

## Analysis

### Primary Analysis

Analyses of the primary outcomes are usually straightforward and involve a simple comparison of incidence rates between the treatment and control groups. Under the assumption that confounding has been controlled by the randomization procedure, complex multivariate analyses are not necessary (and may not be possible because only limited data on potential confounders are available). Descriptive data collected at enrollment should be analyzed by treatment group to test the randomization procedure; any material differences between treatment groups suggest an imbalance despite randomization. As noted above, it is assumed that there is no material interaction between patient characteristics and medication effects, thus eliminating the need for complex statistical analyses to test for effect modification.

### Subgroup Analyses

It is important to remember that confounding factors will be distributed evenly only among groups that were randomized; subgroups which are not random samples of the original randomization groups may not have similar distributions of confounding factors. For example, participants who have remained in the study (i.e. have not dropped out or been lost to follow-up) may not be fully representative of the original randomization groups and may not be comparable with respect to confounders among the different groups. Despite all efforts, complete follow-up is rarely achieved, and because only the original randomization groups can be assumed to be free of confounding, the primary analysis should include all enrolled study subjects regardless of whether or not they adhered to taking the assigned therapy (i.e. an intention-to-treat analysis) should be performed. Also, unless a stratified randomization scheme was used, one cannot be certain that unmeasured confounding variables will be evenly distributed in subgroups of participants, and the smaller the subgroup, the greater the potential for imbalance. Therefore, subgroup analyses will be subject to the same limitations as observational studies (i.e. the potential for uncontrolled confounding).

### Data Monitoring/Interim Analyses

Because of the substantial commitment of resources and large number of patients potentially at risk for adverse outcomes, it is appropriate to monitor the accumulating data during the study. A study may be ended prematurely if participants experience unacceptable risks, if the hypothesis can be satisfactorily tested earlier than anticipated, or if it becomes clear that a statistically significant result cannot be achieved, even if the study were to be completed as planned. A data monitoring committee, independent of the study investigators, should conduct periodic reviews of the data using an appropriate analysis procedure.

## The Future

With accelerated approval of new medications and rapid increases in their use, we may see a greater need for large, randomized postmarketing studies to assess small differences in risk. This is particularly the case for medications considered for over-the-counter switch, because the risks of rare and unknown events that would be acceptable under prescription status might be unacceptable when the drug is self-administered by much larger and more diverse populations. In the absence of techniques that reliably control for confounding by indication in observational studies, there will

be a growing need for LSTs to evaluate larger relative risks. Because of few restrictions on participant eligibility, LSTs are more likely than classical randomized clinical trials to reflect the true benefits and risks of medications when used in actual clinical practice. The generalizability of the results of LSTs and other pragmatic clinical trials makes these studies particularly attractive to regulators and policy-makers and may lead to increased use of these studies.

One possible approach that may improve efficiency in large studies is to conduct trials involving patients who receive care from very large health delivery systems (see Chapters 8 and 10). These data arise from electronic health records (EHRs) with information recorded by clinical staff at the point of care (e.g. in hospitals or outpatient clinics), administrative claims data (e.g. the Veterans Affairs database in the US), national/regional registries (e.g. population-wide databases in Sweden and Denmark), and patient disease/condition/drug registries (e.g. CorEvitas rheumatoid arthritis registry). EHRs and registries have been used in conventional RCTs (e.g. the West of Scotland Coronary Prevention Study, the Scandinavian Simvastatin Survival Study and the EHR4CR project) to identify potential trial participants and collect long-term follow-up data. The most recent development is the use of registries for identification, recruitment and as follow-up for trials, providing an efficient and reusable infrastructure for LSTs. While uncommon, recent simplified trials conducted in the UK Clinical Practice Research Data, the US Veterans Affairs Healthcare System and PCORnet, the National Patient Centered Clinical Research Network, illustrate the approach. Research questions where the study results are directly relevant to patient care offer the most promise for a successful trial in large health delivery systems. With more experience, we anticipate more systems will recognize the potential benefits and efficiencies of this approach, developing the capability to conduct embedded point-of-care LSTs.

It is clear that very large simple controlled trials of drug safety can be successfully carried out. It is less clear, however, how frequently the factors that indicate the need for a very large trial (Table 17.1) will converge with those that permit such a trial to be carried out (Table 17.2). As a discipline, pharmacoepidemiology is well suited to conduct LSTs and to develop more efficient methods of subject recruitment and follow-up data collection that can make these studies a more common option for the evaluation of small but important risks of medication use.

## Key Points

- Randomization usually controls for confounding, including confounding by indication.
- A large study allows assessment of small to modest associations of common events and large associations with rare events and assures that randomization produces balanced treatment groups.
- Large RCTs are feasible if data collection is kept simple and outcome events are objective and verifiable.

## Further Reading

Choudhry, N.K. (2017). Randomized, controlled trials in health insurance systems. *N. Engl. J. Med.* 377: 957–964.

Connolly, S.J., Ezekowitz, M.D., Yusuf, S. et al. (2009). Dabigatran versus warfarin in patients with atrial fibrillation. *N. Engl. J. Med.* 361 (12): 1139–1151.

D'Avolio, L., Ferguson, R., Goryachev, S. et al. (2012). Implementation of the department of Veterans Affairs' first point-of-care clinical trial. *J. Am. Med. Inform. Assoc.* 19 (e1): e170–e176.

DeMets, D.L. (1998). Data and safety monitoring boards. In: *Encyclopedia of Biostatistics* (eds. P. Armitage and T. Colton), 1067–1071. Chichester: Wiley.

Fisher, B., Costantion, J.P., Wickerham, D.L. et al. (1998). Tamoxifen for prevention of breast cancer: report of the National Surgical Adjuvant Breast and Bowel Project P-1 Study. *J. Natl. Cancer Inst.* 90: 1371–1388.

Francis, T. Jr., Korns, R., Voight, R. et al. (1955). An evaluation of the 1954 poliomyelitis vaccine trials: summary report. *Am. J. Public Health* 45 (suppl): 1–50.

Hasford, J. (1994). Drug risk assessment: a case for large trials with lean protocols. *Pharmacoepidemiol. Drug Saf.* 3: 321–327.

Hennekens, C.H. and Buring, J.E. (1989). Methodologic considerations in the design and conduct of randomized trials: the U.S. Physicians' Health Study. *Control. Clin. Trials* 10: 142S–150S.

Hennekens, C.H., Buring, J.E., Manson, J.E. et al. (1996). Lack of effect of long-term supplementation with beta carotene on the incidence of malignant neoplasms and cardiovascular disease. *N. Engl. J. Med.* 334: 1145–1149.

Lee, I.M., Cook, N.R., Manson, J.E. et al. (1999). Beta-carotene supplementation and incidence of cancer and cardiovascular disease: the Women's Health Study. *J. Natl. Cancer Inst.* 91 (24): 2102–2106.

Lesko, S.M. and Mitchell, A.A. (1995). An assessment of the safety of pediatric ibuprofen: a practitioner-based randomized clinical trial. *JAMA* 273: 929–933.

Mitchell, A.A. and Lesko, S.M. (1995). When a randomized controlled trial is needed to assess drug safety: the case of pediatric ibuprofen. *Drug Saf.* 13: 15–24.

ONTARGET Investigators, Yusuf, S., Teo, K.K. et al. (2008). Telmisartan, ramipril, or both in patients at high risk for vascular events. *N. Engl. J. Med.* 358 (15): 1547–1559.

Peto, R., Collins, R., and Gray, R. (1995). Large-scale randomized evidence: large, simple trials and overviews of trials. *J. Clin. Epidemiol.* 48 (1): 23–40.

Reynolds, R.F., Lem, J.A., Gatto, N.M., and Eng, S.M. (2011). Is the large simple trial design used for comparative, post-approval safety research? A review of a clinical trials registry and the published literature. *Drug Saf.* 34: 799–820.

Rothman, K.J. and Michels, K.B. (1994). The continuing unethical use of placebo controls. *N. Engl. J. Med.* 331: 394–398.

Slone, D., Shapiro, S., Miettinen, O.S. et al. (1979). Drug evaluation after marketing. A policy perspective. *Ann. Intern. Med.* 90: 257–261.

van Staa, T.P., Dyson, L., McCann, G. et al. (2014). The opportunities and challenges of pragmatic point-of-care randomised trials using routinely collected electronic records: evaluations of two exemplar trials. *Health Technol. Assess. (Winch. Eng.)* 18 (43): 1–146.

Strandberg, T.E., Pyörälä, K., Cook, T.J. et al. (2004). Mortality and incidence of cancer during 10-year follow-up of the Scandinavian Simvastatin Survival Study (4S). *Lancet* 364 (9436): 771–777.

Strom, B.L., Faich, G.A., Reynolds, R.F. et al. (2008). The ziprasidone observational study of cardiac outcomes (ZODIAC): design and baseline characteristics. *J. Clin. Psychiatry* 69: 114–121.

Strom, B.L., Eng, S.M., Faich, G. et al. (2010). Comparative mortality associated with ziprasidone and olanzapine in real-world use among 18,154 patients with schizophrenia: the ziprasidone observational study of cardiac outcomes (ZODIAC). *Am. J. Psychiatry* 168: 193–201.

Yusuf, S., Collins, R., and Peto, R. (1984). Why do we need some large, simple randomized trials? *Stat. Med.* 3: 409–420.

Yusuf, S. (1993). Reduced mortality and morbidity with the use of angiotensin-converting enzyme inhibitors in patients with left ventricular dysfunction and congestive heart failure. *Herz* 18 (suppl): 444–448.

# 18

# Pharmacoeconomics

Economic Evaluation of Pharmaceuticals

*Kevin A. Schulman*

*Clinical Excellence Research Center, Stanford University, Stanford, CA, USA*

## Introduction

The science of drug development and assessment has been well described throughout this book. The economics of this process brings together concepts of finance, health economics, and behavioral economics in a manner that is truly unique.

## Clinical Problems to be Addressed by Pharmacoeconomic Research

At its core, drug development is about innovation, and bringing the benefits of the science of medicine to patients. Drug development is time consuming, expensive, and risky, so we need to ensure there are adequate financial incentives to bring these new innovations to market, especially for areas of unmet clinical need. At the same time, we need to ensure access to medications, including their affordability to public or private payers. Pharmacoeconomics provides a pathway to understand the conflicts between all of these interests and perspectives.

## The Economics of Drug Development

Drug development starts with an investment in science. Historically, public grant funds through the National Institutes of Health or the National Science Foundation, or private funds through programs like the Howard Hughes Medical Institute, would support fundamental science that might be years or even generations away from translation into medical products. Academic researchers and the pharmaceutical industry would use the insights from this work to begin an effort at translation, moving from fundamental science to specific interventions for specific diseases. This work could still be publicly funded, but might be more likely to be funded through private resources such as pharmaceutical firms, or even applied science efforts such as the Bill and Melinda Gates Foundation. These efforts serve to translate biology into drug targets, identifying potential pathways to alter the target through the identification of small molecules or biologics that have (hopefully) unique effects on the target. The discovery of a candidate drug would lead to the filing of a patent, an opportunity for the inventor to own the rights to the discovery and to preclude others from patenting the invention (under a provision called the Bayh–Dole Act, universities own the patent rights to discoveries even if the work was funded using federal grants).

The patent rights are critical in the next stage of drug development. This is when drug development moves out of the laboratory and into human testing. This is the most expensive step in drug development, and for the most part the work is privately funded. Investors justify their willingness to invest in a molecule given the opportunity for financial returns resulting from their ownership of the molecule through the patent. This transition from public to private support is challenging for many discoveries. The "Valley of Death" is the gap between science that is funded by public grants and the ability to attract private investment to the development of a molecule.

Clinical testing of pharmaceuticals is carefully regulated by the Food and Drug Administration (FDA) and other global regulatory bodies. For most products, regulatory authorities require proof of safety and efficacy of products before they are approved for sale. Clinical testing can require up to a decade to complete and can require more than $1 billion in direct outlays.

At the end of drug development, with product approval by the FDA, the manufacturer can set a price and market the product. Prices set by manufacturers reflect their significant investment in clinical development, and the inherent risk they were required to assume, but also considerations of market access or barriers to full reimbursement for patients. The price can reflect the marginal cost of producing a product, but often this is a relatively minor consideration. The prices of specialty pharmaceutical products can be extraordinary, reaching $475 000 per patient for Novartis's CAR-T therapy. Prices also vary across markets, with a 30-day supply of Janssen's Xarelto® priced at $48 in South Africa, $102 in Switzerland, and $292 in the United States, or 400 mg of Genentech's Avastin® priced at $956 in South Africa, $1752 in

Switzerland, and $3930 in the United States. Not only are drug prices high, but cancer therapies have experienced significant price growth. In one analysis, the monthly cost of oncology products has increased from approximately $100 as recently as 1980 to $10 000 by 2010.

## Health Economics and Health Care Financing

### Health Insurance

Insurance is a mechanism for sharing risk across individuals. Generally, insurance works best when the occurrence being insured is infrequent, can be catastrophic to the individual, and is not influenced by the individual or organization being insured. In insurance markets characterized by these conditions, insurance can be a relatively inexpensive proposition. Health insurance has different characteristics. We use healthcare services frequently, and with medications even more frequently. While some healthcare costs can be catastrophic, not all are. While paying for a monthly medication is not enjoyable, for most people it is not financially catastrophic. Finally, consumption of healthcare services is inherently influenced not only by individuals (do you want to go to the clinician for that bad cold or sprained ankle?), but also by pharmaceutical manufacturers and healthcare systems encouraging you in prime time television advertisements to consume more healthcare resources. As a result, health insurance is often a very expensive insurance product. In truth, most health insurance combines the idea of prepayment for usual healthcare services with a catastrophic medical benefit (to some extent, high-deductible health plans try to separate out these two different elements of healthcare financing).

A lot of attention has been focused on the impact of health insurance on the prices of pharmaceutical products. Historically, prescription drugs were relatively affordable, and so were paid for by patients. As medications became more effective, the concept of prescription drug insurance began to develop. In 1960 in the United States, 96% of prescription drug spending was out of pocket by individuals. By 1980, out-of-pocket spending was still 71% of total spending. By 1990, it was down to 57%, 2000 to 28%, 2010 to 18%, and 2015 to 14%. Prescription drug coverage has led to a transformation of the pharmaceutical market. Over this same period, the prescription drug market in the US has grown from $2.7 billion in 1960 to $479 billion in gross sales in 2018 (resulting in net pharmaceutical sales to manufacturers of $344 billion).

## Moral Hazard

Health economists have long been worried about the economic impact of health insurance on the patterns of consumption of healthcare due to a concept called "moral hazard." Moral hazard describes the change in individual behavior between conditions of self-pay and conditions of third-party payment. Kenneth Arrow was awarded the Nobel Prize in economics for developing this framework, and Mark Pauly further developed the theory to focus on demand.

The basic framework is easy to understand. We all make purchases based on our concept of value. We generally make purchases of goods or products for $1.00 when we perceive that they offer $1.00 worth of value. This concept of value is an individual determination: we all have our own tastes, preferences, and needs which form our assessment of value.

Third-party payment alters this fundamental calculus. Consider going out to dinner with a group of friends. After the menu is passed around, you notice items of lower and higher price, say salad and steak. You can approach payment in one of two ways: individual checks or splitting the check. If you all decide on individual checks before you order, you may decide to purchase the lower-cost salad since you are on a budget. However, what happens if you decide to split the check before you order? You may be worried that everyone else at the table is likely to order the higher-priced steak, and you will have to pay your share of their higher-priced meals. Since you are paying for their steak, why not order your own steak so at least you get the benefit of the higher price you will pay for dinner? In this simple illustration, your behavior changes between self-payment and third-party payment models.

Health insurance is one form of third-party payment. Under health insurance, rather than paying the full cost of medical products, you pay only a co-payment (fixed amount), or co-insurance (a percentage payment) for medical products. As illustrated in Figure 18.1, products 1 through 3 offer at least $1.00 of value for $1.00 of cost. In a self-payment model, you would be expected to purchase only products 1 through 3 since only these products have a value of $1.00. In an insurance model, however, you only pay the co-payment of $0.20. Now,

| | Product 1 | Product 2 | Product 3 | Product 4 | Product 5 | Product 6 | Product 7 |
|---|---|---|---|---|---|---|---|
| **Value** | 1.50 | 1.25 | 1.0 | .75 | .50 | .25 | .10 |
| **Cost (No Insurance)** | $1.00 | $1.00 | $1.00 | $1.00 | $1.00 | $1.00 | $1.00 |
| **Cost (Insurance)** | $0.20 | $0.20 | $0.20 | $0.20 | $0.20 | $0.20 | $0.20 |

**Figure 18.1** Moral Hazard and Product Choice. Note: Cost (No insurance)-assumes only cash payments for the product. Cost (insurance)-assumes the product is covered by an insurance policy with a 20% coinsurance requirement.

products 1 through 6 offer value equal to or greater than the $0.20 copayment, so using the same rule (only buying products that offer value greater than or equal to the price you pay), you would purchase products 1 through 6. Again, behavior changes under conditions of third-party payment. While many economists have argued that health insurance increases the overall cost of healthcare due to these changes in demand, there is also the concept of good moral hazard where people can purchase goods or products through insurance that would otherwise be unaffordable. It is possible to develop a direct estimate of the increase in prescription drug spending between those with and without insurance.

To this point, the discussion has focused on the impact of moral hazard on the demand for healthcare products. However, the impact of moral hazard also extends to the supply side of healthcare. While much of the literature examines the impact of moral hazard on the provision of services, there is also an impact on the price of products. Given insurance, the suppliers of high-value products can realize that products are perceived as being significantly underpriced since insured patients only consider the out-of-pocket costs and not the full cost of therapy. Applying a value framework to pricing can lead manufacturers to raise their prices to meet the value threshold rather than simply developing a price to meet their internal financial expectations. This supply-side moral hazard effect on the price of pharmaceutical products have been much less discussed in the literature.

Again, going back to the basic example of product 1 in Figure 18.1, this product provides great value to patients under conditions of self-payment and even more under conditions of third-party payment. Sophisticated suppliers will notice these conditions. In a competitive market, suppliers will have little ability to influence the welfare surplus enjoyed by patients in this example since the price is determined by the market and is driven by entry and exit of firms. However, there are circumstances when suppliers have power to influence prices, especially in healthcare. Suppliers can have market power when they have a barrier to market entry such as a patent awarded to a pharmaceutical manufacturer or a product developed for a niche category, such as an orphan drug, which is too small to attract competition. In these cases, suppliers can increase the price of product 1 based on value. If they decide to price at the total value of the product, they could raise the price from $1.00 to $1.50 to capture the full value to patients. Under our conceptual model, this pricing strategy would be attractive to patients even in a cash pay market. However, under conditions of third-party payment, suppliers can consider an even more aggressive pricing strategy by considering that patients measure value against their co-insurance, not the full cost of the product. Under these conditions, suppliers can raise the price to $7.50 while consumers would have a cost-share of $1.50, or an amount equal to the value they expect to receive from the therapy. As a result of supply-side moral hazard, the cost increased from $1.00 to $7.50 in this simple example. Co-payment coupons or patient assistance programs can exacerbate this effect by artificially decreasing the amount individuals have to pay. This "discount" on out-of-pocket payments can allow suppliers even more latitude to raise prices under this framework.

### Behavioral Economics

This concept of patients being risk-averse is consistent with the idea of buying health insurance in the first place. Buying health insurance is seen as a risk-averse financial decision. People pay some money annually for health insurance to avoid the potential financial consequences associated with the rare risk of becoming severely ill. Consumers may even buy certain policies with limits on things that are not important to them when they are healthy – narrow networks of providers, for example, or limits on the drug formulary for specialty pharmaceutical products. However, buying health insurance is not the same as buying health care. Whether the risk-averse decision-making approach to buying insurance carry-over to making treatment decisions for health care products or services is an open question.

Let's consider a clinical scenario. Assume an otherwise healthy patient comes into a physician's office. They feel great, have a full social and work life, exercise regularly, and have a lot to look forward to. Given a history of smoking in the past, the physician had ordered a chest X-ray. Unfortunately, the chest X-ray showed that the patient had a spot on their lung. After further work-up, it was found to be lung cancer that had spread. This otherwise healthy person now has a life-threatening condition. Obviously, this is a significant loss in life expectancy for the patient. How do they react to the shock of their diagnosis? They seek treatment for their condition. In this case, the patient will accept a treatment which has any chance of restoring their health, irrespective of the side effects of the therapy. They definitely do not ask about the cost of treatment. Under conditions of loss, the way that patients make decisions changes from how they felt about future potential treatment choices when they bought their health insurance policy.

This idea that people make different decisions under conditions of gains and losses earned Daniel Kahneman the Nobel Prize in Economics in 2002 (he collaborated with Amos Tversky in developing prospect theory, but Amos passed away before the prize was awarded). Under conditions of gains, we are risk-averse, and under conditions of loss we are risk-seeking. When a 70-year-old patient refuses a flu shot because of her concerns that she does not want to get sick from the shot she is under a condition of gain (full health) and is being risk-averse. The unfortunate patient with lung cancer is an example of decision making under conditions of loss. The application of this framework to treatment choices by patients with life threatening diseases helps to explain the apparently risk-seeking behavior of patients. This study of the psychology of decision making in real-world setting has been called behavioral economics.

More recently, Kahneman and others have focused on the role of emotion in decision making. They have developed a framework which considers two different ways of making decisions, System 1 and System 2. System 1 decision processes are autonomous decision-making efforts that represent our "gut" or emotional response to an uncertain situation. System 1 processes easily incorporate societal attitudes and is subject to many systematic flaws. System 2 decision processes are more data driven and analytical, but they have a high cognitive burden. In the normal course of events, we make most decisions using the System 1 framework, despite its limitations, so that we minimize our cognitive burden in making simple choices or completing simple job tasks. However, we have System 2 processes available for more complex decision making. Importantly, in a heightened emotional state, we generally rely on System 1 processes for decision making. This can be critically important in understanding medical decision making, where patients (or their loved ones) can experience significant anxiety from the care process, the diagnosis itself, or can be in a heightened emotional state from the experience of the symptoms of the illness, especially when suffering from a disease with an acute presentation.

While the role of loss can make patients appear to be risk seeking in making treatment choices, we have suggested that the role of emotion can also lead to the same type of decision making by patients.

## Economic Evaluation of Pharmaceuticals

Across the globe, technology assessment agencies have been established to help provide or evaluate economic data as part of the reimbursement process. In light of all of the challenges of third-party payment, the charge to these agencies is to understand the value of new medical therapies (value is the cost in relationship to the benefit), and to make a recommendation about whether they should be included in a benefit package for patients. In the UK, the National Institute for Health and Care Excellence (NICE) provides guidance to the National Health Service. In Germany, the Institute for Quality and Efficiency in Health Care (IQWiG) evaluates the effectiveness of drugs. In the US, the Institute for Clinical and Economic Review (ICER) is a private organization publishing independent economic analyses of new pharmaceutical products.

## Methodological Problems to be Addressed by Pharmacoeconomic Research

In considering economic analysis of medical care, there are three dimensions of analysis, represented by the three axes of the cube in

Figure 18.2 with which readers should become familiar. Along the X-axis are three types of economic analysis – cost identification, cost-effectiveness, and cost–benefit. Along the Y-axis are four points of view, or perspectives, that one may take in carrying out an analysis. One may take the point of view of society in assessing the costs and benefits of a new medical therapy. Alternatively, one may take the point of view of the patient, the payer, or the provider. Along the third axis, the Z-axis, are the types of costs and benefits that can be included in economic analysis of medical care. These costs and benefits, which will be defined below, include direct costs and benefits, productivity costs and benefits, and intangible costs and benefits.

### Types of Analysis

#### Cost–Benefit Analysis

Cost–benefit analysis of medical care compares the cost of a medical intervention to its benefit. Both costs and benefits are measured

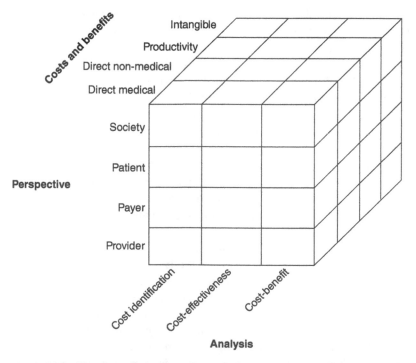

**Figure 18.2** The three dimensions of economic evaluation of clinical care. Reproduced from Bombardier and Eisenberg (1985) with permission from *The Journal of Rheumatology*.

---

**Case Example 18.1    Economic Evaluation of High-Dose Chemotherapy plus Autologous Stem Cell Transplantation for Metastatic Breast Cancer**

---

*Background*

A clinical trial of high-dose chemotherapy plus autologous hematopoietic stem cell transplantation versus conventional dose chemotherapy in women with metastatic breast cancer found no significant differences in survival between the two treatment groups. Thus, the economic evaluation would provide decision makers with important additional information about the two therapies.

*Question*

What were the differences between the two treatment groups with regard to course of treatment and resources consumed?

*Approach*

- The researchers abstracted the clinical trial records and oncology department flow sheets retrospectively to document resource use.
- Each patient's course of treatment and resource use was analyzed in four phases. Based on these clinical phases, patients were grouped into one of three clinical "trajectories."
- Costs were estimated using the Medicare Fee Schedule for inpatient costs and average wholesale prices for medications.
- Sensitivity analyses examined changes in the discount rate, hospital costs, and the number of cycles of the chemotherapeutic drugs paclitaxel and docetaxel.

*Results*

- Patients undergoing transplantation used more resources, mostly due to inpatient care.
- The investigators also found differences by clinical trajectory, and these differences were not consistent between treatment groups.
- High-dose chemotherapy plus stem-cell transplantation was associated with greater morbidity and economic costs with no improvement in survival.
- Results of the sensitivity analyses suggested that the findings were robust even when important cost assumptions varied.

*Strengths*

- By studying resource use and estimating costs, the authors were able to quantify the economic burden associated with the two treatments.
- The study allowed the investigators to provide novel information about the "clinical trajectories" of patients with metastatic breast cancer.
- The economic evaluation did not place any additional data collection burden on investigators, but yielded important secondary findings.
- Economic evaluation allowed the researchers to quantify the economic burden associated with interventions.

*Limitations*

- Collection of resource use data from the clinical trial records may have resulted in underestimation of treatment costs.
- Resource costs were estimated rather than directly observed.

*Key Points*

- By studying resource use and estimating costs, the authors were able to quantify the economic burden associated with the two treatments and to provide information about the "clinical trajectories" of patients with metastatic breast cancer.
- Sensitivity analyses are crucial in studies that rely on numerous estimates and assumptions.
- Economic analysis can provide important additional information to decision makers in cases where no differences were observed between treatment groups on the primary clinical endpoint.

---

**Case Example 18.2    Economic Analysis of a Novel SARS-CoV-2 Vaccine**

*Background*

SARS-CoV-2 emerged in late 2019 and spawned a global pandemic in 2020. Since this was a novel virus, there was no native immunity in infected populations. There was a global rush to develop a vaccine. You are now a member of a national panel looking to determine the appropriate market price for the vaccine.

*Question and Issue*

- What are the economic benefits of the vaccine?
- How would you assess the value of the vaccine based on estimates of the population that have yet to be exposed to the virus?
- How should these economic benefits relate to the price you would agree is a fair market price for the vaccine? For developed countries? For emerging market economies?

*Approach*

- How would your answer differ if you were asked to consider a budget impact analysis,

a cost-effectiveness analysis, or a cost–benefit analysis? What about a benefit pool analysis?

- How does choice of perspective influence your assessment of the question?
- How does societal value relate to the determination of a market price? What other considerations might be in play?
- Would your analysis change if you were risk-averse (someone who survived an asymptomatic infection with SARS-CoV-2), or risk-seeking (high-risk individual who has not been infected with SARS-CoV-2)?
- How would consideration of the role of public vs private investment in vaccine development impact your assessment?

*Key Points*

This analysis of a fair market price for a SARS-CoV-2 vaccine highlights many of the challenges in economic analysis of pharmaceutical products.

---

in the same (usually monetary) units (e.g. dollars). These measurements are used to determine either the ratio of dollars spent to dollars saved or the net saving (if benefits are greater than costs) or net cost. All else being equal, an investment should be undertaken when its benefits exceed its costs. One potential difficulty of cost–benefit analysis is that it requires researchers to express an intervention's costs and outcomes in the same units. Thus, monetary values must be associated with years of life lost and morbidity due to disease and with years of life gained and morbidity avoided due to intervention.

**Cost-Effectiveness Analysis**

Cost-effectiveness analysis provides an alternative approach that avoids the dilemma of assessing the monetary value of health

outcomes as part of the evaluation. While cost generally is still calculated only in monetary terms (e.g. dollars spent), effectiveness is determined independently and may be measured only in clinical terms, using any meaningful clinical unit. For example, one might measure clinical outcomes in terms of number of lives saved, complications prevented, or diseases cured. Alternatively, health outcomes can be reported in terms of a change in an intermediate clinical outcome, such as cost per percent change in blood cholesterol level. These results generally are reported as a ratio of costs to clinical benefits, with costs measured in monetary terms but with benefits measured in the units of the relevant outcome measure (for example, dollars per year of life saved).

When several outcomes result from a medical intervention (e.g. the prevention of both death and disability), cost-effectiveness analysis may consider these two outcomes together only if a common measure of outcome can be developed. Frequently, analysts combine different categories of clinical outcomes according to their desirability, assigning a weighted utility, or value, to the overall treatment outcome. A utility weight is a measure of the patient's preferences for his/her health state or for the outcome of an intervention. The comparison of costs and utilities sometimes is referred to as cost–utility analysis, with the denominator expressed as quality-adjusted life years (QALYs).

## Cost Identification Analysis

An even less complex approach than cost–benefit or cost-effectiveness analysis would be simply to enumerate the costs involved in medical care and to ignore the outcomes that result from that care. This approach is known as cost identification analysis, by which the researcher can determine alternative ways of providing a service. The analysis might be expressed in terms of the cost per unit of service provided. For example, a cost identification study might measure the cost of a course of antibiotic treatment, but it would not calculate the clinical outcomes (cost-effectiveness analysis) or the value of the outcomes in units of currency (cost–benefit analysis). Cost identification studies, which include comparisons among different treatments based upon their costs alone, are appropriate only if treatment outcomes or benefits are equivalent among the therapies being evaluated.

## Sensitivity Analysis

Most cost–benefit and cost-effectiveness studies require large amounts of data that may vary in reliability and validity, and could affect the overall results of the study. This is especially the case when models are developed for the economic analysis using secondary data sources, when data collection is performed retrospectively, or when critical data elements are unmeasured or unknown. Sensitivity analysis

is a set of procedures in which the results of a study are recalculated using alternate values for some of the study's variables in order to test the sensitivity of the conclusions to these altered specifications. Such an analysis can yield several important results by demonstrating the independence or dependence of a result on particular assumptions, establishing the minimum or maximum values of a variable that would be required to affect a recommendation to adopt or reject a program, and identifying clinical or economic uncertainties that require additional research. In general, sensitivity analyses are performed on variables that have a significant effect on the study's conclusions but for which values are uncertain.

## Types of Costs

Another dimension of economic analysis of clinical practice illustrated by Figure 18.2 is the evaluation of costs of a therapy. Economists consider three types of costs: direct, productivity, and intangible.

## Direct Medical Costs

The direct medical costs of care usually are associated with monetary transactions and represent costs incurred during the provision of care. Examples of direct medical costs include payments for purchasing a pharmaceutical product, payments for physicians' fees, salaries of allied health professionals, or purchases of diagnostic tests. Because the charge for medical care may not accurately reflect the resources consumed, accounting or statistical techniques may be needed to determine direct costs.

## Direct Nonmedical Costs

Monetary transactions undertaken as a result of illness or healthcare to detect, prevent, or treat disease are not limited to direct medical costs. There is another type of cost that is often overlooked: direct nonmedical costs. These costs are incurred because of illness or the need to seek medical care. They include the cost of transportation to the hospital or physician's office, the cost of special clothing needed because of the illness, the cost of hotel stays for receiving medical treatment at a distant medical facility, and the cost of special housing (e.g. modification of a home to accommodate an ill individual). Direct nonmedical costs, which are generally paid out of pocket by patients and their families, are just as much direct costs as are expenses that are more usually covered by third-party insurance plans.

### Productivity Costs

In contrast to direct costs, productivity costs, sometimes referred to as indirect costs, do not stem from transactions for goods or services. Instead, they represent the cost of morbidity (e.g. time lost from work) or mortality (e.g. premature death leading to removal from the workforce). They are costs because they represent the loss of opportunities to use a valuable resource, a life, in alternative ways. A variety of techniques are used to estimate productivity costs of illness or healthcare. Sometimes, as with varicella vaccination, the productivity costs of an illness are substantially greater than the direct costs of the illness.

### Intangible Costs

Intangible costs are those of pain, suffering, and grief. These costs result from medical illness itself and from the services used to treat the illness. They are difficult to measure as part of a pharmacoeconomic study, though they are clearly considered by clinicians and patients in considering potential alternative treatments. Although investigators are developing ways to measure intangible costs – such as willingness-to-pay analysis whereby patients are asked to place monetary values on intangible costs – at present these costs are often omitted in clinical economics research.

### Perspective of Analysis

The third axis in Figure 18.2 is the perspective of an economic analysis of medical care. Costs

and benefits can be calculated with respect to society's, the patient's, the payer's, and the provider's points of view. A study's perspective determines how costs and benefits are measured, and the economist's strict definition of costs (the consumption of a resource that could otherwise be used for another purpose) no longer may be appropriate when perspectives different from that of society as a whole are used. For example, a hospital's cost of providing a service may be less than its charge. From the hospital's perspective, then, the charge could be an overstatement of the resources consumed for some services. However, if the patient has to pay the full charge, it is an accurate reflection of the cost of the service to the patient. Alternatively, if the hospital decreases its costs by discharging patients early, the hospital's costs may decrease but patients' costs may increase because of the need for increased outpatient expenses that are not covered by their health insurance plan.

Because costs will differ depending on the perspective, the economic impact of an intervention will be different from different perspectives. To make comparisons of the economic impact across different interventions, it is important for all economic analyses to adopt a similar perspective. It has been recommended that, as a base case, all analyses adopt a societal perspective.

In summary, economic analysis of medical technology or medical care evaluates a medical service by comparing its dollar cost with its dollar benefit (cost–benefit), by measuring its dollar cost in relation to its outcomes (cost-effectiveness), or simply by tabulating the costs involved (cost identification). Direct costs are generated as services are provided. In addition, productivity costs should be considered, especially in determining the benefit of a service that decreases morbidity or mortality. Finally, the perspective of the study determines the costs and benefits that will be quantified in the analysis, and sensitivity analyses test the effects of changes in variable specifications for estimated measures on the results of the study.

## Using Economic Data

Health economics helps to understand both the supply and demand for pharmaceutical products, while pharmacoeconomics provides insight into the value of products to patient, payers, and the marketplace. With all of these elegant data, the next challenge for analysts and policy makers is to relate the results of the economic analysis to purchase decisions for pharmaceutical products. Should a patient, hospital, or payer (public or private) make a decision to approve payments for a therapy (for example, by adding the product to an approved drug list or formulary)?

Generally, if a product is thought to add clinical benefit and save money, it is an easy decision to add the therapy. These types of products are described as cost-saving or dominant (see Figure 18.3). For example, vaccines sometimes fall into this category, as do generic drugs (in comparison with brand-name products). If a product worsens clinical outcomes but raises cost, this is also usually an easy decision to not add the therapy. These types of products are described as dominated but are much less common. The major challenges in making formulary decisions generally relate to therapies that add clinical benefit at additional cost. This analysis requires further discussion on how this decision can be approached.

Outside healthcare environments, we make these types of decisions frequently. The new product on the shelf tastes better but costs more. Should we buy this product? The first question is a budget question – do we have the money to make this purchase? We have not said anything about prices but obviously, this is an important part of our consideration. If the new product is enormously more expensive (it is hand crafted in small batches and infused with gold and sold in a crystal decanter), we may not have the money to afford the new product and so the question becomes moot. This is a budget constraint. This constraint does not have to be so extreme; we can make a budget of $100 for a grocery list, and hold ourselves to meeting our budget in our shopping trip. With this budget, even a modestly priced new item may not meet our budget constraint.

Of course, we may decide we have some room in our budget to increase spending at the supermarket. For simplicity, let's assume we have two choices to consider for our increased spending: products A and B. Product A is the tastier version of one of our shopping staples, while product B is a new item that a friend recommended. Product A costs $5.00 more than our usual item, and product B costs $5.00, so our budget would now be $105 if either is added to the shopping list (a 5% increase in cost). How would you choose between these two? This is a cost-effectiveness question. Given the increase in cost, which product would provide more value to you as a consumer - enhanced flavor

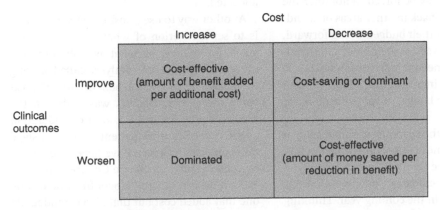

**Figure 18.3** Cost and clinical outcomes.

from A or the novelty of B? We make these types of decisions all the time, and the answer greatly depends on individual taste preferences. So, in this simple case, cost is transparent and value is based on individual preferences.

Now, back to the pharmaceutical market. Budget constraints are built into healthcare spending. National health insurance programs often have a fixed allocation from government for annual spending. In private health insurance markets, health insurers estimate premiums for the coming year before selling policies during open-enrollment season, or as much as 18 months in advance of actual spending. So, the introduction of a new product that adds cost can face real budget constraints depending on the potential magnitude of the spending increase. Sofosbuvir, a drug used to treat hepatitis C, had a list price of $84 000 in the US and a potential market size of 3.2 million people when it was first launched. This would require a staggering budget of $269 billion to treat everyone with the infection. So, while the clinical potential of this therapy was tremendous, the budget constraint resulted in policies to limit its adoption.

As with the shopping example, budget constraints can be absolute. For example, the Medicaid program is jointly funded by federal and state governments, and states are not allowed to run budget deficits by law. Thus, if increased spending on a new therapy would require an increase in outlay by the Medicaid program, states may be forced to not offer the therapy, or to cut back in other areas of spending to stay within their budget. Going forward, if states wanted to add to their Medicaid spending, they would need to raise revenues (taxes) to support this increased spending, or find other parts of the budget to cut (education, for example).

Again, as with the shopping example, budget constraints may not be absolute. Imagine that a health insurance company calculated its premiums to incorporate new spending on drugs to be introduced in the coming year. Thinking about the budget from the perspective of premiums is interesting. We have called this approach the "benefit pool" perspective. It suggests that we can calculate how much additional premium we would all have to contribute for us to have an increase in our pharmaceutical budget. The budget model looks at the issue from the insurer perspective, while the benefit pool perspective looks at the same issue from the perspective of everyone buying insurance (or paying taxes). With an increase in premium, we would still have a budget constraint, but one that allows for growth in pharmacy spending.

With the additional resources, we would need to develop a process for increasing our pharmacy spending. In our cash payment shopping model, the willingness to allocate additional resources to our budget was based on consumers' individual perceptions of value. In healthcare, we do not pay for our medicines directly, so the organization administering the benefit pool (which could be a public or private payer) needs to make this determination. Here, cost-effectiveness analysis can be used to assess the relative value of additional investments in different therapies. From here, one can consider the relative value across products and fund the product that is the most economically attractive (the lowest cost-effectiveness ratio) first. In this way, we will ensure that incremental spending is for the product delivering the most value. You can continue adding therapies in this way until all of your resources are allocated.

Another way to use a cost-effectiveness ratio is to set a criterion of what represents good value for money, or what is "economically attractive." In the US, dialysis care has long been used to provide a benchmark of good value for money. Dialysis was added to the Medicare program in 1972, after consideration of the cost of care for patients with end-stage renal disease. As a result, we have an example of a clinical program where Congress made an explicit decision to add a benefit to Medicare, one that added cost but that also extended life expectancy for beneficiaries who need the service. Since patients on dialysis can cost $50 000 per annum, the benchmark for value as reflected in Congressional approval of this service was seen to be $50 000 per year of life gained. Since dialysis requires treatment three times a week for several hours at a time, the benchmark was thought to be even higher when considering quality-adjusted survival.

Does that mean that we can add therapies to the formulary that offer good value? The answer is, "it depends." Again, while cost-effectiveness analysis does a good job assessing the relative value of different therapies, the ratio itself is not tied to a budget impact or premium. In other words, a product that is not good value for money for a rare condition would have a relatively modest budget impact, while a drug that is good value for money for a common condition could have a significant impact on budgets. The value of a product can also change by indication. For example, since patients with known heart disease have higher risk for cardiovascular events than patients without heart disease, secondary prevention can provide more value for money than primary prevention. To date, efforts such as pricing by indication have been challenging to implement.

Rather than providing an absolute recommendation, the UK has an implicit relative framework for value, with products that have a lower cost-effectiveness ratio more likely to be recommended by NICE.

Returning to the benefit pool perspective can be another way of looking at this question. This analysis looks at the impact on the health insurance premium resulting from the addition of a new product to the formulary. For example, the addition of PCSK-9 inhibitors (used to lower cholesterol), which was initially priced at more than $14 000 annually per patient, was calculated to add $140 to the premium for everyone in the insurance pool under modest adoption assumptions. This perspective can be generalized to the consideration of specialty pharmaceutical products more broadly (Figure 18.4). Here, we can see that health insurance premiums increase $250 for every 0.25% of the population that receives a $100 000 drug for any indication. The relationship of access to innovation and affordability is an area of ongoing debate.

Finally, we have the quadrant where the products save money but at the expense of worse clinical outcomes. Actually, the use of therapies that meet this criterion is relatively common, as long as the amount of money saved is large relative to the loss of health benefits (a cost-effectiveness ratio of savings related to benefits lost where a higher number is the most economically attractive). For example, amoxicillin is recommended for first-line

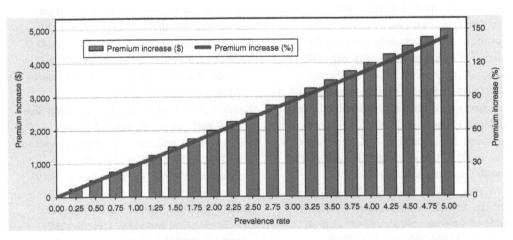

**Figure 18.4** Specialty Pharmaceuticals and Premiums. *Source:* Adapted from Hirsch et al. (2014).

therapy for otitis media, despite the high level of resistance to this antibiotic. This is because of the low cost of the therapy, and the low likelihood of significant complications of failure of this initial treatment.

## The Future

The cost of pharmaceutical products is an important challenge for everyone involved in the healthcare value chain, including patients, physicians, payers, and government. While we all desire innovation in healthcare, it is not clear if it is possible to afford innovation at any price. We have outlined an expanded version of the study of the economics of pharmaceuticals to begin to flesh out a fuller discussion of this fascinating and complex subject.

## Acknowledgements

The author dedicates this chapter to John M. Eisenberg, MD (1946–2002), mentor, friend,

and fellow author in previous editions of this work. The author also acknowledges Henry Glick PhD, Harris Koffer Pharm D, Dan Polsky PhD, and Shelby Reed PhD for contributions to previous versions of this chapter.

## Key Points

- The economics of pharmaceuticals are driven by the value of products, the health condition, and the type of payment model for these products.
- In general, programs that cost more and are more effective (and perhaps even some programs that cost less and have reduced clinical outcomes) are more likely be adopted if both their incremental cost-effectiveness ratios and budget impact from a benefit pool perspective fall within an acceptable range.
- Results of an economic analysis are just one component of the decision-making process regarding the adoption of an intervention; social, legal, political, and ethical issues, among others, are also important.

## Further Reading

Arrow, K.J. (1963). Uncertainty and the welfare economics of medical care. *AER* 53 (5): 141–149.

Bombardier, C. and Eisenberg, J. (1985). Looking into the crystal ball: can we estimate the lifetime cost of rheumatoid arthritis? *The Journal of Rheumatology* 12 (2): 201–204.

DiMasi, J.A., Grabowski, H.G., and Hansen, R.W. (2016). Innovation in the pharmaceutical industry: new estimates of R&D costs. *Journal of Health Economics* 47: 20–33.

Drummond, M.F., Sculpher, M.J., Torrance, G.W. et al. (2005). *Methods for the Evaluation of Health Care Programs*, 3e. New York, New York: Oxford Medical Publications.

Eisenberg, J.M. (1989). Clinical economics: a guide to the economic analysis of clinical practices. *JAMA* 262 (20): 2879–2886.

Hirsch, B.R., Balu, S., and Schulman, K.A. (2014). The impact of specialty pharmaceuticals as drivers of health care costs. *Health Affairs* 33 (10): 1714–1720.

Hlatky, M.A., Owens, D.K., and Sanders, G.D. (2006). Cost-effectiveness as an outcome in randomized clinical trials. *Clinical Trials* 3 (6): 543–551.

Kahneman, D. (2013). *Thinking Fast and Slow*. New York: Farrar, Straus and Giroux.

Lakdawalla, D. and Sood, N. (2009). Innovation and the welfare effects of public drug insurance. *Journal of Public Economics* 93 (3–4): 541–548.

Outlook for Global Medicines Through 2021: Balancing Cost and Value. Quintiles IMS Institute. (2016). http://www.imshealth.com/

en_US/thought-leadership/quintilesims-institute/reports/reports/outlook_for_global_medicines_through_2021 (accessed 6 June 2017.

Pauly, M.V. (1968). The economics of moral Hazard: comment. *AER* 58 (3): 531–537.

The Staffs Of Ranking Member Ron Wyden And Committee Member Charles E. Grassley. (2015). *The Price Of Sovaldi And Its Impact On The U.S. Health Care System,* DECEMBER (2015). US Senate, Committee of Finance. https://www.finance.senate.gov/imo/media/doc/1%20The%20Price%20of%20Sovaldi%20and%20Its%20Impact%20on%20the%20U.S.%20Health%20Care%20System%20(Full%20Report).pdf (accessed 8 July 2017).

Ramsey, S., Willke, R., Briggs, A. et al. (2005). Good research practices for cost-effectiveness analysis alongside clinical trials: the ISPOR RCT-CEA Task Force report. *Value in Health* 8 (5): 521–533.

Rasiel, E.B., Weinfurt, K.P., and Schulman, K.A. (2005). Can prospect theory explain risk-seeking behavior by terminally ill patients? *Medical Decision Making* 25 (6): 609–613.

Reed, S.D., Anstrom, K.J., Bakhai, A. et al. (2005). Conducting economic evaluations alongside multinational clinical trials: toward a research consensus. *American Heart Journal* 149 (3): 434–443.

Reed, S.D., Anstrom, K.J., Ludmer, J.A. et al. (2004). Cost-effectiveness of imatinib versus interferon-alpha plus low-dose cytarabine for patients with newly diagnosed chronic-phase chronic myeloid leukemia. *Cancer* 101 (11): 2574–2583.

Reed, S.D., Friedman, J.Y., Velazquez, E.J. et al. (2004). Multinational economic evaluation of valsartan in patients with chronic heart failure: results from the Valsartan Heart Failure Trial (Val-HeFT). *American Heart Journal* 148 (1): 122–128.

Reed SD, Radeva JI, Weinfurt KP, McMurray JJV, Pfeffer MA, Velazquez EJ, et al. Resource use, costs, and quality of life among patients in the multinational Valsartan in Acute Myocardial Infarction Trial.

Weinstein, M.C. and Stason, W.B. (1982). Cost-effectiveness of coronary artery bypass surgery. *Circulation* 66 (5): 56–68.

# 19

# Patient Engagement and Patient Reported Outcomes

*Esi M. Morgan[1,2] and Adam C. Carle[3,4,5]*

[1] Seattle Children's Hospital, Seattle, WA, USA
[2] University of Washington, Seattle, WA, USA
[3] Cincinanti Children's Hospital Medical Center, Cincinnati, OH, USA
[4] University of Cincinnati, College of Medicine, Cincinnati, OH, USA
[5] University of Cincinnati, College of Arts and Sciences, Cincinnati, OH, USA

## Introduction

*Patient engagement* reflects the effective participation of patients in their own healthcare. The Institute of Medicine's 2001 report on reforming and improving US healthcare identified patient-centeredness as one of six guiding aims for healthcare. Patient centeredness gives rise to the perspective that healthcare is better considered a service rather than a product. As such, achieving the best patient outcomes hinges on co-production. With co-production, the patient (service user) and clinician (service professional) are in a collaborative relationship, sharing creation of the health care service and responsibility for outcomes. This reframing of the patient-clinician relationship elevates the importance of measuring *patient reported outcomes* (PROs).

A PRO is a measure of a patient's health based entirely on reports that come directly from the patient without interpretation by a clinician or anyone else. PROs can be self-reported rating scales, symptoms reports, questionnaires, or structured or unstructured interviews that directly record patients' responses. PROs enable patients to directly communicate information about their status with respect to various domains of health, including: symptoms, function, quality of life, health behaviors, and experience with care. PROs translate the patient experience into data. The use of subjective report in PROs recognizes that a patient's health concerns may not be perceived by the clinician. Further, by failing to elicit direct patient input, clinicians may prioritize topics less valued by patients. Incorporating PROs into clinical care has the potential to enrich clinician patient communication, as well as provide data to anchor clinical decisions and interventions.

Advances in measurement theory and the use of item response theory (IRT) models in measure development have resulted in PROs that are shorter, more reliable, and more precise than previous PROs. Nevertheless, the implementation, interpretation, use and evaluation of PROs pose practical and methodological challenges. In this chapter, we explore these challenges in the context of integration of PROs into pharmacoepidemiology research, including clinical trials and observational studies.

*Textbook of Pharmacoepidemiology*, Third Edition. Edited by Brian L. Strom, Stephen E. Kimmel, and Sean Hennessy.
© 2022 John Wiley & Sons Ltd. Published 2022 by John Wiley & Sons Ltd.

## Patient Reported Outcomes in Clinical Trials

The patient's perspective is important during development of new medication or medical products. PROs serve a variety of functions in new product development. PROs allow one to capture the patient's perspective as a clinical trial outcome. They can help better understand the impact of a medical condition on the patient in the realms of physical, mental, or social health and uncover (unmet) medical needs to be addressed by a new medication. PROs can also be used to enable estimation of the benefit to the patient of use of a medication during the clinical trial and, by extension, can be used to characterize the expected benefit to the end-user in the clinical setting. Adverse effects of treatment, or an estimate of risks of use, may also be captured by PROs. The Food and Drug Administration (FDA), as part of the 2012 reauthorization of the Prescription Drug Use Fee Act (PDUFA V), has been including patient input on the impact of chronic illness to inform which aspects of illness would be most meaningful to target from the patient perspective.

After clinical and PROs that are meaningful drug targets from the patient perspective are identified, it becomes important to be able to determine whether the drug/treatment/intervention under investigation exerts a clinically meaningful effect on the outcomes. Although a statistically significant change in outcome measure scores may be achieved, achieving statistical significance may not correspond to a clinically meaningful benefit. Determination that a change is of clinical meaningfulness rests on the idea that the outcome being measured is of relevance and importance to the patient and that the degree of change exerted creates a clinically appreciable benefit. We briefly describe methods to address this later in the chapter.

## Patient Reported Outcomes in Routine Care

A current challenge to the use of PROs as outcomes in observational studies is that PROs are not routinely collected in clinical care. However, use of PROs in clinical care is starting to increase. Over the past decade, there has been a growing body of published evidence on the benefits of incorporating PROs in clinical care including both process and outcomes improvement. A number of technical solutions for full integration into the electronic health record, used alongside the electronic health record (EHR) or hybrid approaches, have been described. User's guides have been published with step by step instructions for health systems considering adoption of PROs to facilitate incorporation into clinical care.

Published reports of integration of PROs into clinical care have evolved over time from describing acceptability and feasibility, to demonstration of improved care processes and communication, to preliminary evidence of increased clinician satisfaction and even improved outcomes. When PROs are collected and reviewed, patients perceive the clinician to have increased awareness of their symptoms, which otherwise might go unrecognized and unaddressed. Clinicians may be better able to identify and diagnose patient conditions, including mental health concerns, if PRO results are routinely collected. Using PROs may result in increased clinician awareness of the impact of the health condition on the patients' health related quality of life and facilitate patient-clinician discussions. Communication, shared decision making, and collaborative treatment planning is enhanced when PROs are incorporated into patient and clinician conversations. Case Example 19.1 describes the use of PROs to optimize treatment in clinical care.

**Case Example 19.1    Use of Patient Reported Outcomes to Optimize Treatment in Clinical Care**

*Background*
- Clinicians have used a treatment strategy in several chronic conditions to adjust medication to reach a treatment target, known as "treat to target." Examples of possible targets include a lab value (HgbA1c, lipid), a clinical measure (blood pressure, weight), or a measure of disease activity (PROs, or composite measure included PRO).
- A "Treat-to-Target" strategy to gain control of disease relies on regular, standard measurement of disease activity; setting a target for disease control together with the patient; and shared decision making to incorporate patient values and preferences into choice of treatment.

*Questions*
What are some factors that support the use of PROs in patient engagement?

*Approach*
Structured data forms, similar to case report forms, embedded in the electronic medical record enable routine, and regular assessment of patient disease activity at every clinical visit. Disease activity scores can be calculated and scored within the medical record for review with the patient and compared to treatment target. If the patient is not making timely progress toward the target, treatment may be adjusted (this may involve following a clinical decision support, published guideline, or algorithm). Use of standard data elements for collection at point of care of disease activity measures enables data extraction and upload into registries or databases for analysis, coupled with extraction of medications. This feeds analysis of comparative effectiveness of treatments. This approach is exemplified by the PR-COIN (Pediatric Rheumatology Care

and Outcomes Improvement Network) registry (https://pr-coin.org).

*Results*
Incorporating PROs into routine disease assessment that guides decision making and discussing this with the patients can improve patient engagement and patient understanding of how treatment adjustments are made. This could potentially improve adherence to treatment regimens.

*Strengths*
Use of structured data from clinical practice collected on an unbiased sample of patients (every clinic visit, every patient with a given diagnosis) is a resource for understanding comparative effectiveness.

*Limitations*
- There is need for clinician buy-in to collecting and reviewing standard disease activity metrics that include the patient perspectives (via PROs), willingness to share treatment decisions with the patients, and to follow standard treatment guidelines rather than their own style of practice.
- Additional study is needed into downstream effects on outcomes (disease activity, adherence, etc.).

*Key points*
- Incorporation of PROs into measures of disease activity used to inform treatment decisions embeds the patient's perspective into evaluation of treatment effectiveness and review and use of results fosters *patient engagement.*
- Reliable clinical collection of psychometrically sound PROs; integration of scores as discrete, research quality data into the medical record; and establishing MCIDs in PROs will contribute to more efficient, and rigorous observational and pharmacoepidemiologic research.

Much of the literature on the effective use of PROs in clinical medicine has come from the fields of oncology and surgery. For example, a recent compelling report from an oncology randomized trial of PRO use during routine cancer treatment showed that integration of PROs into the care of patients with metastatic cancer was associated with increased survival. This may have been a consequence of expedited medical care team response to patient symptoms, particularly adverse symptoms, and, subsequently, the ability to administer chemotherapy for a relatively longer duration.

Payers recently have begun encouraging PRO collection, including the use of financial incentives for tracking PRO data. For example, PROs are used to evaluate the impact and trajectory of improvement of surgical interventions in the case of Medicare reimbursement for elective joint replacement. The availability of such data can enhance observational studies by providing prospectively collected information on PROs.

# Patient Reported Outcomes as Motivation to Develop New Therapeutic Strategies

Therapeutically, incorporating PROs may contribute to a more targeted conversation on issues that concern the patient, which might otherwise go unaddressed. It may help to quantify the discomfort a patient feels and subsequently trigger the use of a therapeutic intervention. Information on disease control status can focus the visit on topics of most relevance and be a useful measure of disease burden. Having pre-specified and agreed-upon PRO score thresholds that trigger specific evidence-based interventions facilitates action by the clinician. Alternatively, aggregate patient reported data on symptoms, function, quality of life, or experience related to an intervention can be shared with an individual patient as part of a shared decision making discussion.

For example, *self-management support* is a key component of the Chronic Care Model. Patient engagement with informed, activated patients, is key to productive patient-clinician relationships, which affects clinical outcome improvement. Successful self-management support programs have the following elements: (i) clinicians communicate the expectation for the central role of the patient in managing their condition, (ii) patients' self-management skills, confidence in management ability, barriers and supports are assessed regularly, (iii) trained staff employ behavior change interventions, (iv) patients co-develop with health care professionals their own individualized treatment plans, and support is available on an ongoing basis if the patient needs it. Self-management support is a patient-centered, iterative and ongoing process. Due to the fact that the majority of chronic illness care occurs outside of the medical office in the interval (days to months) between office visits, PRO assessment has the potential to become an effective facilitator of in-between visit communication between patients and clinicians and may allow patients to better manage their health conditions.

Further, since medical care at outpatient office visits occurs at relatively infrequent intervals but health events occur on an ongoing basis, the trajectory of illness may not be adequately captured at clinic visits. As a result, medical decision making may not incorporate all relevant health information into treatment decisions. Imagine the situation where a patient, "Patient A," begins a new medication "Drug A" and experiences rapid improvement in signs and symptoms of disease, which gradually return to baseline over time. Patient B experiences gradual improvement following the initiation of "Drug B," then rapid worsening before their condition returns to baseline by time of follow up visit. Both patients have roughly the same disease activity level at the follow-up visit. In this scenario, information is lost about the relative lack of effectiveness and negative impact Patient B experienced being on Drug B, as more time was spent in a flare state than with "Patient A" who took "Drug A."

In the latter example, technology can enable the capture and transmission of both patients' unique experience to the clinical team. Data can be collected at home, on computers, mobile devices, or technology enabled patient generated data (e.g. physiologic monitors), and then shared with the clinical team. Data collection from patient wearable devices requires little or no effort from the patient perspective. This opens the possibility for patient data from in-between patient visits to inform action-oriented interventions. Patients who transmit data will have the expectation that results are reviewed, thus workflows will need to be optimized to allow for reliability of review, and prompt response if deterioration in status or other change is identified.

## Clinical Problems to be Addressed by Pharmacoepidemiologic Research

PROs are directly relevant to pharmacoepidemiology research. They capture information central to evaluating the benefits and adverse effects of medication that may elude physical exam or lab testing. Routine and systematic collection of PROs as part of clinical care will facilitate better understanding the impact of medications on symptoms and quality of life as part of post market surveillance. While PRO collection has benefit to pharmacoepidemiology research, the rationale behind incorporation of the patient voice into clinical care via the use of PROs is to identify unmet needs of patients and to help identify gaps in healthcare and, subsequently, respond to these unmet needs and/or gaps.

### Ensuring PRO Completion and Results Review

It is essential that clinical processes are in place so that research quality data results from clinical

data collection. As the primary motivation for PROs collection may be delivery of optimal patient centered care and better health outcomes, with the ability to use the data for research as secondary, the clinical team – and patients – must be aligned in perceiving the value of quality PRO data collection. To be most useful clinically, and to allow valid inferences in research, PROs must be collected routinely (reliably at regular intervals), uniformly (in a consistent manner), completely (able to be scored), and correctly (patients understand the questions and answers reflect their health status).

Once a decision is made to incorporate PROs into clinical care, there must be a means to achieve reliable review of the results by the clinical team. If clinicians do not understand the PRO measure, the way it is scored, do not feel it relevant to their specialty, or feel there is no intervention or action that can impact the PRO, they may not be inclined to review it. The solution may be cultural and social, and require a clinical champion to motivate the colleagues and gain agreement on selection of PROs (more below). On the other hand, barriers may be technical, related to location and ease of viewing of the reports in the medical record. This may require an information technology solution. Another solution may be to create a workflow in which discussion of PRO completion is an expected part of the clinic visit and is included into process of care quality measures. There are significant consequences of clinicians not reviewing PROs completed by patients. When clinicians do not review PROs it becomes a threat to co-production of care, risks the patient feeling their time and input was not valued and may result in a decreased willingness for PRO completion at subsequent visits. It is also a missed opportunity to check the reliability of the system for PRO administration.

### PRO Selection, Score Interpretation and Interventions

Instrument selection is critical for clinical and research applications to ensure the measure is clinically relevant, addresses an outcome of interest, and is brief and practical to administer. Fundamentally, any measure selected for use should be reliable, valid, and responsive. These and other considerations such as ease of understanding, ability to foster patient-clinician communication, and value in identifying unmet needs should be reviewed with representative patients and clinicians for input and agreement on importance. In order to be actionable, scores on measures for a specific health condition should be known, including the normal range versus when to intervene for an abnormal score. There is need for consensus and standard setting processes on threshold scores to trigger interventions. In order to track longitudinal change, it is helpful if the minimal clinically important difference (MCID) for improvement or worsening has been determined (discussed below). Ensuring these scores and thresholds for action are known, and identifying evidence based interventions or, where such evidence does not exist, gaining consensus agreement among practice clinicians and patient stakeholders on recommended interventions, will facilitate clinicians and patients moving from simple review and discussion of PROs to taking effective action and co-producing treatment plans based in part on PRO scores, which are meaningful to them.

## Patient Engagement and Individualized Assessment and Treatment Plans

Mobile health tracking systems offer the possibility of customized measurement (choice of PROs, timing of administration), and use of individualized measures, which may be of great importance in pharmacoepidemiology outcome studies. In addition, use of PROs for in-between clinic visit care for continuous monitoring and data feedback, with customized reporting and means to detect signals of health status change in a personalized system lends itself to N-of-1 trials. In this type of study an individual can make planned changes to treatment or lifestyle modification, then track changes in symptoms to evaluate for possible effectiveness. By keeping daily journals or other means of annotation, patients can see if other triggers or environmental factors may have led to changes in their health status. This structured type of intervention allows study of the impact of medications with relatively rapid onset and dissipation of effects (e.g. pain medications). In addition, one can study whether patients who are given access to their outcome data become more activated and engaged in their health care.

## Barriers to Measuring PROs in Clinical Practice and Using PROs to Guide Interventions

Barriers to PRO use are varied and start with garnering institutional resources to obtain, store and update electronic data collection tools. Designing integration of PROs into clinical workflow is a necessary step, which first requires gaining clinician consensus on the purpose and value of adding PRO measurement and review to the clinical encounter. Clinicians must understand the ways the use of structured PROs adds value over simply asking the patient about how they feel. Front line staff training on importance of PRO collection and distribution of questionnaires or devices of collection is required for reliability of PRO collection.

Clinician training is required on how to use PROs to facilitate high quality communication with patients. This requires training on how to interpret PRO results and on how to communicate about the results with patients. The process could be facilitated by orientating the patients themselves to use of PROs and their role in their clinical care. For PROs to serve the role in facilitating co-production of care may, in some circumstances, take reframing of the patient-clinician relationship, a complex endeavor in culture and behavior change.

Buy-in may become easier to obtain as more convincing data become available on PRO integration into care resulting in improved outcomes, as barriers to logistics of PRO collection are lowered, as graphical displays become more intuitive, and as interpretation of data and action steps become more familiar and supported with decision aids. Clinicians may have higher interest in use of PROs if they receive feedback on their own patients' scores, relating to outcomes or experience with care (satisfaction) and recognize they can take steps to improve performance.

As use of PROs in clinical trials and pharmacoepidemiology research becomes more prevalent, PRO endpoints may become more widely accepted goals to measure and monitor treatment efficacy. This may serve as positive reinforcement to PRO use for monitoring treatment effectiveness in clinical practice settings.

## Methodologic Problems to be Solved by Pharmacoepidemiologic Research

Just as patient engagement and PROs inform the discussion in the clinical practice setting, they similarly play an increasing role in the research setting. For example, including patient relevant outcomes into clinical trials has become a priority of the FDA and fostering patient engagement in all stages of research has been the genesis of the Patient Centered Outcomes Research Institute (PCORI) and its significant funding portfolio. However, there are methodologic challenges that accompany PROs in pharmacoepidemiologic research and clinical practice. These issues include discordance between raters and measurement of within person change over time.

## Currently Available Solutions

Given the subjective nature of PROs, clinicians', patients', and caregivers' ratings may not agree. One currently available solution to this challenge is to use composite indices, though this is not always a valid approach. Composites aggregate multiple scores into a single summary score. A second challenge is determining whether change across time is clinically meaningful. Although there is no current consensus on the single best approach, using clinical anchors to determine the smallest difference in a score that would prompt a change in patient management is a common solution. Below, we provide further detail regarding these two challenges and current approaches to handling them.

## Discordance in Perspectives between Patients, Clinicians and Researchers

Discrepancies may occur between clinicians' and patients' perceptions of disease activity level and whether there has been improvement or deterioration in the condition. There may also be lack of concordance between composite measures of disease activity used to assess efficacy in clinical trials and measures that use PROs.

Composite indices are helpful to reduce the presentation of information from multiple measures into a single summary score. This approach is most valid when the measures included in an index are highly correlated. When a measure does not correlate, or track well with others, to include it in a composite index would result in lost or obscured information. Studies have found that PROs scores do not always correlate strongly with the composite indices. When PROs are relatively independent predictors of treatment response, their results should be reported separately rather than included in a composite score. In one study, composite indices were better at detecting flare states though worse than PROs at describing low disease activity states.

Composite measures upon which clinicians base their assessment of improvement or deterioration may not necessarily include key aspects of the disease that matter to the patient.

For instance, in the DAS-28 (disease activity score) assessment of rheumatoid arthritis, 28 joints are assessed for tenderness or swelling, but this count does not include the feet or ankles. Therefore, if patients have foot involvement, which can be very painful, it is possible they may not be satisfied with the degree of improvement noted on the DAS-28 because it excludes an important element of their disease experience. Using DAS-28 as an outcome in pharmacoepidemiology studies could therefore miss outcomes important to patients and result in biased measures of association. Further, composite disease activity measures may not always translate to decision making based on the experience of an individual patient.

## Measuring within Person Change

Understanding how to estimate clinically meaningful change using PROs is important to be able to determine the effectiveness of a treatment or intervention. Unfortunately, determining clinically meaningful change is complex. There is no consensus on the best approach, and the topic represents an area of active methodological research. Although there are statistical approaches to analyzing changes in PRO scores over time, the detection of a statistically significant difference may not reflect a meaningful clinical difference. There may be differences in defining a meaningful clinical difference depending on the respondent (e.g. patient, caregiver, or clinician). It may depend on the health condition being studied and whether a patient is experiencing improvement or deterioration in health. Although there is not a uniform consensus, we briefly review some methods for determining meaningful change.

*Statistical methods*: The *minimal important difference* (MID) represents the smallest change in scores that could be determined important. The *MCID* is determined based on clinical anchors, and is generally regarded as the smallest difference in score that would

prompt a change in patient management. In practice, the terms MID and MCID are sometimes used interchangeably, but statistically derived and clinically anchored estimates need not converge. *Anchor-based methods* use external indicators considered to be clinically relevant to the PRO, such as clinical measures (lab tests, clinician ratings) or patient measures (global rating of change) and place subjects on a continuum based on the size of change in the anchor (large negative change, small negative change, no change, small positive change, large positive change). Ideally, multiple relevant anchors should be used, across multiple samples to confirm responsiveness of the PRO measure. Another anchor-based technique to estimate MID employs use of receiver operating characteristic (ROC) curves to evaluate group-level criteria for improvement or worsening of clinical status. *Distribution-based methods* are more strictly based on statistics vs. clinical anchors. The distribution-based approach uses scores from a sample to express the effect in terms of standard-deviation units or standard error of measurement.

*Bookmarking and scale judgement of IRT-based measures:* Alternative approaches to measuring meaningful within-patient change have been developed based on techniques from the field of educational testing. This approach is applicable to PRO measures developed using IRT. The general approach is to develop clinical vignettes representing a continuum of IRT-based scores, present these vignettes to a representative panel of stakeholders (e.g. patients, caregivers, clinicians), and have the panel identify thresholds between scores (delineated by the vignettes), where they would place a "bookmark" separating different levels of severity. Such exercises help to identify clinically meaningful cut-points between scores. Similar qualitative work with panelists can be used to identify minimal clinically meaningful differences by presenting PRO items to stakeholders and asking to note how much response to an item (or items on a scale) would need to change for a change in status to be considered clinically meaningful. Another approach, the "scale-judgement" method, entails having raters compare pre-filled IRT-based PRO questionnaires (for example, considering pre- and post- an intervention) and indicating whether or not the person who completed the questionnaires had experienced an important difference. These types of approaches require qualitative work with patient and other stakeholders across different patient populations (e.g. age, demographics, health conditions) and directions of change in PROs.

*Change in perspective.* Another factor that may complicate the assessment of within-person change over time is when a person's perception and valuation of the domain being measured change over time. This phenomenon, termed *response shift*, means that, across time, an individual may give the same response on a PRO (e.g. "Sometimes pain bothers me") even though their underlying health status has changed. Response shift may occur because a patient's subjective measurement scale may change (e.g. more of the symptom is required before a patient describes it as "sometimes" occurring), a patient's values may change (e.g. a symptom becomes more important over time leading to different responses to questions about the symptom over time), and/or a patient may reconceptualize the construct entirely. Statistical and qualitative methods exist to assess response shift.

### Selection of Patient Reported Outcomes and Implementation into Practice

Publications have begun to offer guidance on training clinicians in use of PROs. Recommendations include: eliciting local barriers and concerns to address during the training (such as how to deal with patient symptoms/concerns outside the specialty, concern about visit time constraints, how to interpret results), inclusion of the stakeholders in PRO selection and format for presentation, keeping the training relatively brief, making

training problem-based and experiential with video examples and case studies, and including relevant treatment decision aids and decision support tools in training.

Considerations for the display and communication of PRO scores have also been published. Display format preferences tend to vary by audience characteristics such as age, education, and role (clinician vs patient). Some studies have identified preferences for line graphs, others for bar graphs. Patients tend to prefer simpler formats, while clinicians prefer more data. Directionality of data has been shown to matter, with better health being portrayed as higher on the chart, and including lines indicating threshold values for normal versus abnormal found to be helpful.

## The Future

Patient engagement in research, advances in PRO measurement, and recognition of the importance of garnering direct patient input will result in increased inclusion of the patient voice in the calculus of medication efficacy in clinical studies. There is growing evidence that electronic PROs may increase the quality of care of processes and clinical outcomes and PROs may become a key part of improving quality of care. PROs may also become increasingly used in comparative effectiveness research. As more is understood about PRO development, effective use, interpretation and potential applications, the use and new use-cases for PROs can be expected to continue to grow.

There is increasing interest in using PRO data from clinical settings and captured in electronic health records as structured outcomes assessment for inclusion in comparative effectiveness research. This could be a powerful data source when combined with other sources of electronic data (see Part II). PROs in EHRs may be particular useful when there are no standardized outcomes assessments provided by clinicians in the clinical note. The complexities of analysis and interpretation of longitudinal PRO data require continued study to best leverage such data to make valid inferences. Cross-cutting PRO measures that could be used across conditions and contexts may confer advantages such as anticipating in clinical trials the expected outcomes in clinical practice. Such PROs, when collected in a clinical setting or with technology to support in-between visit data collection, could be used such that clinical data registries could be combined with administrative claims data to support comparative effectiveness research.

Another area of future development is the use of wearable devices and PROs. Coupling physiologic data with PRO data will aid efforts to determine clinically relevant change in PRO scores. Further, there are open research questions related to the analysis and interpretation of measures used longitudinally. There are interesting and exciting case examples, and it remains to be seen which model will be scalable and generalizable. Ideally, the culture of co-production, patient engagement and self-management will continue to take root and support the shift toward PRO measurement for meaningful application, evidence-generation and shared decision making.

## Key Points

- *Patient engagement* reflects the effective participation of patients in their own healthcare.

- PROs are measures of health from the perspective of the patient and can come in the form of self-reported symptoms, rating scales, questionnaires or interviews.
- PROs measure health domains such as symptoms, function, quality of life and experience with care.
- PROs can be used as clinical trial outcomes to estimate treatment benefits, adverse effects, and impacts on health related quality of life that are not reflected in physical exam or lab data.
- *MCID* is the change in a PRO score that corresponds to a substantive impact on the patient, whereas a statistically significant change in PRO score may not be perceived clinically.
- PROs used in a clinic setting, if reviewed with patient and used to inform care decisions, can facilitate patient engagement in care.
- Reliable clinical collection of psychometrically sound PROs and integration of scores as discrete, research quality data into the medical record can support EHR based observational and pharmacoepidemiologic research.
- PROs have the potential to support remote and asynchronous patient monitoring, when direct observation of the patient isn't possible (e.g. telemedicine, between visit measurement).

## Further Reading

Bantug, E.T., Coles, T., Smith, K.C., et al. (2016). Graphical displays of patient-reported outcomes (PRO) for use in clinical practice: what makes a pro picture worth a thousand words? *Patient Educ. Couns.* 99 (4): 483–490.

Basch, E. (2017). Patient-reported outcomes - harnessing Patients' voices to improve clinical care. *N. Engl. J. Med.* 376 (2): 105–108.

Bantug, E.T., Coles, T., Smith, K.C., et al. (2016). Symptom monitoring with patient-reported outcomes during routine cancer treatment: a randomized controlled trial. *J. Clin. Oncol.* 34 (6): 557–565.

Cella, D., Gershon, R., Lai, J., et al. (2007). The future of outcomes measurement: item banking, tailored short-forms, and computerized adaptive assessment. *Qual. Life Res.* 16 (Suppl 1): 133–141.

Detmar, S.B., Muller, M.J., Schornagel, J.H., et al. (2002). Health-related quality-of-life assessments and patient-physician communication: a randomized controlled trial. *JAMA* 288 (23): 3027–3034.

Fung, C.H. and Hays, R.D. (2008). Prospects and challenges in using patient-reported outcomes in clinical practice. *Qual. Life Res.* 17 (10): 1297–1302.

Greenhalgh, J. and Meadows, K. (1999). The effectiveness of the use of patient-based measures of health in routine practice in improving the process and outcomes of patient care: a literature review. *J. Eval. Clin. Pract.* 5 (4): 401–416.

Institute of Medicine (2001). *Crossing the Quality Chasm: A New Health System for the 21st Century*. Washington, DC: National Academies Press.

Jayadevappa, R., Cook, R., and Chhatre, S. (2017). Minimal important differences to infer changes in health-related quality of life - a systematic review. *J. Clin. Epidemiol.* 89: 188–198.

Lavallee, D.C., Chenok, K.E., Love, R.M., et al. (2016). Incorporating patient-reported outcomes into health care to engage patients and enhance care. *Health Aff. (Millwood)* 35 (4): 575–582.

Morgan, E.M., Mara, C.A., Huang, B., et al. (2017). Establishing clinical meaning and defining important differences for patient-reported outcomes measurement information system (PROMIS(R)) measures in juvenile idiopathic arthritis using standard setting with patients, parents, and providers. *Qual. Life Res.* 26 (3): 565–586.

Patient Reported Outcomes (PROs) in Performance Measurement. (2012) Author: National Quality Forum. https://www. qualityforum.org/Publications/2012/12/ Patient-Reported_Outcomes_in_ Performance_Measurement.aspx.

Reeve, B.B., Hays, R.D., Bjorner, J.K., et al. (2007). Psychometric evaluation and calibration of health-related quality of life item banks: plans for the Patient-Reported Outcomes Measurement Information System (PROMIS). *Med. Care* 45 (5 Suppl 1): S22–S31.

Revicki, D., Hays, R.D., Cella, D., et al. (2008). Recommended methods for determining responsiveness and minimally important differences for patient-reported outcomes. *J. Clin. Epidemiol.* 61 (2): 102–109.

Rotenstein, L.S., Huckman, R.S., and Wagle, N.W. (2017). Making patients and doctors happier - the potential of patient-reported outcomes. *N. Engl. J. Med.* 377 (14): 1309–1312.

Santana, M.J., Haverman, L., Absolom, K., et al. (2015). Training clinicians in how to use patient-reported outcome measures in routine clinical practice. *Qual. Life Res.* 24 (7): 1707–1718.

Snyder, C.F., Smith, K.C., Bantug, E.T., et al. (2017). What do these scores mean? Presenting patient-reported outcomes data to patients and clinicians to improve interpretability. *Cancer* 123 (10): 1848–1859.

Thissen, D., Liu, Y., Magnus, B., et al. (2016). Estimating minimally important difference (MID) in PROMIS pediatric measures using the scale-judgment method. *Qual. Life Res.* 25 (1): 13–23.

User's Guide to Implementing Patient-Reported Outcomes Assessment in Clinical Practice. (2015). International Society for Quality of Life Research (prepared by L. Aaronson, T. Elliott, J. Greenhalgh, et al.). https://www. isoqol.org/wp-content/uploads/2019/ 09/2015UsersGuide-Version2.pdf

User's Guide to Integrating Patient Reported Outcomes in Electronic Health Records. (2017) Prepared for the Patient Centered Outcomes Research Institute (PCORI) by Johns Hopkins University. (Eds. C. Snyder and A.W. Wu). http://www.pcori.org/ document/users-guide-integrating- patient-reported-outcomes-electronic- health-records.

U. S. Department of Health and Human Services, F.D.A., Center for Drug Evaluation and Research, Research Center for Biologics Evaluation and, Center for Devices and Radiological Health. Guidance for Industry. (2009). Patient Reported Outcome Measures: Use in Medical Product Development to Support Labeling Claims.

Wu, A.W., Kharrazi, H., Boulware, L.E., et al. (2013). Measure once, cut twice--adding patient-reported outcome measures to the electronic health record for comparative effectiveness research. *J. Clin. Epidemiol.* 66 (8 Suppl): S12–S20.

The National Institutes of Health (NIH) supported the development and distribution of various IRT-based PROs, including the Patient Reported Outcomes Measurement Information System (PROMIS). A useful reference for PROs developed and evaluated with NIH funding, including PROMIS is the Health Measures website. Available at: http://www.healthmeasures.net/explore-measurement-systems/promis

## 20

# The Use of Meta-analysis in Pharmacoepidemiology

*Brenda J. Crowe[1], Stephen J.W. Evans[2], H. Amy Xia[3], and Jesse A. Berlin[4]*

[1] *Eli Lilly and Company, Indianapolis, IN, USA*
[2] *The London School of Hygiene and Tropical Medicine, London, UK*
[3] *Amgen, Thousand Oaks, CA, USA*
[4] *Johnson & Johnson, Titusville, NJ, USA*

## Introduction

Good science seeks to consider *all* the evidence related to a question of interest. The first step is assembling all the available evidence and the second is, if appropriate, to provide a numerical summary. While both are very important, this chapter concentrates on statistical methods for providing numerical summaries.

We use the definition of meta-analysis from Working Group X of the Council for International Organizations of Medical Sciences (CIOMS):

> The statistical combination of quantitative evidence from two or more studies to address common research questions, where the analytical methods appropriately take into account that the data are derived from multiple individual studies.

Meta-analysis in medicine has mainly used data from randomized trials (we will use "trials" to refer to randomized clinical trials), but in pharmacoepidemiology, evidence from observational studies is also relevant. A meta-analysis itself may be regarded as an observational study.

There are dangers with meta-analysis of non-randomized studies, because of inherent biases. Nevertheless, they can provide evidence beyond that from trials. The Cochrane Collaboration maintains systematic reviews and meta-analyses of trials publicly available. Efficacy of treatments is best tested using randomization but studying harms may require non-randomized studies to detect effects not seen in trials. Given the greater diversity of designs, heterogeneity of patients and wide possibilities of bias in non-randomized studies, there will be more disagreement than among trials.

Increased precision is a motivation for meta-analysis of trials having small sample sizes, unable to provide convincing evidence of the presence or absence of harms. In contrast, observational studies usually have dramatically larger sample sizes so precision is not often the focus, but uncontrolled and unknown bias and confounding can have a large impact. The exploration of reasons for variability of results across observational studies can become a main focus of the meta-analysis.

This chapter addresses conceptual and methodological issues for meta-analysis, especially for observational studies.

## Clinical Problems to be Addressed by Pharmacoepidemiologic Research

The clinical problems to be addressed by pharmacoepidemiologic research are usually estimating efficacy (or effectiveness) and safety parameters that are unable to be addressed or have too much uncertainty in trials. Requirements around the regulatory assessment for new therapies or new indications for existing therapies, considering overall benefit/harm balance, can be especially relevant. Investigating harms using nonexperimental studies is a major challenge because of confounding (see Chapter 22). Also, rare events will not generally have standardized assessment or validation, which makes their evaluation difficult. Comparing results for a particular drug on particular harms may then yield conflicting results because of different study designs or different databases, leaving a confusing picture for clinicians and policy makers. Meta-analysis using *randomized* studies may be better than relying on potentially biased non-randomized studies, but whether randomized or non-randomized studies are used, meta-analysis can also help to explain disagreements. Disagreements may arise from differences in endpoints, exposure, patient inclusion and exclusion criteria, protocols and study designs, analysis methods or other reasons related to the susceptibility of the constituent studies to bias. For example, separating studies by whether or not there is possible recall bias in drug exposure measurement allows assessment of whether recall bias is a problem for a particular therapeutic question. For example, this applies with congenital anomalies where ascertainment of exposure prior to birth and potential recall bias is important.

In drug development, data on harms are often summarized in an "Integrated Summary of Safety" or similar report just prior to submitting an application for marketing authorization. If some type of aggregate safety review, which could include formal data integration, is only done when all trials have been completed, it is a missed opportunity to understand evolving safety. Crude pooling, summing numbers with and without the harm, by treatment, then analyzing as if the data came from a single trial, can be misleading and biased. While the crude approach gives some information, doing a proper meta-analysis will always be more informative.

For regulatory purposes, periodic aggregate safety reviews are extremely important. It is recommended though, that sponsors plan repeated, cumulative meta-analyses, with clear definitions of adverse events of interest, and to the extent possible, use standardized data collection and study designs (at least from the perspective of safety data collection). During development, ongoing review of blinded trials is helpful for understanding *potential* safety issues that may require additional data capture or unblinding to determine if additional action is required to protect patients and satisfy regulatory requirements. Typically, determination of causal adverse reactions begins after data are unblinded. Better understanding of the safety profile, following a proactive approach during development, including periodic updating of cumulative meta-analyses, may identify potential harms earlier.

The exploration of subgroups of patients in whom therapy may be more or less effective is a controversial question and, rather than focusing on individual trials, meta-analysis can be used. A pre-specified protocol is important in this context.

Evidence-based medicine (EBM) uses the best evidence available in making decisions. Meta-analyses have been a key component of EBM but generally focus on placebo-controlled trials, and thus head-to-head comparisons between therapeutic alternatives are often unavailable. However, consumers, health care providers and policy makers require comparative effectiveness evidence to make better informed decisions – each specific pharmacologic treatment for a condition/disease should be compared with others in terms of safety and efficacy.

There are further techniques such as indirect comparisons and network meta-analyses (also known as mixed treatment comparisons) that can combine evidence in a single analysis. These techniques can allow ranking of treatments in terms of efficacy and safety and enable better decisions because they are based on more data, but they also require assumptions that may not be testable.

# Methodological Problems to be Solved by Pharmacoepidemiologic Research

The most important problem in studying medicines is obtaining the correct estimates of their effects on outcomes related to medical health. Biases can arise in many areas, especially in non-randomized studies and there is always statistical uncertainty in the estimates of effects, especially if they involve rare outcomes. Meta-analysis should always address issues of statistical uncertainty and may help with bias. It may be able to address the effect of applying different methods of studying drug effects. Results from randomized and non-randomized data may give different insights. However meta-analysis itself has many methodologic issues. The problems relate to the process of combining diverse studies and the methods to obtain estimates of effect from all the studies. Dealing with the original studies in their differing aspects of design, protocol, analysis, reporting in addition to their overall quality, is not a trivial task; this section addresses some of the main challenges.

## Susceptibility of the Original Studies to Bias

The most important aspect of quality is susceptibility to bias, and guidelines such as the Preferred Reporting Items for Systematic Reviews and Meta-analyses (PRISMA) reflect this. The Cochrane Collaboration developed a "Risk of Bias Tool" for assessment of the trials in a meta-analysis. The "ROBIS" tool assesses the risk of bias in a meta-analysis itself. A similar approach has been applied to "Risk of Bias in Non-randomized Studies – of Interventions," ROBINS-I.

There are many such tools and while no single method of assessing bias is accepted by everyone, those doing and interpreting meta-analyses in pharmacoepidemiology should be aware and assess potential bias using one of the methods.

Combining poorly done studies can produce a summary result with misleading precision, which may have undue credibility and should not be used as a basis for formulating clinical or policy strategies. Judgment about susceptibility to bias of a study can be subtly influenced by its results, so excluding them using subjective judgment can result in a different, potentially serious, bias.

## Combinability of Studies

Different studies have different designs, outcomes, treatments and patients. Combining extremely diverse studies can be nonsensical. Combining studies of breast cancer with those on coronary heart disease would obviously not be appropriate; the outcomes are not expected to show the same effect of the same exposure. However, it is not always simple. How different can studies on different patient populations, or different regimens for the same treatment, be before combining them is wrong? For example, it may be relevant to look at all hormone preparations as a single group, but for some purposes it will be important to distinguish types, or even different doses and durations of treatment for a single product. In pharmacoepidemiology, risks of adverse effects will often vary notably with duration of treatment and length of follow-up. At the very least, it is necessary to explore possible variation in the size of the effect, especially in terms of how that variability in effects might relate to aspects of study design, populations included, etc.

For example, combining all statin trials but looking just at patients with low LDL (low-density lipoprotein) levels at baseline may be reasonable to see if effects are present in that patient group. A more difficult question is whether non-randomized studies should be combined with randomized studies. There are challenges combining nonrandomized studies in a meta-analysis and this is discussed later. The treatment of randomized and non-randomized evidence as equivalent in a single analysis is a mistake; some distinction should be made. Although some have used Bayesian methods to combine evidence from both sources in a single analysis, there is not wide agreement on this approach. Results should be reported for both sources separately, even if later combined. Within non-randomized studies, studies with different designs, e.g. case-control and cohort, also should be evaluated separately (and possibly later combined).

## Publication Bias

Unpublished material cannot be retrieved by literature searches and is likely to be difficult to find. *Publication bias* occurs when study results are not available to be included at the time when the meta-analysis is conducted, and there are differences between the available and unavailable data. Registration of randomized trials, with protocols and other information, being done prior to results being available should reduce the problem. Many journals and regulators require clinical trials to be listed in a public registry. Some registers also contain observational study protocols and results, notably at the

European Medicines Agency under the auspices of the European Network of Centres for Pharmacoepidemiology and Pharmacovigilance (ENCePP®). However, there is no guarantee that observational studies will appear in any registry.

While not including unpublished studies is usual, unpublished data can represent a large proportion of all relevant data. Published results generally are a biased sample. Statistically significant, "positive" results (the intervention works) are more likely to be published, published rapidly, published in English, published more than once, published in high impact journals, and cited. The contribution made to the totality of the evidence in systematic reviews by studies with non-significant results is as important as those with the statistically significant results. If unpublished studies are systematically different from published studies in the magnitude and/or direction of the findings, but they are similar in terms of risk of bias, omitting them yields a biased summary estimate.

There is no guarantee that either a published trial or a published meta-analysis will follow the protocol, and bias toward finding "interesting" results is pervasive. Choosing outcomes to report after the data are available and analyzed is one common way of obtaining biased results in trials. Investigators do not always keep to the protocols when publishing. It is one thing to have the trial data biased, but then the systematic reviewers may add to the problem. Even in the highly regarded Cochrane Reviews there is evidence that reviewers do not keep to their own protocols and it seems harms are especially likely to be affected by publication bias (i.e. studies reporting statistically significant increased risk of harms are more likely to be published).

It is clear that the published literature may not be as reliable as it should be and it has been found that review by regulatory authorities may be more reliable, and at the very least should also be searched for in any meta-analysis based on published data.

## Bias in the Abstraction of Data

Meta-analysis, being retrospective research, is subject to the potential biases inherent in extracting data from reports. It has been shown that when more than one meta-analysis of a treatment for a disease has been done, there can be differences between them, especially in the inclusion and exclusion of papers to be analyzed. While the results were similar in some cases, they had occasional extreme disagreement regarding efficacy and some variation in whether results were statistically significant or not. These disagreements were not easily explainable. In some instances, even though the same papers are included, the data extracted can vary, and this can lead to different conclusions about the efficacy of therapy. Despite efforts to make meta-analysis an objective, reproducible activity, there is evidently some judgment involved.

One other important aspect of meta-analysis is the use of aggregate-level data (usually from published studies) compared with using individual patient data (IPD). Meta-analyses based on IPD have several advantages, including the ability to conduct proper time-to-event analyses (not always possible from published data) and the ability to perform appropriate subgroup analyses. Sharing of such data, provided confidentiality can be preserved, is increasing. The Yale University Open Data Access (YODA) Project is one such example.

Most of the interest in this area is around randomized trials, but there are also issues around the availability of observational data. Platt and Lieu have noted that there are challenges to overcome despite enthusiasm of the research community for wider availability of IPD. They identify three reasons for the challenges: (i) confidentiality and proprietary concerns, (ii) the cost in terms of time and effort, required to make raw data usable for analyses, and (iii) the need to create incentives for data holders that outweigh the disadvantages.

# Currently Available Solutions

There are many guidelines on reporting and conducting systematic reviews and meta-analyses and these should be consulted for details. Here we give general principles relevant to pharmacoepidemiology.

## Steps Involved in Performing a Meta-analysis

The main steps in performing a meta-analysis are given in this section.

### Define the Purpose

The primary and secondary objectives of a meta-analysis should be defined precisely. A well-formulated question includes a clearly defined Patient Population, Intervention, Comparator, and Outcome.

An example could be "What is the magnitude of the increased risk of gastrointestinal side effects with NSAIDs (nonsteroidal anti-inflammatory drugs) used for the treatment of pain, compared with placebo?" For NSAIDs, estimating the absolute risk difference (RD) (and, thus, the public health implications) as well as the relative risk (and, thus, the etiologic implications) might be a secondary objective. Too broadly defined questions could "mix apples and oranges" and too narrow a focus could lead to finding no, or limited data, or the inability to generalize.

### Perform the Literature Search

It is important to have a search strategy sensitive enough to identify most of the studies to be included. Just using a computer system may not be enough, and it may find too many irrelevant studies – i.e. the specificity is very low. Searching for the text word "random*" in MEDLINE will retrieve all randomized controlled trials (RCTs) but will find many that are not RCTs and excluding publication types such as commentaries, editorials, meta-analyses, reviews, or practice guidelines removes many non-relevant citations, without losing any of the relevant trials. The Cochrane Handbook has a chapter devoted to searching for randomized trials, including a section on ongoing studies and unpublished data. It also has guidance on searching for nonrandomized studies, but in practice this is more difficult. Publication bias is a major problem for observational studies since they are not necessarily registered, may not require ethical review, and may be untraceable. It seems likely that searching for particular adverse event terms is likely to be better than using terms related to methods. "Hand" searching, using reference sections of relevant retrieved publications or whole searches of relevant journals, may help.

### Establish Inclusion/Exclusion Criteria

Rules for including and excluding studies should be defined when the meta-analysis is planned. Limiting to randomized studies with at least 100 patients has been done where many large trials on a topic have been performed. With non-randomized studies, one might include studies of incident cases only, when the relationship between exposure and outcome differs between incident and prevalent cases. Practical considerations may force changes: e.g. there may be no randomized studies of a new indication for an existing therapy.

If broad inclusion criteria are used, then a broad hypothesis may be tested. This may permit examination of the association between design and outcome (e.g. do randomized and nonrandomized studies tend to show similar effects?) or the exploration of subgroup effects. For example, with aspirin given following myocardial infarction, restriction to studies using more than 75 mg aspirin would not permit comparison of dose–response effects.

A priori considerations of original study design and features should determine inclusion and exclusion criteria, not their results. The temptation to justify exclusions post hoc may be strong, making clinically plausible arguments. However, such exclusions, made after having seen the data and the effect of individual studies on the pooled result may form the basis for legitimate sensitivity analyses (comparing combined results with and without that particular study included), but should not be viewed as primary exclusion criteria.

Readers often cannot assess whether the exclusion criteria were defined after seeing study results, but registration of systematic review protocols helps reduce this problem. Registration has also helped with the realization that both reporting of trials and of systematic reviews is often altered by authors even after a protocol has been recorded, thus the potential for bias is considerable. A registry specifically for systematic reviews is "PROSPERO" (International **Prospe**ctive **Re**gister **Of** systematic reviews). Key features from the review protocol are recorded and maintained as a permanent record. There also is a registry of studies, maintained by the European Medicines Agency, under the auspices of the ENCePP.

Studies may generate more than one published paper and choosing which of multiple papers to include and ensuring that there is no double-counting requires care.

### Collect the Data

When the relevant studies have been identified and retrieved, typically, data abstraction forms are developed, pilot tested and revised. A balance is needed between the completeness and time needed to extract that information. Careful specification in the protocol may help avoid over- or under-collecting information. For randomized trials, it is generally advisable to collect raw data on outcomes by group rather than derived measures such as odds ratios (ODs). In contrast, for observational studies, estimates from each of the studies adjusted for confounding are best, along with information about what and how confounding factors were included in the adjustment.

In terms of study quality, it is best to collect data on the individual aspects of study design that affect potential bias, such as whether, for example, there was concealment of randomized allocation or "blinded" outcome assessment. Such explorations clearly need to be guided by common sense. For example an outcome of total mortality is less likely to be biased than an outcome such as recurrent chest pain.

### Perform Statistical Analyses

#### Odds Ratio, Risk Ratio or Risk Difference, Does It Matter?

There are three summary measures of effect size that can be used in meta-analysis when the outcome of interest is binary (e.g. proportion of subjects with pain relief): risk ratio (RR), OR, or RD. Although the summary measure used often does not greatly affect the statistical significance of the results, the choice can affect applicability and interpretability in clinical practice. These measures are described in detail in Chapter 2 on study design.

RR and RD are easier to interpret than ORs. When the baseline (untreated) risk is constant across studies, the RD also allows calculation of relevant public health measures (e.g. a number of events prevented or caused by a given treatment). A disadvantage of using RDs in meta-analysis is that it cannot be constant at all levels of baseline risk. If the summary measure suggests a decrease of say 10% on an absolute scale, perhaps when the average baseline risk in the studies is say 30%, in a group with a baseline risk of 10% or less, an absolute decrease of 10% will be impossible.

ORs have better mathematical properties than RRs; switching the roles of event and non-event does not alter ORs; one is the reciprocal of the other (unlike RRs when events are common).

#### Choice of Statistical Method

In most situations, the statistical method uses some form of weighted average of within-study results. Intuitively it is clear that large studies should contribute more than small studies. Using weights proportional to the inverse of the variance of the within-study OR may introduce bias with rare binary outcomes because the weights depend not only on study size, but on the event rates themselves.

The usual basic principle is that within study comparisons between treated and untreated are made prior to combination across studies. With randomized trials, this preserves randomization.

Some methods, called "fixed-effect" models, assume there is a single, common effect. Any variability among study results is assumed to be random and is ignored in producing a summary estimate of the treatment effect. Methods that do not assume this are called "random-effects" models. Between-study variability in estimates of treatment effect is taken into account by random-effects models, incorporating variability into the weighting scheme for the summary estimate.

Random-effects models produce wider confidence intervals than fixed-effect methods but are not a panacea for unexplained heterogeneity. Random-effects models tend to assign relatively higher weights to small studies than fixed-effect models, which may have unwanted consequences, particularly when published small studies show relatively larger effect sizes than unpublished small studies or when there are a large number of small studies that then have a combined weight greater than the large ones. For example, consider an analysis of 10 trials that all have sample sizes of 500 in both the treated and control groups. Suppose nine studies have event rates of 28% in the treated groups compared with 30% in the control groups. In this same analysis, a single study has event rates of 3% in the treated group versus 1% in controls. For an inverse-variance weighted analysis of RDs, which are −2% in the nine studies and +2% in the single study, the single study with the low event rates would get 54% of the weight in the meta-analysis, compared with 5.1% of the weight for each of the other nine studies. For an analysis of (log) relative risks, the single study would get 0.4% of the weight, compared with 11.1% of the weight for each of the other nine studies.

The random-effects model is often implemented with DerSimonian and Laird (DL) methodology but this method of weighting is known to be suboptimal in several situations and is not to be recommended in general. Another random-effects method that is worth considering is the Hartung-Knapp-Sidik-Jonkman (HKSJ) method. While it is straightforward and can outperform the standard DL method, extra caution is needed when there are ≤5 studies of very unequal sizes.

Recently, Stanley and Doucouliagos challenged the two core conventional meta-analysis methods (fixed- and random-effects) and proposed a weighted least squares method that is neither fixed nor random-effects and has some good properties with small numbers of events. However, unlike the Peto method, which is described in more detail below, it is unable to deal with zero events in one of the comparison arms.

Bayesian statistical methods can take into account the investigator's prior beliefs about the size of an effect or about the factors biasing the observed effects. They are particularly appealing for meta-analyses that attempt to synthesize evidence from multiple sources under a unified framework, to make direct probability statements about any hypotheses, and to handle complex problems. Askling and colleagues used the Bayesian hierarchical piecewise exponential survival model to investigate the cancer risk for the anti-tumor necrosis factor ("TNF") drug class. All 74 RCTs of TNF inhibitors of at least four weeks duration were provided to a team of independent investigators, for events indicating a possible cancer. A Bayesian "piece-wise" exponential model was used to analyze the individual patient-level data. One hundred thirty (0.84%) individuals (of 15 418) randomized to anti-TNF therapy were diagnosed with cancer, compared to 48 (0.64% of 7486) randomized to comparators. The overall

relative risks associated with anti-TNF were 0.99 (95% confidence interval (CI) 0.61–1.68) for cancers excluding non-melanoma skin cancer (NMSC), and 2.02 (95%CI 1.11–3.95) for NMSC. Relative risks were heterogeneous across the anti-TNF drug groups. The authors concluded that, despite a reassuring overall short-term risk, they could neither refute nor confirm either an increased or unchanged risk. Despite the large numbers of studies and patients included, statistical precision, differences in baseline cancer risk, and incomplete reporting detail between trials limited the ability to detect or dismiss increases in risk. The authors noted that this example illustrates the challenges in safety-assessments using meta-analyses of RCTs and suggested that long-term risk assessment requires observational studies.

### *Combinability of Results from Diverse Studies: Heterogeneity*

A key question is whether it is clinically and statistically reasonable to estimate an average effect of therapy, either positive or negative. Being too inclusive with studies may mean that the average effect may not apply to any particular subgroup of patients. On the other hand, it may be desirable to allow for some heterogeneity in study design and analysis to increase the generalizability of the results and to permit the exploration of various factors as modifiers of the treatment effect. We can distinguish between aspects affecting variability related to modifiable aspects of the conduct and analysis of studies such as choice of summary measure (e.g. RR vs. RD) or study design features (e.g. blinding in the evaluation of endpoints), and real biological or clinical variation in treatment effect. The latter represents the potential to target therapy to the appropriate patient populations.

The $I^2$ statistic quantifies among-study variability by estimating the proportion of variability in point estimates due to heterogeneity rather than sampling error. $I^2$ is recommended because:

- it focuses attention on the effect of any heterogeneity on the meta-analytic result;
- its interpretation is intuitive, i.e. the percentage of total variation across studies due to heterogeneity;
- it can be accompanied by an uncertainty interval;
- it is simple to calculate and can usually be derived from published meta-analyses;
- it does not inherently depend on the number of studies in the meta-analysis; and
- it may be interpreted similarly irrespective of the type of outcome data (e.g. time to event, quantitative, or dichotomous) and choice of effect measure (e.g. odds or hazard ratios).

While significant heterogeneity, or a large value for $I^2$, means the studies are not all estimating the same parameter, the magnitude of difference may not be great when the component studies themselves are large (and the within-study variability is small). The Cochrane Handbook (Section 9.5.2) has qualitative guidelines for interpreting the magnitude of $I^2$.

In searching for sources of heterogeneity one might stratify the studies by patient characteristics or design features and investigate heterogeneity within and across strata. If stratification explains the heterogeneity, the combined results will differ between strata and heterogeneity within each stratum would be reduced. For example, if the full set of trials includes some studies with severely ill patients and others with mildly ill patients, one could observe heterogeneity of treatment effects. Stratification on disease severity could (hypothetically) show that treatment effects are large in severely ill patients and small in less ill patients. Regression methods, such as weighted least squares linear regression, can also be used to explore sources of heterogeneity. Graphical methods for meta-analysis can augment analytical approaches when the focus is on issues related to heterogeneity. Statistical tests of heterogeneity often suffer from lack of

statistical power, especially with a small number of studies.

It has been argued that because of the potential for bias in observational epidemiologic studies, exploring heterogeneity should be the main point of meta-analyses of such studies, rather than producing a single summary measure.

As an example of the type of analysis that could be used to investigate study design issues, Hennessy and colleagues performed a meta-analysis of nonexperimental studies comparing third generation oral contraceptives (those containing gestodene and desogestrel) to second generation pills (those containing levonorgestrel) with respect to the risk of venous thromboembolic events. A major issue in these studies has been the possibility of depletion of susceptibles. Specifically, the concern is that users of the newer drugs might tend to be new users of any oral contraceptives, whereas users of the older, second generation drugs, would tend to be established users. The risk of venous events tends to be highest for new users, who have events soon after beginning pill use. These susceptible individuals, the argument goes, would be depleted from the ranks of users of second-generation pills, but not from among the third-generation pill users, thereby leaving a more susceptible population of third generation pill users. The authors found several studies that had performed subgroup analyses of new users in their first year of use. When combined, these subgroups still demonstrated an increased risk from third generation pills. The power to look within subgroups was only available within the context of the meta-analysis, not within any of the individual studies.

Exploratory analyses of meta-analyzed data may provide insights into biology and/or may generate hypotheses. Figure 20.1 shows a "forest plot." It is a useful graphical picture of studies, even when no single summary statistic is derived. This figure shows four observational studies on the effect of hydroxychloroquine on death or serious outcomes

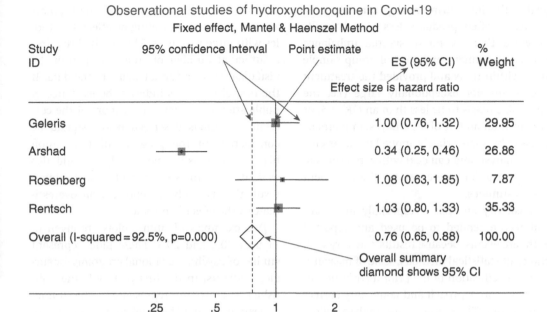

**Figure 20.1** Forest plot of four recent observational studies on the effect of hydroxychloroquine on death or serious outcomes from COVID-19. Features of a forest plot are indicated. *Source:* Data are taken from Arshad et al. (2020), Geleris et al. (2020), Rentsch et al. (2021), and Rosenberg et al. (2020).

from COVID-19. It is not based on a systematic review. There is variation in the settings, the detailed outcomes, and some heterogeneity in the results. Showing the actual values of the results with their confidence intervals is always helpful, even if a summary value is inappropriate. The sizes and numbers of events (deaths) in the different studies means that the small studies contribute less (lower "weight") and larger studies contribute more. The size of the box showing the central estimate is proportional to the weight.

### Analysis of Rare Events
By combining results of trials meta-analysis can help address challenging problems with rare events, but many methods for combining data are based on large sample approximations so may be unsuitable leading to variations in the overall result depending on the method used. Recommendations are based on simulation studies in which the "truth" is generated by the investigators and show that fixed-effect models should be used over random-effects

methods and that the inverse-variance-average should be avoided.

With rare events, studies may have no events in one or both of the arms, and relative measures such as relative risk or ORs cannot be calculated, so those studies will be automatically excluded. RDs can be estimated but in the presence of rare events produce biased results and have very limited power. In cases when there are no events in *one* arm, relative measures can be calculated. Some methods, including the commonly used Mantel-Haenszel method add "continuity corrections," typically adding 0.5 to all cells in a two-by-two table. This leads to bias in the presence of rare events, and is not necessary, even for the Mantel-Haenszel method. It is better to use the reciprocal of the sample size of the opposite treatment arm.

The Peto method, also known as the "one-step" model, is a fixed-effect model that focuses on the observed number of events in the experimental intervention and compares it with the expected number; this has the effect that it can deal with single arms having zero observed events. It often produces less biased results provided there is no substantial imbalance between treatment and control group sample sizes within trials and provided the treatment effects are not exceptionally large (i.e. the effect size needs to be less than an OR of 5, or greater than an OR of 0.2). Bayesian methods can also be appropriately applied to rare events meta-analysis and can deal with zero events to derive posterior inferences for the treatment effect estimates.

Sensitivity analysis is especially important and recommended to be used and reported with rare events, because results may vary with choice of statistical methods, scale of measurement, specification of the prior distribution in the Bayesian approach and continuity correction factors. These sensitivity analyses allow readers to assess the robustness of the results.

### Formulate Conclusions and Recommendations

The conclusions of a meta-analysis should be clearly summarized, with appropriate interpretation of the strengths and weaknesses and generalizability. Suggestions for future research and hypotheses generated should be distinguished from conclusions.

### Publication Bias

As discussed above under Methodological Problems, when the primary source is published data, these may represent a biased subset of all the studies that have been done. Generally, "significant" studies are more likely to be published than non-significant ones. The "funnel plot," plotting the effect size (e.g. the RD) against a measure of study size, such as the sample size or the inverse of the variance of the individual effect sizes, can help. With no publication bias, the points produce a funnel shape, with scattered points centered around the true value, and with the degree of scatter narrowing as the variances decrease. If publication bias exists, the funnel would show

asymmetry, with very few (if any) points around the point indicating no effect, for studies with large variances. This method requires a sufficient number of studies to permit the visualization of a funnel shape to the data. If the funnel plot does indicate the existence of publication bias, then one or more of the correction methods described below should be considered. In the presence of publication bias, the responsible meta-analyst should also evaluate the ethics of presenting a summary result that is likely to represent an overestimate of the effect in question.

Two examples of funnel plots are given in Figures 20.2 and 20.3. These plots represent studies of psychoeducational programs for surgical patients. In the first plot, only the published studies are represented. The funnel appears to have a "bite" taken out of it where the small studies showing no effect of these programs should be. In the second plot, the unpublished studies, including doctoral dissertations, are included, and the former "bite" is now filled with these unpublished studies.

Sterne and Egger provide guidelines for the choice of axes in funnel plots of studies with dichotomous outcomes, recommending that the standard error of the treatment effect (e.g. the standard error of the log OR) be used as the measure of study size and that relative measures (relative risk, as opposed to RD) be used as the treatment effect measures. These same authors and a colleague point out that publication bias is only one possible explanation for funnel plot asymmetry, so that the funnel plot should be seen as estimating "small study effects," rather than necessarily publication bias.

Several methods to deal with potential unpublished studies have been developed. These include formal methods to test for the presence of publication bias and methods to adjust summary estimates to account for unpublished studies, but these methods make fairly strong assumptions about the specific mechanism producing the publication bias. A method called "trim-and-fill" has a fair amount

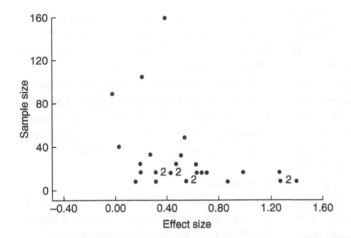

**Figure 20.2**  Funnel plot for published 34 studies only: analysis of data from Devine and Cook's review of psychoeducational programs for surgical patient. *Source:* Reprinted by permission of the publishers from Light and Pillemer (1984) by the President and Fellows of Harvard College.

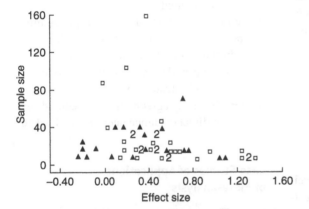

**Figure 20.3**  Funnel plot for published 34 studies (open boxes) and unpublished (closed triangles): analysis of data from Devine and Cook's review of psychoeducational programs for surgical patients. *Source:* Reprinted by permission of the publishers from Light and Pillemer (1984) by the President and Fellows of Harvard College.

of intuitive appeal, although it, too, relies on assumptions about the missing studies. It is based on the funnel plot, focusing on the studies that lead to the appearance of funnel plot asymmetry. Under this approach, a mirror image of the studies producing the asymmetry is imputed, using a carefully defined statistical algorithm to determine which studies to mirror, and the impact of adding those mirror image studies to the pooled analysis is assessed.

As noted earlier, one solution to the problem of publication bias is the use of prospective registration of studies at their inception, prior to the availability of results. Others have suggested obtaining unpublished data from the Food and Drug Administration (FDA), an approach used by Turner and colleagues. These authors obtained reviews from FDA for studies of 12 antidepressant agents, conducted a systematic literature search to identify matching publications, and compared the results based on published studies with the results based on the FDA data. The analysis restricted to published literature showed that

94% of the trials were positive. In contrast, the analysis of FDA data showed that only 51% were positive. A further review in looking at other indications for anti-depressants found a similar bias in the literature. Although the estimate of effect size was only increased marginally, "reporting biases led to significant increases in the number of positive findings in the literature". The "Open Trials project" and the Yale project "YODA" cited above are attempts to reduce the bias from using only published literature. Now there is an online tool (https://fda.opentrials.net/search) that allows FDA documents to be retrieved more easily.

Going one step further, meta-analyses that are prospectively planned, with complete protocols, including proposed tests of subgroup effects, prior to having knowledge of the results of any of the component studies, can be conducted. More on the topic of prospective meta-analysis is presented below.

## Indirect Comparison and Simultaneous Comparison of Treatments Available for Specific Conditions

Decision-makers need to make informed decisions on head-to-head comparisons of treatments, but relevant trials may not exist. When the treatments have been compared to a common comparator, for example placebo, it is possible obtain indirect evidence synthesis – also known as network meta-analysis.

Indirect evidence involves using data from trials that have compared medication "A" vs medication "B", and from trials that have compared medication "A" vs medication "C", to draw conclusions about the effect of medication "B" relative to medication "C." It is crucial that when an indirect comparison is estimated, the analysis respects the randomization. This means that the analysis must be based on treatment differences within each trial. Simply collapsing results by treatment arm ignores randomization producing biased and overly precise estimates. To correctly compare B with C, we obtain appropriate meta-analytic OR for the comparisons A-B and A-C and obtain OR (B vs. C) = OR (A vs. B) / OR (A vs. C).

Multiple-treatment comparison techniques can easily deal with multiple arms and account for correlation between them. They also permit assessment of inconsistency – disagreement between direct and indirect evidence.

### Assumptions

Indirect comparison methodologies have similar assumptions to traditional meta-analysis. The following are the main assumptions.

i) homogeneity: each of the A-B, B-C and other comparisons should be homogeneous enough for those specific comparisons to be combined.
ii) similarity: factors affecting response must be similarly distributed across the trials (similar patient characteristics, settings, follow up, and outcomes and methodologically similar trials).
iii) consistency: agreement between direct and indirect evidence needs to be checked.

## Case Studies of Applications of Meta-analysis

### Saving Time and Resources by Using Meta-analysis

Meta-analysis can shorten the time between research findings and implementation of change in clinical practice or policy and regulation. A simple but elegant example of the use of meta-analysis in the approval context was the use of meta-analysis of ECG data from several clinical pharmacology studies for two drug application submissions. They calculated a pooled estimate for the difference between active doses and placebo on QT prolongation, avoiding the need for a new study to address the question.

"Cumulative meta-analysis," i.e. performing a new meta-analysis each time new RCT results are available for a given treatment has been advocated. As an example, Antman and colleagues analyzed data from 17 trials of β-blockers for the prevention of death in the years following a myocardial infarction. In the left-hand side of Figure 20.4, reproduced from their paper, the data are presented as a traditional meta-analysis, with individual study results presented along with the summary OR arbitrarily estimated after 17 trials had been completed. In the right-hand side of Figure 20.4, the same data are presented as a cumulative meta-analysis, with an updated summary estimate calculated after the completion of each new trial. The cumulative meta-analysis clearly shows that the updated pooled estimate became statistically significant in 1977 and has remained so ever since.

Caution is advisable in interpreting cumulative meta-analyses because multiple statistical tests can generate false positive findings (type 1 error) and this is often ignored. To address that concern, sequential analysis methods have been applied, but some suggest that the most natural approach is Bayesian, as continuous learning and updating our knowledge over time fits the Bayesian philosophy. Existing data form the basis for the prior distribution and new studies update this forming a posterior distribution, which then becomes the new prior distribution. Multiplicity is handled naturally in this framework and conclusions (usually in the form of "credible intervals") are expressed as probabilistic statements about findings (which can be flexible in terms of different treatment effect sizes under different scales), not as statements about hypotheses.

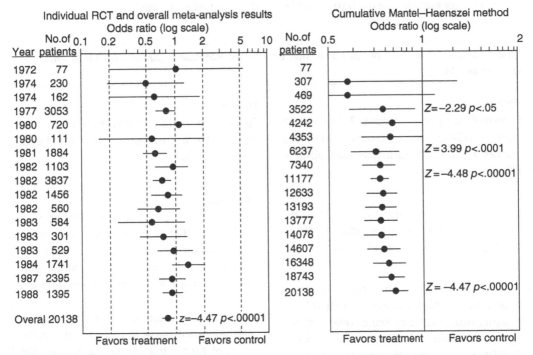

**Figure 20.4** Results of 17 RCTs of the effect of oral beta-blockers for secondary prevention of mortality in patients surviving a myocardial infarction presented as two types of meta-analyses. On the left is the traditional one, revealing any trials with nonsignificant results but a highly significant estimate of the pooled results on the bottom of the panel. On the right, the same data are presented as cumulative meta-analyses, illustrating that the updated pooled estimate became statistically significant in 1977 and has remained so up to the present. Note that the scale is changed on the right graph to improve clarity of the confidence intervals. *Source:* Reproduced from Antman et al. (1992) with permission from the American Medical Association.

There is no consensus on the multiplicity problems in cumulative meta-analysis, so some use it mainly as an exploratory tool, providing caveats about the number of analyses performed without a formal correction. This approach is analogous to that for many conventional safety analyses, for which nominal $P$ values from hypothesis tests are often provided without adjustment, when there are a limited number of pre-specified outcomes.

Another consideration is that estimates of treatment effect may not be stable over time, perhaps due to changing clinical environments. In the $\beta$-blocker example, treatment appears to be less effective in the most recent studies. Thus, it may be important to re-evaluate therapies as other treatment strategies evolve.

A final caution relates to the continuing need for well-designed RCTs. New indications for existing therapies, for example, are often suggested by nonexperimental studies, but are not always confirmed by subsequent, properly designed randomized trials. Consider the case of beta-carotene in the prevention of cancer. A series of observational studies examined the relation between dietary intake of foods rich in $\beta$-carotene and the risk of lung cancer. Overall, they showed a relatively consistent association between diets rich in $\beta$-carotene and reduced risk of lung cancer. Subsequent randomized trials of this specific nutrient as a supplement have failed to confirm a protective effect against lung cancer.

### Cumulative Meta-analysis as a Tool to Detect Harm Signals earlier

Cumulative meta-analysis also could be used as a tool to detect safety signals earlier. Case Example 20.1 illustrates some of the potential methodological issues (that are shared by traditional meta-analysis).

---

**Case Example 20.1    Risk of Cardiovascular Events and Rofecoxib: Cumulative Meta-analysis (Juni et al. 2004)**

*Background*
Rofecoxib, a cyclo-oxygenase-2 inhibitor (a type of NSAID), was withdrawn from the market because of cardiovascular adverse effects.

*Question*
Can cumulative meta-analysis of RCTs establish whether evidence on the adverse effects of rofecoxib was available before its removal?

*Approach*
The authors searched bibliographic databases and FDA files and included all RCTs in patients with chronic musculoskeletal disorders that compared rofecoxib with other NSAIDs or placebo. Myocardial infarction was the outcome assessed.

*Results*
The adverse cardiovascular effects of rofecoxib could have been identified several years earlier.

*Strengths*
Cumulative meta-analysis potentially can detect harm earlier than traditional meta-analysis.

*Limitations*
- The validity of pooling of trials that were not clinically homogeneous is questionable. The authors combined the results of trials with dissimilar control arms (placebo, naproxen and non-naproxen NSAIDs).
- The authors excluded trials that evaluated Alzheimer's disease. In this case, the inclusion of such a trial would have made the early signal disappear.

*Key Points*
Cumulative meta-analysis is a tool to evaluate the safety of health interventions.

First, one might question, or at least require justification for, the validity of pooling of trials that are not clinically homogeneous. For example, the authors combined the results of trials with dissimilar control arms (placebo, naproxen and non-naproxen NSAIDs).

Second, excluding trials assessing an intervention in other indications may be questioned. In Case Example 20.1, trials in chronic musculoskeletal pain were the focus, and trials in Alzheimer's disease were excluded. Clearly, one would not combine trials for different indications to assess efficacy, but it is less clear with harms, although harms could also vary by indication. An approach often used in the regulatory setting may seem appropriate by including all indications but stratifying by indication.

Third, one can ask whether efficacy and safety should be evaluated similarly. For efficacy, multiple looks at data can lead to false positive results and have serious consequences. For safety, it could be argued that adjustments should not be as large, if done at all (in the interest of remaining sensitive to safety issues that might arise).

Fourth, it is uncertain whether cumulative meta-analysis can systematically detect harm earlier. Rare adverse events, or those occurring late after exposure may not be seen during drug development, so cumulative meta-analysis may not always help (or may work best if large post-approval studies are conducted).

Ryan and colleagues conducted a meta-analysis of 22 RCTs studying the effects of anti-IL-12/23 therapies. These are anti-inflammatory agents used to treat conditions such as psoriasis (the initial indication). The studies included 10 183 patients. The primary outcome measure was major adverse cardiac events (MACE). MACE definitions can vary; in this analysis it was defined as a composite of myocardial infarction, cerebrovascular accident, or cardiovascular death during the placebo-controlled portions of the included trials. They chose absolute RDs as their effect measure, using the Mantel-Haenszel fixed-effect method. They found that 10 of 3179 patients receiving anti–IL-12/23 therapies experienced MACEs compared with no events in 1474 patients receiving placebo (Mantel-Haenszel risk difference, 0.012 events/person-year; 95% CI, −0.001 to 0.026; P = 0.12). (NOTE: in the original paper, the authors use the term "risk difference" but report results in terms of person-time, which would usually require use of rate differences). They concluded that there was no significant difference in the rate of MACEs associated with anti–IL-12/IL-23 antibodies, but that even the meta-analysis may have been underpowered to identify a significant difference (because there were only 10 events).

In a second meta-analysis, Tzellos and colleagues also studied anti-IL-12 / 23 biological agents (ustekinumab and briakinumab) with respect to risk of MACE, specifically in the setting of treatment of chronic plaque psoriasis. Studies of psoriatic arthritis were excluded, as in the Ryan meta-analysis. These authors used the Peto fixed-effect method to estimate ORs. They found a "possible higher risk of MACEs" in patients treated with IL-12/23 antibodies compared with placebo-treated patients (OR = 4.23, 95% CI: 1.07–16.75, P = 0.04).

### Indirect Comparisons: Network Meta-analysis and Simultaneous Evaluation of Treatment Therapies for the Same Indication

Network meta-analysis has a number of specific issues. This is illustrated by an analysis of the efficacy and acceptability of new generation antidepressants, performed by Cipriani and colleagues. In one study the authors excluded placebo groups where present, after a careful search for trials that included asking pharmaceutical companies, regulatory agencies, and study investigators to supply information about details of study design and related factors.

Efficacy was evaluated as the proportion of patients who had a reduction of at least 50% from the baseline score on standard depression rating scales or the proportion who scored "much" or "very much" improvement on the clinical global impression. Acceptability of therapy was evaluated as the proportion of patients who terminated the study early for any reason during the first eight weeks of treatment. The authors calculated the ORs for each of the drugs compared to fluoxetine, using a random-effects model within a Bayesian framework, resulting in an estimated probability that each antidepressant was the most efficacious, or the most acceptable, the second, the third, etc. ranking treatments in terms of efficacy and acceptability. They also assessed the consistency between direct and indirect evidence.

With 117 trials with 25928 participants and 12 antidepressants included in the analyses, there was generally consistency between direct and indirect evidence, but not all the antidepressants were equally efficacious or equally well tolerated; they were able to report a ranking for efficacy or acceptability.

There was both enthusiasm for, and criticism of, this study. Exclusion of placebo-controlled data and publication bias were the main concerns. Another study found that 95% of published trials were "positive" compared to only 51% of FDA-registered studies (some of which were unpublished) so relying primarily on published data may overestimate benefits.

### Regulators' Role

The U.S. FDA routinely obtains IPD for new drug applications and may also request such data for other issues. The consequence is that they are able to do IPD meta-analyses. This has rarely been done by other regulators, but the situation is changing and there are signs that other regulators are interested in following the FDA example.

In recent years, the FDA has used meta-analysis to investigate adverse events associated with the use of certain drugs. While publication bias is often a major concern in conducting a meta-analysis, regulatory authorities like the FDA have authority to request sponsors to submit all published or unpublished data and the FDA can use patient-level data. The findings from those meta-analyses have been used to support regulatory decisions to mandate labeling changes.

For example, the FDA examined antiepileptic drugs and suicidality events. Their review of 199 placebo-controlled trials from 11 antiepileptic drugs found that there were 1.9 per 1000 (95% CI: 0.6, 3.9) more antiepileptic drug patients than placebo patients who experienced suicidal behavior or ideation compared to the placebo patients. Based on the findings, the FDA requested updates to product labels.

Not only does meta-analysis sometimes support the decision to change or update the current labeling of approved drugs, it can also provide evidence as to whether or not to keep a drug on the market or withdraw its use for a particular indication. For example, the FDA's patient-level meta-analysis for rosiglitazone found about a 40% increase in myocardial ischemia among diabetes patients taking insulin or those using nitrates but less evidence when compared with metformin or a sulfonylurea.

## The Future

The examples above have raised several important issues for the future. When evaluating safety during drug development there is problem with multiplicity. Trials have hundreds of different adverse events and if cumulative meta-analyses are updated for each trial completed, repeated testing yields further multiplicity problems. Focusing on p-values, ignoring magnitude and clinical importance is unwise. More work is needed on sensible ways to deal with the problem.

The current situation with respect to registration of clinical trial protocols and results is that there is a wide array of registries making it difficult to find all relevant studies. What would be useful is a dedicated search engine, with low false positive and false negative rates, that would be able to find all trials with given characteristics. This would improve meta-analysis by using *all* relevant randomized evidence and would improve the science.

When hundreds of categories of events are tabulated, specific events will be seen in very small numbers. Work to date suggests that more targeted definitions can sometimes lead to stronger signals (larger relative risks) and may actually make it more likely that signals will be detected, despite observing fewer events with narrower definitions.

Results of a meta-analysis when there is substantial heterogeneity are difficult to interpret. If the heterogeneity is adequately explained in the analysis in terms of subgroup effects, or trial quality, meta-analysis might still be an acceptable part of demonstrating effectiveness or harm. Work is needed to establish transparent criteria by which to evaluate situations where inconsistency in results suggests benefit (or harm) in some but not others. This can be just chance but might have other explanations.

As the focus of policy and clinical decisions moves in the direction of comparative effectiveness, which also includes comparative safety, one might wish to make direct comparisons across all drugs for a given indication, but this is not easy to implement. Work is needed, however, to explore in practice, the conditions under which indirect comparisons may be both valid and useful.

The inclusion of observational studies in meta-analyses, particularly of serious but uncommon adverse events, will almost certainly be a necessity, but reliability of answers is not guaranteed. Methodological considerations need to be addressed (e.g. by examining how methodology relates to study results) to help with interpretation.

Distributed data networks have been established within and outside the US and are being used for large drug safety studies. Using multiple sources of data for these may mean that analysis is best done using meta-analytic approaches. The Sentinel network is used by FDA to address questions of interest through specific queries sent to participating data partners. CNODES, in Canada, is a similar kind of network (see Chapter 9). OHDSI (Observational Health Data Sciences and Informatics) is a global collaboration of investigators performing studies in a distributed network but also developing methodology for conducting such studies. It is unclear whether current meta-analytic methods, e.g. doing separate analyses in each database, then using an inverse-variance weighted average, are best suited to this distributed network environment. New methods of distributed analysis, which do a better job of mimicking the results one would get by having one large dataset with data from ALL datasets, need further investigation.

In conclusion, while there are no easy answers to many of the questions presented above, it is clear that meta-analysis will play an increasingly important role in the formulation of treatment and policy recommendations. Thus, the design and analytical attributes of the meta-analyses performed, and of the included studies, are of the utmost importance and need to be reviewed by the scientific community in an open, published forum. Meta-analyses, if they are carefully interpreted in view of their strengths and weaknesses, should prove to be extremely helpful in pharmacoepidemiologic research.

## Key Points

- Meta-analysis, if carefully done, is a powerful method that can be used to identify sources of variation among studies and provide an overall measure of effect.
- Combining evidence across diverse study designs and study populations may lead to generalizable results.
- Much care is needed in the interpretation of meta-analyses, due to issues such as publication bias and flaws in the design of component studies.

- Meta-analysis plays an increasingly important role in safety assessment. It might be necessary to consider non-randomized studies, separately from randomized trials, for questions about uncommon adverse events.

- Extended meta-analytic techniques that can handle indirect treatment comparisons and more than two interventions in a network meta-analysis can strengthen the inference regarding a treatment.

## Further Reading

Antman, E.M., Lau, I., Kupelnick, B. et al. (1992). A comparison of results of meta-analyses of randomized control trials and recommendations of clinical experts. Treatments for myocardial infarction. *JAMA* 268 (2): 240–248.

Arshad, S., Kilgore, P., Chaudhry, Z.S. et al. (2020). Treatment with hydroxychloroquine, azithromycin, and combination in patients hospitalized with COVID-19. *Int. J. Infect. Dis.* 97: 396–403.

Askling, I., Fahrbach, K., Nordstrom, B. et al. (2011). Cancer risk with tumor necrosis factor alpha (TNF) inhibitors: meta – analysis of randomized controlled trials of adalimumab, etanercept, and infliximab using patient level data. *Pharmacoepidemiol. Drug Saf.* 20 (2): 119–130.

Baigent, C., Keech, A., Kearney, P.M. et al. (2005). Efficacy and safety of cholesterol-lowering treatment: prospective meta-analysis of data from 90,056 participants in 14 randomised trials of statins. *Lancet* 366 (9493): 1267–1278.

Bender, R., Friede, T., Koch, A. et al. (2018). Methods for evidence synthesis in the case of very few studies. *Res. Synth. Methods* 9 (3): 382–392. https://doi.org/10.1002/jrsm.1297.

Berlin, I.A. and Colditz, G.A. (1999). The role of meta-analysis in the regulatory process for foods, drugs, and devices. *JAMA* 281 (9): 830–834.

Cipriani, A., Furukawa, T.A., Salanti, G. et al. (2009). Comparative efficacy and acceptability of 12 new-generation antidepressants: a multiple-treatments meta-analysis. *Lancet* 373 (9665): 746–758.

De Angelis, C., Drazen, I.M., Frizelle, E.A. et al. (2004). Clinical trial registration: a statement from the International Committee of Medical Journal Editors. *N. Engl. J. Med.* 351 (12): 1250–1251.

DerSimonian, R. and Laird, N. (1986). Meta-analysis in clinical trials. *Control. Clin. Trials* 7 (3): 177–188.

Devine, E.C. and Cook, T.D. (1983). Effects of psycho – educational interventions on length of hospital stay: a meta – analytic review of 34 studies. In: *Evaluation Studies Review Annual*, vol. 8 (ed. R.I. Light), 417–432. Beverly Hills, CA: Sage.

Duan, R., Boland, M.R., Liu, Z. et al. (2020). Learning from electronic health records across multiple sites: a communication-efficient and privacy-preserving distributed algorithm. *J. Am. Med. Inform. Assoc.* 27 (3): 376–385.

Geleris, J., Sun, Y., Platt, J. et al. (2020). Observational study of hydroxychloroquine in hospitalized patients with Covid-19. *N. Engl. J. Med.* 382 (25): 2411–2418.

Hartung, J. (1999). An alternative method for meta-analysis. *Biom. J. J. Math. Methods Biosci.* 41 (8): 901–916.

Hartung, J. and Knapp, G. (2001a). A refined method for the meta-analysis of controlled clinical trials with binary outcome. *Stat. Med.* 20 (24): 3875–3889.

Hartung, J. and Knapp, G. (2001b). On tests of the overall treatment effect in meta-analysis with normally distributed responses. *Stat. Med.* 20 (12): 1771–1782.

Hartung, J. and Makambi, K.H. (2003). Reducing the number of unjustified significant results in meta-analysis. *Commun. Stat.Simul. Comput.* 32 (4): 1179–1190.

Hennessy, S., Berlin, I.A., Kinman, I.L. et al. (2001). Risk of venous thromboembolism from oral contraceptives containing gestodene and desogestrel versus levonorgestrel: a meta – analysis and formal sensitivity analysis. *Contraception* 64 (2): 125–133.

Higgins, I.P. and Green, S. (eds.) (2011). *Cochrane Handbook for Systematic Reviews of Interventions Version 5.1.0*. Oxford: Cochrane Collaboration.

IntHout, J., Ioannidis, J.P., and Borm, G.F. (2014). The Hartung-Knapp-Sidik-Jonkman method for random-effects meta-analysis is straightforward and considerably outperforms the standard DerSimonian-Laird method. *BMC Med. Res. Methodol.* 14: 25.

Juni, P., Nartey, L., Reichenbach, S. et al. (2004). Risk of cardiovascular events and rofecoxib: cumulative meta-analysis. *Lancet* 364: 2021–2029.

Kearney, P.M., Baigent, C., Godwin, I. et al. (2006). Do selective cyclo-oxygenase – 2 inhibitors and traditional non-steroidal anti-inflammatory drugs increase the risk of atherothrombosis? Meta-analysis of randomised trials. *BMJ* 332 (7553): 1302–1308.

Light, R.J. and Pillemer, D.B. (1984). *Summing Up: The Science of Reviewing Research*. Cambridge, MA: Harvard University Press.

Makambi, K.H. (2004). The effect of the heterogeneity variance estimator on some tests of treatment efficacy. *J. Biopharm. Stat.* 14 (2): 439–449.

Metelli, S. and Chaimani, A. (2020). Challenges in meta-analyses with observational studies. *Evid. Based Ment. Health* 23 (2): 83–87.

Page, M.J., McKenzie, J.E., and Higgins, J.P.T. (2018). Tools for assessing risk of reporting biases in studies and syntheses of studies: a systematic review. *BMJ Open* 8 (3): e019703.

Platt, R. and Lieu, T. (2018). Data enclaves for sharing information derived from clinical and administrative data. *JAMA* https://doi. org/10.1001/jama.2018.9342.

PROSPERO: https://www.crd.york.ac.uk/ prospero

Rentsch, C.T., DeVito, N.J., MacKenna, B. et al. (2021). Effect of pre-exposure use of

hydroxychloroquine on COVID-19 mortality: a population-based cohort study in patients with rheumatoid arthritis or systemic lupus erythematosus using the OpenSAFELY platform. *Lancet Rheumatol.* 3: e19–e27.

Rosenberg, E.S., Dufort, E.M., Udo, T. et al. (2020). Association of treatment with hydroxychloroquine or azithromycin with in-hospital mortality in patients with COVID-19 in New York State. *JAMA* 323 (24): 2493–2502.

Roest, A.M., de Ionge, P., Williams, C.D. et al. (2015). Reporting bias in clinical trials investigating the efficacy of second – generation antidepressants in the treatment of anxiety disorders: a report of 2 meta – analyses. *JAMA Psychiat.* 72 (5): 500–510.

Rover, C., Knapp, G., and Friede, T. (2015). Hartung-Knapp-Sidik-Jonkman approach and its modification for random-effects meta-analysis with few studies. *BMC Med. Res. Methodol.* 15: 99.

Ryan, C., Leonardi, C.L., Krueger, I.G. et al. (2011). Association between biologic therapies for chronic plaque psoriasis and cardiovascular events: a meta-analysis of randomized controlled trials. *JAMA* 306 (8): 864–871.

Sidik, K. and Jonkman, J.N. (2002). A simple confidence interval for meta-analysis. *Stat. Med.* 21 (21): 3153–3159.

Sidik, K. and Jonkman, J.N. (2006). Robust variance estimation for random-effects meta-analysis. *Comput. Stat. Data Anal.* 50 (12): 3681–3701.

Spiegelhalter, D.J., Abrams, K.R., and Myles, J.P. (2004). *Bayesian Approaches to Clinical Trials and Health-Care Evaluation*. Wiley.

Stanley, T.D. and Doucouliagos, H. (2015). Neither fixed nor random: weighted least squares meta-analysis. *Stat. Med.* 34 (13): 2116–2127.

Sterne, I.A.C., Egger, M., and Smith, G.D. (2001). Investigating and dealing with publication and other biases in meta-analysis. *BMJ* 323: 101–105.

Sweeting, M.I., Sutton, A.I., and Lambert, P.C. (2004). What to add to nothing? Use and avoidance of continuity corrections in meta – analysis of sparse data. *Stat. Med.* 23 (9): 1351–1375.

Sweeting, M.I., Sutton, A.I., and Lambert, P.C. (2006). Correction. *Stat. Med.* 25: 2700.

The Yale University Open Data Access (YODA) Project. http://yoda.yale.edu/welcome-yoda-project

Training materials available freely on the internet for using risk of bias tools from the Cochrane Collaboration (https://training.cochrane.org/resource/rob-20-webinar).

Turner, E.H., Matthews, A.M., Linardatos, E. et al. (2008). Selective publication of antidepressant trials and its influence on apparent efficacy. *N. Engl. J. Med.* 358 (3): 252–260.

Tzellos, T., Kyrgidis, A., and Zouboulis, C. (2013). Re-evaluation of the risk for major adverse cardiovascular events in patients treated with anti – IL – 12/ 23 biological agents for chronic plaque psoriasis: a meta-analysis of randomized controlled trials. *J. Eur. Acad. Dermatol. Venereol.* 27 (5): 622–627.

Valsecchi, M.G. and Masera, G. (1996). A new challenge in clinical research in childhood ALL: the prospective meta – analysis strategy for intergroup collaboration. *Ann. Oncol.* 7 (10): 1005–1008.

Verde, P.E. and Ohmann, C. (2015). Combining randomized and non-randomized evidence in clinical research: a review of methods and applications. *Res. Synth. Methods* 6 (1): 45–62.

Ziegler, R.G., Mayne, S.T., and Swanson, C.A. (1996). Nutrition and lung cancer. *Cancer Causes Control* 7 (1): 157–177.

# 21

# Studies of Medication Adherence

*Julie Lauffenburger[1], Trisha Acri[2], and Robert Gross[3]*

[1] *Brigham and Women's Hospital and Harvard Medical School, Boston, MA, USA*
[2] *Courage Medicine, Philadelphia, PA, USA*
[3] *University of Pennsylvania Perelman School of Medicine, Philadelphia, PA, USA*

## Introduction

The underuse of essential medications imposes significant clinical and financial burdens on healthcare systems. As many as half of patients do not take their medications as prescribed, resulting in an estimated $100 billion in excess annual spending in the US alone. Without accurate measurements of adherence for research and practice, the problem will remain underappreciated and poorly addressed. In this chapter, we describe the importance of adherence in pharmacoepidemiologic research, methods for measuring adherence, methodologic issues that arise once adherence has been measured, and future directions. We focus here on examples from HIV and cardiometabolic diseases because these areas have been major focuses of adherence research.

Despite its importance, medication adherence is difficult to define. Earlier research has used the term *Compliance*, or "the extent to which the patient's dosing history conforms to the prescribed regimen." However, this term implies that patients passively "conform" to the prescriber's directions, so the term *adherence* is now strongly preferred. *Adherence* better conveys the idea of a patient–provider relationship where the patient implements the provider's recommendations.

Another reason that adherence has been difficult to define is that it is not a single behavior but instead encompasses a set of behaviors over time. One common taxonomy developed by a scientific consensus group classifies adherence along three phases: (i) initiation, (ii) implementation, and (iii) persistence (**see** Figure 21.1).

*Initiation* describes initial engagement with the prescribed medication. As many as 30% of newly-prescribed therapies are never actually filled by patients, which is often referred to as primary non-adherence. *Implementation* represents how well patients follow the prescribed regimen after they have begun treatment. While varying greatly across diseases, approximately 50% of patients are thought to not correctly follow prescribed regimens. *Persistence* refers to how long the patient continues to follow the regimen. Poor adherence can occur along any of these phases.

This taxonomy helps distinguish between patients who never initially fill a prescription from patients who occasionally forget to take doses and those who take a medication regularly at first but then later discontinue.

*Textbook of Pharmacoepidemiology*, Third Edition. Edited by Brian L. Strom, Stephen E. Kimmel, and Sean Hennessy.
© 2022 John Wiley & Sons Ltd. Published 2022 by John Wiley & Sons Ltd.

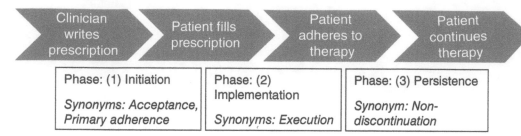

**Figure 21.1** Phases and taxonomy of adherence.

Classifying all these patients simply as "non-adherent" ignores that they may differ with respect to treatment outcomes and likely have different adherence barriers requiring different interventions.

## Clinical Problems to be Addressed by Pharmacoepidemiologic Research

Adherence research confronts the truism attributed to former US Surgeon General C. Everett Coop, MD that "drugs don't work in patients who don't take them." Measuring adherence is essential to address several issues in the interpretation of studies of beneficial and adverse effects of medications. In randomized trials, poor adherence to the drug being tested can lead to underestimates of drug efficacy. Information about adherence also allows for a more accurate assessment of drug safety because those who do not take the drug cannot experience its toxicity. Poor adherence may itself also be a marker of toxicity or adverse events.

Once a medication is marketed, information from clinical trials gives only a limited view of how drugs are used by patients. Patients who volunteer for clinical trials are often more motivated than those in usual care, so assessing adherence in observational studies provides a more "real world" estimate of adherence. Finally, because adherence itself is a major determinant of treatment outcomes, it

can also be the specific focus of pharmacoepidemiologic research.

Non-adherence can be intentional or unintentional. Studies have identified many potential barriers to adherence, broadly categorized as patient, system, and medication-specific factors. Common patient barriers consist of forgetting to take the medication, lack of knowledge or health literacy, and psychosocial factors such as depression and lack of social support. System barriers include costs of the medication as well as logistical difficulty in obtaining medication, including drug shortages in some settings. Key medication-specific factors include regimen complexity and adverse effects. "Pill fatigue" can also occur, in that adherence can decrease over time. This may be due to, for example, being emotionally overwhelmed by taking medication or no longer having a sense of urgency about the medical issue, particularly when patients are observed for periods longer than in typical trials and they have not experienced disease complications prevented by the medications themselves. It is also common that the optimal adherence seen early in therapy may decrease over time.

While missed doses are a more common adherence problem, taking extra doses can also occur. Extra doses of drugs with a narrow therapeutic window, such as warfarin for anticoagulation, may result in toxicity. Patients may also take extra doses of opioids prescribed for the treatment of pain because of inadequate relief or for recreational purposes.

Measuring adherence can also be useful for determining thresholds of how much medication must be taken to obtain desired clinical outcomes, which likely differ by drug and disease. In hypertension, taking at least 80% of prescribed medication has been an acceptable standard for blood pressure control. However, in HIV, higher thresholds are often necessary. Even though 80% of doses taken may not be the optimal universal cut-point for acceptable adherence, this threshold persists across research and quality measures. Therefore, the default adherence goal should be to encourage the patient to take as many prescribed doses as possible, and future research should focus on identifying more empiric and robust dose–response thresholds for various drug-disease settings.

## Methodological Problems to be Addressed by Pharmacoepidemiologic Research

While the gold standard for measuring adherence to pharmacotherapy is directly observed therapy, this approach is only practical in limited settings, such as the administration of a novel agent in a controlled environment. There are many different methods for measuring medication adherence, and each method has strengths and weaknesses. The most appropriate method depends upon the situation and precision needed for the measurement. Some methods require more intensive patient-level contact while others provide more granular data about timing of dose-taking. For example, prospective clinical trials can use many different methods. However, options are more limited in retrospective studies using databases. Thus, the use of multiple measures or sources of data may be useful to confirm findings.

For all approaches, the interpretation of adherence findings may also change depending on whether incident users or prevalent users of medication are examined, as adherence tends to be higher among prevalent users, in part because discontinuation is highest

shortly after initiation. Many studies focus on incident users, but there are situations in which studying prevalent users is more important because new initiators are only a small proportion of all patients on a therapy at a given time. Regardless of measurement approach, as discussed later, the discovery of non-adherence in clinical settings can be embarrassing for patients. Thus, knowledge that one's adherence is being monitored risks influencing the behavior it is measuring (i.e. a Hawthorne effect). When selecting a method and describing results, it is highly recommended to use standardized reporting approaches based on the adherence taxonomy presented in Figure 21.1.

## Currently Available Solutions

### Specific Techniques for Measuring Adherence

#### Self-Reports

The most common adherence measurement method has been patient self-report or asking respondents about their adherence behaviors. Self-reported metrics are simple, relatively inexpensive, quick and feasible and can be obtained over the telephone, in person, or with paper or electronic surveys. Several validated methods for assessing self-reported adherence are described below.

Self-reported adherence measures range from one-item questions inquiring about the frequency of missed doses to longer multi-item assessments evaluating beliefs associated with adherence and identifying barriers to non-adherence. Most self-reported measures involve count or estimation-based recall focused on the implementation phase, in which respondents report the number of doses missed or taken within an interval or to estimate their overall execution of adherence.

Numerous validated self-reported adherence scales exist in the English language. Perhaps the most common self-reported adherence tool historically used is the eight-item Morisky Medication Adherence Questionnaire (MMAS-8), but it requires licensing fees. The adult AIDS Clinical Trials Group (ACTG) adherence questionnaire, three-item tool by Wilson et al., and the Brief Medication Questionnaire are other examples of common, publicly-available tools that explore both behaviors and barriers to adherence. Overall, the choice of measure may depend on its purpose (e.g. clinical use or research), burden to patients, and disease states in which it has been validated. Self-report may also be the easiest method for clinicians to administer and best way to identify reasons for poor adherence for targeting interventions.

Self-reported adherence measures are moderately correlated with methods using electronic drug monitors (EDM) or pharmacy dispensing data (described later), though concordance can vary depending on the patient's level of adherence or the measurement window. However, because of potential over-reporting, self-reported measures generally have high specificity and low sensitivity; that is, self-reported non-adherence is generally accurate, while high self-reported adherence may not be accurate.

Self-reported adherence measurements have other limitations, such as being limited by the ability to recall missed doses and being subject to social desirability bias (i.e. over-reporting adherence to please providers or researchers), which can be potentially reduced by administering questions at a kiosk or tablet/computer. Reading instructions and questions aloud and including photographs of medicines can reduce literacy barriers. Self-report is also unlikely to provide a precise measurement of timing or patterns of dose-taking.

### Pharmacy Dispensing Data

Pharmacy dispensing measurement was pioneered in the late 1980s with wide use in chronic diseases and is one of the most commonly used modalities for measuring adherence in pharmacoepidemiology. Data can be obtained from health insurers (i.e. administrative claims data) or from pharmacies or patients directly. Pharmacy dispensing data are generally considered to be accurate measures of drug dispensing because the dispenser (e.g. a pharmacy) would not receive insurance reimbursement if the medication fills are not recorded and guilty of fraud if billing for medications not actually dispensed.

There are several different methods for measuring adherence using pharmacy dispensing data. In all approaches, adherence is measured indirectly based on patterns of medication dispensings (using medication name, dispensing date, and days supplied) by generating a "drug supply diary" that strings together consecutive medication dispensings based on the dates on which medication are dispensed to the patient and the duration of the supply dispensed. This supply diary can adjust for overlapping fills (e.g. truncating the days supplied for medications which are refilled before the medication supply from the prior dispensing would have been exhausted) and any known interruptions that may have occurred (e.g. by hospitalization). When generating the supply diary, researchers generally consider medications that are chemically related and not intended for use in combination to be interchangeable (e.g. two beta-blockers). For example, patients may initiate one beta-blocker and later switch to a different beta blocker. In this case, beta-blocker adherence is often measured continuously, rather than separately measuring adherence to each medication, to generate one continuous exposure episode. Sometimes, medications within the same disease state but chemically different (e.g. beta-blockers and calcium channel blockers) could be considered interchangeable.

Several types of adherence metrics can be calculated using these data, including implementation and persistence measures (see Figure 21.2). In the most common approach, the proportion of days that patients had an available supply of medication, or the

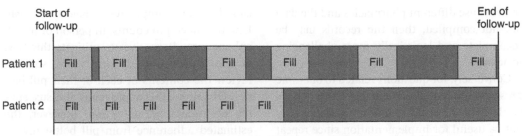

*Assume here each fill is 30 days, follow-up is 365 days, and supply diary is adjusted for overlap*

**Measuring implementation (e.g., Proportion of Days Covered [PDC])**
- Patient 1: PDC = (30 + 30 + 30 + 30 + 30 + 30)/365=0.49 or 49.3%
- Patient 2: PDC = (30 + 30 + 30 + 30 + 30 + 30)/365=0.49 or 49.3%

**Measuring persistence**
> Refill gap method (90-day)
> - Patient 1: "Persistent"
> - Patient 2: "Non-persistent"
> Treatment anniversary method
> - Patient 1: "Non-persistent"
> - Patient 2: "Non-persistent"

**Figure 21.2** Example of implementation and persistence measures in pharmacy dispensing data.

proportion of days covered (PDC), is calculated. The PDC is calculated by dividing the number of days with an available supply of medication by the number of days in the interval. Other approaches include calculating the medication possession ratio (MPR). MPR is calculated as the quotient of the total number of days supplied of all dispensings in each interval for the medication under investigation and the total number of days in the interval. The primary difference between PDC and MPR adherence metrics is how overlapping days supplied of the same medication are handled; the MPR focuses on days supplied while PDC focuses on days covered. The specific approach is typically determined by researcher preference; however, PDC is becoming increasingly recommended by healthcare quality organizations and may be more accurate for measuring adherence to multiple medications. Regardless, the different approaches yield similar results and are similarly associated with clinical outcomes.

Approaches for persistence include evaluating whether clinically-meaningful treatment gaps or discontinuations are observed in the dispensing data. Approaches include evaluating

whether a dispensation overlaps with the end of a follow-up period (i.e. the "treatment anniversary method") or a "refill gap method" that measures the availability of drug supply at a fixed time after the last dispensing (e.g. whether patients have a gap of at least 30 or 60 days with no medication after the supply is exhausted). Whichever method is chosen, investigators should conduct sensitivity analyses of the "gap rule." However, it is difficult to disentangle clinically-directed medication discontinuation from discontinuation against provider recommendation.

Compared with self-report, pharmacy dispensing data are not biased by poor recall and can be obtained from computerized records. Another advantage is that the data are available on large numbers of patients (often millions in a single database). However, the quality of data may be less accurate when tracking is less crucial for reimbursement or if prescriptions are obtained outside of insurance plans. To overcome this, some approaches compile data from pharmacies directly to capture all medications dispensed to patients and not just those paid by insurers. However, if patients use different pharmacies and the data are not compiled, then the records may be incomplete and logistically more challenging to acquire.

Conversely, for questions related to one-time prescriptions (e.g. short courses of antibiotics), while viable to study initiation, these data may not be useful for implementation since repeat dispensings are required to calculate the amount of medication consumed. Also, in the US, pharmacy dispensing data are generally only accurate for outpatient medications, because medications are not paid for separately during hospitalizations. Furthermore, pharmacy dispensing data also do not measure actual pill consumption, so they cannot be used when the timing of missed doses is pivotal. However, the estimation of adherence with pharmacy dispensing data has been shown to be valid for chronic medications where measuring overall exposure between refills is clinically relevant. Moreover, pharmacy dispensing measures of adherence have also been shown to be strongly associated with clinical outcomes.

## Pill Counts

While less commonly used, adherence can also be measured indirectly by pill counts, which involves counting the number of pills available for a patient. Pill counts are like pharmacy dispensing data in that percent adherence is calculated by dividing the days' supply consumed by the number of days observed. Data collected include the dispensing date, quantity dispensed, number of pills per dose, and number of pills left in the bottle, adjusted for doses taken that day and any additional pills left over from the last count.

Like adherence measures estimated using the medication dispensing date and days supplied (e.g. PDC), pill count data cannot determine if the medication was consumed. However, they do provide direct evidence that the medication was not taken when pills are left over. Pill counts are susceptible to deception since "dumping" pills is simple and can be done impulsively before a visit. Unannounced pill counts, in person or by telephone, are alternatives to mitigate this type of misclassification. During visits, subjects review the contents of each of their pill bottles. Of course, this approach is also susceptible to intentional deception; however, the estimated adherence from pill bottle review has been shown to be associated with treatment response. The time for both staff and participants is a potential disadvantage of pill counting and additional source of error. In addition, missing data can result when patients do not bring in their pill bottles or have them available during telephone calls. Reinforcing the importance of accuracy with staff is vital to ensure validity.

## Medication Diaries

Although the measures described above summarize how much medication was taken over a specified time period, they provide no detail on the timing of missed doses. Missing doses may have different consequences depending on whether they were missed consecutively or if they were missed at separate times (see Figure 21.2). One solution is medication diaries where participants keep a record of the date and time of each dose of medication and its timing with food. These data can be collected handwritten or electronically. Diaries are regularly used in pediatric patients and are particularly useful for medications like insulin or inhalers that are otherwise difficult to measure. However, diaries are susceptible to both overreporting and underreporting of adherence. Social desirability results in patients listing doses even though they were not taken, but the potential is lessened somewhat by the burden of creating a detailed falsified record. In fact, the risk of underreporting may be greater because of the burden of tracking each dose. It is also not easy to employ this method at scale for larger studies. Newer approaches are exploring the use of apps on enabled smart phones to track more nuanced medication-taking patterns.

### Electronic Drug Monitoring Technology

Electronic drug monitors (EDMs) have similar advantages as medication diaries but are less susceptible to deception or forgetting to document doses taken, because they provide time-stamped data about doses taken. While there are several different hardware options, EDMs employ electronic date/time stamp technology triggered by opening a container (i.e. pill bottle), puncturing a blister pack, or ingesting a dose, and data are uploaded to a computer or smartphone via hardwire or wireless linkage.

While EDMs are less susceptible to deception than self-report, they could theoretically be more susceptible than pharmacy dispensing data. However, it is highly unlikely that subjects will open and close the monitor to record doses over long periods of time without actually taking the medication, though this does occasionally happen accidentally. Though EDM technology is advancing rapidly, the packaging and cost of EDMs can still be burdensome and expensive. For example, they often preclude the use of pillboxes by generally requiring that the medication remain in the package until taken. However, EDMs could be used even when the medication is not kept in the container, where participants are asked to open the empty bottle whenever they take medications from a pillbox. Newer approaches integrate EDMs with text messaging technology to remind patients when they miss doses.

In 2015, the US Food and Drug Administration approved the first ingestible sensor technology that measures actual intake time through ingestion of a medication that communicates with an adhesive patch and sends a signal to the team monitoring adherence. Other research is exploring the utility and accuracy of adherence measures in which patients take date and time stamped photographs of themselves or their pills each time they take a dose.

### Drug Concentrations

Identifying the presence of a drug in plasma or other tissues provides direct evidence of drug ingestion. However, the use of drug concentrations to measure adherence is limited by variability across patients (i.e. absorption, distribution, metabolism, and clearance) and the need to potentially collect concentrations frequently to gain a fuller picture of adherence behaviors. Measurement of drug concentrations in hair using liquid chromatography and confirmed by mass spectrometry can be a useful indicator of long-term medication exposure. Unfortunately, many assays are unavailable commercially. Furthermore, serum drug levels may not be the relevant measure for many drugs when the site of action is elsewhere (e.g. intracellularly rather than in serum or hair). Cost and patient inconvenience may also be limitations.

### Measuring Primary Adherence

Each of the approaches described above have focused on later adherence phases (e.g. implementation and persistence). Without linkage to other types of data (e.g. electronic health records that include provider medication orders), it can be difficult to evaluate medication initiation (primary adherence) in dispensation data without knowledge of what was prescribed. Newer approaches are beginning to link these data sources to allow better assessment of the full cascade. On their own, electronic health record data limited to physician orders are not useful at evaluating adherence because they do not provide information about actual patient behaviors. By contrast, self-report may allow for easier study of primary adherence.

### Measuring Adherence to Non-pill Formulations

Measuring adherence to non-pill formulations can be difficult, largely because they are generally administered with a variable dosing schedule. Injectable medications like insulin may be administered on a sliding scale, with doses adjusted as needed, so measuring adherence using indirect dispensing data may be imprecise. For these, persistence-based measures may presenting be the most accurate. For inhaled medications, dispensing data could be used for ones with specific schedules (e.g. tiotropium). Medication diaries and self-report could theoretically be used but have the same issues as pill formulations. EDMs have been used for metered dose inhalers and ophthalmic solutions; while the monitors increase the size of packaging, the devices cannot be taken out of the package unlike pill formulations. For transdermal formulations in patches (e.g. nicotine, testosterone), adherence based on dispensation data is a viable option because the supply is typically fixed. However, for creams and ointments, because the amount used at each application varies by the size of the lesion being treated or the size of the individual, self-reports and medication diaries may be the only currently viable options. Measuring adherence will continue to be a challenge for newer non-pill formulations, including biologics, and in disease states in which both oral and injectable formulations are used interchangeably (e.g. osteoporosis).

## Analysis Issues in Adherence

### Use of Adherence Data in Clinical Trials and Comparative Effectiveness Studies

In analyzing trials, the standard approach remains intention-to-treat. This approach limits the introduction of bias and makes the results more generalizable. In clinical trials, adjusting results for adherence is complicated by the fact that the behavior of being adherent itself is associated with better outcomes (i.e. a healthy user effect). While clinical trial participants may be more motivated to adhere to treatments than those in clinical practice, non-adherence occurs for all types of self-administered therapies. Missed doses will typically make the active drug less effective and diminish observed differences versus placebo

in intention-to-treat analyses. To compensate, Phase III trials may inflate sample sizes to account for variability in drug exposure or incorporate run-in periods to minimize poor adherence. Of course, medication adherence itself can also be a primary or secondary outcome in randomized trials, particularly for studies of interventions. The inclusion of adherence data in analyses of trials is particularly important when a treatment fails. Reasons for failure might be attributable to either lack of biological effect or non-adherence, so unless adherence is measured, the results of the trial will be only partly useful. (See Case Example 21.1)

Similarly, observational studies of comparative effectiveness and safety of medications often benefit from measuring the relationship between adherence and treatment response. "As-treated" analyses of safety evaluations often censor follow-up in patients who discontinue therapies for reasons other than toxicity to decrease bias toward the null. Secondly, marginal structural modeling approaches often include adherence as a time-varying exposure. Exploring the relationship between adherence observed between comparators may enrich the conclusions from these studies.

### Selecting Adherence Intervals

For all adherence measures, one must choose a pre-specified window for assessing and evaluating adherence. While the choice of interval length depends on the research goals, in general, monitoring adherence over shorter intervals would be desirable, because interventions can be more rapidly implemented. Selecting the interval depends on two important factors: pharmacokinetics/pharmacodynamics and granularity of the adherence measurement. For drugs with short half-lives and onset of action, short intervals are likely to be more clinically relevant than when drugs have longer half-lives and onsets of action. Shorter intervals can be calculated for techniques that can accurately assess adherence over short

---

**Case Example 21.1    Non-adherence as a Key Factor for the Success of HIV Pre-Exposure Prophylaxis Trials**

*Background*
- Pre-exposure prophylaxis (PrEP) may prevent HIV transmission, especially in serodiscordant couples (e.g. HIV-positive patients with HIV-negative partners).
- Several antiretroviral-based PrEP drug therapies, including oral and vaginal gel formulations, have been studied since the late 2000s in clinical trials in sub-Saharan Africa and other regions of clinical need.

*Question*
Four early trials of antiretroviral-based PrEP showed success in reducing HIV transmission and were also well-tolerated by patients. However, three subsequent trials found surprisingly negative results of no effect of PrEP, including some that were stopped for futility.

*Approach*
Researchers in 2012 reviewed these seven trials' data on adherence to PrEP therapies and determined the degree of variation in adherence and potential explanations for the mixed findings.

*Results*
- Adherence to PrEP was found to vary substantially depending on the trial. In trials that demonstrated effectiveness, adherence was 84% or greater and was measured by pill counts and self-report.
- Trials with lower success had lower adherence rates or did not report adherence.
- Variations in adherence patterns (such as in Figure 21.2) or administration preferences, such as for oral or gel therapies, was also thought to influence adherence.

*Strength*
This was a comprehensive summary of factors for observed results across trials.

*Limitations*
Different techniques of measuring adherence (e.g. pill counts and self-report) limited the ability to make clear comparisons across trials.

*Key Points*
- Non-adherence resulted in surprisingly negative trials of a therapy that was ultimately found to be efficacious, which almost halted efforts to continue to study PrEP.
- Efforts to ensure optimal adherence appear critical to the success of PrEP.
- Additional efforts to expand PrEP formulations, such as injectables, are underway; these options may help reduce non-adherence once trials are completed.

---

periods of time, such as electronic data monitors. By contrast, for measures derived from dispensing data, adherence analysis intervals must be longer because adherence is based on evaluating patterns between medication dispensing dates in conjunction with the days supplied per dispensing (e.g. 30 days, like in Figure 21.2). The vast majority of dispensings for chronic medications in the United States are for 30-day supplies, and increasingly 90 days. Accordingly, measuring adherence in intervals shorter than 180 days make it difficult to observe variation since, by definition, patients are classified as fully adherent (100%) for the first 30 or 90 days. In general, choices for an adherence interval should be made based on pharmacokinetic/pharmacodynamic data.

**Statistical Analysis**

The simplest approach to summarizing adherence is the percent of doses taken (or missed). For electronic monitors, because the timing of each dose is available, percent of doses taken "on time," standard deviation of time between doses, or maximum time gap between doses can be calculated. For metrics in pharmacy dispensing data, analyses focus on percentage of available medication or gaps between dispensations. Self-report typically focuses on the proportion of doses the patients have taken. Whichever metric is used, one must choose whether to include adherence as a continuous or dichotomous variable. As previously described, dichotomous thresholds must consider both the likelihood of failure and clinical consequences of treatment failure. Few thresholds have been established based on evidence, yet in research and quality improvement efforts, to dichotomize these adherence variables, patients are often defined as fully adherent if they take ≥80% of prescribed doses. So, for example, both patients in Figure 21.2 would be "non-adherent" because they had a PDC < 80%. Often, evaluating differences in adherence on a continuous scale would be clinically more meaningful than binary measures, although adherence measures are typically not normally distributed. In addition, the presence of non-adherence values of zero will make it impossible to log transform continuous adherence data. Alternatively, when neither dichotomous nor continuous measures capture the clinically-relevant dose–response relationship, assigning ordinal adherence categories (e.g. <60%, 60–<80%, 80–<100% etc.) may be sometimes preferable. Other researchers have sometimes used quantile regression to overcome assumptions of linearity.

In addition, evaluating regimens with multiple medications poses analysis challenges. A final consideration is how to accurately characterize adherence to multiple medications for the same condition (e.g. anti-hypertensives). Some classify adherence based on optimal adherence to at least one medication for that disease state (e.g. hypertension) to be fully adherent, although this misclassifies individuals who are non-adherent to some but not all

components of the regimen. Another common approach is to measure adherence at the therapeutic class levels individually (e.g. measuring adherence to beta-blockers and calcium channel blockers separately) and then "average" adherence across the entire chronic condition for patients exposed to any medication for that disease state (e.g. hypertension).

## Time-Varying Nature of Adherence and Trajectory Modeling

Adherence is a non-static behavior, and methods are needed to capture changes in adherence over time. This phenomenon has historically been ignored in studies that measure adherence only once or over short intervals. Even when measured longitudinally, adherence data are often averaged. However, patients may experience substantial increases and decreases in adherence not fully captured by composite measures. Consider, for example, the two patients presented in Figure 21.2, where Patient One takes the medication regularly but with intermittent gaps while Patient Two takes the medication perfectly for the first six months but then discontinues. Both patients had the same calculated adherence (~50%) but very different medication use patterns. Composite, cross-sectional measures obfuscate the potential for each patient to experience different health outcomes and require different adherence interventions.

Advanced statistical methods are beginning to take advantage of repeated measurements in adherence data, particularly in dispensing data, to enhance analysis beyond composite measures. One such method applied is group-based trajectory modeling which estimates changes in an outcome that is measured repeatedly over time and identifies individuals with similar longitudinal patterns. This approach fits a semiparametric (discrete) mixture model and assigns groupings in longitudinal data (e.g. monthly PDC) based on probability distributions for a pre-specified number of groups. The probability of belonging to each potential group is modeled as a multinomial logistic regression, and within each group, adherence is modeled as a function of time. The statistical output includes each individual's estimated probabilities of group membership and estimated trajectory curve of adherence over time for each group. However, trajectories provide general patterns for adherence behaviors; that is, no one individual follows the exact pattern described by the trajectory of the group to which they are assigned.

## Prediction of Adherence for Interventions

Unfortunately, low rates of adherence have persisted despite extensive efforts to identify and predict patients at risk of poor adherence with the goal of developing interventions to improve adherence. Despite the expansion of databases with rich patient data, prediction of future adherence remains poor. Traditional approaches have focused on clinical and demographic factors at the time of medication initiation, with discriminative ability that is modest at best even with dozens of predictor variables (e.g. c-statistics generally ranging between 0.60–0.75). Even machine learning, with the capability of measuring complex interactions among predictor variables, has not led to drastically improved prediction, likely because the true factors associated with poor adherence are usually not observable in databases. One of the more successful approaches has been evaluating patterns of medication filling shortly after initiation. For example, in pharmacy dispensing data, researchers have found that failing to refill in the second and third months after initiation is highly predictive of poor adherence over the following year (i.e. past adherence predicts future adherence). Predictions of adherence by providers has also been shown to be no better than chance, so they should not be used routinely in adherence studies or in practice.

## The Future

Adherence studies are likely to advance in several ways. Because optimal adherence thresholds may differ across individuals and diseases, researchers are beginning to explore personalized adherence targets. Novel approaches using other types of data are likely to emerge as well, including the use of more advanced microelectronic technology, often linked with communication systems that both identify and report non-adherence, or the enhancement of mobile and smartphone technology for tracking and intervening on adherence. Refinements to currently available electronic monitors will also likely include more convenient packaging that can both help with adherence (e.g. a reminder or organizer system) and provide two-way personalized communication with patients.

Hopefully, with greater recognition of the importance of non-adherence, more research will be conducted over the next several decades to solve some of these problems as well as develop better approaches to improving adherence so that evidence-based medications can be optimally used.

## Key Points

- Nonadherence occurs in as many as half of patients, resulting in avoidable costs and adverse clinical outcomes. Accurate adherence measurement must be incorporated into research and clinical practice or the problem will remain underappreciated and poorly addressed.
- While missing doses is the more common adherence problem, taking extra doses can also be an issue in some settings, such as anticoagulation and pain medication.
- Potential barriers to adherence include patient-level factors, system-level factors, and medication-specific factors.

- Currently available techniques for measuring adherence include self-report, pharmacy refill measures, pill counts, medication diaries, electronic drug monitors, and drug concentrations. Measuring adherence to multiple medications and non-pill formulations has special challenges.
- Measurement of adherence can be used to determine the threshold of how much medication must be taken to obtain the desired clinical outcome.
- Because adherence behavior varies over time, analysis of data requires consideration of the appropriate duration, time period, and metrics for adherence.
- Adherence is a non-static behavior, and methods are needed to capture changes in adherence over time.
- The inclusion of adherence data in analyses of clinical trials and studies of comparative effectiveness is particularly important when a treatment fails.
- The effectiveness of existing adherence interventions remains modest. Better methods for detecting and addressing nonadherence will be welcome developments.

## Further Reading

Acri, T., Grossberg, R., and Gross, R. (2010). How long is the right interval for assessing antiretroviral pharmacy refill adherence? *JAIDS* 54 (5): e16–e18.

Alfin, S.D., Pradipta, I.S., Hak, E., and Denig, P. (2019). A systematic review finds inconsistency in the measures used to estimate adherence and persistence to multiple cardiometabolic medications. *J. Clin. Epidemiol.* 108: 44–53.

Conn, V.S. and Ruppar, T.M. (2017). Medication adherence outcomes of 771 intervention trials: systematic review and meta-analysis. *Prev. Med.* 99: 269–276.

Choudhry, N.K., Shrank, W.H., Levin, R.L. et al. (2009). Measuring concurrent adherence to multiple related medications. *Am. J. Manag. Care* 15: 457–464.

De Geest, S., Zullig, L.L., Dunbar-Jacob, J. et al. (2018). ESPACOMP medication adherence reporting guideline (EMERGE). *Ann. Intern. Med.* 169: 30–35.

Franklin, J.M., Shrank, W.H., Lii, J. et al. (2016). Observing versus predicting: initial patterns of filling predict long-term adherence more accurately than high-dimensional modeling techniques. *Health Serv. Res.* 51: 220–239.

Franklin, J.M., Shrank, W.H., Pakes, J. et al. (2013). Group-based trajectory models: a new approach to classifying and predicting long-term medication adherence. *Med. Care* 51: 789–796.

Gross, R., Bilker, W.B., Friedman, H.M., and Strom, B.L. (2001). Effect of adherence to newly initiated antiretroviral therapy on plasma viral load. *AIDS* 15: 2109–2117.

Gross, R., Bellamy, S.L., Chapman, J. et al. (2013). Managed problem solving for antiretroviral therapy adherence: a randomized trial. *JAMA Intern. Med.* 173: 300–306.

Grossberg, R., Zhang, Y., and Gross, R. (2004). A time-to-prescription-refill measure of antiretroviral adherence predicted changes in viral load in HIV. *J. Clin. Epidemiol.* 57: 1107–1110.

Lauffenburger, J.C., Balasubramanian, A., Farley, J.F. et al. (2013). Completeness of prescription information in US commercial claims databases. *Pharmacoepidemiol. Drug Saf.* 22: 899–906.

Lauffenburger, J.C., Isaac, T., Bhattacharya, R. et al. (2020). Prevalence and impact of having multiple barriers to medication adherence in nonadherent patients with poorly controlled cardiometabolic disease. *Am. J. Cardiol.* 125: 376–382.

Lo-Ciganic, W.H., Donohue, J.M., Thorpe, J.M. et al. (2015). Using machine learning to examine medication adherence thresholds and risk of hospitalization. *Med. Care* 53: 720–728.

Mehta, S.J., Asch, D.A., Troxel, A.B. et al. (2019). Comparison of pharmacy claims and electronic bottles for measurement of medication adherence among myocardial infarction patients. *Med. Care* 57: e9–e14.

Nguyen, T.M., La, C., and Cottrell, N. (2014). What are validated self-report adherence scales really measuring?: a systematic review. *Br. J. Clin. Pharmacol.* 44: 427–445.

Osterberg, L. and Blaschke, T. (2005). Adherence to medication. *N. Engl. J. Med.* 353: 487–497.

Steiner, J.F., Koepsell, T.D., Fihn, S.D., and Inui, T.S. (1988). A general method of compliance assessment using centralized pharmacy records: description and validation. *Med. Care* 26: 814–823.

Van der Straten, A., Van Damme, L., Haberer, J.E., and Bangsberg, D.R. (2012). Unraveling the divergent results of pre-exposure prophylaxis trials for HIV prevention. *AIDS* 26: F13–F19.

Vrijens, B., De Geest, S., Hughes, D.A. et al. (2012). A new taxonomy for describing and defining adherence to medications. *Br. J. Clin. Pharmacol.* 73: 691–705.

Wilson, I.B., Lee, Y., Michaud, J. et al. (2016). Validation of a three-item self-report measure for medication adherence. *AIDS Behav.* 20: 2700–2708.

## 22

# Advanced Approaches to Controlling Confounding in Pharmacoepidemiologic Studies

*Sebastian Schneeweiss[1] and Samy Suissa[2]*

[1] *Harvard Medical School and Brigham & Women's Hospital, Boston, MA, USA*
[2] *McGill University and Jewish General Hospital, Montreal, Quebec, Canada*

## Introduction

The past two decades have witnessed advances in the design and analysis of epidemiologic studies. In this chapter, we introduce some of these approaches with a focus on confounding control, one of the major methodological challenges in pharmacoepidemiology.

## Clinical Problems to be Addressed by Pharmacoepidemiologic Research

Pharmacoepidemiologic analyses are in principle not different from analyses in other subject areas within epidemiology. They are typically concerned with valid estimation of the causal effects. Some issues specific to pharmacoepidemiology stem from the constraints of secondary data sources, in particular large electronic longitudinal healthcare databases (see Chapter 10). Another difference is the close interdependency of treatment choice with health status, severity of disease, and prognosis. Pharmacoepidemiologists try to reduce bias by appropriate choices of study design and analytic strategies. This chapter provides an overview of selected options that fit typical pharmacoepidemiologic data sources and study questions.

## Methodological Problems to be Addressed by Pharmacoepidemiologic Research

The availability of large longitudinal patient-level healthcare databases make the new-user cohort design a natural design choice as a starting point that mimics the classical parallel group controlled trial, except of course for the randomized treatment assignment (Figure 22.1). Efficient sampling within such cohorts, including case–control, case-cohort, and 2-stage sampling designs are important extensions.

Bias can be reduced by appropriate design choices. Considerations about the sources for exposure variation will lead to decisions on the appropriate study design. In a hypothetical causal experiment, one would expose a patient to an agent and observe the outcome, then rewind time, leave the patient unexposed, and keep all other factors constant to establish a

**Figure 22.1** Principle of the new user design and its variations when studying second line therapies. *Source:* Reproduced from Schneeweiss (2010) with permission from John Wiley & Sons Ltd.

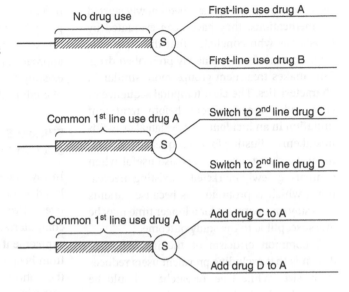

**Figure 22.2** Study design choice by source of exposure variation. *Source:* Reproduced from Schneeweiss (2010) with permission from John Wiley & Sons Ltd.

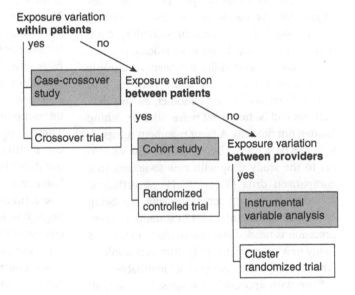

counterfactual experience. Since this experiment is impossible, the next logical expansion is to randomly introduce or observe exposure variation within the same patient but over time (Figure 22.2). If we observe sporadic drug use resulting in fluctuations of exposure status within a patient over time, if that drug has a short washout period, and if the adverse event of interest has a rapid onset, then we may consider a case-crossover design or related approach (see below). Another option is random

allocation of treatments between different patients. For most pharmacoepidemiologic studies, we utilize variation in exposure among individual patients, and we will therefore use a cohort study design. Exposure variation among higher-level entities (provider, region, etc.) can be exploited using instrumental variable (IV) analyses (described below).

In a cohort design, there are several advantages to identifying patients who start a new drug. As patients in both the study group and the comparison group have been newly started on medications, they have been evaluated by physicians who concluded that these patients might benefit from the newly prescribed drug. This makes treatment groups more similar in characteristics. The clear temporal sequence of confounder ascertainment before treatment initiation in an incident user design also avoids mistakenly adjusting for consequences of treatment. Studying new users is also useful when comparing newly marketed to existing medications, which is prone to bias because patients who stay on treatment for a longer time may be less susceptible to the study outcome.

A common criticism of the incident user design is that excluding prevalent users reduces study size. While true, researchers should be aware that by including prevalent users they might gain precision at the cost of validity. Identifying incident users in secondary databases is not costly. In some situations, particularly studies of second-line treatments in chronic conditions, we can only study patients who switch from one drug to another, as very few patients will be treatment naive. Such switching is often not random. A fairer treatment comparison may be achieved by comparing new switchers to the study drug with new switchers to a comparison drug (Figure 22.1). Nevertheless, prevalent new-user cohort designs are being developed to minimize bias in situations where precision is needed and one needs to include as many new users of the study drug as possible or when a comparison drug is not identifiable.

Even with appropriate designs, however, all observational pharmacoepidemiologic studies still must consider carefully how to approach potential confounding.

# Currently Available Solutions

The solutions available to minimize confounding in pharmacoepidemiologic database studies can be broadly categorized into: (i) approaches that collect more information on potential confounders and apply efficient sampling designs to reduce the time and resources it takes to complete the study, and (ii) analytic approaches that try to make better use of the existing data with the goal of improved control of confounding.

## Efficient Sampling Designs within a Cohort Study

In any cohort study, the resources needed to collect data on all cohort members can be prohibitive. Even with cohorts formed from computerized databases, there may be a need to supplement and validate data with information from hospital records and other sources. When the cohort size is large, such additional data gathering can become a formidable task. Moreover, even if no additional data are needed, the data analysis of a cohort with multiple and time-dependent drug exposures can be technically infeasible, particularly if the cohort size and number of outcome events are large.

To counter these constraints, designs based on sampling subjects within a cohort exist. These designs are based on the selection of all cases with the outcome event from the cohort, but differ in the selection of a small subset of "non-cases." Generally, they permit the precise estimation of relative risk measures with negligible losses in precision. Below, we discuss structural aspects of cohorts and present three sampling designs within a cohort: nested case– control, multi-time case–control, and case–cohort.

### Structures of Cohorts

Figure 22.3 illustrates a hypothetical cohort of 21 newly diagnosed diabetics over the period 1995–2010. This cohort is plotted in terms of *calendar time*, with subjects ranked according to their date of entry, which can correspond to the date of diagnosis or treatment initiation. An alternative depiction of this same cohort could be based on disease onset. In this instance, the illustration given in Figure 22.4 for the same cohort, using follow-up time as

**Figure 22.3** Illustration of a *calendar-time* cohort of 21 subjects followed from 1995 to 2010 with 4 cases (•) occurring and related risk-sets (–).

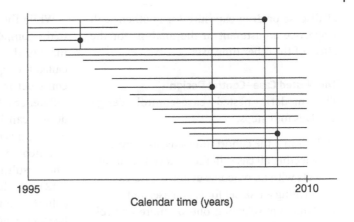

1995            2010

Calendar time (years)

**Figure 22.4** Illustration of *follow-up-time* cohort representation after rearranging the cohort in Figure 22.1, with the new risk-sets (–) for the 4 cases.

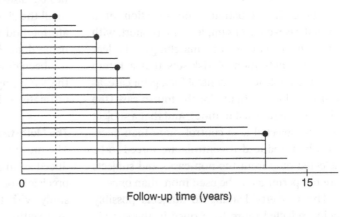

0            15

Follow-up time (years)

the new time axis, is significantly different from the previous one. In these *follow-up-time* cohorts, the same subjects are ranked according to the length of follow-up time in the study with zero-time being the time of diagnosis or treatment start.

The question of which of the two forms one should use rests on one's judgment of the more relevant of the two time axes. This decision is important, since it affects the demarcation of "risk-sets," which are fundamental to the analysis of data from cohorts and consequently the sampling designs within cohorts. A risk-set is formed by the members of the cohort who are at-risk of the outcome event at a given point in time, namely they are free of the outcome and members of the cohort at that point in time called the index date. Drug exposure measures are then anchored at this index date. It is clear

that Figures 22.3 and 22.4 produce distinct risk-sets for the same cases in the same cohort, as illustrated by the different sets of subjects crossed by the vertical broken line for the same case under the two forms of the cohort. In Figure 22.3, for example, the first chronological case to occur has in its risk-set only the first six subjects to enter the cohort, while in Figure 22.4, all 21 cohort members belong to its risk-set at the time that the first case arises. While the second form based on disease duration is often used, because drug exposure can vary substantially over calendar time, the first form may be as relevant for the formation of risk-sets and data analysis as the second form. Regardless, an advantage of having data on the entire cohort is that the primary time axis can be changed according to the study question, using calendar time for one analysis, duration of disease or drug exposure for another, with respective adjustment in the analysis for the effect of the other time axis.

### The Nested Case–Control Design

The modern nested case–control design involves four steps:

1) Defining the cohort time axis, as above,
2) Selecting all cases in the cohort, i.e. all subjects with an outcome event of interest,
3) Forming a risk-set for each case, and
4) *Randomly* selecting one or more controls from each risk-set.

Figure 22.5 illustrates the selection of a nested case–control sample from a cohort, with one control per case (1 : 1 matching). It is clear from the definition of risk-sets that a future case is eligible to be a control for a prior case, as illustrated in the figure for the fourth case (the circle occurring last in time), and that a subject may be selected as a control more than once. Bias is introduced if controls are forced to be selected only from the non-cases and subjects are not permitted to be used more than once.

The property leading to subjects possibly being selected more than once in the sample may be challenging when the exposure and covariate factors are time-dependent, particularly when the data are obtained by questionnaire where the respondent would have to answer questions regarding multiple time points in their history (see also Chapter 13).

While the nested case–control design leads to the computation of the odds-ratio as an estimate of the rate or hazard ratio, its extension called the "quasi-cohort approach," provides a construct to estimate crude and adjusted rate differences. Moreover, the nested case–control design can be used to contrast exposure to a drug versus no exposure by comparing the rate of outcome to that of an external population. The resulting standardized incidence ratio (SIR) calculation must take into account that cohort members with the longest follow-up have a greater chance of being selected in the nested case–control sample, since they belong to all the risk-sets (Figure 22.5). The appropriate method to perform external comparisons using data from a nested case–control design has been developed and uses knowledge about the sampling structure to yield an unbiased estimate of the standardized rate.

### The Multi-time Case–Control Design

The multi-time case–control design was introduced as an alternative strategy to improve the precision of the odds ratio in a case–control study with transient time-varying exposures, in a setting where increasing the number of control subjects is too costly. This approach is based on increasing the number of observations per control subject, by measuring drug exposure at many different points in time. Indeed, several case–control studies will collect extensive data on time-dependent expo-

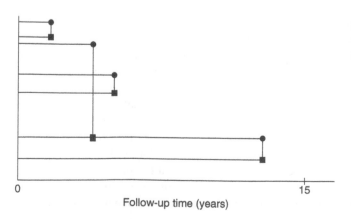

**Figure 22.5** Nested case–control sample of one control (■) per case (•) from cohort in Figure 22.4.

Follow-up time (years)

sures but use only a portion of these data in estimating the rate ratio.

For example, the International Agranulocytosis and Aplastic Anemia Study (IAAAS) assessed the risk of agranulocytosis associated with the use of analgesics using a case–control study of 221 cases of agranulocytosis and 1425 controls. While the study collected data on exposure for four weeks prior to the index date, only one week's worth of data was used in the analysis. The multi-time case–control approach allows the use of all available exposure data during the four weeks (i.e. four control person-moments) rather than only one week (i.e. one control person-moment) to improve the precision of the odds ratio estimate, which must however be corrected for within-subject correlation.

This design increases the number of control observations per case, thus potentially also increasing the power of the study without adding additional subjects. For example, in a nested case–control study within a cohort of 12 090 patients with chronic obstructive pulmonary disease (COPD), there were 245 incident cases of acute myocardial infarction (AMI) that occurred during follow-up, for whom 1 and 10 controls per case were identified. The rate ratio of AMI associated with use of antibiotics in the month prior to the index date was 2.00 (95% CI: 1.16–3.44) with one control per case, with improved precision with

10 controls per case (rate ratio 2.13; 95% CI: 1.48–3.05). Alternatively, keeping only one control patient per case, but increasing the number of control time windows per subject from 1 to 10 months (prior to the index date) also improved the precision, with a rate ratio of 1.99 (95% CI: 1.36–2.90).

### The Case–Cohort Design

The case–cohort design involves two steps:

1) selecting all cases in the cohort, i.e. all subjects with an adverse event; and
2) randomly selecting a sample of predetermined size of subjects from the cohort, irrespective of case or control status.

Figure 22.6 depicts the selection of a case–cohort sample of six subjects from the illustrative cohort. Note it is possible that some cases selected in step 1 are also selected in the step 2 sample, as illustrated in the figure for the third case.

The case–cohort design resembles a reduced version of the cohort, with all cases from the full cohort included. The method of analysis for a case-cohort sample takes into account the overlap of cohort members between successive risk-sets induced by this sampling strategy.

The first advantage of the case–cohort design is its capacity to use the same sample to study multiple types of events. In contrast, the nested case– control design requires different control

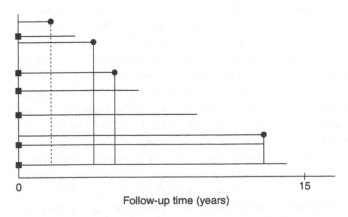

**Figure 22.6** Case-cohort sample with six controls (■) from cohort in Figure 22.4.

groups for each type. For example, a nested case–control study of the risks of β-agonists had two distinct control groups, one of size 233 for the 44 asthma deaths, the other of size 422 for the 85 asthma near-deaths. Another useful advantage is that the case–cohort design permits one to change the primary time axis of analysis from calendar to disease time and vice versa, depending on either the assumed model or the targeted outcome. This is not possible with the nested case–control study, where the primary time axis must be set a priori to permit the risk-set construction. Yet another advantage is its simplicity in sampling, which has benefits in both comprehensibility and computer programming.

The nested case–control design does have some advantages over the case–cohort design. The first is the simplicity of statistical power calculation. The nested case–control design is independent of the size of the cohort, while for the case–cohort design knowledge about overlap in risk-sets is essential, thus greatly complicating these calculations. Second, data on time-dependent exposure and covariates need only be collected up to the time of the risk-set for the nested case–control study, while the collection must be exhaustive for the case–cohort.

### Prevalent New-User Cohort Designs

A common situation in pharmacoepidemiology involves the study of the effect of a new drug entering the market, with the best comparator being an older drug. Most often, patients prescribed the new drug will have been switched from the older comparator drug. An incident new-user cohort design based on incident new users of the study and comparator drugs, including only patients who were treatment-naïve to both drugs, would be optimal. However, it would exclude the possibly large number of subjects who switched from the older to the new drug, a clinically relevant subset. The prevalent new-user cohort design provides an approach to include these switchers.

A prevalent new-user cohort is formed from the base cohort of all users of the comparator drug and of the drug under study, which inherently includes the subjects who switched from the comparator to the study drug as well as those who initiated the study drug de novo. These latter subjects can be directly matched to contemporaneous initiators on covariates or propensity scores (PSs). For the subjects who switched from the comparator to the study drug, comparators can be selected from the base cohort by matching conditional on exposure sets. Time-based exposure sets are defined by the time from the first prescription of the comparator drug up to the point of switching (with a time interval such as ±1 month), while prescription-based exposure sets are defined by the number of prescriptions of the comparator drug received up to the point of switching. Thus, each switcher to the study drug will belong to an exposure set that includes subjects of similar duration or prescription history with a dispensing of the comparator drug. The importance of the exposure sets is that a visit occurred where the physician decided to either continue the comparator treatment or switch to the new study drug, providing equivalent time points in the disease course at which confounding patient characteristics can be measured and controlled for.

Time-conditional propensity scores (TCPS) can be used to identify and match, within the exposure sets, the comparator drug users most similar to the patients who switched to the study drug. The time-dependent Cox proportional hazards model or, alternatively, conditional logistic regression if the exposure sets are too large, can be used to compute the "propensity" of switching to the study drug, versus continuing on the comparator drug, as a function of the time-varying patient characteristics measured at the point of the exposure set, thus conserving the matching induced by the exposure set and avoiding adjusting for causal intermediates. For the purposes of the positivity assumption, the TCPS of the switcher should lie within the range of the TCPS of the members of the corresponding exposure set. To emulate the randomized trial, the selection process can be initiated with the first chronological index study drug subject and repeated sequentially. Thus, each subject who initiated the study drug will have a comparator user, matched on the TCPS. Cohort entry is taken as the date of the first prescription of the study drug and the corresponding date for the matched comparator.

This approach is also useful for studies having a "non-use" comparator, by using a physician visit or prescription for any drug other than the study drug as the comparator. Several questions remain regarding this design, in particular the potential bias from using the prevalent users as comparators, which should be investigated by stratification on the incident/prevalent new-user status.

## Within-Subject Designs

When dealing with the study of transient effects on the risk of acute adverse events, Maclure asserts that the best representatives of the source population that produced the cases would be the case subjects themselves: this is the premise of the case-crossover design. This is a design where comparisons between exposures are made within subjects, thus removing confounding by factors that remain constant within subject. An extension to the case-crossover design, the case–time–control design is also presented here.

### The Case-Crossover Design

The case-crossover study is simply an observational crossover study *in the cases only*. The subjects alternate at varying frequencies between exposure and non-exposure to the drug of interest, until the adverse event occurs, which happens for all subjects in the study sample, since all are cases by definition. With respect to the timing of the adverse event, each case is investigated to determine whether exposure was present within the presumed effect period. This occurrence is then classified as having arisen either under drug exposure or non-exposure on the basis of the presumed effect period. Thus, for each case, we have either an exposed or unexposed status, which represents for data analysis the first column of a $2 \times 2$ table, one for each case. Since each case will be matched to itself for comparison, the analysis is matched and thus we must create separate $2 \times 2$ tables for each case (see Maclure 1991 for further details).

With respect to control information, the data on the average drug use pattern are necessary to determine the typical probability of exposure during the time window of effect. This is done by obtaining data for a sufficiently stable period of time. For example, we may wish to study the risk of ventricular tachycardia in association with the use of inhaled beta-agonists in asthma, where prolonged Q-T intervals were observed in patients in the four-hour period following drug absorption. Table 22.1 displays data for 10 cases of ventricular tachycardia, including the average number of times a day each case has been using β-agonists in the past year. Note that there are six four-hour periods (the duration of the effect period) per day. Such data determine the proportion of time that each asthmatic is usually spending in the effect period and thus potentially "at risk" of ventricular tachycardia. This proportion is then used to obtain the expected exposure on the basis of time spent in these "at risk" periods, for comparison with the actual exposure in the cases observed during the last four-hour period. This is done by forming a $2 \times 2$ table for each case, with the corresponding control data as defined above, and combining the tables using the Mantel–Haenszel technique.

To carry out a case-crossover study, three critical points must be considered. First, the study outcome must be an acute event that is hypothesized to be the result of a transient drug effect. Thus, drugs with chronic or regular patterns of use which vary only minimally between and within individuals are not amenable to this design. Nor are latent adverse events. Second, since a transient effect is under study, the presumed effect period must be precisely stated. For example, in a study of the

**Table 22.1** Hypothetical data for 10 subjects with ventricular tachycardia included in a case-crossover study of the risk of ventricular tachycardia in asthma associated with the four-hour period after β-agonist exposure.

| Case # | β-agonist use in last 4 hours[a] ($E_i$) | Usual β-agonist use in last year | Periods of exposure ($N_{1i}$) | Periods of no exposure ($N_{0i}$) |
|---|---|---|---|---|
| 1 | 0 | 1/day | 365 | 1825 |
| 2 | 1 | 6/year | 6 | 2184 |
| 3 | 0 | 2/day | 730 | 1460 |
| 4 | 1 | 1/month | 12 | 2178 |
| 5 | 0 | 4/week | 208 | 1982 |
| 6 | 0 | 1/week | 52 | 2138 |
| 7 | 0 | 1/month | 12 | 2178 |
| 8 | 1 | 2/month | 24 | 2166 |
| 9 | 0 | 2/day | 730 | 1460 |
| 10 | 0 | 2/week | 104 | 2086 |

*Note:* Rate ratio estimator is $(\sum E_i N_{0i})/(\sum (1 - E_i) N_{1i})$
[a] Inhalations of 200 mcg: 1 = yes, 0 = no.

possible acute cardiotoxicity of inhaled β-agonists in asthmatics, this effect period can be hypothesized to be four hours after having taken the usual dose. An incorrect specification of this time window can have important repercussions on the relative risk estimate. Third, one must be able to obtain reliable data on the usual pattern of drug exposure for each case, over a sufficiently long period of time.

### The Case–Time–Control Design

One of the limitations of the case-crossover design is the assumption of the absence of a time trend in the exposure prevalence. An approach that adjusts for such time trends is the case–time–control design, an extension of the case-crossover analysis that uses, in addition to the case series, a series of control subjects to adjust for exposure time trends. By using cases and controls of a conventional case–control study as their own referents, the *case–time-control design* addresses the time trend assumption.

The approach is illustrated with data from the Saskatchewan Asthma Epidemiologic Project, conducted to investigate the risks

associated with the use of inhaled β-agonists. Using a cohort of 12 301 asthmatics followed during 1980–1987, 129 cases of fatal or near-fatal asthma and 655 controls were identified. The amount of β-agonist used in the year prior to the index date was used for exposure. Table 22.2 displays the data comparing low (<12 canisters per year) with high (>12) use of β-agonists. The crude odds ratio for high β-agonist use was 4.4 (95% CI: 2.9–6.7). Adjustment for all available markers of severity lowered the odds ratio to 3.1 (95% CI: 1.8–5.4).

To apply the case–time–control design, exposure to β-agonists was obtained for the one-year current period and the one-year reference period prior to the current period. First, a case-crossover analysis was performed using the discordant subjects among the 129 cases, namely the 29 who were current high users of β-agonists and low users in the reference period, and the 9 cases who were current low users of β-agonist and high users previously. This analysis is repeated for the 655 controls, of whom there were 90 discordant in exposure; that is, 65 were current high users of β-agonists and low users in the reference period, and 25 were

**Table 22.2** Illustration of a case-time-control analysis of data from a case–control study of 129 cases of fatal or near-fatal asthma and 655 matched controls, and current beta-agonist use.

| | Cases | | Controls | | OR | 95% CI |
|---|---|---|---|---|---|---|
| | High | Low | High | Low | | |
| Current beta-agonist use (case–control) | 93 | 36 | 241 | 414 | 3.1[a] | 1.8–5.4 |
| Discordant[b] use (case-crossover) | 29 | 9 | | | 3.2 | 1.5–6.8 |
| Discordant[b] use (control-crossover) | | | 65 | 25 | 2.6 | 1.6–4.1 |
| Case-time-control | 29 | 9 | 65 | 25 | 1.2 | 0.5–3.0 |

[a] Adjusted estimate from case–control analysis.
[b] Discordant from exposure level during reference time period.

current low users of β-agonists and high users previously. The case–time–control odds ratio, using these discordant pairs frequencies for a paired-matched analysis, is given by (29/9)/(65/25) = 1.2 (95% CI: 0.5–3.0). This estimate, which does not account for potential confounding by asthma severity that varies over time, indicates a minimal risk for these drugs.

The case–time–control approach can provide an unbiased estimate of the odds ratio in the presence of confounding by time-invariant factors, including indication, despite the fact that the indication for drug use (in our example, intrinsic disease severity) is not measured, because of the within-subject analysis. It also controls for time trends in drug use. Nevertheless, its validity is subject to several assumptions, including the absence of time-varying confounders, such as increasing asthma severity over time (an important problem, since new drugs may be more likely to be implemented when disease is most severe), so that caution is recommended in its use.

## Analytic Approaches for Improved Confounding Control

### Balancing Patient Characteristics
Confounding caused by imbalance of patient risk factors between treatment groups is a known threat to validity in nonrandomized studies. Many analytic options for reducing

confounding are available. Several approaches fit key characteristics of longitudinal healthcare databases well and address important concerns in pharmacoepidemiologic analyses.

### Propensity Score Analyses
Propensity score analysis has emerged as a convenient and effective tool for adjusting large numbers of confounders. In an incident user cohort design, a PS is the estimated probability of starting medication A versus starting medication B, conditional on all observed pretreatment patient characteristics. Propensity scores are a multivariate balancing tool that balance large numbers of covariates in an efficient way even if the study outcome is rare, which is frequent in pharmacoepidemiology. Estimating the PS using logistic regression is uncomplicated, and strategies for variable selection are well described. Variables that are only predictors of treatment choice but are not independent predictors of outcome will lead to less precise estimates and in some extreme situations to bias. Selecting variables based on p-values is not helpful as this strategy depends on study size. Once a PS is estimated based on observed covariates there are several options to utilize it in a second step to reduce confounding. Typical strategies include adjustment from quantiles of the score with or without trimming, regression modeling of the PS, or matching on PSs. Matching illustrates the working of PSs well.

Fixed ratio matching on PSs like 1 : 1 matching has several advantages that may outweigh its drawback of not utilizing the full dataset in situations where not all eligible patients match. Such matching will exclude patients in the extreme PS ranges where there is little clinical ambivalence in treatment choice (Figure 22.7). These tails of the PS distribution often harbor extreme patient scenarios that are not representative for the majority in clinical practice and may be due to residual confounding. Trimming these extreme PS values will gener-

ally reduce residual confounding. Another advantage is that the multivariate balance of potential confounders can be demonstrated by cross-tabulating observed patient characteristics by actual exposure status after fixed ratio matching. Matching with a fixed ratio in cohort studies does not require matched analyses, but variable ratio matching does. Analytic techniques that condition on the matching sets and may be used in this setting include conditional logistic regression or stratified Cox regression, depending on the data model.

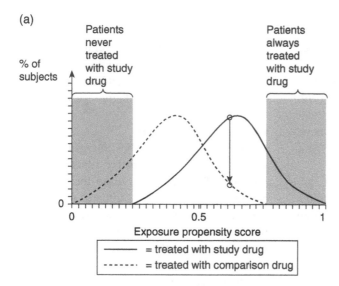

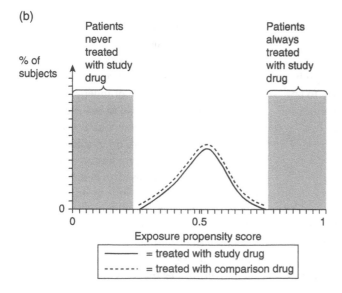

**Figure 22.7** Two hypothetical propensity score distributions before and after matching. (a) Before matching: two propensity score distributions partially overlap indicating some similarities between the comparison groups in a multivariate parameter space. (b) After 1 : 1 matching on propensity score: Not all patients found matches that were similar enough in their multivariable characteristics. Areas of non-overlap between PS distributions drop out entirely. *Source:* Reproduced from Schneeweiss (2010) with permission from John Wiley & Sons Ltd.

In summary, PS analyses are convenient tools to adjust for many covariates when study outcomes are rare. Extensive confounding adjustment is central in most pharmacoepidemiologic applications, and in secondary healthcare databases we can often define many covariates. In contrast to traditional outcome models, PS matching allows the investigator to achieve covariate balance achieved in the final study sample. PS estimation is well developed for comparing two agents using logistic regression to predict treatment choice. When more than two agents or several dose categories are compared, multinomial regression models are used to estimate the PS and either pragmatic pairwise matching to a common reference group or multidimensional matching is applied. Of importance, PS analyses still can only adjust for measured variables, although they can be used to adjust for many at the same time. Further, one loses the ability to see the effects of adjusting for one variable at a time.

In situations where exposure is rare, disease risk scores, an alternative to PS analysis, might be more suitable. They estimate the association between patient factors and the study outcome in an unexposed population using multivariate regression and summarize the relationship in each patient's estimated probability of the outcome independent of exposure.

### Focusing on the Analysis of Comparable Patients

Restriction is a common and effective analytic tool to make drug user groups more comparable by making populations more homogeneous, which leads to less residual confounding. Some restrictions are quite obvious since they are made by explicit criteria, for example, limiting the study population to elderly patients with dementia to study the safety of antipsychotic medications used to control behavioral disturbances in this population. Other restrictions are more implicit and blur the line between design and analytic strategies.

**Choice of comparator group:** picking a comparator group is arguably the most fundamental choice in a pharmacoepidemiologic study design and may influence results dramatically. Ideally, we want to restrict the comparison population to patients who have the identical indication as the users of the study agent. Rosiglitazone and pioglitazone are such a medication pair. They were marketed around the same time, were both indicated for second line treatment of diabetes, come from the same class of compound, and in the early marketing phase were thought to have a similar effectiveness and safety profiles. This should make treatment choice largely random with regard to patient characteristics and treatment groups comparable by design, resulting in almost overlapping PS distributions and little confounding.

**Limiting to incident users:** By restricting the study population to new users of the study agent or a comparator agent we implicitly require that both groups have been recently evaluated by a physician. Based on this evaluation, the physician has decided that the indicating condition has reached a state where a pharmacologic treatment should be initiated. Therefore, such patients are likely to be more similar in observable and unobservable characteristics than comparing incident users versus non-users or versus ongoing users of another drug.

**Matching on patient characteristics:** Multivariate PSs demonstrate areas of non-overlap where no referent patients with comparable baseline characteristics can be identified. It is recommended to remove those patients from the analysis as they do not contribute to the estimation and may introduce bias. Such a restriction can be achieved by trimming these patients from the study population (see Figure 22.7b) or by matching patients on the PS or on specific key patient characteristics of importance.

While restriction is an important tool to improve internal validity it will reduce generalizability of findings. However, in pharmacoepidemiology we usually place higher value on internal validity even if that comes at the price of reduced external validity. Investigators need to be aware of this tradeoff and make choices accordingly.

## Unobserved Patient Characteristics and Residual Confounding

Once a study is implemented, strategies to reduce confounding further are limited to observable disease risk factors. Secondary data, like electronic healthcare databases often lack critical details on health state and risk factors, which can lead to residual confounding.

## Proxy Adjustment

Longitudinal electronic health care databases are as much a description of medical sociology under financial constraints as they are records of delivered health care and can be analyzed as a set of proxies that indirectly describe the health status of patients. This status is presented through the lenses of health care providers recording their findings and interventions via coders and operating under the constraints of a specific health care system. For example, old age serves as a proxy for many factors including comorbidity, frailty, and cognitive decline; use of an oxygen canister is a sign of frail health; having regular annual check-ups is indicative of a health-seeking lifestyle and increased adherence. Adjusting for a perfect surrogate of an unmeasured factor is equivalent to adjusting for the factor itself. Frequently used proxies in pharmacoepidemiologic analyses are the number of prescription drugs dispensed, the number of physician visits, and hospitalizations before the index drug exposure. Such measures of healthcare intensity, while not perfect surrogates, are useful proxies for general health and access to care and have been shown to meaningfully help adjust for confounding.

Proxy adjustment can be exploited by algorithms that systematically search through recorded codes for diagnoses, procedures, equipment purchases, and prescription drug dispensings before the initiation of study drug use to identify potential confounders or proxies thereof. The hundreds of proxies that will be identified can then be adjusted for in a large PS model. Collinearity may likely occur but is irrelevant, as the individual parameters estimated in the large PS regression will not be interpreted but only used for predicting treatment. Such a high-dimensional PS approach has been shown empirically to improve confounding adjustment in many settings, although it is not yet fully evaluated. Although adjusting for variables that are only related to the exposure and not to the outcome (an IV) could theoretically introduce bias, in practical scenarios the advantage of adjusting for potential confounders outweighs the risk of adjusting for the rare instrument.

## Exploiting Random Aspects in Treatment Choice Via Instrumental Variable Analysis

As explained above, we are interested in identifying residual random exposure variation after adjusting for observable confounders to more completely account for confounding. However, in secondary data, not all clinically relevant risk factors of the outcome may be recorded. To attempt to address this limitation, we can try to identify naturally occurring quasi-random treatment choices in routine care. Factors that determine such quasi-random treatment choices are called IVs, and IV analyses can result in unbiased effect estimates even without observing all confounders if several assumptions are fulfilled.

An instructive example of an instrument is a hospital drug formulary. Some hospitals list only drug A for a given indication and other hospitals list only drug B. It is a reasonable assumption that patients do not choose their preferred hospital based on its formulary but rather based on location and recommendation. Therefore, the choice of drug A versus drug B should be independent of patient characteristics in the hospitals with these restricted formularies. Thus, comparing patient outcomes from drug A hospitals with patient outcomes from drug B hospitals should result in unbiased effects of drug A versus drug B, using the appropriate analytic tools. An example of such a study is a study on the risk of death from aprotinin, an antifibrinolytic agent given to reduce bleeding during cardiac surgery. The study identified surgeons who always used aprotinin and compared their outcomes to surgeons who always used aminocaproic acid, an alternative drug. If physician skill level and performance are on average equal between institutions, independent of drug use, this will result in valid findings. On the other hand, of course, such an assumption may not be valid, e. g., if academic hospitals allow less restrictive formularies, are more likely to see sicker patients, and have skilled physicians, all of which may be true.

Instrumental variable analyses rely on the identification of a valid instrument, a factor that is assumed to be related to treatment, but neither directly nor indirectly related to the study outcome. As such, an IV is an observed variable that causes (or is a marker of) variation in the exposure similar to random treatment choice. Typically, the following three assumptions need to be fulfilled for valid IV estimation: (i) an IV should affect treatment or be associated with treatment choice by sharing a common cause. The strength of this association is also referred to as the instrument strength, (ii) an IV should be a factor that is as good as randomly assigned, so that it is unrelated to patient characteristics, and (iii) an IV should not be related to the outcome other than through its association with treatment. As such, an IV analysis sounds very much like a randomized trial with noncompliance. The flip of a coin determines the instrument status (treat with A vs. treat with B) and the amount of random noncompliance determines the strength of the instrument. In nonrandomized research, however, identifying valid instruments is difficult and successful IV analyses are infrequent. In principle, treatment preference can be influenced by time if treatment guidelines change rapidly and substantially. A comparison of patient outcome before versus

after a sudden change in treatment patterns may then be a reasonable instrument.

### Sensitivity Analyses

A series of sensitivity analyses can help investigators to better understand how robust a study's findings are to a set of structural assumptions. Some of the sensitivity analyses suggested below are generic and others are specific to database analyses.

An important but underutilized diagnostic tool for the impact of unobserved confounders on the validity of findings in nonrandomized studies is quantitative sensitivity analyses. Basic sensitivity analyses of residual confounding try to determine how strong and how imbalanced a confounder would have to be among drug categories to explain the observed effect. Such an "externally" adjusted relative risk ($RRadj$) can be expressed as a function of the unadjusted relative risk ($RRunadj$), the independent RR of the unmeasured confounder on the disease outcome ($RRCD$), and the prevalence of the confounder in both drug exposure categories ($PC|E$):

$$RR_{adj.} = \frac{RR_{unadj}}{\left[\frac{P_{C|E=1}\left(RR_{CD}-1\right)+1}{P_{C|E=0}\left(RR_{CD}-1\right)+1}\right]}$$

As an example, a recent cohort study could not find the expected association between use of TNF (tumor necrosis factor) alpha inhibitors, an immunomodulating agent, in treating rheumatoid arthritis, and the incidence of serious bacterial infections. There was a concern that physicians may have prescribed the agent selectively in patients with more progressive disease. A sensitivity analysis demonstrated the direction and strength of any such bias and concluded that it would be unlikely to change the clinical implications of the study. This type of sensitivity analysis is particularly helpful in database studies, but is underutilized. Spreadsheet software is available for easy implementation of such sensitivity analyses (drugepi.org). Lash and Fink proposed an approach that considers several systematic errors simultaneously, allowing sensitivity analyses for confounding, misclassification, and selection bias in one process.

As another example: When using retrospective databases, it is usually cumbersome or impossible to contact patients and ask when they began using a drug for the first time in order to implement an incident user cohort design. Therefore, incident users are identified empirically by a drug dispensing that was not preceded by a dispensing of the same drug for a defined time period. This washout period is identical for all patients. A typical length is six months. In sensitivity analyses, this interval could be extended to 9 and 12 months. In a study on the comparative safety of antidepressant agents in children in British Columbia, this interval was extended from one year to three years to ensure that the children in the study were treatment-naïve before their first use, which helped balance comparison groups and reduce confounding. Although increasing the length of the washout increases the likelihood that patients are truly incident users, it also reduces the number of patients eligible for the study. This tradeoff is particularly worth noting in health plans with high enrollee turnover.

There is often uncertainty about the correct definition of the exposure risk window based on the clinical pharmacology of the study agent. This is further complicated in healthcare databases, since the discontinuation date is imputed through the days' supply of the last dispensing/prescription. Varying the exposure risk window is therefore insightful and easy to accomplish in cohort studies.

## Conclusion

Minimizing confounding in pharmacoepidemiologic research is an ongoing development that is context and data-source specific. While great progress has been made in analyzing longitudinal healthcare databases, much remains to be improved to reliably achieve unbiased estimates of causal treatment effects that will carry the weight of medical decision making. Several developments are promising. One is the use of IV analyses utilizing the multilevel structure of healthcare systems. Another is the expanded use of PS methods including its combination with machine learning for high-dimensional proxy adjustment. A development that is gaining importance is the enrichment of existing data environments with supplemental clinical data linked from electronic medical records, from disease registries, from patient surveys, and/or from laboratory test result repositories. While this information will provide an opportunity for improved confounding adjustment, it comes with equally large methodological challenges, as information is collected in routine care and may have been requested/recorded selectively in patients who were thought to benefit most. Clearly there is still plenty of work to be done to find satisfactory and scalable solutions for the control of confounding.

## Key Points

- Pharmacoepidemiologic studies must be efficient by offering rapid information of the utmost validity.
- Computerized databases provide valuable data sources for pharmacoepidemiologic studies with unique methodological challenges.
- Target trial thinking and study design choices, like the new-user active-comparator cohort design, are paramount in limiting the effect of confounding and other biases.
- Epidemiologic designs such as nested case–control and case-crossover are efficient approaches to assess the risks and benefits of drugs if additional data are collected.
- Confounding bias can be assessed efficiently using subsets of the data with enriched information.

---

**Case Example 22.1   (Confavreux, C. et al.)**

*Background*

The occurrence of relapses in multiple sclerosis is highly variable and unpredictable. Vaccines, particularly for hepatitis B, have been suspected to induce relapses in multiple sclerosis.

*Question*

Does vaccination increase in the rate of relapse in multiple sclerosis?

*Approach*

A case-crossover study within the European Database for Multiple Sclerosis network. Cases with a relapse after a 12-month relapse-free period were questioned on vaccinations. Exposure to vaccination in the two-month risk-period immediately preceding the relapse was compared with that of the four previous two-month control periods to estimate the relative risk.

*Results*

• The prevalence of exposure during the two-month risk period was similar to that of the four control periods.
• The relative risk of relapse associated with exposure to any vaccination was thus unity.

*Strengths*

• Large clinical population with extensive computerized information.
• Efficient study design using only cases for this acute event and transient drug exposure.
• Confounding factors that do not change over time are inherently controlled for by the within-subject matched analysis.

*Limitations*

• Low vaccination prevalence in this clinical population does not permit assessment of the risk for shorter effect periods, such as a week.
• Confounding by factors that change over time, such as infections, could not be controlled for.

*Key Points*

• Multiple sclerosis is highly variable over time and thus not easily amenable to cohort or case–control study designs.
• The case-crossover design is an efficient approach to study vaccine safety.

---

**Case Example 22.2   (Schneeweiss S., Patrick AR., et al.)**

*Background*

A meta-analysis of randomized placebo-controlled trials has shown an increased risk of suicides among children initiating antidepressants (AD), however, the study could not elucidate the comparative safety, i.e. whether this risk varies meaningfully between antidepressant agents.

*Question*

Do tricyclic AD have similar risk of suicidal actions including completed suicide compared with selective serotonin reuptake inhibitors (SSRIs).

*Approach*

A PS-matched new user cohort study of children and young adults (10–18 years of age) using health care utilization databases from the province of British Columbia linked with vital statistics information. Suicidal actions were defined as emergency hospitalizations for intentional self harm and completed suicides. First exposure to a tricyclic AD with no AD exposure in previous three years was compared to new use of fluoxetine. Follow-up started the day after the first AD dispensing

*(Continued)*

**Case Example 22.2 (Continued)**

and ended 14 days after their last exposure to the cohort-qualifying drug exposure.

*Results*
- Unadjusted and insufficiently adjusted analyses showed a spurious up to 50% relative risk decrease for tricyclic ADs compared with SSRIs, suggesting that tricyclic agents are avoided in patients with suicidal thoughts as they are known to be poisonous in high doses.
- There was no difference in the risk for suicidal actions between tricyclic ADs and fluoxetine after nonparsimonious high-dimensional PSs matching.

*Strengths*
- Large stable population of children and young adults with information on all health service encounters and vital statistics.
- The new users design ensures that all patient characteristics are assessed before exposure starts and that suicidal actions shortly after initiation will be accounted for and the duration of use-dependent risk function can be plotted and illustrate the depletion of the most susceptible patients.

- Confounding factors may bias results due to strong channeling of sicker patients to the safer SSRIs but nonparsimonious adjustment with high-dimensional PSs can remedy the issue in this example.

*Limitations*
- Despite the large population size, the number of outcomes remains limited, leading to less precise estimates and making adjustment for many potential confounders in outcome regression models perilous.
- Confounding by outcome risk factors that channel patients into the treatment groups can be strong and hard to control.

*Key Points*
- Two major antidepressant classes have similar risks of suicidal actions in newly treated children and young adults.
- The new user cohort design is a flexible and robust approach for studies that rely entirely on secondary healthcare databases when combined with nonparsimonious PS adjustment.

# Further Reading

Blais, L., Ernst, P., and Suissa, S. (1996). Confounding by indication and channeling over time: the risks of beta-agonists. *Am. J. Epidemiol.* 144: 1161–1169.

Brookhart, M.A., Rassen, J.A., and Schneeweiss, S. (2010). Instrumental variable methods in comparative safety and effectiveness research. *Pharmacoepidemiol. Drug Saf.* 19: 537–554.

Brookhart, M.A., Schneeweiss, S., Rothman, K.J. et al. (2006). Variable selection for propensity score models. *Am. J. Epidemiol.* 163: 1149–1156.

Collet, J.P., Schaubel, D., Hanley, J. et al. (1998). Controlling confounding when studying large pharmacoepidemiologic databases: a case study of the two-stage sampling design. *Epidemiology* 9: 309–315.

Confavreux, C., Suissa, S., Saddier, P. et al. (2001). Vaccinations and the risk of relapse in multiple sclerosis. *New Engl. J. Med.* 344 (5): 319–326.

Lash, T.L., Fox, M.P., MacLehose, R.F. et al. (2014). Good practices for quantitative bias analysis. *Int. J. Epidemiol.* 43: 1969–1985.

Maclure, M. (1991). The case-crossover design: a method for studying transient effects on the risk of acute events. *Am. J. Epidemiol.* 133: 144–153.

Ray, W.A. (2003). Evaluating medication effects outside of clinical trials: new-user designs. *Am. J. Epidemiol.* 158: 915–920.

Rothman, K.J., Greenland, S., and Lash, T.L. (eds.) (2008). *Modern Epidemiology*, 3rde. Philadelphia, PA: Lippincott Williams & Wilkins.

Schneeweiss, S., Patrick, A.R., Solomon, D.H., Dormuth, C.R., Miller, M., Mehta, J., Lee, J.C., and Wang, P.S. (2010). Comparative safety of antidepressant agents for children and adolescents regarding suicidal acts. *Pediatrics.* 125 (5): 876–88.

Schneeweiss, S. (2018). Automated data-adaptive analytics for electronic healthcare data to study causal treatment effects. *Clin. Epidemiol.* 10: 771–788.

Schneeweiss, S. and Avorn, J. (2005). A review of uses of health care utilization databases for epidemiologic research on therapeutics. *J. Clin. Epidemiol.* 58: 323–337.

Schneeweiss, S. (2010). A basic study design for expedited safety signal evaluation based on electronic healthcare data. *Pharmacoepidemiol. Drug Saf.* 19: 858–868.

Schneeweiss, S., Patrick, A.R., Sturmer, T. et al. (2007). Increasing levels of restriction in pharmacoepidemiologic database studies of elderly and comparison with randomized trial results. *Med. Care* 45 (10 Suppl 2): S131–S142.

Schneeweiss, S., Seeger, J.D., Maclure, M. et al. (2001). Performance of comorbidity scores to control for confounding in epidemiologic studies using claims data. *Am. J. Epidemiol.* 154: 854–864.

Spitzer, W.O., Suissa, S., Ernst, P. et al. (1992). The use of beta-agonists and the risk of death and near death from asthma. *N. Engl. J. Med.* 326: 501–506.

Sturmer, T., Rothman, K.J., Avorn, J., and Glynn, R.J. (2010). Treatment effects in the presence of unmeasured confounding: dealing with observations in the tails of the propensity score distribution–a simulation study. *Am. J. Epidemiol.* 172: 843–854.

Suissa, S. (1995). The case–time–control design. *Epidemiology* 6: 248–253.

Suissa, S. (2015). The quasi-cohort approach in pharmacoepidemiology: upgrading the nested case–control. *Epidemiology* 26 (2): 242–246.

Suissa, S., Dell'aniello, S., and Martinez, C. (2010). The multitime case–control design for time-varying exposures. *Epidemiology* 21 (6): 876–883.

Suissa, S., Edwardes, M.D., and Boivin, J.F. (1998). External comparisons from nested case–control designs. *Epidemiology* 9: 72–78.

Suissa, S., Moodie, E.E., and Dell'Aniello, S. (2017). Prevalent new-user cohort designs for comparative drug effect studies by time-conditional propensity scores. *Pharmacoepidemiol. Drug Saf.* 26 (4): 459–468.

Wacholder, S. (1991). Practical considerations in choosing between the case–cohort and nested case–control designs. *Epidemiology* 2: 155–158.

Walker, A.M. (1996). Confounding by indication. *Epidemiology* 7: 335–336.

**Part IV**

**Special Applications and the Future of Pharmacoepidemiology**

# 23

# Special Applications of Pharmacoepidemiology

David Lee[1], Björn Wettermark[2], Christine Y. Lu[3], Stephen B. Soumerai[3], Robert T. Chen[4], Sharon-Lise T. Normand[5], Art Sedrakyan[6], Danica Marinac-Dabic[7], Daniel B. Horton[8], Sonia Hernandez-Diaz[9], Tamar Lasky[7], Krista F. Huybrechts[10], Claudia Manzo[7], Emil Cochino[11], Hanna M. Seidling[12], David W. Bates[10], Bennett Levitan[13], Rachael L. DiSantostefano[13], and Scott Evans[14]

[1] (Retired) Center for Pharmaceutical Management, Management Sciences for Health, Arlington, VA, USA
[2] Disciplinary Domain of Medicine and Pharmacy, Uppsala University, Uppsala, Sweden
[3] Harvard Medical School and Harvard Pilgrim Health Care Institute, Boston, MA, USA
[4] Brighton Collaboration, Task Force for Global Health, Decatur, GA, USA
[5] Harvard Medical School and Harvard School of Public Health, Boston, MA, USA
[6] New York Presbyterian Hospital and Weill Cornell Medical College, New York, NY, USA
[7] US Food and Drug Administration, Silver Spring, MD, USA
[8] Rutgers Robert Wood Johnson Medical School, Rutgers Center for Pharmacoepidemiology and Treatment Science, Rutgers School of Public Health, New Brunswick, NJ, USA
[9] Harvard T.H. Chan School of Public Health, Boston, MA, USA
[10] Brigham and Women's Hospital, Harvard Medical School, Boston, MA, USA
[11] European Medicines Agency, Amsterdam, The Netherlands
[12] Cooperation Unit Clinical Pharmacy, University of Heidelberg, Heidelberg, Germany
[13] Department of Epidemiology, Janssen Research & Development, Titusville, NJ, USA
[14] Biostatistics Center, The George Washington University, Rockville, MD, USA
Note: The views expressed in this section are those of the authors, and not necessarily those of the US Food and Drug Administration or the European Medicines Agency.

In this chapter, we will present selected special applications of pharamcoepidemiology, which include studies of drug utilization; evaluating and improving prescribing; special methodological issues in pharmacoepidemiologic studies of vaccine safety; epidemiologic studies of implantable medical devices; research on the effects of medications in pregnancy and in children; risk management; the pharmacoepidemiology of medication errors; and benefit–risk assessments of medical treatments. We present this information using a standard format, focusing on clinical and methodological problems, examples of solutions, and perspectives on the future. Each application section then ends with a case example and key points.

## Studies of Drug Utilization

### Introduction

Drug utilization was defined by the World Health Organization (WHO) as the "marketing, distribution, prescription and use of drugs in a society, with special emphasis on the resulting medical, social, and economic consequences." Studies of drug utilization address not only the medical and nonmedical aspects influencing prescribing, dispensing, administration, and taking of medication, but also the effects of drug utilization at all levels of the health care system.

Drug utilization research (DUR), in the more recent European literature, refers to an "eclectic collection of descriptive and analytical methods for quantifying, understanding, and evaluating the processes of prescribing, dispensing, and consumption of medicines and for testing interventions to enhance the quality of these processes." This new definition was introduced to illustrate that DUR may include both qualitative and quantitative studies and emphasize the importance of intervention studies to promote quality use of medicines. In North America, DUR usually refers to drug utilization review (discussed in a separate section). In drug utilization studies, the objective is to quantify the present state, developmental trends, and time course of drug usage at various levels of the health care system, whether national, regional, local, or institutional. Routinely compiled *drug statistics* or drug utilization data that result from such studies can be used to estimate drug utilization in populations by age, sex, social class, morbidity, and other characteristics, and to identify areas of possible over- or underutilization. They also can be used as denominator data for calculating rates of reported adverse drug reactions (see Chapter 7); to monitor the utilization of specific therapeutic categories where particular problems can be anticipated (e.g. narcotic analgesics, hypnotics and sedatives, and other psychotropic drugs); to monitor the effects of informational and regulatory activities (e.g. adverse events alerts, delisting of drugs from therapeutic formularies); as markers for very crude estimates of disease prevalence (e.g. anti-Parkinsonian drugs for Parkinson's disease); to plan for drug importation, production, and distribution; and to estimate drug expenditures. Such studies can

either be descriptive or analytical assessing factors influencing drug utilization. Some drug utilization studies may also be qualitative to gain a deeper understanding of drug prescribing, dispensing, or consumption of medicines.

*Drug utilization review studies* assess the appropriateness of drug utilization, usually by linking prescription data to the reasons for drug prescribing. Explicit predetermined criteria are created, which aspects of the quality, medical necessity, and appropriateness of drug prescribing may be compared. Drug use criteria may be based upon such parameters as indications for use, daily dose, and length of therapy, or others such as: failure to select a more effective or less hazardous drug if available, use of a fixed combination drug when only one of its components is justified, or use of a costly drug when a less costly equivalent drug is available. In North America, these studies are also known as *drug use evaluation (DUE) studies*. For example, a large number of studies have documented the extent of inappropriate prescribing of drugs, particularly antibiotics, and the associated adverse clinical, ecological, and economic consequences. Other studies have been conducted in the elderly (e.g. using Beers criteria for Potentially Inappropriate Medication Use in Older Adults).

*Quantitative DUR and DUE studies*, aimed at detecting and quantifying problems, combined with methods to understand their underlying factors, are usually one-time projects (rather than routinely conducted), provide for only minimal, if any, feedback to the involved prescribers and, most importantly, do not include any follow-up measures to ascertain whether any changes in drug therapy have occurred (see Table 23.1). A DUR or DUE *program*, on the other hand, is an intervention in the form of an authorized, structured, and ongoing system for improving the quality of drug use within a given health care institution (see Table 23.1). DUR studies may then be used

**Table 23.1** Drug utilization studies in perspective: operational concepts.

|  | Drug statistics | Drug utilization study | Drug utilization review program |
|---|---|---|---|
| Synonyms (therapeutic) | Drug utilization data | Drug utilization review or drug utilization review study | Drug audit |
| Descriptive quantitative methods | Yes | Yes | Usually |
| Analytic quantitative methods | No | Yes | Maybe |
| Qualitative methods | No | Maybe | No |
| Continuous (ongoing) | Usually | No | Yes |

after the implementation of the program to assess its effectiveness.

*Qualitative drug utilization studies* apply qualitative methods. Such studies originate from social science and gather information that may not be compiled in numerical form. These studies include focus-group discussions, open-ended questionnaires, in-depth interviews, and observations. They are valuable to explore the perceptions of prescribers, pharmacists, and patients dealing with medicines in gaining a deeper understanding of social phenomena in drug utilization.

## Clinical Problems to be Addressed by Pharmacoepidemiologic Research

For a drug to be approved for market, it must be shown that it can effectively modify the natural course of disease or alleviate symptoms when used appropriately– that is, for the right patient, with the right disease, in the proper dosage and intervals, and for the appropriate length of time. Used inappropriately, drugs often fail to live up to their potential, with the potential for consequent morbidity and mortality. Even when used appropriately, all drugs have the potential to cause harm. However, many of their adverse effects are predictable and preventable.

Adverse drug reactions and nonadherence to therapy are important causes of preventable adult and pediatric hospital admissions. The situations that may lead to preventable adverse drug reactions and drug-induced illness include the use of a drug for the wrong indication; the use of a potentially toxic drug when one with less toxicity risk would be as effective; the concurrent administration of an excessive number of drugs, thereby increasing the possibility of adverse drug interactions; the use of excessive doses, especially for pediatric or geriatric patients; and continued use of a drug after evidence becomes available concerning important toxic effects. Many contributory causes have been proposed: excessive prescribing, failure to define therapeutic endpoints, the increased availability of potent prescription and non-prescription drugs, increased public exposure to information and marketing about drugs, the availability of illicit preparations, and prescribers' lack of knowledge of the pharmacology of the prescribed drugs. Medication error (discussed in the "Medication Errors" section of this chapter), poor patient adherence (see Chapter 21), discontinuation of therapy, and problems in communication resulting from modern day fragmentation of patient care also may contribute to increased morbidity and mortality.

Therapeutic practice, as recommended by relevant professional bodies, academic researchers, and opinion leaders is initially based largely on data from premarketing clinical trials. Complementary data from clinical experience and studies in the post-marketing period may result in changes in therapeutic indication (e.g. an antibiotic becoming no longer a choice because of antimicrobial resistance), treatment duration (e.g. short-course antibiotic treatment of community-acquired pneumonia in children under five years old), regimen (e.g. changes due to tolerance to oral hypoglycemic agents), and precautions and contraindications (e.g. gastrointestinal bleeding with nonsteroidal anti-inflammatory agents) among others. As therapy recommendations are updated through guidelines and other approaches, drug utilization studies must address the relationship between therapeutic practice as recommended and actual clinical practice.

## Methodological Problems to be Addressed by Pharmacoepidemiologic Research

DUR may be quantitative or qualitative. Quantitative studies aim to establish quantities, presented in numeric figures in categories or rank order and measured in various units. These studies collect data to determine associations between variables and differences between categories, using different statistical methods. On the other hand, qualitative studies attempt to examine, analyze, and interpret observations for the purpose of discovering underlying meanings and patterns of relationships. Drug use data may be obtained from several sources, and their usefulness depends on the purpose of the study at hand. All have certain limitations in their direct clinical relevance. For quantitative studies, the ideal is a count of the number of patients in a defined population who ingest a drug of interest during a particular time frame. The drug utilization data available are only approximations of this, and raise many questions about their presentation and interpretation. For studying the quality of medicine use, one ideal is a count of the

number of patients in a defined population who use a drug inappropriately during a particular time frame among all those who received the drug in that population during that time frame. There has been a large growth in databases in all countries, but available drug exposure and diagnosis data are still suboptimal in most settings. Also, the criteria to be used to define "appropriate" are often arbitrary.

Since most drug consumption statistics were compiled for administrative or commercial reasons, the data are usually expressed in terms of cost or volume. Data on drug utilization can be available in several different quantities: One is *total costs or unit cost*, such as cost per package, tablet, dose, or treatment course. Although such data may be useful for measuring and comparing the economic impact of drug use, these units do not provide information on the amount of drug exposure in the population. Moreover, cost data are influenced by price fluctuations over time, distribution channels, inflation, exchange rate fluctuations, price control measures, etc. Official data on drug expenditures in hospitals may also be false if there are separate rebates and risk-sharing arrangements between payers and pharmaceutical companies.

Another quantity, *volume data*, are available from manufacturers, importers, or distributors, as the overall weight of the drug sold or the unit volume sold (e.g. the number of tablets, capsules, or doses sold). This is closer to the number of patients exposed. However, tablet sizes vary, making it difficult to translate weight into the number of tablets. Prescription sizes also vary, so it is difficult to translate number of tablets into the number of exposed patients.

The *number of prescriptions* is the measure most frequently used in drug utilization studies. However, different patients receive a different number of prescriptions in any given time interval and there may be large differences between countries in prescription regulations and reimbursement. To translate the number of prescriptions into the number of patients, one must divide by the average number of prescriptions per patient, or else distinctions must be made between first prescriptions and refill prescriptions. The latter is, of course, better for studies of new drug therapy, but will omit individuals who are receiving chronic drug therapy. Additional problems may be created by differences in the number of drugs in each prescription. Finally, it should be noted that all these units represent approximate estimates of true consumption. The latter is ultimately modified by the patients' actual drug intake (see degree of adherence, Chapter 21).

From a quality of care perspective, to interpret drug utilization data appropriately, it is necessary to relate the data to the reasons for the drug usage. Data on morbidity and mortality may be obtained from national registries (general or specialized); national samples where medical service reimbursement schemes operate; ad hoc surveys and special studies; hospital records, physician records; and patient or household surveys. Appropriateness of use must be assessed relative to indication for treatment, patient characteristics (age-related physiological status, sex, habits), drug dosage (over- or under-dosage), concomitant diseases (that might contraindicate or interfere with chosen therapy), and the use of other drugs (interactions). However, no single source is generally available for obtaining all this information. Moreover, because of incompleteness, the medical record may not be a very useful source of drug use data.

## Examples of Currently Available Solutions

### Current Data Sources

Drug utilization studies have been conducted using a large variety of data sources, including sales registries, procurement records, reimbursement/claims databases, medical records, pharmacy dispensing records, pharmacy stock records, disease-based registries, and population health surveys. The availability of such data varies substantially between countries, but there has been a large growth in access to them over time everywhere.

Aggregated sales data have been used in drug utilization research (DUR) for decades. Today, most countries in Europe keep some records of drug sales, at a regional or national level. These data can be obtained from health authorities as well as from private companies such as IQVIA, a well-known commercial source of drug utilization data. The Pharmacoepidemiological Research on Outcomes of Therapeutics by a European ConsorTium (PROTECT) indicates that aggregate sales data are widely collected across Europe. In the US, the IQVIA National Sales Perspective database documents sales data for prescription drugs, over-the-counter (OTC) products, and some self-administered diagnostic products. Data collected include volume of dollars and quantities moving from manufacturers in various outlets within all states. In Canada, the IQVIA CompuScript database contains data on prescriptions sold from about two-thirds of Canadian retail pharmacies. Sales data collected by authorities or by companies such as IQVIA may be the only secondary source available in studies conducted in regions where other databases are not yet established or more accessible. This is the case in most low- and middle-income countries, but it is important to acknowledge that large scale databases are created also in many of these countries.

Individual-level dispensing databases are increasingly available. These administrative claims databases may be kept by pharmacy chains, health authorities or reimbursement agencies. An example of such a dispensing database is the Swedish Prescribed Drug Register, which contains data with unique patient identifiers for the entire population of 10 million inhabitants for all dispensed prescriptions in ambulatory care. This registry includes data on the patient (age, sex, personal identification number, place of residence), dispensed drug (Anatomic Therapeutic Chemical [ATC] classification code, defined daily dose

[DDD] number, prescribed dose, package, reimbursement, date of prescribing and dispensing), prescriber (profession, specialty, workplace), and pharmacy (identifier, location). It can often be linked to many other registers, including clinical quality registers with diagnoses and outcome data as well as socio-economic data on migration, family situation, income, education, and country of birth.

Large databases are also derived from electronic health records. For example, the General Practice Research Database (GPRD) in the United Kingdom is based on medical records from general practitioners (GPs). Hundreds of GPs contribute anonymized patient information to a central database that now contains millions of patients. Included are prescriptions issued by the GP but with no information from the pharmacy to permit assessment of adherence. Although primarily used for studying drug safety, such databases have also been used to study drug utilization.

Although the use of health insurance databases has also been reported in countries outside North America, Europe and East Asia, medical and pharmaceutical databases are generally not available in most low- and middle-income countries. The International Network for Rational Use of Drugs (INRUD) and WHO have developed approaches that use standardized criteria/indicators to measure changes in medicines prescribing, dispensing, and patient care, which has facilitated the study of drug utilization in low- and middle-income countries, including adherence to chronic therapy. The approaches include recommendations on core and complementary indicators, minimum sample sizes, sampling methods, and data collection techniques, depending on study objectives.

**Units of Measurement**

The DDD methodology was developed in response to the need to convert and standardize readily available volume data from sales statistics or pharmacy inventory data to medically meaningful units and to make crude estimates of the number of persons exposed to a particular medicine or class of medicines. The DDD is the assumed average daily maintenance dose for a drug for its main indication in adults. Expressed as DDDs per 1000 inhabitants per day (DDD/TID), for chronically used drugs, it can be interpreted as the proportion of the population that may receive treatment with a particular medicine on any given day. For use in hospital settings, the unit is expressed as DDDs per 100 bed-days (adjusted for occupancy rate); it suggests the proportion of inpatients that may receive a DDD. For medicines that are used for short-term periods, such as antimicrobials, the unit is expressed as DDDs per inhabitant per year; this provides an estimate of the number of days for which each person is treated with a particular medication in a year.

The DDD methodology is useful for working with readily available gross drug statistics and is relatively easy and inexpensive to use. However, the DDD methodology should be used and interpreted with caution. The DDD is not a recommended or a prescribed dose, but a technical unit of comparison; it is usually the result of literature review and available information on use in various countries. Thus, DDDs may be high or low relative to actual prescribed doses. For example, children's doses are substantially lower than the established DDDs. If unadjusted, this situation will lead to an underestimation of population exposures, which may be significant in countries with a large pediatric population. Pediatric DDDs have also been proposed, but the concept and its application have not yet been incorporated into the WHO methodology. Finally, DDDs do not take into account variations in adherence.

The prescribed daily dose (PDD) is another unit, developed as a means to validate the DDDs. The PDD is the average daily dose prescribed, as obtained from a representative sample of prescriptions. Problems may arise in calculating the PDD due to a lack of clear and exact dosage indication in the prescription and dosage alteration via verbal instructions between prescribing events. For certain groups of drugs, such as the oral anti-diabetes medicines, the mean PDD may be lower than the corresponding DDDs. Up to twofold variations in the mean PDD have been documented in international comparisons. Although the DDD and the PDD may be used to estimate population drug exposure "therapeutic intensity," the methodology is not useful to estimate incidence and prevalence of drug use or to quantify or identify patients who receive doses lower or higher than those considered effective and safe.

The Infectious Diseases Society of America and the Society for Healthcare Epidemiology of America (IDSA/SHEA) have recommended days of therapy (DOT) for expressing antimicrobial drug use. DOT is the number of days when at least one dose of a medication was administered irrespective of dose or route of administration. They are not affected by dose adjustments and can be used in both adult and pediatric populations. Similar to PDDs, expressing drug use in the number of DOTs requires patient level use data, which may not be feasible at every facility.

## Classification Systems

Classification systems are used to categorize drugs into standardized groups. For example, the ATC classification system is generally used in conjunction with the DDD methodology. The ATC system consists of five hierarchical levels: a main anatomical group, two therapeutic subgroups, a chemical–therapeutic subgroup, and a chemical substance subgroup. Medicinal products are classified according to the main therapeutic indication for the principal active ingredient. Use of the ATC classification system is recommended for reporting drug consumption statistics and conducting comparative DUR. The WHO International Drug Monitoring Program uses the system for drug coding in adverse drug reaction monitoring, and some developing countries have begun to use the ATC system to classify their essential drugs, which may

eventually lead to preparation of drug utilization statistics.

The US uses the Iowa Drug Information System (IDIS), which is a hierarchical drug coding system based on the three therapeutic categories of the American Hospital Formulary Society (AHFS), to which a fourth level was added to code individual drug ingredients. Other coding systems, such as the National Drug Code and the Veterans' Administration Classification, do not provide unique codes for drug ingredients.

In the United Kingdom, British National Formulary (BNF) codes are widely used for drug utilization studies. The BNF provides monographs for drugs available in the UK. The numbering system is produced by NHS Prescription Services, part of the NHS Business Services Authority in England.

The International Classification of Diseases is a system of diagnostic codes for classifying diseases and other health problems. The ICD is published by the WHO and used worldwide in morbidity and mortality statistics, drug reimbursement systems, and automated decision support in healthcare. The system includes categories relating to medicinal substances, but in the context of adverse outcomes, and often in quite broad terms. It does not include codes suitable for recording and classifying drug utilization.

The Systematized Nomenclature of Medicine (SNOMED) provides a core general terminology for use in various medical fields. SNOMED clinical terms (CT) contain more than 311 000 active concepts in clinical settings, organized in different hierarchies. An individual number represents each concept, and several concepts can be used in combination to describe a complex situation. Clinical finding/disorder and procedure/ intervention are examples of the main levels in SNOMED CT. Substance and pharmaceutical/ biologic product hierarchy was also introduced as a top-level hierarchy in order to distinguish drug products from their chemical constituents (substances). It contains multiple levels of granularity, used to support a variety of purposes, including electronic prescribing and formulary management (See www.ihtsdo.org).

## The Future

DUR has expanded in all countries across the globe, ranging from early descriptive studies to advanced studies combining different data sources to further understand medicine use in the population. Addressing the medical, social, and economic aspects of drug utilization remains relevant for future research. However, the types of drugs in focus will differ, with 42% of the substances in drug development being biologics, compared to 8% on the market currently. The growing pressures on all healthcare systems with aging populations, rising patient expectations, stricter clinical targets, and expensive new medicines will further increase the need for drug utilization studies to monitor that resources are used wisely and that new medicines are prescribed to those who may benefit most from them.

From a public health perspective, the observed differences in national and international patterns of drug utilization require much further study. The medical consequences and the explanations for such differences are still not well documented. Analysis of medicine use by gender and age group may suggest important associations. The increasing availability of population-based data resources will facilitate studies of incidence and prevalence of medicine use by age and gender.

Numerous studies have addressed factors influencing drug prescribing. However, the relative importance of the many determinants of appropriate prescribing still remains to be adequately elucidated. Many strategies aimed at modifying prescribing behavior have been proposed and adopted. Current evidence indicates that mailed educational materials alone are not sufficient to modify prescribing behavior. For interventions shown to be effective in improving drug prescribing, there is a need to further define their relative efficacy and proper role in a comprehensive strategy for optimizing drug utilization. Questions yet to be addressed through proper methods deal with the role of printed drug information such as drug bulletins; the duration of effect of educational interventions such as group discussions, lectures, and seminars, each in the outpatient and inpatient settings; and the generalizability of face-to-face methods. We also need more research on whether the benefits and savings achieved with intervention strategies outweighed the costs of performing the intervention.

More clinically applicable approaches to drug utilization review programs, such as the computerized screening of patient-specific drug histories in outpatient care to prevent drug-induced hospitalizations, still require further development and assessment. Patient outcome measures and process measures of quality of drug utilization have to be included in such studies.

The availability of large computerized databases that allow the linkage of drug utilization data to diagnoses is contributing to expand this field of study. The WHO/INRUD indicator-based approach to drug utilization studies facilitates the conduct of DUR in low- and middle-income countries. Drug utilization review programs, particularly approaches that take into primary consideration patient outcome measures, merit further rigorous study and improvement. Opportunities for the study of drug utilization are still underexplored, but the political issue regarding the confidentiality of medical records and limitations in funds and manpower will determine the pace of growth of DUR.

## Key Points for Studies of Drug Utilization

- Drug utilization studies can be performed to quantify, identify problems in drug utilization, monitor changes in utilization patterns, understand their determinants, or evaluate the impact of interventions.
- Drug utilization studies may be conducted on an on-going basis in programs for improving the quality use of medicines.

---

**Case Example 23.1    Prevalence of Potentially Suboptimal Medication Use in Older Men and Association with Adverse Outcomes**

*Background*

Medication-related symptoms often underlie presentations to primary care services and emergency departments and are a common cause of hospital admission, morbidity and mortality. Among frail older people, falls and confusion (geriatric syndromes) and hip fractures may be medicine-use related. Adverse drug reactions and polypharmacy are also common in the elderly.

*Question*

How prevalent is suboptimal use of medicines in men over 65 years old and is this associated with adverse outcomes?

*Approach*

- Prospective cohort study of community-dwelling older men.
- Use of a comprehensive population-based data linkage system, combined with self-reported retrospective data from a health-in-men survey that included biochemical and hormone analysis of blood samples.
- Adverse outcomes included self-reported or documented history of falls and database-recorded hospital admissions due to geriatric syndromes, cardiovascular events, and death.
- Markers of suboptimal medication use were defined for potential over-utilization, potential under-utilization, and potentially inappropriate medicines use.

*Results*

- Use of potentially inappropriate medicines (48.7%), polypharmacy ($\geqslant 5$ medications, 35.8%), and potential under-utilization (56.7%) were highly prevalent, and overall 8.3% of participants reported some form of potentially suboptimal medication use.
- Polypharmacy was associated with all cause admission to hospital, cardiovascular events, and all cause mortality over 4.5 years of follow-up.
- Potential medication under-utilization was associated with subsequent cardiovascular events.

- Reported use of one or more potentially inappropriate medicines was associated with greater hazard of admission to hospital.
- Hospital admissions for falls were not associated with any of the markers of suboptimal prescribing.

*Strengths*

- Community-based sampling of study population.
- Large sample size.
- Reliable data on selected morbidity and mortality endpoints captured through comprehensive data linkage system.

*Limitations*

- Study was based on volunteers, recruited from randomly selected subjects of a previous population-based study.
- Potential underestimation of adverse events; e.g. falls that do not result in hospitalization were not captured in the comprehensive database, and may not be recalled in self-reports.
- Accuracy of self-reported medication histories was not validated.
- Unavailability of medication dosage data limits determining inappropriateness due to excessive dosing.
- Potential underutilization focused only on certain cardiovascular conditions and treatments.
- Medication use variables did not account for all valid medication indications/contraindications.

*Key points*

- Additional data collection approaches may be combined with use of comprehensive data linkage systems.
- Study results suggest that both medication overuse and underuse occur frequently in older men and may be associated with significant adverse clinical outcomes.
- Reducing under-utilization is just as important as reducing over-utilization and inappropriate medication use.

- Assessing appropriateness of drug utilization requires data on indication for treatment, patient characteristics, drug regimen, concomitant diseases, and concurrent use of other medications. Even then, the criteria to be used to define "appropriate" are arbitrary.
- When assessing quality of care, drug utilization studies must often rely on multiple sources of data.

## Evaluating and Improving Prescribing

One of the most important, but perhaps underappreciated, goals of pharmacoepidemiology is to foster ways to improve evidence-based prescribing. It is clear, however, that there is a significant disconnect between the available evidence for treatment ("what we know") and everyday clinical practice ("what we do"). This so-called *care-gap* in prescribing needs to be urgently addressed. If physicians and other health practitioners fail to update their knowledge and practice in response to new and clinically important evidence on the outcomes of specific prescribing patterns, then the "fruits" of pharmacoepidemiologic research may have little impact on clinical practice. Thus, the science of assessing and improving clinical practices has grown rapidly in importance. The rapid growth of this new field (sometimes referred to as translation research) is based on the recognition that passive knowledge dissemination (e.g. publishing articles, distributing practice guidelines) is generally insufficient to improve clinical practices without supplemental behavioral change interventions based on relevant theories of diffusion of innovations, persuasive communications, adult learning theory or social cognitive theory.

### Clinical Problems to be Addressed by Pharmacoepidemiologic Research

Issues related to underuse, overuse, and misuse of medications all contribute to the suboptimal utilization of pharmaceutical therapies.

Some of the factors responsible for suboptimal prescribing include the failure of clinicians to keep abreast of important new findings on the risks and benefits of medications; excessive promotion of some drugs through pharmaceutical company advertising, sales representatives, or other marketing strategies; simple errors of omission; patient and family demand for a particular agent, even when it is not scientifically substantiated; and clinical inertia. These diverse influences suggest the need for tailoring intervention strategies to the key factors influencing a given behavior based on models of behavioral change and knowledge translation. Poor adherence to medications is another important factor contributing to the care-gap (discussed in see Chapter 21).

### Methodological Problems to be Addressed by Pharmacoepidemiologic Research

#### Internal Validity

Poorly controlled studies (e.g. one-group post-only or pre– post designs without a control group) produce misleading (and usually exaggerated) estimates of the effects of a variety of medication prescribing interventions. Many nonintervention factors can affect medication use over time. Indeed, the "success" of many uncontrolled studies is often due to the attribution of preexisting trends in practice patterns rather than to the studied intervention. Because randomized controlled trials (RCTs) are sometimes not feasible (e.g. because of contamination of controls within a single institution) or ethical (e.g. unacceptability of withholding quality assurance programs from controls), other quasi-experimental designs (e.g. interrupted time-series with or without comparison series, pre–post with concurrent comparison group studies) should be used instead of weak one-group post-only or pre–post designs that do not generally permit valid causal inferences.

#### Regression Toward the Mean

The tendency for observations on populations selected on the basis of exceeding a predetermined threshold level to approach the mean on subsequent observations is a common and insidious problem. This argues once again for the need to conduct RCTs and well-controlled quasi-experimental studies to establish the effectiveness of interventions *before* they become a routine part of quality improvement programs.

## Unit of Analysis

A common methodological problem in studies of physician behavior is the incorrect use of the patient as the unit of analysis. This violates basic statistical assumptions of independence because prescribing behaviors and outcomes for individual patients are likely to be correlated within each physician's practice. Such hierarchical "nesting" or statistical "clustering" often leads to accurate point estimates of effect but inappropriately low p-values and narrow confidence intervals compared with the correct unit of analysis, such as the physician or practice or facility. Consequently, interventions may appear to lead to "statistically significant" improvements in prescribing practices because of mistakenly inflated sample sizes. Fortunately, methods for analyzing clustered data are available that can simultaneously control for clustering of observations at the patient, physician, and facility levels.

## Ethical and Legal Problems Hindering the Implementation of Randomized Clinical Trials

It has been argued that there are ethical and legal problems related to "withholding" interventions designed to improve prescribing. This explicitly assumes that the proposed interventions will be beneficial. In fact, the effectiveness of many interventions is the very question that should be under investigation. Others have argued that mandating interventions without adequate proof of benefit and lack of unintended consequences is unethical. What is important is to demonstrate that such interventions are safe, efficacious, and cost-effective *before* widespread adoption.

## Detecting Effects on Patient Outcomes

Few large well-controlled studies have linked changes in prescribing to improved patient outcomes (e.g. a link between improvements in processes of care and patient outcomes such as adverse clinical events). Sample sizes may need to be enormous to detect even modest changes in patient outcomes. However, process outcomes (e.g. use of recommended medications for acute myocardial infarction from evidence-based practice guidelines) are often sensitive, clinically reasonable, and appropriate measures of the quality of care, and improvements in processes of care may be important in and of themselves, and some are associated with better clinical outcomes.

## Examples of Currently Available Solutions

### Conceptual Framework

A useful starting point for designing an intervention to improve prescribing is to develop a framework for organizing the clinical and non-clinical factors that could help or impede desired changes in clinical behaviors. The "Theory of Planned Behavior" or "PRECEDE" (Predisposing, Reinforcing, and Enabling Constructs in Educational Diagnosis and Evaluation) is an example of such a framework. This model – PRECEDE – was developed for adult health education programs, and proposes factors influencing three sequential stages of behavior change: predisposing, enabling, and reinforcing factors. *Predisposing* variables include such factors as awareness of a guideline, knowledge of the underlying evidence, or beliefs in the efficacy of treatment. However, while a mailed drug bulletin or e-mail alert may predispose some physicians to new information (if they read it), behavior change may be impossible without new *enabling* skills (e.g. skills in administering a new therapy, or overcoming patient or family demand for unsubstantiated treatments). Once a new pattern of behavior is tried, multiple and positive *reinforcements* (e.g. through peers, reminders, and feedback) may be necessary to fully establish the new behavior. Such a framework explains a common observation: namely, that multifaceted interventions that encompass all stages of behavior change are more likely to improve physician prescribing than are uni-dimensional interventions that only predispose, enable, or reinforce.

### Empirical Evidence on the Effectiveness of Interventions to Improve Prescribing

There are numerous research syntheses that have evaluated the effectiveness of the most commonly studied interventions, including: educational interventions; monitoring and feedback; multimedia campaigns; and formulary interventions and financial incentives; and so on.

Distributing printed educational materials aimed at improving prescribing practice remains the most ubiquitous form of prescribing education. Unfortunately, use of disseminated educational materials *alone* may affect some predisposing variables (e.g. knowledge or attitudes), but have minimal effect on actual prescribing practice.

Academic detailing involving face-to-face visits by pharmacists, physician counselors or peer-leaders have been shown to be effective in promoting evidence-based practice and improving patient outcomes. Reinforcement is needed to sustain improvement. What sets academic detailing apart from industry detailing is that the messengers and the messages of the former are presumably independent, objective, and evidence-based.

Group education methods such as small group discussions conducted by clinical leaders have been shown to improve prescribing. Traditional large-group, didactic continuing medical education seminars have not been as successful, by themselves, in improving physician practice.

Identifying local opinion leaders is another approach to help in the adoption of new pharmacological agents. In addition to opinion-leader involvement, this approach includes brief orientation to research findings, printed educational materials, and encouragement to implement guidelines during informal "teachable moments." However, opinion leader studies have shown mixed results and their cost-effectiveness remains to be determined.

Another popular approach to improving physician performance is providing physicians with clinical feedback regarding their prescribing practices, either in the form of comparative practice patterns with peers or predetermined standards such as practice guidelines. Most types of feedback have a clinically minimal effect on prescribing and are unlikely to offset the costs of the programs themselves.

Drug utilization review programs attempt to review the appropriateness of medication prescribing for individual patients (e.g. drug interactions and dosage). Results from controlled trials do not support the effectiveness of this approach.

Computerized reminders can enable physicians to reduce errors of omission by issuing alerts to perform specific actions in response to patient-level information such as laboratory findings or diagnoses. However, excessive reminders may create "reminder-fatigue." Computerized decision support systems (CDSS) integrated with electronic health records, a major component of health information technology, succeed beyond a "secretarial reminder" function. They can support physicians' prescribing decisions in more complex areas such as dosage, schedule, suboptimal choices, and prevention of adverse drug events. CDSS might moderately improve process of care such as rates of lab monitoring and prescribing decisions, and they may help reduce the length of hospital stay compared with routine care while comparable or better cost-effectiveness is achieved, but there is no evidence that CDSS have fulfilled their promised effect on healthcare costs, mortality or other clinical adverse events. (See Case Example 23.2.)

Studies have shown that a broader warning campaign involving the medical and popular

---

**Case Example 23.2    For Evaluating and Improving Physician Prescribing**

*Background*

Because many experts have assumed that computerized decision support will be the magic bullet that improves physician prescribing, vast resources are being committed to widespread implementation before rigorous evaluation.

*Question*

Can computerized decision support improve quality of ambulatory care for chronic conditions such as ischemic heart disease or asthma?

*Approach*

- Cluster randomized controlled trial of 60 primary care practices in the United Kingdom; 30 practices randomized to heart disease and 30 to asthma, with each practice acting as a control for the non-assigned condition. Practices already had computerized health records and many had electronic prescribing.
- Compared about 40 measures of guideline adherence (prescribing, testing, patient reported outcomes) between intervention and control practices one year after implementation of decision support.

*Results*

- No effect of computerized decision support on any measure of guideline adherence for either heart disease or asthma.
- Hypothesized reason for lack of effect was extremely low levels of use of, and dissatisfaction with, the decision support tools by physicians.

*Strengths*

- Cluster randomized trial design eliminated selection and volunteer bias, while controlling for any secular improvements in quality of care.
- Overcomes almost all of the flaws in design and analysis of previous studies of computerized decision support.
- Conducted in a "real world" setting rather than with house-staff or within academic practices or in the hospital setting.

*Limitations*

- Newer technologies or better delivery systems may be more acceptable to primary care physicians.
- Inadequate attention may have been paid to the nontechnological factors that influence the acceptability and use of an intervention (e.g. lack of up-front buy in from end-users, lack of incentives for using the system, lack of participation in the actual guideline development process).

*Key points*

- Just as with any drug or device, interventions to improve prescribing should be tested in controlled studies before widespread adoption.
- Results of interventions (including decision support) conducted at specialized academic centers or in the hospital setting may not necessarily be applicable to the "real world" of busy primary care practice.

---

press, internet, newspapers, television, and radio may be effective in changing prescribing patterns in large populations. However, because information may be oversimplified and distorted when communicated in the media, this type of intervention should probably be used when the adverse effects of marketed drugs are severe and preventable, alternative agents exist, and the messages are simple enough to convey in mass communications.

Finally, in response to escalating health care spending, formulary interventions (such as preferred drug lists) and financial incentives (e.g. pay for performance) have been used to change the way that physicians practice medicine. Numerous quasi-experimental studies suggest such interventions are associated with little cost-savings or improvements in quality of care but may have unintended consequences (e.g. treatment discontinuity).

## The Future

In general, the achievement of long-term changes in practice depends on inclusion of multiple strategies that predispose, enable, and reinforce desired behaviors. The following characteristics recur in successful interventions:

- Use of theoretical or conceptual frameworks to help identify key factors that influence prescribing decisions, informed by surveys, focus groups, or interviews.
- Targeting physicians in need of education (e.g. review of prescribing data).
- Recruitment and participation of local opinion leaders.
- Use of credible and objective messengers and materials.
- Face-to-face interaction, especially in primary care settings.
- Repetition and reinforcement of a limited number of messages at one time.
- Provision of acceptable alternatives to the practices that are to be extinguished.
- Use of multiple evidence-based strategies to address multiple barriers to best practice.
- Emphasis on the goal of improvement in the quality of prescribing and patient safety, not just cost minimization in the guise of quality improvement.

Although we know that prescribing problems exist, we still know surprisingly little about their prevalence or determinants. This paucity of data is all the more remarkable considering that three-quarters of all physician visits end in the prescription of a drug. Future research efforts need to describe in greater detail the nature, prevalence, rate of prescribing, and severity of prescribing problems associated with the overuse, misuse, and underuse of medications (as discussed in the previous section on "Drug utilization" in this chapter). Finally, studies examining the economic outcomes of interventions as well as studies that include patient reported outcomes would advance the field.

There is also a tremendous need for carefully controlled research of interventions to improve prescribing, and how best to combine various strategies to allow for rapid and effective implementation of prescribing guidelines. New models are needed to predict the most effective types of intervention for specific problem types and various broader questions still need to be answered, including issues related to opportunity costs and cost-effectiveness.

Important effects of medications on many health outcomes have been demonstrated in clinical trials; therefore, it is reasonable to hypothesize that more appropriate use of some medications could reduce morbidity and mortality, increase patient functioning, and improve quality-of-life. Whether improved prescribing is a surrogate measure, or an outcome that directly leads to improved health outcomes, it remains a critically important area for future study.

## Key Points for Evaluating and Improving Prescribing

- Quality problems in prescribing exist at the level of medication overuse (e.g. antibiotics for viral respiratory tract infections), misuse (e.g. nonsteroidal anti-inflammatory drugs without gastric protection for patients at very high risk of upper gastrointestinal bleeding), and underuse (e.g. bisphosphonates in the secondary prevention of osteoporosis-related fractures or inhaled corticosteroids for reactive airways disease).
- Passive interventions, such as dissemination of printed or emailed guidelines, drug utilization reviews, or traditional continuing medical education lectures, are unlikely to improve practice.
- More active interventions (e.g. one-to-one education, point-of-care reminders, achievable

benchmarks with audit and feedback), especially when combined together to overcome barriers at the level of the system, the physician, and the patient, are able to modestly improve the quality of prescribing.

- Interventions (e.g. financial incentives) may have unintended consequences that need to be investigated.
- For most interventions that aim to change prescribing, there is little evidence on their economic outcomes or patient-reported outcomes.
- Just as with the adoption of drugs and devices, interventions to improve physician prescribing need to be tested in rigorous controlled trials before widespread and expensive implementation. In particular, investigators should consider "mixed-method" evaluations (i.e. quantitative data, prescriber surveys, qualitative inquiry about barriers and facilitators to adoption) of their interventions to better understand what works or does not work -and why.

# Special Methodological Issues in Pharmacoepidemiologic Studies of Vaccine Safety

Vaccines are among the most cost-effective public health interventions available. However, no vaccine is perfectly safe or effective. Concerns over adverse events following immunizations (AEFIs) can result in vaccine hesitancy and destabilize immunization programs. As immunization programs "mature" with high vaccine coverage and near elimination of target vaccine-preventable diseases, there may be increased prominence of vaccine-induced and vaccine-coincidental AEFI's, particularly in the modern media.

## Clinical Problems to be Addressed by Pharmacoepidemiologic Research

The tolerance for AEFI's to vaccines given to healthy persons – especially healthy babies – is lower than for medical products administered to persons due to ill health. A higher standard of safety is required for vaccines because of the large number of persons who are exposed, some of whom are compelled to do so by law or regulation for public health reasons. These issues are the basis for strict regulatory control and other oversight of vaccines by the Food and Drug Administration (FDA) and the WHO. These concerns also often lead to investigation of much rarer adverse events following vaccinations than for pharmaceuticals. However, the cost and difficulty of studying AEFI's increase with their rarity, and it is difficult to provide definitive conclusions from epidemiologic studies of such rare events. Furthermore, high standards of accuracy and timeliness are needed because vaccine safety studies may have important impacts on vaccination policies.

Unlike many classes of drugs for which other effective therapy may be substituted, vaccines generally have few alternative choices, and the decision to withdraw a vaccine from the market may have wide ramifications. Establishing whether an AEFI is causally due to a vaccine or not, and if so, a prompt definition of the attributable risk are critical in placing AEFI's in the proper risk/benefit perspective. Vaccines are relatively universal exposures. Therefore, despite the relative rarity of serious true vaccine reactions, ~50 000 reports of AEFI's are received annually in the US (~8% are serious), few reports can be causally linked to vaccination. Recommendations for immunization requires a dynamic balancing of risks and benefits. As vaccine preventable diseases approach eradication, information on complications due to vaccination relative to that of the wild disease (that the vaccine prevents) may lead to a perception that the vaccine complications outweigh the benefits and therefore lead to a discontinuation or decreased use of the vaccine.

Research in vaccine safety can help to distinguish true vaccine reactions from coincidental events, estimate an attributable risk, facilitate vaccine injury compensation, identify risk factors that can inform the development of valid precautions and contraindications, and if the pathophysiologic mechanism becomes known, develop safer vaccines.

All of these issues have been highlighted during the COVID19 pandemic. An unprecedented number of new vaccines have been developed (many using technologies with limited or no prior use in humans) and approved for emergency use within ~300 days (vs. typical decade) of identification of the target SARS Coronavirus 2 pathogen. New adverse events of special interest [AESI; e.g., thrombosis with thrombycytopenia syndrome] have been identified after certain vaccines and are under study. In the meantime, challenging benefit-risk policy decisions for various subpopulations have had to be made as the entire global population likely needs to be immunized, possibly periodically. The heterogeneity in quality of pre- and post-introduction safety data available for each COVID19 vacine presents opportunities and challenges for pharmacovigilance, especially in low- and middle-income countries.

## Methodological Problems to be Addressed by Pharmacoepidemiologic Research

An Institute of Medicine (IOM) review of vaccine safety in 1991 found that the US knowledge and research capacity has been limited by: (i) inadequate understanding of biologic mechanisms underlying adverse events, (ii) insufficient or inconsistent information from case reports and case series, (iii) inadequate size or length of follow-up of many population-based epidemiologic studies, and (iv) limitations of existing surveillance systems to provide persuasive evidence of causation. These limitations were cited again in a more recent IOM review (2011), *Adverse Events of Vaccines: Evidence and Causality*. This report noted that even very large epidemiologic studies may not detect or rule out rare events, and that using case reports is complicated by the wide variation of available information often

insufficient to rule out other potential causes of the adverse event. To overcome these limitations, epidemiology and creative methodology have been vital in providing a rigorous scientific approach for assessing the safety of vaccines.

### Signal Detection

High profile vaccine adverse events, such as intussusception following rotavirus vaccination (see Case Example 23.3), demonstrate the need for surveillance systems able to detect potential aberrations in a timely manner. However, some factors make identification of true signals difficult; for example, many vaccines are administered early in life, at a time when the baseline risk for many adverse health outcomes is constantly evolving. Until the recent advent of systematic analyses of automated data including data mining of spontaneous reports, identification of a vaccine safety signal occurred as much due to a persistent patient as from data analysis.

### Assessment of Causality

Assessing whether any adverse event was actually caused by vaccine is generally not possible unless a vaccine-specific clinical syndrome (e.g. myopericarditis in healthy young adult recipients of smallpox vaccine), recurrence upon rechallenge (e.g. alopecia and hepatitis B vaccination), or a vaccine-specific laboratory finding (e.g. Urabe mumps vaccine virus isolation) can be identified. When the adverse event also occurs in the absence of vaccination (e.g. seizure), epidemiologic studies are necessary to assess whether vaccinated persons are at higher risk than unvaccinated persons. The latter is complicated by limited unvaccinated populations (particularly among children), potential confounding due to differences between those vaccinated and not vaccinated, and determining whether events are attributable to particular vaccines since frequently combination vaccines or more than one vaccine are administered together.

---

**Case Example 23.3    For Special Methodological Issues in Pharmacoepidemiologic Studies of Vaccine Safety**

*Background*
- Five cases of intussusception occurred among 10 054 recipients from three phase three trials [each with its own data safety monitoring board] of a rhesus-human rotavirus reassortant-tetravalent vaccine (RRV-TV), vs one case in 4633 controls, a difference that was not statistically significant. However, this analysis failed to take into account that three of the five vaccinated intussusception cases had their onset within one week of vaccination.
- RRV-TV was licensed on 31 August 1998 with intussusception listed as a potential adverse reaction needing post-licensure surveillance.

*Question*
Does a vaccine containing four live viruses, a rhesus rotavirus (serotype 3) and three rhesus-human reassortant viruses (serotypes 1, 2, and 4), increase the risk of intussusception in RRV-TV vaccine recipients?

*Approach*
- Conduct post-licensure vaccine safety surveillance with both passive and active systems.
- Analyze Vaccine Adverse Event Reporting System (VAERS) spontaneous reporting surveillance for reports of intussusception (new code need to be added).
- Conduct active surveillance on large populations with two studies (a case–control and a cohort study) on RRV-TV recipients and controls.
- Quantify risk associated with RRV-TV receipt and intussusception.

*Results*
- 15 initial VAERS reports (total of 112 VAERS intussusception reports from licensure on 31 August 1998 to 31 December 1999) with 95 confirmed intussusception cases following RRV-TV (confirmed by medical record review).
- Case–control study found infants receiving RRV-TV were 37 times more likely to have intussusception three to seven days after the first dose than infants who did not receive RRV-TV (95% confidence interval [CI] = 12.6–110.1).
- Retrospective cohort study using large linked databases (LLDB) among 463 277 children in managed care organizations from the Vaccine Safety Datalink (VSD) project demonstrated that those receiving the vaccine, 56 253 infants, were 30 times more likely to have intussusception three to seven days after the first dose than infants who did not receive the vaccine (95% CI = 8.8–104.9).
- Causal link between RRV-TV receipt and intussusception suggested in the postmarketing period at a frequency detectable by current surveillance tools (approximately 1/5000–1/10000 vaccinees).
- On 16 July 1999, CDC recommended temporarily suspending use of RRV-TV following initial 15 VAERS reports. When the VAERS findings were substantiated by preliminary findings of the more definitive studies, the manufacturer voluntarily recalled the vaccine. The US Advisory Committee on Immunization Practices recommendations for RRV-TV vaccination were withdrawn in October 1999.

*Key Points*
- Safety assessment during pre-licensure trials can benefit from oversight by a single data safety monitoring board with at least one member with rare disease epidemiology skills.
- Passive surveillance systems such as VAERS are subject to multiple limitations,

*(Continued)*

---

**Case Example 23.3    (Continued)**

including underreporting and biased reporting, reporting of temporal associations or unconfirmed diagnoses, lack of denominator data, and unbiased comparison groups; VAERS alone cannot usually assess causality.

- VAERS can successfully provide a timely vaccine adverse event alert (hypothesis generation) and overcome its limitations when paired with rigorous hypothesis testing active surveillance systems that can assess causality. Both contribute to a functional vaccine safety surveillance system.
- Similar results for both active surveillance studies help confirm the causal relationship between RRV-TV and intussusception.
- The hypothesis testing results from the VSD project using pre-organized LLDBs

was available more quickly and efficiently than the traditional case–control study (teams sent to 19 states to manually collect data). Pre-organized LLDB's are now the preferred mode for routine post-licensure pharmacovigilance.

- A "rapid cycle" initiative for more timely detection of vaccine safety signals has been formed by the CDC VSD project; this project successfully simulated and retrospectively "detected" the RRV-TV intussusception signal within the VSD by mid-May 1999.
- Subsequent clinical trials and post-marketing studies of next generation rotavirus vaccine used standardized Brighton Collaboration case definition for intussusception to show these new vaccines are safer than RotaShield.

---

### Measurement Accuracy

Misclassification of exposure status (vaccination) may occur if there is poor documentation of vaccinations. Documentation of exposure status has been fairly good through school age, but difficulty has been encountered in ascertaining vaccination status in older persons. Misclassification of outcomes can also occur in observational studies that rely on ICD-9 codes from computerized databases. Such diagnosis codes are often validated with a manual medical records review. Vaccines in the US (and some other countries) are now routinely shipped with 2D barcodes to help solve this problem.

### Sample Size

Because adverse health events of concern (e.g. encephalopathy) are often extremely rare, it may be a challenge to identify enough cases for a meaningful study. The difficulty with adequate study power is further compounded in assessing rare events in populations less fre-

quently exposed (e.g. subpopulations with special indications). For studies of rare outcomes, case–control and self-control designs are the most efficient. Case–control designs typically sample the source population of cases, identify an appropriate control group, and assess the exposure status of both groups to estimate the risk associated with exposure (see Chapter 2). Self-controlled designs usually find vaccinated cases in the source population and compare incidence rates of post-vaccination adverse events during defined periods following vaccination (also known as the risk interval) with the rates of the adverse event in the same person during varying control periods (either pre- or post-vaccination), which do not occur in close relationship to the time of vaccination.

### Confounding and Bias

Because childhood vaccines are generally administered on schedule and children may have developmental dispositions to particular events, age may confound exposure-outcome relations, e.g. MMR vaccine with febrile seizures or pneumococcal vaccine with sudden infant death syndrome (SIDS). Consequently, such factors must be controlled in the study design and analysis, which is often done by matching.

More difficult to control are factors leading to delayed vaccination or non-vaccination. Such factors (e.g. low socioeconomic status) may confound studies of AEFIs and lead to underestimates of the true relative risks. Those who have not been vaccinated may differ substantially from the vaccinated population in risks of AEs and thus be unsuitable as a reference group in epidemiologic studies. The unvaccinated may be persons for whom vaccination is medically contraindicated, or they may have other risks for the outcome being studied (e.g. they may be members of low socioeconomic groups). Similarly, vaccinated persons may be preferentially targeted for vaccination because of their underlying medical condition, potentially over-estimating the true relative risk. In addition, some children may be unvaccinated due to parental choice. These children may have different health care utilization patterns than fully vaccinated children, which in turn could bias study results.

## Examples of Currently Available Solutions

### Signal Detection

Identifying a potential new vaccine safety problem ("signal") pre- or post-licensure requires a mix of clinical and epidemiologic expertise. Hypothesis clarification via standardized case definitions or clinical case series may be needed. Data mining is often used to assess disproportional reporting in spontaneous reporting systems. One disproportionality assessment tool for comparing safety profiles of vaccines involves comparing the proportions of particular symptoms out of the total number of symptoms reported for a given vaccine to that observed among reports for another vaccine or group of vaccines. Because of the

ease of implementation and interpretation, this proportional reporting rate ratio (PRR) has been widely used for vaccine safety signal detection in spontaneous reporting systems such as the US VAERS, (see Chapter 7). Of course, any signals need to be confirmed in formal epidemiologic studies.

### Epidemiologic Studies

Historically, ad hoc epidemiologic studies have been employed to assess potential AEFIs. However, automated, large-linked databases provide a more flexible framework for hypothesis testing than ad hoc epidemiologic studies. The Centers for Disease Control and Prevention (CDC) initiated the VSD project in 1990 and has since become a standard for vaccine safety surveillance and research. The VSD project prospectively collects vaccination, medical outcome (e.g. hospital discharge, outpatient visits, emergency room visits, and deaths), and covariate data (e.g. birth certificates, census) under joint protocol at multiple managed care organizations (MCOs). The VSD project also provides safety signals near-real time using "rapid cycle" data sets that are updated weekly or monthly. This surveillance is usually employed to monitor newly licensed vaccines and existing vaccines that may have new recommendations. Pre-specified events of interest (usually chosen based on pre-licensure clinical trials, signals from other sources, or historical concerns, such as Guillain-Barre Syndrome) are tested at regular intervals (weekly or monthly) for increased risk of an event following the vaccine under surveillance using an appropriate comparison group, either historical data or a concurrent cohort. New "Tree Scan" methods also allow real time surveillance for unspecified outcomes. The VSD can also validate surveillance findings and test new ad hoc vaccine safety hypotheses using traditional epidemiologic methods and recently more frequent use of self-control designs that can avoid potential confounding from person-level factors and comorbidities (assuming they do not change over time). Due to the high coverage attained in the MCOs for most vaccines, few unvaccinated controls are available, and thus the VSD is limited in its capacity to assess associations between vaccination and adverse events with delayed or insidious onset (e.g. neurodevelopmental or behavioral outcomes).

The VSD provides an essential, powerful, and relatively cost-effective complement to ongoing evaluations of vaccine safety in the US. Similar systems have since been developed in other high income countries such as Denmark, the UK, and Taiwan. Similar capacity is needed in low and middle-income countries, where first introduction of new vaccines targeting locally prevalent pathogens are increasingly occurring.

### The Future

Although considerable progress has been achieved in vaccine safety monitoring and research, there are still several challenges, both scientific and non-scientific. One analytic challenge is identifying optimal risk windows following vaccination, which requires understanding the biologic mechanisms of the AEFI but can be somewhat arbitrary; data-driven approaches to defining risk intervals are underway. Detecting lifetime dose responses to multiple exposures of the same vaccine or vaccine components, determining the feasibility of studying vaccine safety of combined and simultaneous vaccinations, and data-mining for unknown AEFI using electronic medical records are all challenging areas in vaccine safety research. Vaccine safety science also faces the challenge of credibility; as vaccine preventable diseases continue to decline, many are skeptical about the need for vaccination and are suspicious of the motives of both governments (since many vaccines are mandated) and manufacturers. The VSD is studying health outcomes after "alternative" (vs routine) vaccination schedules. Faulty research may arise from those seeking to prove that the motives for vaccination are questionable.

Furthermore, proving that an AEFI may be coincidental can be difficult, particularly when the event is rare. On the other hand, combining adversomics, systems biology, and Big Data may allow eventual shift from "one size fits all" to personalized vaccinations. Vaccine safety surveillance and research requires persistence in providing rigorous science, educating the public, and providing reassurance that robust vaccine safety systems are in place.

### Key Points for Special Methodological Issues in Pharmacoepidemiologic Studies of Vaccine Safety

- There are still substantial gaps and limitations to our knowledge of many vaccine safety issues.
- A high standard of safety is required for vaccines due to the large number of persons who are exposed, some of whom are compelled to do so by law or public health regulations.
- New research capacity, such as the Vaccine Safety Datalink, provides powerful tools to address many safety concerns. Similar capacity needs to be expanded globally, especially for new vaccines (e.g. COVID-19).

## Epidemiologic Studies of Implantable Medical Devices

Recent decades have seen an explosion in medical device technologies worldwide. The global medical devices market reached a value of nearly $423.8 billion in 2018 and is expected to grow to nearly $521.64 billion by 2022 and $612.7 billion by 2025. Groundbreaking innovations in the areas of transcatheter interventions, nanotechnology, telemedicine, robotic procedures, sophisticated health information technology software, and smart applications continue to offer new diagnostic and therapeutic options to patients and clinicians. Recent approvals of the medical devices that use artificial intelligence to aid in diagnosis are good examples of the dynamic landscape where software as a medical device will play a more prominent role in the delivery of health care.

## What Is a Medical Device and how Is it Different from a Drug?

The US government defines a medical device as an instrument, apparatus, implement, machine, contrivance, implant, *in vitro* reagent or other similar or related article, including any component part or accessory which is: (i) recognized in the official National Formulary or United States Pharmacopeia or any supplement of them, (ii) intended for use in the diagnosis of disease or other conditions or in the cure, mitigation, treatment or prevention of disease in men or other animals, or (iii) intended to affect the structure or any function of the body of man or other animals, and which does not achieve its primary intended purposes through chemical action within or on the body of man or other animals and which is not dependent upon being metabolized for the achievement of any of its principal intended purposes.

There are many similarities regarding medical device definitions and classifications, but differences exist in requirements for approval. International Medical Device Regulators Forum (IMDRF) emerged in 2011 as a driver of harmonization and convergence efforts among regulatory authorities on medical devices. This voluntary organization brings together regulators from Australia, the European Union, Canada, the United States, Singapore, China, Japan and Brazil. IMDRF has made major steps toward the convergence of activities in the area of adverse event reporting, patient registries, software as a medical device, and implementation of Unique Device Identification (UDI), among other efforts.

In this section, we concentrate on implantable devices because of their significant clinical and public health impact, high risk for adverse events, and uncertainties surrounding the effects of long-term exposure. Implantable medical devices comprise an important device category in the very heterogeneous world of medical devices. As true of other devices, implantables share characteristics that distinguish them not only from other devices, but also from regulated drugs. Implantable devices, most of which are in US class III (highest risk), can be further differentiated.

Implantable devices often have a long (years or even decades) product life cycle (from design to device removal) although incremental changes occur over time. Implantable devices may consist of multiple components (such as a total hip implant) or a single component (such as a pacemaker lead). Exposure to such devices is typically chronic, with the onset of exposure clearly defined at time of implantation. Exposure typically ends at the time of device removal, but in practice may continue if part of the device remains in the human body (e.g. silicone leakage from ruptured breast implants).

Outcomes associated with implantable devices are affected not only by underlying patient factors and device factors (such as biomaterials), but also by user interface (e.g. operator technique, operator experience). Adverse effects of implantable devices are typically localized but may sometimes be systemic (e.g. secondary to toxic, allergic, auto-immune effects). Additional hazards may be related to human factors (e.g. improper programming of pacemakers) and interference (e.g. magnetic resonance imaging interaction with deep brain stimulator leads). Lastly, malfunctions may derive from several sources, including manufacturing problems, design-induced errors, and anatomic or engineering effects.

## Clinical Problems to be Addressed by Implantable Medical Device Epidemiologic Research

The following key issues should be considered when planning and conducting medical device epidemiologic research: (i) assessment of benefits and harms in real world settings, and (ii) assessment of long-term outcomes.

### Benefits and Harms Profile in a Real-Word Setting

Real-world implantable device evaluation relies predominantly on observational research methods. One of the main reasons for such focus is related to limitations of RCTs. In the RCTs of surgical devices, the participating operators are typically early adopters, highly skilled, and quick learners, which affects the learning curve. Traditionally, the learning curve is studied using observational studies of the volume-outcome relationship. In the past, some volume-outcome studies have demonstrated that increased surgical volume has an inverse linear relationship with the incidence of adverse outcomes; while others have identified a volume threshold for procedures above which increasing volume is no longer associated with improved outcomes. There are three distinct components of the volume-outcome relationship that can be studied: (i) lifetime experience (operator's volume), (ii) operator's volume per unit of time (e.g. year), and (iii) hospital volume where operators practice. Other factors related to learning curve might include type of procedure and practice setting (e.g. academic hospital). Adequate study of learning curves can establish thresholds for proficiency based on background expertise related to physicians' specialties. For example, thresholds for stenting of carotid artery vary by operator across specialties (e.g. radiologists, cardiologists, and neurosurgeons).

In addition to highly selected clinicians, RCTs often involve homogeneous, nonrepresentative patient populations. Pre-marketing device trials often lack sufficient representation of important patient populations (women, children, elderly, racial and ethnic minorities, etc.), which diminishes the generalizability of results. Well-designed observational studies can provide more information on device performance in the sub-populations of interest in routine care. The utility of observational studies has been increasing with advances in medical device data capture in medical records, electronic databases, and prospective registries, and with the development of and dissemination of analytical tools.

### Long-Term Safety and Effectiveness

Premarket device clinical trials are typically of short duration (e.g. one to two years), and generate limited information on long-term safety and effectiveness. Due to the inherent complexity of implantable devices, it is often difficult to predict fully their long-term safety and effectiveness based solely on the preclinical testing and premarket clinical trials. Postmarket attention is therefore increasingly directed toward ensuring that studies/surveillance of enough size and length of follow-up are conducted in the postmarket setting to better illustrate and assess problems occurring long-term. Many countries have established national registries of procedures involving implanted medical devices that collect long-term patient outcomes and device performance (e.g. orthopedic registries in Sweden, the United Kingdom, Australia, Canada and other countries). During the past decades the US had seen a growth in the number of national registries (e.g. National Cardiovascular Data Registry [NCDR], Kaiser Permanente National Joint Replacement Registry [NJRR], American Joint Replacement Registry [AJRR], National Breast Implant Registry [NBIR], and Vascular Quality Initiative [VQI].

### Methodological Problems to be Solved by Implantable Medical Device Epidemiologic Research

Evidence generation for implantable medical devices requires accounting for unique issues that typically do not arise when evaluating benefits and risks of drugs. Key issues arise from the interaction of device, operator, patient and the setting (e.g. hospital, outpatient clinic) in which the device is being used. Furthermore, device design, complexity, and its specific biomaterial and mechanical characteristics, can be as important to outcomes as the device's clinical applications such as type of the lesion being treated, severity of the disease, and concomitant therapy. In commonly used device epidemiologic research databases, these details are often only partially available, and sometimes are missing.

## Challenges in Individual Patient Exposure Assessment

The UDI captures critical device information, such as the name of the manufacturer, brand, version or model, and device group terms. The UDI system has only recently been established, and the UDI is now entering data systems within the US, unlike pharmaceuticals where the National Drug Code (NDC) Directory has a long history and is broadly used. Consequently, many databases still lack specific device identifiers, making exposure assessments challenging. For example, procedure codes may capture device groups (such as hip implants or types of hip articulation systems), but lack specificity to the manufacturer-level. Characterization of the sensitivity and specificity of device identifiers found in medical records, clinical registries, or insurance claims databases will be important to understand errors in device exposure. Promoting routine documentation of UDIs in medical records and in other health databases will contribute to a better understanding of device-specific performance. Another challenge associated with medical device epidemiology relates to device complexity – devices are frequently approved or used as systems involving several components. Device components are often used in combination with components of the same or different brands. Thus, experience with capturing complete device exposure information is far more complex for devices than it is for drugs. Once completely adopted, such a robust, widely incorporated medical device nomenclature will significantly further safety surveillance and epidemiologic studies of medical devices.

## Challenges in National Population Exposure Assessment

The challenges include incorporation of UDIs into data systems, including electronic health records, and routine documentation of device use and patient problems associated with that use. In the US, population medical device exposure data must be derived from a variety of sources including electronic health records, administrative claims data, registries and coordinated registry networks, national surveys, nationally representative samples of health providers, and marketing data. These data sources differ in their level of device specific granularity, design (retrospective versus prospective), and data collection (patient reports, sales, etc.). While these sources differ in the level of completeness and reliability, they may complement each other.

## Challenges in Comparative Studies

Epidemiologic research relies on non-experimental data to develop evidence about the safety and effectiveness of medical products. While limitations of non-randomized studies are well-known, two facts must be recognized. First, of the methodological approaches that are recognized as key components of high internal validity in pharmaceutical studies (e.g. randomization, allocation concealment, masking/blinding, withdrawal/follow-up, and intention-to-treat analyses), not all can be applied to evidence development for medical devices. Aside from recognized limitations of clinical trials (e.g. select study subjects, small sample sizes, short duration), the need for data observed in routine care arises because of learning curve issues, product modifications, and risks of unexpected adverse events related to mechanical failure of the products.

### Addressing Sample Size and Real World Performance Issues

Premark clinical trials are designed to have sufficient statistical power for effectiveness outcomes. Powering the RCTs for less common or rare but serious side effects is not feasible in most instances. RCTs of devices, because of small sample size and participant selection, often lack *generalizability (or external validity)*, which is defined as the extension of research findings and conclusions from a study conducted on a sample population to the population at large.

Systematic reviews with meta-analyses attempt to capitalize on the detailed data collection within each study. Systematic reviews are one mechanism to address the small study problems of the RCTs. Systematic reviews with meta-analysis assume that most of the individual RCTs of devices and surgery carefully record relevant clinical outcomes and offer a good opportunity to conduct evidence appraisal and synthesis when a reasonable number of studies are available.

Well-designed observational studies are often large and involve consecutive patient enrollment and comprehensive data collection. They are the best suited tools to evaluate the safety and effectiveness of devices in routine care. With large observational studies, one can evaluate relevant subgroup effects as well as rare safety and effectiveness endpoints that cannot usually be captured by RCTs.

### Ensuring Comparability of Study Groups

Cohort designs offer the opportunity to create groups of patients exposed to different devices of interest. Optimally, these designs are based on prospective and consecutive patient enrollment, prospective data collection, and a study that is hypothesis driven. Such observational studies should use statistical approaches to adjust for measured confounders and methods that help characterize the impact of unmeasured confounding on results.

We have good tools to address unequal distribution in observed baseline patient characteristics. Several analytical methods are available to handle selection factors and confounding. These methods involve stratification, regression models, or a combination of the two using propensity scores. Machine learning approaches are promising as they can accommodate many more confounders than traditional models and are less reliant on parametric assumptions. Each approach relies on a set of statistical assumptions that may or may not be appropriate in the setting. When it is felt that there is unmeasured confounding present beyond that accounted for in the collected information, another potential approach is that of *instrumental variable-based methods* which have assumptions and limitations of their own.

## Examples of Currently Available Solutions

### Adverse Event Reporting Systems

Once approved, manufacturers must monitor the safety of their products, including forwarding reports of adverse events to regulatory authorities. In the US, manufacturers are required to submit reports of device-related deaths, serious injuries, and malfunctions to the FDA. Healthcare providers and consumers submit reports voluntarily. These reports, obtained through passive surveillance are housed in the Manufacturer and User Facility Device Experience (MAUDE) database, established in 1996. Most reports in MAUDE are from manufacturers, with a small percentage from user facilities, voluntary sources, and importers.

Passive reporting systems have notable weaknesses including: (i) data may be incomplete or inaccurate and are typically not independently verified, (ii) data may reflect reporting biases driven by event severity or uniqueness or by publicity and litigation, (iii) causality generally cannot be reliably inferred from any individual report, and (iv) events are generally underreported and this, in combination with lack of denominator (exposure) data, precludes determination of event incidence or prevalence. The latter point is particularly important for implantable devices, because reports may capture device-associated events (such as thrombosis, infection, stroke, revision or replacement) for which estimation of incidence is of paramount importance.

To enhance the usefulness of reported data, statistical tools are used to assist in detecting safety signals. Bayesian and other data mining methods are employed to estimate the relative frequency of specific adverse event-device combinations as compared to the frequency of the event with all other devices in the same group.

In addition to MAUDE, the Medical Product Safety Network (MedSun) was established to provide additional reporting system based on the subset of 350 user facilities in the US. The MedSun network helps promote dialogue between the FDA and clinical community, refine potential safety signals in real time through targeted surveys, problem solving, and posting of reports.

### Signal Detection/Outlier Identification Using Variety of Methodologies

In many countries, national registries of procedures involving implanted medical devices have significantly augmented their national surveillance efforts using a variety of methodologies. For example, a likelihood-based scoring method of calculation of CUSUM is used by the Scottish\ Orthopedic registry described as part of International Consortium of Orthopedics (ICOR) series. In another example, the Australian orthopedic registry process identified the ASR artificial hip as outlier device using this method followed by proportional-hazards modeling to calculate the hazard ratios and adjust for age and sex in order to conduct a comparative analysis of revision rate between groups.

### Automated Surveillance

Automated surveillance using Data Extraction and Longitudinal Time Analysis (DELTA) has been used to monitor device outcomes. The DELTA was validated and applied in the surveillance of a spectrum of medical devices including medical devices, coronary stents, peripheral vascular stents, and other implantable devices. The system is compatible with a broad array of potential data sources and supports a variety of statistical methods, allowing for both unadjusted and risk-adjusted safety monitoring for prospective and retrospective analyses.

### Mandated Post Marketing Studies

The FDA has a unique statutory authority to mandate postmarketing studies either as a condition of approval or "for cause" later in the postmarketing period. A major regulatory/ public health challenge the FDA is facing is to find appropriate balance for obtaining clinical data premarketing to prevent delays in device approval and ensure that only safe and effective devices enter the marketplace. The appropriate postmarketing questions answerable in a mandated post-approval study include long-term safety and effectiveness, a real-world experience of the device as it enters broader user populations (clinicians and patients), effectiveness of training programs and learning curve effects, and the device performance in certain subgroups of patients not well studied in the premarketing clinical trials. Designing scientifically sound but practical studies, and then achieving adequate patient and physician recruitment rates can be challenging for implantable device studies.

### Registries

Recognition that RCTs cannot fill all the gaps in clinical evidence for implantable devices is not new, but has garnered renewed interest as registries have emerged as powerful resources to harness a full potential of observational studies. The International Medical Device Regulator's Forum (IMDRF) definition of medical device registry system is as follows: "Registries are organized systems with a primary aim to increase the knowledge of medical devices contributing to improve the quality of patient care that continuously collect relevant data, evaluate meaningful outcomes, and comprehensively cover the population defined by exposure to particular device(s) at a reasonably generalizable scale (e.g. international, national, regional, and health system)." Registries provide important infrastructure for conducting large-scale medical device studies. In the absence of a unique device identification code, the added value of registries for medical devices surveillance include capturing brand/model specific information crucial for signal identification and comparative effectiveness/safety studies. The complexity and scientific rigor of a registry can vary from those designed to evaluate quality of health care delivered, those specifically established to study sustained effectiveness and safety of a specific procedure, and those designed to systematically collect long-term data on many different types of treatment including risk factors, clinical events, and outcomes in a defined population. Once the framework of a registry is in place, studies with various designs can be performed using the registry data (e.g. cohort, case–control, cross sectional, quasi-experimental).

Major limitations of the registries include their often voluntary nature and the short duration of follow-up of patients. For implantable medical devices in particular, the modes of follow-up are critical. These registries can be linked to other databases including administrative billing data. The linkage of clinically rich procedural and intra-hospital data captured by the registry to the follow-up data from administrative databases (such as Medicare and Medicaid databases) can substantially augment the value of registries.

## Administrative Claims Data

The use of administrative databases for epidemiologic research has the strengths of studying large numbers of patients with diverse characteristics and wide varieties of clinical settings, as well as inclusion of longitudinal data from the real-world clinical care, and good representation of vulnerable populations, leading to increased external validity (generalizability). The large number of diverse patients present the opportunities to study device effect heterogeneity and to advance methods such as high-dimensionality propensity scores and instrumental variables. Current limitations of administrative databases include the lack of UDIs, potential inaccuracy of coding of diagnosis, difficulty separating comorbidity from complications, and type of revision procedure performed. The lack of clinical information in the administrative billing data can be supplemented by linking the billing data to data from registries or other clinically rich data from other data sources including electronic health records.

## Coordinated Real-World and Registry Networks (CRNs)

In 2015 the US National Medical Device Registry Task Force (NMDRTF) recommended the strategically Coordinated Registry Networks (CRNs) as an approach to build the national system for medical devices. To implement that recommendation, Medical Device Epidemiology Network (MDEpiNet), through cooperative agreement with the FDA, has been advancing various sources of real-world data and addressing the needs of device research and surveillance for multiple stakeholders. The CRN approach circumvents the limitations of traditional registries, claims, EHRs, and other relevant data by promoting interoperability and harmonization and by building linked data systems from these multiple sources. MDEpiNet has been developing the CRN-based learning healthcare communities to speed the development and maturity of the networks. CRNs are facilitated and supported by the MDEpiNet Coordinating Center at Weill Cornell Medicine which is establishing working groups charged with advancing multiple maturity domains through developmental work and implementation. Each CRN focuses on broad and balanced stakeholder participation which leads to strong stakeholder engagement and sustainability. Within the community, the CRN leaders can leverage medical device ecosystem stakeholders currently engaged with the MDEpiNet.

## Methodological Framework for Implantable Medical Device Outcome Evaluation

A methodological framework for implantable device epidemiology and surveillance involves understanding factors impacting the decision to implant the device, identifying the comparison group(s), and estimating the safety and effectiveness of the device compared to the alternative strategies. In the context of multiple clinical issues and methodological challenges noted previously, a critical issue in addressing these goals relates to the multiple sources of variability that exist with implantable devices: systematic and random variation due to the patient, to the surgeon or operator, to the healthcare center, and to the device itself.

Measurable patient characteristics may predict what type of device is implanted as well as clinical and device outcomes (*patient variation*). For instance, in the case of total hip replacements, advanced age, comorbidities such as heart failure and diabetes, and non-elective admissions are associated with inferior patient outcomes. However, advanced age is also associated with increased use of metal-on-polyethylene hip systems compared to hip systems constructed from other bearing surfaces.

Surgeon and surgical center skills (*provider variation*) may have a large impact on the type of implantable device used, such as the type of hip replacement surgery and clinical outcomes. Several features of the surgical procedure in which the device is implanted can also vary. For example, some orthopedic surgeons may use less invasive approaches/access when implanting a total hip replacement system than other surgeons. Complications and device failures can increase if the surgeon is early in his/her learning curve and annual surgical volumes of the surgeon and of the center may be associated with procedural success.

Several measurable characteristics of devices have been shown to be predictive of device use and outcome (*device variation*). For instance, the types of weight bearing surface in hip replacement systems are related to revision rates. In particular, hard on hard bearing surfaces, such as metal-on-metal or ceramic-on-ceramic, result in higher revision rates. Additionally, large diameter femoral head size may result in lower dislocation rates. The process of implantation fixation to the bone also results in variations in clinical outcomes. Hip systems can be implanted with bone cement that helps position the implant within the bone or the systems may have a porous surface that permits bone to grow into its surface.

## The Future

### Epidemiology, Digital Health and Patient-Generated Health Data

The broad scope of digital health includes categories such as mobile health (mHealth), health information technology (IT), wearable devices, telehealth and telemedicine, and personalized medicine. These technologies open new opportunities for patients and consumers to better manage and track their health and wellness through greater access to information. The interface of these devices and health care will continue to open new opportunities for medical device epidemiology to lead patient-centered evidence generation, synthesis and appraisal.

### Epidemiology and Evidence-Informed Practice and Policy

Epidemiology is becoming the essential link between an exploding demand for the knowledge derived from diverse evidence and the decisions made in health care policy and practice settings. In the larger public health context, the imminent future of device epidemiology will be to integrate and infer from massive amounts of heterogeneous and multidimensional data available from disparate data sources. In doing so, medical device epidemiology will continue to draw from advances in electronic health records, electronic data capture, standard taxonomy, unique device identifiers, global patient identifiers, integrated security, and privacy services. Contemporary device epidemiology will be able to mobilize the advances of translational health research sciences through new methods that combine basic science and clinical data, leading to the choice of best available treatment targeted for specific groups of patients.

### Translational Epidemiology

Epidemiologic data have an enormous potential to help guide basic science investigations (e.g. guiding the development of biomarkers for detection of patient risks for development of adverse responses to implantable devices). In addition, when combined with preclinical and other data sources (e.g. genetic, histology, explant retrieval), epidemiologic findings could significantly broaden evidence synthesis. In addition, epidemiology could leverage pre-existing implant-related data from observational data sources, in individuals with and without implant-related adverse outcomes to improve our understanding of implant safety and effectiveness. These types of interdisciplinary application of epidemiology could lead to more effective identification of candidate biomarkers predictive of certain implant-related responses (both local and systemic) in different patient subgroups. For instance, in silico approaches could combine epidemiologic and other data sources to help guide development of biomarkers.

### Epidemiology and Public–Private Partnerships

Public–private partnerships will continue to bring together expertise and diverse data sources such as registries, electronic health records, and patient generated health data,

which provide new and promising opportunities for the epidemiologic study of medical devices. The intent is to have a comprehensive, up-to-date risk–benefit profile of specific medical devices at any point in its life cycle so that optimally informed decisions can be made and provide more useful information to practitioners, patients, and industry. Evolution of public–private partnerships will drive the collaborative knowledge sharing between members of the ecosystem.

### Epidemiology and International Infrastructure

The accelerating pace of emerging medical technologies worldwide will continue, and the information science applications are expected to further shape IT-based health care dealing with new demands for storage, transmission, management, and analysis of patient data. The future global impact of epidemiology on our understanding of implantable devices will depend on technological and policy solutions for international collaboration to achieve consistency between global data sources, regulations, and methodologic approaches for various medical device implant applications.

Collaborative research efforts can particularly help to fill a major gap via international consortia. One such example of a collaborative effort is ICOR, International Consortium of Vascular Registries (ICVR) and International Coalition of Breast Registries Associations (I-COBRA). Development of international infrastructure creates opportunities for novel methods developments for epidemiologic studies. The methods for harmonization, sharing, and combining data are not well developed and require innovative approaches. Such international collaborations coupled with increasing regulatory convergence driven by IMDRF present unprecedented opportunity for influencing the clinical and policy decision making with enormous public health implications.

---

**Case Example 23.4    For epidemiologic Studies of Implantable Medical Devices (See Chughtai et al. BMJ)**

---

*Background*

- Surgical mesh is approved for treatment of pelvic organ prolapse (POP) since 1996 and its use has been increasing over time.
- In 2008 and 2011 FDA issued safety communications and highlighting fivefold growth of adverse event reports over time.
- The evidence mostly came from analyses of Manufacturer and User Facility Device Experience (MAUDE) database and extensive literature review.
- The safety of surgical mesh has been scrutinized by the media and led to an unprecedented number of lawsuits worldwide.

*Issues*

- No major studies of mesh outcomes were conducted, and due to the relatively low chance of complications large scale and real-world study is needed.
- Determine the risk complications after mesh use when compared to control group at 90 days.
- Determine the risk of repeat operations (re-operations) after mesh use when compared to control group at one year after surgery.
- Hospital claims data analyses can provide good evidence but the code for erosion was introduced in 2008.

*Approach*

- Mesh use is frequent but there are many surgeons who are able to avoid the "shortcut" and use native tissues for POP repairs. Most of these operations are conducted in the hospitals and the exposure information appears in US hospital claims data since 2008. Repeat surgery also requires hospitalization and is expensive: hence this outcome information appears in US longitudinal hospital claims data.

- New York State longitudinal records of hospitalization are available. Limiting data to New York State residents enables good follow-up particularly for short-term outcomes.
- Repeat operation is likely reliably coded for patients receiving outpatient or inpatient procedures.
- Propensity score matching enabled adjustment of differences in baseline characteristics between mesh and no mesh groups.

*Results*

- There were 27991 women undergoing POP repairs during the three-year study period (2008–2011). More than 24% of patients received mesh and mesh use did not decrease over time.
- 90-day complications related to urinary retentions occurred more after mesh-based repairs (risk ratio 1.33; 95% CI, 1.18–1.51).
- The risk of repeat operation was also significantly higher after mesh-based repairs at one year (risk ratio, 1.47; 95% CI, 1.21–1.79).
- There was interaction of surgery with age (cutoff at 65 years). Mesh use was not associated with statistically significant risk urinary retention among the younger women but led to much higher risk of repeat operation in this age group

*Strengths*

- Large and diverse real-world patient population.
- Ability to specify the exposure groups and outcomes.
- Billing codes facilitated reasonable risk classification of patients despite some limitations.

*(Continued)*

---

**Case Example 23.4   (Continued)**

*Limitations*
Reliability and completeness of outcome codes unknown but bias should be equally distributed.

POP disease severity and vaginal and abdominal mesh is hard to determine using codes but use of mesh is known to be related surgeon training/preference and the impact of unmeasured confounding is limited

*Key points*
- Claims data can be used for medical device research when codes are available and

longitudinal records are released by data owners.
- It is important to focus exposures and outcomes of interest that are codes using billing claims. Collaboration with surgeons trained in research, robust study design and analytic approaches can reduce the impact of measured and unmeasured confounders.
- Claims data can be used for medical device research when codes are available and longitudinal records are released by data owners.

---

**Key Points for epidemiologic Studies of Implantable Medical Devices**

- Medical devices are of great public health importance.
- Medical devices and their users have diverse and unique characteristics, creating different challenges compared with studying pharmaceuticals.
- Existing data sources have limited utility for medical device epidemiology because complete documentation of device use is not routine.
- The lack of a detailed identification system (analogous to the National Drug Code) for medical devices presents a barrier to understanding device performance.
- Due to increasing availability of electronic data sources, methodology for extracting and assessing the information from diverse data sources will be required.

# Research on the Effects of Medications in Pregnancy and in Children

Note: This section reflects the views of the authors and should not be construed to represent FDA's views or policies.

The historical exclusion of pregnant women and children from clinical trials leave these populations more susceptible to the potential risks of drugs used off-label and without high-quality evidence of efficacy, effectiveness, or safety. Pharmacoepidemiology has an important role in supplying critical missing evidence about the beneficial and harmful effects of drugs in pregnant women and children.

However, pharmacoepidemiologic research in these populations presents numerous methodologic and practical challenges related to changing disease epidemiology and treatment patterns in different stages of pregnancy and childhood; infrequent uses of medications, rare outcomes, and subgroup considerations requiring large sample sizes; and bias from confounding and other sources.

## Clinical Problems to be Addressed by Pharmacoepidemiologic Research

### Unique Biology and Epidemiology
*PREGNANT WOMEN:* Biologic processes in pregnancy lead to rapid changes in baseline risks of maternal conditions, including indications for treatment (e.g. nausea). Moreover, some outcomes are unique to pregnant women (e.g. pre-eclampsia) or their offspring (e.g. birth defects), and their etiologically sensitive

period changes throughout gestation (e.g. critical portions of organogenesis occur in the first trimester). Therefore, investigators must consider the fluctuating timelines of both the need for and the potential effects of treatment.

*CHILDREN:* The timing of birth and biologic changes due to the growth and development of children from infancy through adolescence influence their risks of disease (e.g. necrotizing enterocolitis, chlamydial infection) and patterns of treatment. Some medical conditions exclusively affect children or specific subgroups (e.g. retinopathy of prematurity), while others manifest and are treated differently from adults (e.g. depression). The states and rates of growth and development provide critical windows into pediatric health and can represent or influence key variables (e.g. exposures, outcomes).

### Treatment Responses and Patterns

*PREGNANT WOMEN:* The physiological changes associated with pregnancy can alter pharmacokinetics. Extrapolating conclusions regarding dosing, efficacy and safety from non-pregnant populations will therefore often be incorrect. Drug utilization patterns and medication adherence also vary more markedly around pregnancy. Some medications may be discontinued due to perceived or real risks associated with use during pregnancy (e.g. lithium, valproate), while others are indicated specifically during pregnancy (e.g. treatment for hyperemesis gravidarum). Nonadherence could lead to under-treatment of diseases (e.g. asthma) that could adversely affect outcomes of pregnancy; and to misclassification of exposure (e.g. if drug use is assessed solely based on prescriptions) that could bias studies.

*CHILDREN*: Pharmacokinetics change rapidly in childhood as various organs needed to absorb, distribute, metabolize, and excrete drugs mature. Children differ from adults in body composition, skin surface area, and other factors that affect drug absorption and metabolism. While children are mostly healthy and use fewer medications than adults, chronic medication use in children (e.g. for asthma,

attention deficit/hyperactivity disorder) has risen over time. Drug formulation and adherence may also affect drug effectiveness and safety in children.

### Evidence to Inform Clinical Practice, Role of Pharmacoepidemiology

Because of the typical exclusions of pregnant women and children from pre-approval clinical trials, there is usually very little premarket information on drug safety and effectiveness in pregnant or pediatric populations. Given that a drug's safety can rarely be predicted based on its structure and function alone, animal studies are often used to identify pregnancy-related or pediatric toxicity. However, animal studies can be poor predictors of teratogenic and other toxic effects in humans. Therefore, most information regarding the benefit/risk profile of drugs in these populations is collected after a drug's initial approval; post-approval controlled observational studies provide the primary approach for identifying potential teratogenic and toxic effects in pregnant and pediatric populations.

### Methodological Problems to be Solved by Pharmacoepidemiologic Research

#### Defining the Population

*PREGNANT WOMEN:* The peculiarities of pregnancy research start when defining the target population, since the unit of observation may be the mother, the pregnancy (sibling clusters within mother), or the fetus (multifetal clusters within pregnancy). Sometimes parity or twinning are outcomes of interest themselves; when they are not the outcome, the analysis needs to account for the correlation within mother and within pregnancy. Moreover, restriction of the study population to livebirths may have consequences for risk and relative risk estimation and interpretation.

*CHILDREN:* The age definition for pediatric populations varies across countries, organizations, and agencies, with cutoffs mostly around ages 17–22. Additionally, age-related developmental changes and heterogeneity of pediatric populations require consideration of study-specific subgroups in pediatric research, such as infants (premature and term), children (preschool and school age), and adolescents. Varying definitions of pediatrics and pediatric sub-groups make comparisons across studies and regulatory bodies more challenging. While birthdate is sometimes withheld from large databases as an identifier, precise age measurements are vital for studying children in the earliest months and years of life. Researchers studying infants and young children may need special waivers or permissions to access birthdate data.

## Sample Size Requirements and Challenges

An important practical hurdle when studying the effects of medications in pregnancy and in children is the ability to attain adequate sample sizes because, often, the use of specific medications is uncommon, and diseases and outcomes of interest are correspondingly uncommon. Therefore, in the absence of large effects, the study size needed rapidly becomes prohibitive.

## Exposure Ascertainment, Timing, and Misclassification

To ascertain exposures, we can either rely on secondary data (such as records of medication dispensings) or primary data collection (such as interviews). Users of secondary data sources should be aware of the potential disconnect between prescribed, dispensed, and consumed medications. Studies with primary data collection may rely on interviews for drug exposure information, which is often the only feasible way to obtain information on OTC drug use and verify the intake of medications. This approach raises concerns about the overall accuracy of recall. Moreover, researchers often conduct such interviews retrospectively after the outcome of interest has occurred (e.g. birth anomalies, pediatric cancer), raising concern

about recall bias or differential misclassification of exposure. In theory, the birth of a malformed child or a severe pediatric condition may affect recall of prior, remote exposures (e.g. during pregnancy or infancy). More complete exposure recall among mothers of cases would create a false positive association between the drug and the birth anomaly or pediatric condition, or overestimate an association if it exists. One approach to reducing this bias is improving accuracy by using well-designed interviews with highly structured questions to maximize recall and minimize errors in exposure assessment.

Pregnancy and childhood are highly dynamic times in medication management, including use of OTC medications. It is therefore important for investigators to define exposure during the etiologically relevant window (e.g. the first few weeks after conception for neural tube defects) with high specificity since misclassifying subjects who are unexposed during the transient sensitive periods as exposed would dilute the association, if one truly existed.

*PREGNANCY*: Given the variability of exposures and risks across stages of pregnancy, identification and consideration of gestational age is important for many research questions. Moreover, not all pregnancies are 40 weeks in duration, and outcomes of interest may be associated with shorter gestational length (e.g. spontaneous abortion). In those instances, one must avoid defining the exposure window in a way that creates *differential opportunity for exposure* in affected and unaffected pregnancies (e.g. exposure during the first trimester would be less likely for miscarriages), as this will bias the association measure. A few different strategies are available to avoid this bias, including defining exposure at start of follow-up (e.g. use at conception) and using a time-varying exposure definition (e.g. use in last 30 days).

*CHILDREN:* Because pediatric dosing is frequently weight-based, studies of dose effects in younger children may be more challenging in secondary data sources without weight data. One may categorize dose based on dose distributions within suitable age groups or from estimated dose per weight imputed from appropriate pediatric growth charts (e.g. national, WHO). However, imputed weight-based doses may be less valid in children with conditions (e.g. malnutrition) whose weight distributions substantially deviate from the source population or when granular dosage is desired.

Researchers ascertaining exposures through interviews or surveys should understand that parents do not always know what medications adolescent children are or are not taking.

### Outcome Definition and Ascertainment

Validation of outcomes in pregnant and pediatric populations may involve consultation with expert clinicians, patients, and families. As with other populations, studies using administrative claims or EHR data may use restrictive algorithms or validate outcomes using medical records.

Differential misclassification of outcomes with respect to exposure leads to additional analytic challenges. Diagnostic bias may occur if exposed pregnant women or children receive more testing because of suspicion of drug-induced effects, resulting in more complete diagnosis or over-diagnosis of subclinical conditions (e.g. minor anomalies or viral illnesses).

Evaluation of long-term outcomes following prenatal or early life exposures (e.g. neuropsychiatric disorders) is particularly challenging for outcomes that are rare (e.g. pediatric malignancies), have less readily available measures (e.g. cognitive impairment), do not consistently come to medical attention (e.g. autism spectrum disorders), or in settings that limit long-term follow-up (e.g. certain automated databases, transitions to adult care). Loss to follow-up could compromise statistical power and lead to bias if dropout is not random and informative censoring is not appropriately handled. Evaluations of the effects of prenatal or early life drug exposure on child development and other long-term outcomes also face multiple potential sources of confounding (see Chapter 22).

*PREGNANCY*: While teratogenesis has received special attention as a rare but dramatic outcome, pregnancy researchers and regulators more recently have expanded their attention to include other obstetric and neonatal outcomes such as fetal losses and long-term consequences in the child. Major birth defects are typically defined as those that are life threatening, require major surgery, or present a significant disability. Depending on inclusion criteria and ascertainment windows, the risk can range from 1% to greater than 10%. Therefore, investigators should strongly consider including an internal reference group with consistent outcome definition and data collection for major malformations. Moreover, given the etiologic heterogeneity of malformations, combining multiple malformations into a single outcome may lack a sound embryologic basis. A more appropriate approach may be to create categories that reflect the embryologic tissue of origin or teratogenic mechanism, when known. However, researchers sometimes lump together various fetal malformations, partially for conservation of statistical power. Of note, birth certificates can be inaccurate records of birth anomalies and are not recommended as gold standards.

*CHILDREN*: Conceptualization and operationalization of study outcomes may differ in pediatric populations because of differences in disease manifestation, symptoms, and diagnostic findings. The sensitivity, specificity, and predictive values of outcome definitions will also be different in children than in adults because of differences in disease prevalence. Growth (e.g. height velocity, weight z-score) and development (e.g. motor, behavioral, or pubertal milestones) can serve as important outcomes in pediatric studies.

### Confounding

Confounding can occur if children or pregnant women who receive a drug are more likely to have risk factors for the outcome. Available approaches to minimize confounding include (i) restricting to individuals with the indication(s) and using an alternative therapeutic strategy as the reference, (ii) adjusting for potentially unbalanced risk factors for the outcome(s) of interest (e.g. severity of the underlying condition), (iii) comparing continuers with discontinuers of the medication of interest, and (iv) sibling discordance study to control for stable family factors (see also Chapter 22).

*PREGNANCY*: Although many treatment indications are not traditional risk factors for adverse outcomes of pregnancy, certain indications may be confounders due to strong associations with other conditions or behaviors that are risk factors for the outcome. For example, women treated with antidepressants for depression or anxiety may also be more likely to have comorbidities or habits predisposing to adverse pregnancy outcomes. In addition, women with anxiety utilize more health care resources, including fetal or early-life testing (e.g. echocardiography), than unaffected counterparts. Hence, anxious women are more likely to have infants diagnosed with mild cardiac malformations that might have gone clinically undetected in children of other women, such as small muscular ventricular septal defects. Failure to account for such sources of confounding and surveillance bias when studying the safety of psychotropic medications might bias results.

*CHILDREN:* Potentially important sources of confounding in pediatric studies may be difficult to ascertain in certain settings, such as administrative claims. Such confounders include second-hand smoke exposure, parental income and occupation (e.g. measures of socioeconomic status or environmental exposure), parenting behaviors (e.g. seeking testing or antibiotics), early childhood feeding (e.g. breastmilk or formula), familial medical conditions (genetics), and vaccinations. Birth weight and gestational age at birth, also missing in some databases, can be particularly

important to understanding the indications and effects of treatment in early life, especially in premature infants. States of growth (e.g. underweight or obesity) and development (e.g. skeletal turnover, pubertal stage) could also be sources of confounding or effect modification.

### Selection Bias

When selection into or retention in the study is directly or indirectly affected by the exposure and the outcome, selection bias may distort estimates of risk.

*PREGNANCY*: The ideal pregnancy cohort begins at or before conception, if not at the time of first exposure. Most studies enroll women after pregnancy is confirmed, which may underestimate risks of early pregnancy events (e.g. miscarriages). Follow-up of exposed and unexposed pregnancies should start at comparable gestational ages to avoid bias. Similarly, in studies of birth defects, women should be enrolled before prenatal screening for major malformations is completed to avoid biased selection.

Unique to the study of birth anomalies is the possibility of pregnancy losses, whether spontaneous or induced. Studies of liveborn infants underestimate the risk of lethal and prenatally detectable anomalies resulting in termination. Bias may occur in instances where exposed and reference groups have different proportions of terminations of affected fetuses. Sensitivity analyses can be used to assess the uncertainty around the relative risk estimates due to this potential selection bias.

Case–control studies are susceptible to selection bias resulting from inappropriate control selection. In some studies of birth anomalies, controls comprise infants with malformations besides those affecting cases, in order to reduce the opportunity for differential recall of exposure. This approach is valid as long as the exposure being evaluated does not increase the risk of the control malformations. Whether malformed or not, controls should be sampled from the same population that gave rise to the cases, e.g. same hospital catchment area.

Lastly, one can introduce selection bias during the analysis by adjusting for variables that share common causes with the outcome or are affected by it. For example, adjustment for low birth weight is unwarranted when the analytic goal is to estimate the total effect of prenatal variables, such as maternal drug use, on infant mortality, or when the goal is to estimate the direct effect but there is an unmeasured common cause of low birth weight and mortality.

*CHILDREN:* Among pediatric populations, research in very premature infants, who are at high risk of poor outcomes, may be particularly subject to selection bias. For instance, in studies of infants within highly specialized neonatal intensive care units, selection bias may result when referral relates to both the risk of exposure (e.g. indomethacin) and outcomes (e.g. intraventricular hemorrhage). Furthermore, in the most medically fragile neonatal populations, failure to account for mortality risk in the first weeks of life (e.g. through time-varying or competing risk models) may lead to survivor treatment selection bias (immortal time bias).

## Examples of Currently Available Solutions

Below we review the main pharmacoepidemiologic designs used for pregnant and pediatric populations to quantify the risk/benefit profile of medication exposure during pregnancy, infancy, or childhood, and the solutions they offer to common forms of bias.

### Prospective Cohorts

Prospective inception (or follow-up) cohorts offer the advantage of identifying drug exposure before adverse outcomes are recognized. For pregnancy cohorts, women are identified at the time of pregnancy planning or shortly after conception; the periodic collection of information on demographics, exposures, and potential confounders; as well as formal evaluation of offspring at birth (or fetal death) and ideally throughout childhood. A similar approach can be applied to newborns (e.g.

premature birth inception cohorts) or children with new-onset disease, particularly rare pediatric diseases. Unfortunately, even large inception cohorts are often too small to examine the risks of less common outcomes (e.g. specific birth anomalies) related to specific exposures.

### Registries

*PREGNANT WOMEN:* For new or infrequently used drugs, it is more efficient to assemble cohorts of exposed women and follow them to determine outcomes including maternal, obstetric, fetal, and infant outcomes (known as exposure pregnancy registries). While critically important for the detection of major adverse effects (e.g. isotretinoin teratogenicity), the small size of most registries prohibits identification or disproof of small to moderate effects involving rare outcomes. Selective inclusion or retention may affect the generalizability of absolute risk estimates and may bias the relative risk if related to both exposures and outcomes. To avoid selection bias, women should be enrolled into a pregnancy registry before pregnancy outcomes are known. In any pharmacoepidemiologic study, reference groups should be comparable. Pregnancy registries should therefore compare women exposed to a drug of interest with other women with similar indications, whether untreated or treated with alternative drugs. When feasible, multi-drug pregnancy registries allow comparisons among drugs from the same class or indication.

*CHILDREN:* Like other prospective disease cohorts, pediatric registries of rare pediatric diseases can serve as settings for drug safety and effectiveness research, providing rich information about study variables. Rare pediatric disease registries may also collect biologic specimens that facilitate molecular pharmacoepidemiology. Population-based pediatric registries that comprehensively ascertain affected children minimize selection bias and yield generalizable knowledge. In contrast, registries relying on voluntary participation may be subject to selection bias and reduced external validity.

### Retrospective Cohorts and Nested Case–Control Studies within Automated Health Care Databases

Population-based automated healthcare databases (e.g. national registries, administrative claims and EHR databases) offer detailed, longitudinal real-world data on health care utilization, diagnoses, procedures, and treatments across various healthcare settings. Clinical care reflects real-world practices, and study populations may include minorities and other marginalized populations often excluded from volunteer-based studies. While their size makes them excellent settings to study rare exposures or outcomes, some automated databases have substantial limitations due to lack of child–mother linkages or routinely collected data on OTC drugs and other potentially important variables (see Chapter 22). When only a small fraction of pregnant women or children are exposed to treatments of interest, even large cohorts may be insufficient. Multi-site collaborations may allow identification of exposed pregnancy or pediatric cohorts nested in multiple large databases with the goal to conduct surveillance and/or etiologic research on medication safety. Examples include the Medication Exposure in Pregnancy Risk Evaluation Program (MEPREP), the International Pregnancy Safety Study (InPreSS) consortium, the Comparative Effectiveness Research through Collaborative Electronic Reporting (CER2) Consortium, and PEDSnet.

### Case–Control Studies

Case–control studies identify individuals with the outcome of interest (e.g. specific birth anomaly) and compare their frequency of exposures to that in a control group without this outcome. This design can facilitate evaluation of associations between prenatal or early life exposure to relatively common medication and risks for rare events. However, important challenges include retrospective ascertainment of exposure, inability to evaluate infrequently used medications, potential for inappropriate control selection, limited focus on one outcome, and inability to estimate absolute risks (unless studies are nested within defined cohorts). Case–control studies on birth anomalies are often based on interviews, allowing collection of information often missing from other data sources (e.g. nonprescription drugs, lifestyle variables). Examples include the Birth Defects Study to Evaluate Pregnancy exposureS (BD-STEPS) and EUROmediCAT.

### Newer Designs

Epidemiologists continue to explore more valid and efficient approaches to study pregnant women and children. In specific circumstances, when carefully conducted with clearly stated assumptions and interpretation of estimates, novel designs may bring advantages to the field.

To avoid between-person confounding, one might study the risk of birth anomalies using a self-controlled design or a sibling discordance study. For example, to study whether flu vaccines triggers miscarriage, one could conduct a self-controlled study comparing the frequency of vaccinations during the month before miscarriage and a one-month control window three months before miscarriage. In sibling discordance studies, one compares outcomes in siblings born to the same parents but who differ with respect to exposure status during pregnancy or early childhood, therefore accounting for unmeasured genetic and environmental factors.

### The Future

Professional organizations and governments have increasingly supported policies and regulations that prioritize research on medicines and devices for pregnant women and children. Large-scale, longitudinal, collaborative research using multiple data sources across multiple countries will become increasingly common and important for generating generalizable, actionable evidence for these understudied populations. Collaborative networks and pooled resources, potentially through distributed data models and sharing of protocols, data, and analytic code and tools, will enable the conduct of robust research on rare exposures and rare outcomes in pregnant women and children. Linkages between complementary data types – e.g. automated databases, registries, patient-generated data, genomic and other -omic data – will enable discovery and validation of personalized treatment regimens, as well as outcome validation and better confounding control (e.g. propensity-score calibration). Given the limits of large health care databases to address all research questions about pregnant and pediatric populations, we should continue to use, improve, and teach field methods for primary

data collection (including biospecimens for pharmaco-omic studies) from patients and families. Future efforts must help build capacity, expertise, and infrastructure to conduct pharmacoepidemiologic studies in underserved settings and low- and middle-income countries. Such approaches will be necessary to address the changing epidemiology of diseases affecting pregnant women and children, including the rise in obesity and associated ailments, emerging infectious diseases (e.g. Zika virus, SARS-CoV-2), improving survival from life-threatening diseases (e.g. cystic fibrosis, inborn errors of metabolism), and many others. More research and better methods are also needed for pharmacoepidemiologic research in lactating mothers and breastfed infants.

---

**Case Example 23.5   For Studies of Drug-Induced Birth Defects (see Huybrechts et al, JAMA 2018)**

*Background*
- Prior experiences with thalidomide (delayed regulatory action in response to safety signal) and other antiemetic drugs (including potential over-reactions) raised important questions about the potential teratogenicity of treatments for nausea and vomiting in pregnancy.
- By 2009, ondansetron was the most frequently prescribed drug for nausea and vomiting in pregnancy in the US.

*Issue*
- Available evidence on the risks of cleft palate and heart defects following ondansetron exposure in early pregnancy was limited and conflicting, with concerns about systematic errors in prior research.
- Ondansetron can cross the placenta and disrupt serotonin pathways by blocking $5\text{-HT}_3$ receptors, making an association biologically plausible.

*Approach*
- Researchers conducted a cohort study nested in the nationwide Medicaid Analytic eXtract to evaluate the association between ondansetron exposure during the first trimester of pregnancy and the risk of cardiac malformations and oral clefts; using propensity score (PS) stratification to control for treatment indications and other potential confounders.

*Results*
- Among 1 816 414 pregnancies, 88 467 women filled prescriptions for ondansetron during the first trimester.
- Absolute risks of cardiac malformations were 94.4 and 84.4 per 10 000 exposed and unexposed liveborn infants, respectively.
- Absolute risks of oral clefts were 14.0 and 11.1 per 10 000 exposed and unexposed liveborn infants respectively.
- PS-adjusted relative risks were 0.99 (95% CI, 0.93–1.06) for cardiac malformations

*(Continued)*

**Case Example 23.5    (Continued)**

and 1.24 (95% CI, 1.03–1.48) for oral clefts (corresponding to three additional cases of oral cleft per 10 000 women treated).

- Findings persisted across multiple sensitivity analyses.

*Strengths*
- Large cohort size allowing associations to be estimated with great precision.
- Prospective exposure ascertainment based on filled prescriptions, free of recall bias.
- Estimation of absolute risks and risk differences.
- Rich patient-level information allowing for extensive confounding control.
- Additional comparisons of ondansetron-exposed women with women exposed to other antiemetics, yielding consistent results.
- Use of validated outcome definitions with high positive predictive value.
- Robustness of findings tested across multiple sensitivity analyses.

*Limitations*
- Differences between filled prescriptions and medication consumption; sensitivity analyses limited to women with ≥2 filled prescriptions or intravenous administration led to similar results.

- Concerns about residual confounding, mitigated through use of high-dimensional propensity scores, alternate reference groups, and a negative control analysis.
- Severe congenital malformations resulting in pregnancy losses or terminations are missed in cohorts restricted to livebirths; quantitative bias analysis was conducted.

*Key points*
- Healthcare utilization databases are increasingly being used to complement exposure pregnancy registries and case–control studies.
- Cohorts nested in healthcare utilization databases facilitate the study of rare exposure and outcomes.
- Large population-based cohorts ensure representation of populations that are frequently underrepresented in clinical trials and volunteer cohort studies but are most at risk of adverse pregnancy outcomes.
- Rich information on potential confounders (e.g. underlying indication and severity, maternal comorbidities, and concomitant medication use) allow for extensive confounding control.
- Sensitivity analyses can address potential limitations and test robustness of findings.

## Key Points for Research on the Effects of Medications in Pregnancy and in Children

- Because pregnant women and children are often excluded from clinical trials, pharmacoepidemiologic research is an important source of real-world evidence on the use, effectiveness, and safety of drugs used during pregnancy and childhood.
- In addition to random error and confounding, methodological challenges for pharma-

coepidemiologic studies in pregnant and pediatric populations include changing patterns of drug utilization and adherence during pregnancy and childhood, rapid changes in risks of outcomes and etiologically sensitive periods, timing of enrollment relative to critical events (e.g. conception, prenatal screening, birth), selection of survivors when only livebirths are included, missing information (e.g. structural malformations in fetal losses, referral patterns of neonates), and differential opportunities for drug exposure due to variable durations of pregnancies.

- Exposure pregnancy registries (small ad hoc cohorts that oversample exposed) are useful to evaluate the safety to new drugs, identify high-risk teratogens, and can collect real use, sociodemographic information and biologic samples, but are underpowered to identify lesser risks.
- Pediatric disease registries can facilitate research on drug safety and effectiveness in rare diseases but may be subject to selection bias and reduced external validity if enrollment is voluntary.
- Large cohorts nested within large healthcare databases may provide adequate power for less frequent exposures or outcomes and contain detailed clinical information on population-based samples but frequently lack information on OTC drugs, adherence, outcomes that do not trigger claims, and important covariates such as BMI, smoking, early childhood feeding, and pediatric growth parameters.
- Case–control studies can efficiently estimate associations with the outcome collected, provided drugs are relatively commonly used, selection of controls is valid, and retrospective collection of information is not biased by differential recall.
- Under certain assumptions, self-controlled designs and sibling discordance studies may be valuable alternative study designs.

## Risk Management

For medicines, risk management is used to ensure that the potential benefits of a medicine exceed its potential risks, and to minimize those risks throughout the lifecycle of the product. Current understanding of the risks of medicines is based on the premise that the risk of a medicine derives not only from the inherent properties of the medicine, but also from how the medicine is used in actual clinical practice.

In the context of human medicines in the United States, the FDA has defined risk management as:

> an iterative process of (1) assessing a product's benefit-risk balance, (2) developing and implementing tools to minimize its risks while preserving its benefits, (3) evaluating tool effectiveness and reassessing the benefit-risk balance, and (4) making adjustments, as appropriate, to the risk minimization tools to further improve the benefit-risk balance. This four-part process should be continuous throughout a product's lifecycle, with the results of risk assessment informing decisions regarding risk minimization.

In the European Union (EU), the concept of risk management is established in legislation. Article 1 (28b) of Directive 2001/83 EC as amended, defines a risk management system as: "a set of pharmacovigilance activities and interventions designed to identify, characterize, prevent or minimize risks relating to a medicinal product including the assessment of the effectiveness of those interventions." Thus, in the EU, risk management incorporates (i) the identification or characterization of the safety profile of the medicinal product, with emphasis on important identified potential risks and missing information, and also on which safety concerns need to be managed proactively or further studied (the "safety specification"), (ii) the planning of pharmacovigilance activities aimed at characterizing and quantifying clinically relevant risks, and identifying new adverse reactions (the "pharmacovigilance plan"), and (iii) the planning and implementation of risk minimization measures, including the evaluation of the effectiveness of these activities (the "risk minimization plan"). As a result, both in the US and the EU, risk management measures are iterative processes frequently leading to the generation of similar data needs and conceptually similar risk management tools.

## Clinical Problems to be Addressed by Pharmacoepidemiologic Research

All medicines have risks. The traditional tools used to manage the risks of prescription medicines have been the prescription status itself (i.e. whether the drug was approved for prescription only use or whether it could be obtained without a prescription), professional labeling, and the requirement that manufacturers monitor and report to regulatory authorities adverse events that occur with use of the medicine once it is marketed. In the past few decades, additional minimization strategies have been undertaken to manage more proactively the risks of certain medicinal products. These measures have included increased communication to patients as well as to healthcare professionals, and measures to restrict, in various ways, the usage of certain medicines.

### The Complexities of the Medication Use System

The medication use system is a complex network of stakeholders, including patients, their families, physicians, nurses, pharmacists, other health professionals, health care organizations and healthcare facilities, payors, manufacturers, and regulatory agencies. Not only does each stakeholder have a role in ensuring the safe use of a medicine, the interactions among them do as well.

In this context, the approach to risk management must consider all environments of where the medicine will be used (e.g. hospitals, long-term healthcare facilities, physicians' offices, outpatient home care).

### The Sources of Risk from Medical Products

There are several sources of risks from medical products. The known risks of a product are based on prior experience or, in some cases, on the pharmacologic or other properties of the medicine.

Preventable risks can occur when a product is administered under a condition of use that imparts a risk that would not be present under a different condition of use. For example, if drug A, when used in combination with drug B, results in an unacceptable risk that is not present when either drug is used alone, this unacceptable risk is preventable by ensuring that drug A and drug B are never coadministered. Other sources of preventable adverse events are medication errors and, occasionally, injury from product quality defects. Because they are preventable, medication errors are well suited to risk management efforts. Because medication errors can occur anywhere in the medication use system, efforts to minimize the risk of medication error must involve multiple stakeholders.

Unavoidable risks are those that might occur when all the known necessary conditions for safe use of a product are followed. In these circumstances, risk minimization activities might be directed toward identifying the adverse consequences as early as possible with the aim of preventing more serious harm. For example, a drug may be known to cause liver damage but its occurrence in a specific patient may not be predictable or preventable. In this case, risk minimization activities might be directed toward regular monitoring of liver enzyme levels to identify any hepatic damage as early as possible and thus to stop or modify the treatment to prevent serious hepatitis or hepatic failure.

Removing all risks from the use of all medicines is not the overall goal of managing the risks of medicines. Rather, careful consideration of benefit–risk balance both for the individual patient and for the target population is an important consideration of risk management.

### Risk Management Strives to be Scientifically Driven

The scientific approach to risk management requires integrating data from various studies and disciplines that, when taken together, can promote the safe and effective use of a medicine. The scientific approach also compels manufacturers and regulators to examine the critical gaps in knowledge that exist. Such gaps may concern the pharmacologic properties of the medicine, clinical outcomes related to its use, including that in higher risk populations, or the way the medicine is used in actual practice. Any of these areas could lead to further post-approval studies, the results of which would lead to changes in labeling or other changes that could enhance the safe and effective use of the medicine.

## Risk Management Proceeds throughout a product's Lifecycle

Knowledge about a product's safety profile is limited to some extent at the time of product approval, because of recognized practical limitations in the drug development process. Even after a product has been marketed for a decade or more, uncertainties will remain. For example, a study of new molecular entities approved for use by the US FDA between 2002 and 2014 indicated that safety-related labeling changes were being made as long as 13 years after the products were approved. Because of this lifecycle approach, all stakeholders – patients, practitioners, manufacturers, and regulators – must remain vigilant about the benefit–risk profile of a medicine. Such vigilance is critical for informed decision making, which is an important component of the safe and effective use of medicinal products.

## Risk Management Applies to all Medicines

All medicines have risks. The magnitude, frequency, and severity of risks vary from medicine to medicine. For example, at one end of the spectrum, neutropenia is commonly associated with chemotherapy and other immunosuppressive agents and is a major risk factor for development of infections. Strategies to monitor, prevent, and manage these infections can lead to improved outcomes and will ensure the benefits of these drugs continue to outweigh the risk. At the other end of the spectrum, many topical OTC medicines have very few side effects. The management of these risks is clearly much less intense. In the middle of this spectrum are the vast majority of medicines, mainly prescription medicines, for which a measured approach to risk management must be taken.

For most prescription medicines, the most common side effects are generally not life-threatening. Rather, many are mild and self-limited. Others are bothersome, and some are so clinically significant that they require the medicine to be discontinued. OTC medicines have been found to be safe and appropriate for use without the supervision of a health care provider, and they can be purchased by consumers without a prescription. When OTC medicines are taken properly, most of their side effects are generally mild. However, there can be serious, even life-threatening or fatal, side effects of OTC medicines when they are not taken properly. For example, acetaminophen (paracetamol), one of the most widely used OTC analgesics, is generally very safe when taken as recommended on the product's label. Overdose, however, can result in acute severe liver injury, which can lead to acute liver failure, and sometimes the need for liver transplantation or even death.

## Risk Management Is a Proactive Process

Risk management must be proactive to be optimally effective. The ability to identify risks in the pre-approval period allows manufacturers to work with regulators on risk management planning during the drug development phase. A proactive approach in the post-approval phase demands that manufacturers, regulators, and practitioners agree on a system to identify new risks, manage known risks, assess the effectiveness of the risk management efforts, and modify them as needed. A carefully designed risk management plan can identify or further characterize risks, communicate and manage risks using evidence-based tools when possible, and assess the effectiveness of these efforts in a proactive way. The proactive nature of risk management planning demands the constant vigilance of all stakeholders.

### Risk Management Activities

Managing the risks of medicines is not a single activity or the province of a single profession or stakeholder group. Rather, it is an iterative process that involves a set of inter-related activities, including risk assessment, risk minimization, and evaluation of risk minimization strategies with adjustments, as appropriate, to the risk minimization strategies to optimize the benefit–risk balance of the medicinal product.

### Risk Assessment

Risk assessment occurs throughout a product's lifecycle and consists of identifying, characterizing, and quantifying the risks associated with the use of a medicine, and evaluating their importance in relation to the benefit–risk balance. Pre-approval risk assessment is an extensive process that involves preclinical safety assessments, clinical pharmacology assessments, and clinical trials. Animal toxicology studies are performed prior to the first human exposure to a new medicine to establish the general toxicity profile of the drug and to guide initial human dosing. Clinical pharmacologic studies establish the pharmacokinetic profile of the medicine, exposure-response relationships, and can be used to assess drug–drug interactions. Pre-approval clinical trials provide the efficacy and safety information that form the basis for an approval decision. The pre-approval safety assessment generally quantifies and characterizes the common adverse events associated with a medicinal product. Depending on the number of subjects exposed prior to approval, less common adverse events might also be detected.

Because even large clinical development programs cannot identify all risks associated with a product, it is imperative that risk assessment continue in the post-approval period, when large numbers of persons will be exposed to the medicine, including many with comorbid conditions or on concomitant medications not present in clinical trials. Post-approval risk assessment can be based on either non-experimental data or on clinical trial data. Non-experimental data include individual case reports of suspected adverse drug reactions (spontaneous reports), case series of such reports, databases of spontaneous reports, disease-based registries, drug-based registries, electronic medical records systems, administrative claims databases, drug utilization databases, poison control center databases, and other public health databases that track usage of the medicine.

It is also important for risk assessments to identify medication errors. Proactive risk assessments that reflect human and environmental factors in medicine's use should be employed from the earliest stages of product design to help anticipate potential medication errors. After approval, the identification of medication errors must focus on identifying the specific reasons for, or causes of, the event.

New risks of a medicine will continue to be recognized after the drug is on the market. Some of these risks will be sufficiently serious to alter the benefit–risk balance of the medicine, such that post-approval regulatory action will be needed.

### Risk Minimization

Risk minimization or mitigation refers to a set of interventions intended to prevent or reduce the occurrence, or the severity of adverse events associated with exposure to a medicine. The range of risk mitigation activities varies from one country or region to the next, but certain common themes emerge.

The very fact that a medicine must be reviewed before approval is, in many ways, the most fundamental risk mitigation activity, in that it prohibits the marketing of medicines that have not been judged to be safe and effective, thus virtually eliminating the risks of medicines being legally marketed for which there is no demonstrated benefit. The requirement that certain medicines be available only by prescription is another form of risk mitigation. The premise underlying the prescription-only status of a medicine is that some medicines are potentially harmful, or the method of their use is not safe without the involvement of a health care provider, whose judgment can be used to ensure that, for a particular patient, the potential benefits outweigh the potential risks.

### Risk Communication

Communicating information about the benefits and risk of medicines is central to minimizing the risks of medicines. The principal form of communication to healthcare professionals in the US is the product's approved professional labeling. In the EU, this professional information is known as the Summary of Product Characteristics (SmPC).

Additional communications to healthcare professionals come in the form of so-called "Dear Health Care Provider Letters" or "Direct Healthcare Profession Communication." These letters, typically issued by a medicine's manufacturer, are usually one to a few pages in length, and generally focus on specific, newly-identified safety information.

Labeling directed to patients and consumers is also a risk communication tool in that it highlights basic information necessary for the safe use of the product, and often provides instructions for actions that patients should take when certain symptoms are present. In the US, FDA-approved patient labeling includes a Medication Guide, a Patient Package Insert, or instructions-for-use. In the EU, all medicines are required to have a patient information leaflet, which must be provided to the patient as part of the product packaging, or in exceptional circumstances as a separate leaflet or even as online information. This leaflet is based upon the information provided in the SmPC but written in patient-friendly language.

If additional communication measures are utilized, they are generally designed to address one, or at most a few, specific important risks associated with a medicine and may include focused risk information targeted to practitioners that are likely to prescribe the medicine or to care for patients that are treated with the medicine. Specific risk information may also be targeted to healthcare professional societies to share with their members. The types of communication tools can include letters, prescriber checklists, or educational brochures. Communication tools for patients can include a dosing card for medicines with complicated dosing instructions or a patient alert card. In certain cases, these additional communication measures may be required as part of a formal Risk Minimization Plan in the EU or risk evaluation and mitigation strategy (REMS) in the US.

Regulatory agencies have also been engaging in increasing efforts to communicate the risks of medicines. FDA's primary tool for communicating important new and emerging safety information about a medicine is through a Drug Safety Communication or DSC. In the EU, the competent regulatory authorities communicate drug safety information using different methods, which depend upon what has been established for the individual country. The European Medicines Agency (EMA) plays a central role in coordinating the communications.

### Additional Risk Minimization Strategies

A variety of other minimization strategies can be employed when product labeling and other forms of risk communication are not sufficient. In the US, FDA reviews proposed proprietary names of medicinal products to ensure that these names are not similar in spelling or pronunciation to the proprietary or established names of other medicines. In addition, FDA reviews the proposed container labels, carton labeling, packaging, and product design to ensure that these do not have features that could cause or contribute to medication errors. Similarly, in the EU, medicines authorized through the centralized procedure have their invented (or brand) name approved by the (invented) name review group who checks that there are no products licensed with similar names in the EU, which could lead to confusion. The layout, format, and wording on the immediate and outer packaging of the product are also reviewed as part of the evaluation procedure of the medicine and these form part of the authorization.

There are a variety of other strategies that can be used to mitigate risks associated with a medicine. For health care providers, this might include specialized training or materials that facilitate discussions between health care providers and patients about the risks and safe use of medicine such as prescriber-patient agreements. For teratogenic medications, these may include strategies to prevent fetal exposure to a medicine, including required pregnancy testing prior to prescribing or dispensing the medicine to individuals that could become pregnant, as well as contraceptive counseling. Some medicines may require patient monitoring or periods of observation by a healthcare professional after administration or it may require that a medicine is administered in a certain type of healthcare setting that is equipped to manage the serious adverse event.

In the EU and the US, a controlled distribution system may be used to minimize an important risk. The patients' access to the medicine in such a system is contingent on fulfilling strict requirements before the medicinal product is used. Since a controlled access program has large implications for all stakeholders, the use of these types of programs are generally limited and are guided by a clear therapeutic need for the product based on its demonstrated benefit, the nature of the associated risk, and the likelihood that this risk can be managed by such program.

### Evaluation of Risk Minimization and Mitigation Measures

Evaluation of risk minimization and mitigation activities is a critical component of a risk management system; this aims to ensure that the objectives of the risk mitigation measures are fulfilled and that the activities in place are proportionate. Such evaluation is closely related to the risk assessment activities, but it also differs in the way that enables modifica-

tions of the initial measures, if warranted, to improve the risk minimization strategy in the context of an iterative process of evaluation, correction, and re-evaluation throughout the lifecycle of a medicinal product.

In the EU, the pharmacovigilance legislation explicitly requires the active monitoring of the outcome of risk minimization activities. In the US, the metrics of a REMS assessment plan is approved in advance of REMS implementation, and assessment reports are submitted by the manufacturers at pre-defined intervals and additionally, if needed.

The following principles apply to measuring the effectiveness of risk minimization:

- Robust risk minimization evaluation is longitudinal in nature.
- A multi-faceted assessment is needed for a comprehensive risk minimization evaluation. There are some key elements aimed to evaluate the implementation of the risk minimization, such as:
  1) enablers and barriers for optimal program delivery and success.
  2) stakeholders' knowledge, attitudes and perception of risk.
  3) intended and observed clinical behavior.
- Safety outcome data define the ultimate success of a risk minimization program.
- The unintended consequences of a risk minimization measures should be taken into account.

First, evaluation of risk mitigation activities can assess if risk mitigation recommendations are being followed (e.g. the proportion of patients who receive the required information, are aware of it, or using the tools provided). This can be measured using target audience surveys or via proxy indicators such as healthcare professionals' requests for refills of consumable tools (e.g. checklists and forms).

Second, the evaluation can focus on understanding of the purpose of the risk minimization tools and their key messages (e.g. the proportion of correct responses in a test on such risk minimization tools). Scientifically rigorous survey methods should be applied; comprehensive guidelines for research are available in published literature.

Next, the evaluation can determine if recommended behaviors are being followed (e.g. if patients that have read the information they are given, do the specific actions the information recommends). Questionnaire-based surveys are not well suited to assess behavioral modification because they rely on the respondent's self-reporting, which have a large impact on the validity of the study findings. Therefore, this evaluation could rely on time-trends analyses of data from electronic medical records.

The ultimate measures of success of a risk minimization program are the safety outcomes. This evaluation can demonstrate whether the introduction of a risk mitigation strategy leads to a decrease in frequency or the severity of the adverse events. Incidence rates or cumulative incidence are most appropriate to be used, while reporting rates should only be used with caution (e.g. for rare events), due to the well-known underreporting. The incidence of the adverse events can be evaluated in cohort studies using information from healthcare databases or registries. Disease registries may be more suitable to evaluate the risk minimization measures as they may contain comparator groups, which could provide background rates for the events.

It is also important, while challenging, to identify potential barriers to patient access to the medicine related to the risk minimization strategies (e.g. providers in the patient's area may choose not to prescribe the drug because they may be unwilling to follow the risk minimization recommendations).

Pharmaceutical manufacturers usually fund and/or conduct the evaluations of risk mitigation strategies, and regulators review the results of those evaluations. In some instances, regulators may conduct independent assessments of drug safety.

## Methodological Problems to be Addressed by Pharmacoepidemiologic Research

### The Roles of Pharmacoepidemiology in Risk Management

Pharmacoepidemiology can play several roles in risk management. The most fundamental role is to identify and quantify the risks of a medicine using a variety of pharmacoepidemiologic techniques, including clinical trials, spontaneous reports, case series, and observational pharmacoepidemiologic studies. Use of these techniques for risk assessment is described in Parts I and II of this book.

An important use of pharmacoepidemiology is to measure how medications are used in practice, especially if they are used under conditions that can lead to adverse outcomes. Examples of pharmacoepidemiologic findings that could signal that a product is not being used appropriately include a finding that a medication is being prescribed concomitantly with a contraindicated medication, a finding that a drug is being used in a population of patients for whom the potential benefits do not outweigh the potential risks, and a finding that a medication is frequently prescribed for a duration of treatment that is associated with an increased risk of serious adverse events. For these analyses, drug utilization databases, electronic medical record systems, and other administrative healthcare data, especially those with longitudinal patient-level data, are often useful.

A third application of pharmacoepidemiology is to provide population-based assessments of the causes and contexts in which known harm from medications can occur. For these analyses, one or more public health databases may be helpful to estimate the burden of a given drug-related toxicity in the population. Because they are designed for the public health purposes of quantifying health and harm in society, projected national level estimates are often available. They are especially useful for characterizing and quantifying known drug risk, rather than identifying new risks.

A fourth emerging role of pharmacoepidemiology in the field of risk management is the assessment of risk mitigation efforts. For an effective evaluation, the risk mitigation activity must have a clearly defined goal that is relevant and measurable. Goals that are based on vague or imprecise metrics generally cannot be measured, and even if they are measurable, interpretations of the findings would be difficult. As noted above, assessing the effectiveness of a risk mitigation strategy can be conducted at several levels, including processes, behaviors, and health outcomes. While the traditional methods of pharmacoepidemiology may be used to assess the observed behavior and health outcomes, it is quite likely that additional methods, such as those used in social sciences and health policy and management fields, may be needed to assess process and behavior. It is important to understand the relationship between each component of the risk mitigation strategy and the desired health outcomes. It is possible that practitioners and patients adhere to the processes and exhibit the behaviors desired by the risk mitigation strategy, but that the health outcome of interest is not improved or is difficult to measure. Alternatively, it is possible that practitioners and patients do not adhere to the processes or exhibit the desired behaviors, but the desired health outcome (e.g. a reduction in the specific risk) is achieved, perhaps because of other interventions or factors that were not part of the risk mitigation strategy. In either case, a critical examination of the risk mitigation strategy would be necessary.

Another role for pharmacoepidemiology is in the area of assessing risk communication. Approaches may include a survey of patients' and healthcare providers' understanding of the risks and safe use of a medicine. Other approaches may include focus groups, questionnaires, interviews, and other methods used to assess readability and/or understanding.

## Examples of Currently Available Solutions

In both the US and the EU, specific legislation has been enacted to formalize managing the risks of medicines. The legal and regulatory frameworks in each of these jurisdictions are beyond the scope of this chapter. In the US, the legislation specifies that FDA can require a REMS when certain criteria are met. In the EU, a Risk Management Plan (RMP) is required for all medicinal products. Despite their differences, REMS and RMPs share the common features of being able to use, as appropriate, and allowed by law or regulation, communication to patients, communication to healthcare professionals, and certain restrictions to manage the risks of medicines. In the US, it is required that REMS be assessed to ensure that they are meeting their goals. In the EU, measuring the effectiveness of risk minimization activities and interventions is included in the definition of a risk management system.

## The Future

Managing the risk of medicinal products is an evolving area involving multiple stakeholders in the complex medication use system.

One critical area for future development is to continue to improve the way risk mitigation activities are being implemented. Many of the risk mitigation tools have relied in whole or in part on communicating a risk associated with a medicinal product to increase the stakeholders' awareness and knowledge. The goal being that awareness of a particular risk will impart knowledge and influence prescribing practices of the medicinal product or how the practitioners will monitor patients once treatment with the product has begun.

Risk management plans are designed to work within a complex medication use system. A current challenge for risk management systems is that they be developed in ways that can integrate, with minimal difficulty, into the current medication use systems and in a manner that is least burdensome for healthcare providers. Risk mitigation strategies that require documentation of safe use conditions need refinement. A future challenge is to develop a quality systems approach to implementing this type of risk mitigation strategy in a manner that is seamless for practitioners and within the scope of their usual clinical practice.

Another area for future refinement is to continue to gather evidence of the impact of risk mitigation strategies. Measurement of this impact is important, because it allows policy makers and other stakeholders to determine if the goals of the strategy are being met. The challenges for this field include developing models to relate risk mitigation strategies to health outcomes, as well as ways to identify the contribution of individual components of the strategy to the overall outcome. A further challenge is to assess if there are negative consequences of risk mitigation strategies.

---

**Case Example 23.6    For Pharmacoepidemiology and Risk Management**

*Risk Management Example in the EU – Bupropion/Naltrexone (Mysimba)*

*Background*
Bupropion/naltrexone (Mysimba) was authorized in the EU in March 2015. Mysimba is a medicine used together with diet and exercise to treat obesity; it can also be given to very overweight patients who have weight-related complications.

*Issue*
The main safety and tolerability concerns were related to central nervous system, gastrointestinal adverse events, and longer-term cardiovascular outcomes. Both additional pharmacovigilance and risk minimization activities were required.

*Approach*
*Additional pharmacovigilance activities*: The manufacturer agreed to conduct two phase-4 randomized clinical trials, evaluating major adverse cardiovascular events, a drug utilization study, and a physician survey, looking at the real-world use and the potential off-label use.

*Risk minimization activities*: The main risk minimization strategy was to prevent Mysimba use by patients with an increased risk of seizures and suicide. In addition to the SmPC, a Physician Prescribing checklist was implemented to help:

- use Mysimba only as approved, considering any risk factors
- consider concomitant conditions when evaluating individual risk–benefit balance, before the treatment decision.

*Results*
Post-marketing, a review of all data for hepatotoxicity led to regulatory actions: product information recommendations updates. The additional risk minimization activities continued, with re-evaluation planned integrating results from the drug utilization study and physician survey.

*Strengths*
The comprehensive set of actions addressed limitations in safety data at approval and managed identified risks. Additional data collected, including spontaneous reporting, informed further regulatory decisions in an iterative process.

*Limitations*
Additional activities focus on most important risks of the product considering the limited time available to prescribers in the treatment act, as well as striking a balance between the need to know more and what is reasonable to request from a manufacturer.

## Key Points for Risk Management

- The risks of a medicine derive both from its inherent pharmacological properties as well as from the way the medicine is used.
- Because the risks of medicines can occur at any point in the complex medication use system, managing the risks of medicines requires that the entire medication use system be involved.
- Risk management is an iterative process involving multiple, related activities that proceed throughout the product's lifecycle.
- Risk mitigation refers to a set of activities designed to minimize the risks of a medicine while preserving its benefits.
- Risk communication is an important component of risk management.
- It is critical that risk management activities be evaluated.

# The Pharmacoepidemiology of Medication Errors

Medications are the most commonly used form of medical therapy today. For adults, about 75% of office visits to GP and internists are associated with the continuation or initiation of a drug, while in the hospital multiple medication orders tend to be written for each patient daily. Medication errors have been defined as "any error in the process of ordering, dispensing, or administering a drug" regardless of whether an injury occurred or the potential for injury was present. Mechanistically, medication errors are triggered from errors in planning actions (i.e. knowledge-based mistakes or rule-based mistakes) or errors in executing correctly planned actions (i.e. action-based slips or memory-based lapses). In clinical practice, a medication error may occur at any stage of drug therapy, including drug prescribing, transcribing, manufacturing, dispensing, administering, and monitoring. Medication errors with potential for harm are called near-misses or potential

adverse drug event (ADE), and these errors may be intercepted before they reach the patient, or may reach the patient without consequence. However, a small fraction of medication errors indeed reaches the patient and result in patient harm, typically described as an ADE. An ADE would be considered preventable if a medication error is associated with the ADE.

Given the prevalence of prescription medication use, it is not surprising that preventable ADE are one of the most frequent types of preventable iatrogenic injuries. The IOM report, *To Err Is Human* suggested at least 44 000–98 000 deaths in the US are from iatrogenic injury. If accurate, this would mean that there are about 8000 deaths yearly from ADE and 1 million injuries from drug use.

## Safety Theory

One prominent theory for human errors that also applies for medicine was promoted by James Reason. He differentiated the person approach from the system approach for which he made use of the image of the Swiss cheese ("Swiss cheese model"). In the Swiss cheese model, a system has set in place several barriers, defenses and safeguards – pictured as cheese slices – that should prevent errors. However, every defense has its shortcomings ("holes in the cheese"), which is why there are usually several combined, and under unfavorable circumstances, the barriers might fail altogether, allowing an error to arise and slip through the defenses. Hence, Reason emphasizes, that an error likely always results from "active failures and latent conditions." Over the years, this model has been adopted and refined for specific situations in medicine, e.g. for administration errors. In summary, it highlights that although "human errors" occur commonly, the true cause of accidents is often the underlying systems that allow a person error to result in an accident. *Root cause* analysis can be used to define the cause of the defect. Only relatively infrequently are individuals responsible for clusters of errors, and, most often, errors resulting in harm are made by workers whose overall work is good. To make the hospital a safer place, a key initial step is to eliminate the culture of blame, and instead build a culture of safety. Errors and adverse outcomes should be treated as opportunities for improving the process of care through system changes, rather than a signal to begin disciplinary proceedings.

Indeed, systems changes for reducing errors can greatly reduce the likelihood of error, and probably in turn, of adverse outcomes. Within medicine, much of the research has come from anesthesia, which has made major improvements in safety. Examples of successful systems changes in medication delivery include implementation of safer working conditions that allow for concentrate and efficient work (e.g. staffing, facilities) but also implementation of system changes by use of information technology such as computerized physician order entry (CPOE), clinical decision support systems (CDSS), unit dosing, barcoding of medications, and implementation of "smart pumps" that can recognize what medication is being delivered. These technologies can track medication use, and more importantly, the frequencies and types of warnings as they alarm.

Overall, the area of safety has a different philosophy and several different tools than classic epidemiology. For improving safety, culture is extremely important, and tools such as root cause analysis and failure mode and effects analysis – which can be used to project what the problems with a process may be before they occur – are highly valuable. When combined with epidemiologic data, such tools may be extremely powerful for improving the safety of care.

## Patient Safety Concepts as Applied to Pharmacoepidemiology

While pharmacoepidemiology techniques have most often been used to study the risks and benefits of drugs, they can also be used to study medication errors and preventable ADEs (i.e. those due to errors). Approaches to detecting medication errors include manual or automatic screening of claims data, administrative databases, medical records, electronic health records, incident reports mostly by providers in hospitals, patient monitoring, direct observation often by pharmacists, and spontaneous (self-reporting) approaches. All of these approaches have inherent advantages and pitfalls and there is no single approach that is considered the gold standard for detecting medication errors or ADEs. Factors which might influence the identification of medication errors and ADEs include the setting (ambulatory vs inpatients; routine care vs research studies), the expected types of medication errors (prescribing vs administration errors), and the projected costs of detection. In addition, the type of detection method influences which types of medication errors are found (e.g. only those resulting in patient harm) and with which frequency.

Screening of claims data, administrative databases, medical records, and electronic health records is used to evaluate large data sets, but is generally done retrospectively. The quality of the available information, however, varies between different data sources (see Chapters 8, 9, and 10) which restricts opportunities to comprehensively detect medication errors, more of some types than others. Especially in the outpatient setting, claims data can be obtained for very large numbers of individuals. Weaknesses include that it cannot be determined with certainty whether or not the patient actually consumed the medication, and, if not linked to other information sources, clinical detail is often limited (e.g. information on weight or renal function but also information on dosage is typically missing), making it hard to answer questions that relate to a patient's clinical condition.

In the inpatient setting, manual chart review is a well-established method to detect ADEs and medication errors. With most relevant patient information at hand, the appropriateness of drug prescribing and administration can be assessed, although documentation may still be incomplete, especially for assessing issues such as appropriateness. The main problems with chart review are that it is time-consuming and expensive. When electronic health records are in place, the manual screening of paper-based information can be replaced by semi-automated approaches. The level of standardization and the extent to which clinical information is stored by using controlled vocabulary determines the feasibility and effectiveness of automated, algorithm-based data analyses of ADEs and medication errors.

When electronic health records include electronic prescribing applications with clinical decision support, data from these applications can readily be used to detect many types of medication errors at the stage of prescribing. However, the specificity of these systems will also depend on the availability of information accessible via the electronic health records.

Spontaneous reporting (self-reported) of medication errors is comparatively easy to be set in place and to maintain, both in inpatient and outpatient settings. However, both ADEs, medication errors and also critical incidents (i.e. near misses) are substantially underreported (see also Chapter 7). This may be due to the fact that a certain situation must first be recognized and evaluated as an incident, that reporting takes time, and that despite a nonpunitive policy of the hospital, reporting is feared to be associated with disciplinary actions. Thus, spontaneous reporting is useful for getting samples of errors and learning about error etiology, but cannot be used to assess the underlying rate of medication errors in a sample. However, patient monitoring using their self-reporting for ADEs has been successful, and can identify more ADEs than chart review.

Direct observation is primarily done during research studies at inpatient sites and offers a comprehensive assessment of medication dispensing and administration errors. While being both cost and personnel intensive, direct observation has been successfully and reliably used to classify complex medication errors, and it is particularly useful at stages that are not sensitive to other detection methods (e.g. drug preparation and drug administration).

Many of the early medication error and ADE studies were performed in the hospital setting. In the inpatient adult setting, patients are vulnerable to medication errors because of the severity of their illness, the complexity of their disease process and medication regimens, and at times because of their age (e.g. the elderly are particularly susceptible). In pediatric drug use, the system-based factors that may contribute to a higher rate of near misses include the need for weight-based dosing and dilution of stock medicines, as well as decreased communication abilities of young children.

Knowledge about errors in the ambulatory setting is increasing (see Case Example 23.7), although research lags behind the inpatient setting due to the difficulties of accessing patients once they leave a doctor's office. Increasingly, pharmacies are used for medication safety studies, and a lot of research has been done about errors at the point of transition from hospitals to ambulatory settings and vice versa. Overall, comparisons among studies are challenging because of variations in data quality and methodology.

Of note, it is important to acknowledge that while every setting has its particular risk for medication errors, new risks might also arise when new systems or processes are implemented in a specific environment. Hence, while it is the obvious motivation of implementation of medication safety strategies to mitigate the risk of medication errors, one must bear in mind that also new errors might become evident due to new risks.

## Clinical Problems to be Addressed by Pharmacoepidemiologic Research

Medication errors can occur at any stage of the medication use process, including prescribing, transcribing, dispensing, administering, and

---

**Case Example 23.7    For the Use of Pharmacoepidemiology to Study Medication Errors**

*Background*

Most of the data on the frequency of adverse drug events have come from the inpatient setting, and many outpatient studies have relied on chart review or claims data to detect ADEs. Gandhi's 2003 study on the frequency of adverse drug events in a community-living population used a different approach.

*Issue*

The goal of the study was to assess the frequency of adverse drug events in an ambulatory primary care population.

*Approach*

The frequency of adverse drug events was assessed by calling patients after a visit at which medications were prescribed, to determine whether or not an adverse drug event had occurred, and in addition to review the chart at three months.

*Results*

- Adverse drug events occurred at a rate of 20.9 per 100 patients.
- About eight times as many adverse drug events were identified by calling patients as by reviewing charts.
- While the severity of the ADEs overall was fairly low, about a third were preventable, and 6% were both serious and preventable.

*Strengths*

The key strength of this approach was that, by calling patients, it was possible to identify many adverse drug events that were not noted in the chart.

*Limitations*

The key weakness of this approach is that many of the effects patients attributed to their medications may not have been due to the medications at all, but due to other things such as their underlying conditions. The authors attempted to address this by asking the patient's physician in each instance whether they believed the symptoms related to the medication.

*Key points*

- Calling patients – though expensive and time-consuming – identifies many adverse drug events that are not identified through chart review.
- Almost none of the visits was associated with an ICD-9 code suggesting the presence of an ADE, suggesting that claims data should not be used to estimate the frequency of ADEs of all types in the outpatient setting.
- More work is needed to facilitate assessment of whether a specific patient complaint is related to a medication.

---

monitoring. Of these stages, prescribing errors in the hospital have been documented to cause the most harm, although errors at any stage can do so, and monitoring errors (i.e. errors caused by lack of proper monitoring) are quite prominent outside the hospital. The greater proportion of harmful errors at the drug prescribing stage may be a consequence of the data collection methods employed in these studies, which were multipronged but excluded direct observation, the most sensitive technique for administration error detection.

Important types of errors include dosing, route, frequency, drug-allergy, drug–drug interaction, drug–laboratory (including renal dosing), drug–patient characteristic, and drug administration during pregnancy. Although these errors occur most frequently at the drug ordering stage, they can occur at any stage in the medication use process.

In several studies, *dosing errors* have represented the most frequent category. To determine whether or not a dosing error is present, most often some clinical context is needed, for example the patient's age, gender, weight, level of renal function, prior response to the medication (if it has been used previously), response to other similar medications, clinical condition, and often the indication for the therapy. While many of these data elements can be obtained from review of the medical chart, many are not typically available from claims data alone.

*Administration errors* also represent a common type of error. Many drugs can be given by one or a few routes and not by many others. Some such errors – such as giving benzathine penicillin that contains suspended solids intravenously instead of intramuscularly – would often be fatal, and though they have caused fatalities, are fortunately very rare. Other route errors – such as grinding up a sustained released preparation (which can negate the slow release properties of the drug) to give it via a tube – are much more frequent, and can have serious consequences. Route errors are especially problematic at the administration stage of the medication use process and often happen in the context of patient-administered drugs. Unfortunately, administration errors are both difficult to detect and much less often intercepted than prescribing errors.

*Frequency errors* can occur either at the prescribing, dispensing, or administration stage. While these errors probably cause less harm cumulatively than dose or route errors, they can be problematic. Some frequency errors at the prescribing or dispensing stage can be detected even with claims or prescription data. Such errors have greater potential for harm when drugs are given with a greater frequency than intended. However, the therapeutic benefit may not be realized when given with too low frequency, and extremely negative effects can occur for some drugs, for example with antiretrovirals, to which resistance develops if they are given at a low frequency.

*Allergy errors* represent a particularly serious type of error, even though most of the time when a drug is given to a patient with a known allergy, the patient does well. Allergy errors typically cannot be detected with claims data, since allergy information on patients is not available. Thus, these errors have to be detected either through chart review, which is laborious, or more often through electronic medical record data.

*Drug–drug interaction exposures* represent an interesting and difficult area, both for research and interventions, to decrease errors. While many interactions have been reported, the severity varies substantially from minor to life-threatening. If a conscious decision is made to give patients two medications despite the knowledge that they may interact, this cannot be considered an error except in very limited circumstances, for example with meperidine and monoamine oxidase inhibitors. Also, it is legitimate to give many medications together despite clear interactions with important consequences if there are no good alternatives, or if dose alterations are made, or if additional monitoring is carried out (for example, with warfarin and many antibiotics). However, the necessary alterations in dosing or additional monitoring are often omitted, which can have severe consequences. It is possible in large claims data sets to detect situations in which simultaneous exposures appear to have occurred, but not possible to determine if this actually occurred, as a physician may give patients instructions to cease the use of one of the drugs.

*Drug–laboratory errors* (e.g. monitoring of potassium) represent an important category of errors, but can be difficult to detect electronically because of poor interfaces between laboratory and pharmacy information. Such errors are relatively straight-forward to identify when large pharmacy and laboratory databases can be linked, although again assessment of clinical outcomes is difficult unless these data are also available.

*Renal dosing errors* represent a specific subtype of drug–laboratory errors and are especially important; these errors can also be and often are considered dosing errors. In one large inpatient study (Chertow et al. 2001), nearly

40% of inpatients had at least mild renal insufficiency, and there are many medications that require dosing adjustment in the presence of decreased glomerular filtration. In that study, without clinical decision support, patients received the appropriate dose and frequency of medication only 30% of the time.

Many studies of drug–patient characteristic checking have focused on the use of medications in the presence of specific diseases. However, in the future, genomic testing will undoubtedly dominate, as many genes have profound effects on drug metabolism (see Chapter 14). Currently, few large data sets can be linked with genotype information, but this is becoming increasingly frequent in clinical trials and a number of cohorts are being established as well.

## Methodological Problems to be Addressed by Pharmacoepidemiologic Research

### Information Bias

In performing drug analyses, the present conventions preclude the determination of total daily dose in several ways. Physicians may prescribe a greater amount of medicine than is required for the time period prescribed. For example, if a patient requires 50 mg of atenolol per day, the doctor may actually write a prescription for 100 mg of atenolol per day and verbally convey instructions to the patient to divide the pills. This is particularly problematic with drugs that must be titrated to the appropriate therapeutic dose (e.g. warfarin). If either physicians or pharmacists were required to document an accurate total daily dose, this would improve the ability to perform research.

Another important methodological issue is measurement of patient adherence to medications (see also Chapter 20). Since prescribing and dispensing data are seldom jointly available, determining patient adherence is extremely difficult. Improving clinician access to data from pharmacy benefit managers might be very useful, as might availability of electronic prescription data to pharmacies.

Many medications are contraindicated in pregnancy. Here, the greatest difficulty for the investigator is assessing whether or not the patient is actually pregnant at the time of the exposure, although this can be assessed retrospectively by identifying the date of birth, assuming a term pregnancy, and then working backward. The outcomes of interest are often not represented in ways that make it easy to perform analyses, although data on medication exposures and on births are readily available and can often be linked.

Another important piece of clinical information for pediatrics is a child's weight. Most pediatric medications are dosed on the basis of weight. Standardized documentation of this information is unavailable, hindering not only analyses of pediatric dosing but also actual dosing by pediatricians.

A final issue is the coding of allergies. It is important for both clinical care and research that allergies are differentiated from sensitivities or intolerances through codes rather than free text. Continued drug use in the presence of drug sensitivity may be perfectly appropriate, whereas the same treatment in the presence of an allergy is likely an error. It is particularly important that severe reactions, such as anaphylaxis, are clearly coded and identifiable in the medical records. New allergies need to be captured in better ways. The eventual aim is to have one universal allergy list in an electronic format for each patient, rather than multiple disparate lists.

### Sample Size Issues

Sample sizes are often small in medication error and ADE studies if direct observation is used as detection method (high costs of data collection). Electronic databases will be an important tool to improve sample sizes in a cost effective manner. Computerized physician order entry systems, electronic health records, test result viewing systems, computerized pharmacy systems, bar-coding systems, pharmacy benefit managers, and claims systems will all be important sources of such data.

There will be important regulatory issues that will need to be addressed before actual construction and use of these systems.

### Generalizability

Many existing medication error studies have limited generalizability due to setting or methods. For example, many studies have been performed in tertiary care academic hospital settings. It is unclear how findings from this setting translate to other settings. Also, methodologies vary widely from study to study, hindering comparisons.

### The Future

The future of pharmacoepidemiologic research will include large databases that allow linking of prescription information with clinical and claims data. These types of databases will facilitate the studies of medication errors and ADEs. They will also be critical for detecting rare ADEs. Sources of data for these databases will include systems of computerized physician order entry, computerized pharmacy, barcoding, pharmacy benefit managers, and electronic health records. Standardized coding of data, that is, the uniform coding of drug names, as well as doses and concentrations, will be an important advancement to allow easy analysis.

Other important issues that must be addressed are representing prescriptions in ways that allow determination of total daily dose, joint documentation of prescriptions and dispensing data to allow determination of patient adherence, clear documentation of conditions like pregnancy or weights of pediatric patients, and improved coding of allergies.

### Key Points for the Pharmacoepidemiology of Medication Errors

- Medication errors are very common, compared to adverse drug events, and relatively few result in injury.

- In most studies, about one to two third of adverse drug events are preventable.
- The epidemiology of medication errors and adverse drug events has been fairly well described for hospitalized adults, but less information is available for specific populations, and for the ambulatory setting.
- It is possible now to detect many medication errors using large claims databases, and as it becomes possible to link these data with more types of clinical data including especially laboratory and diagnosis data, it will be feasible to more accurately assess the frequency of medication errors across populations.
- The increasing use of electronic health records potentially linked to data collected from wearables should have a dramatic effect on our ability to do research in this area using pharmacoepidemiologic techniques.

# Benefit–Risk Assessments of Medical Treatments

### Introduction

Assessing the benefit–risk (B-R) balance of medical treatments has always been an integral part of drug development, regulatory, and public health decisions. However, methodology and regulatory policies for B-R have advanced considerably in the last decade. Advancements include the application of structured B-R frameworks and consideration of the patient perspective in regulatory submissions and review. In parallel, numerous B-R initiatives have been led by pharmaceutical and device trade organizations, patient advocacy groups, public–private partnerships, and academic groups.

While definitions vary, benefit–risk is generally defined as weighing the benefits of a treatment against its harms for its expected use. The term "risk" is ambiguous in the field of benefit–risk and may refer to the general nature of the harmful effect, its frequency, its severity or a combination of these concepts. To lessen this ambiguity, the terms "harm" or "unfavorable effect" and the analogs of "benefit" or "favorable effect" are used, however, the phrase "benefit-risk" is still used due to its ubiquity. The goals for benefit–risk assessments vary. Examples include go/no-go decisions by a medical product development company, reviews by Institutional Review Boards and data monitoring committees, regulatory reviews by a health authority, reconsideration of a treatment after gaining new information post-approval, and therapeutic decisions by clinicians and patients. B-R assessments are applied to pharmaceuticals, vaccines and medical devices, and consumer health products, and they are a critical component of point-of-care decision making by a patient and physician.

## Clinical Problems to be Addressed by Pharmacoepidemiologic Research

### Systematic Approach to B-R Assessment

Varying approaches to B-R assessment have been used, resulting in considerable differences in the depth, transparency, and clarity of the assessment. What has emerged in recent years is the use of structured, framework approaches to rationally and defensibly frame, conduct and communicate a B-R assessment. We describe these frameworks and their application.

### Incorporating the Patient Perspective

Traditionally, the judgments required in the design and conduct of clinical research have been the province of physicians, scientists, and regulators. Increasingly, regulatory agencies, patient advocacy groups and industry have advocated for patient engagement. While the idea of patient-focused benefit–risk is well-accepted, the challenge is to determine what information should be obtained from patients, how it should be obtained, and how it can be used. There are numerous techniques for

assessing the patient perspective, ranging from qualitative focus groups and structured interviews through quantitative preference studies. We address patient preference studies and their application in B-R decision making.

## Methodological Problems to be Addressed by Pharmacoepidemiologic Research

Methods for gathering, synthesizing, and communicating a B-R assessment based on available data are the key tools for decision-making.

### Identifying Appropriate Data for Benefit–Risk Assessment

The considerations for data source selection and good pharmacoepidemiology practices apply to B-R assessment. Data for B-R assessment come from a variety of sources including randomized controlled trials (see Chapter 17), spontaneous reports and observational data sources (see Part II Sources of Pharmacoepidemiologic Data, Chapters 7–11). When there are multiple data sources, this can result in discordant findings, differences in outcome definitions and ascertainment, important differences between populations, and different treatment comparators. The validity in identifying and characterizing the important benefits and harms must be carefully evaluated through assessment of confounding, bias, study design, and generalizability. The principles for choosing among the available data sources in pharmacoepidemiology are discussed in Chapter 12. The validity of exposure and diagnostic data is further discussed in Chapter 13. Design-based and analytic approaches to adjust for confounding and bias in observational studies are discussed in Chapter 22.

### Integrating Benefits and Risks

Synthesizing the evidence in a structured manner is challenging. Typical research studies can have multiple efficacy and safety endpoints of interest. Some outcomes may favor one treatment, while others may favor the comparator. Approaches that integrate benefits and harms should be sufficiently inclusive to account for the frequency, clinical impact and uncertainty of potentially many benefits and harms considered under multiple conditions including important patient subgroups.

### Communicating Benefit–Risk Assessment

Communicating information about the benefits and risk of medicines is central to both B-R assessment and risk management. This can be challenging due to its complexity and the diversity of stakeholders who will receive this information. Structured B-R frameworks improve the ability to communicate in a clear and consistent manner.

### Currently Available Solutions

#### Structured Approaches to B-R : B-R Frameworks

The most significant recent advance in B-R has been the introduction of B-R frameworks. B-R frameworks are a set of principles, processes and tools to guide decision-makers in selecting, organizing, analyzing and communicating evidence for B-R decisions. Frameworks lead to transparency, consistency and discipline in B-R decisions.

There are several well-known B-R frameworks: the FDA B-R framework, the Pharmaceutical Research and Manufacturers of America Benefit–Risk Action Team (BRAT) framework, the Multi-criteria Decision Analysis (MCDA) framework suggested by EMA for complex B-R decisions, and the framework embedded in the International Council for Harmonisation's (ICH) PSUR/PBRER and Clinical Overview templates. While the frameworks differ in focus and methodology, they share many steps similar to those in the BRAT framework presented in Table 23.2.

Given the ubiquity of B-R frameworks and their incorporation into the regulatory guidance, we structure this currently available solutions section based on these framework steps.

**Table 23.2** Steps in the BRAT benefit–risk framework.

| Step | Definition |
| --- | --- |
| 1) Define decision context | Summarize the nature of disease, medical need for treatment, disease and treatment epidemiology, study treatment, dose/formulation, indication(s), patient population, critical subgroups, comparator(s), time horizon for outcomes, relevant decision-making bodies. |
| 2) Identify and define outcomes | Identify and define all important outcomes, define a preliminary set of measures for each outcome, document rationale for outcomes to be included and excluded. |
| 3) Identify and summarize source data | Determine and document all data sources, extract raw data, summarize over data sources, assemble effects table. |
| 4) Customize the framework | Modify the outcome list and their definitions based on review of the data and clinical expertise. May include tuning of outcomes not considered relevant to a particular B-R assessment or stakeholder group. |
| 5) Assess importance of outcomes | If applicable, assess outcome clinical impact, weight or preferences from the perspective of patients, decision makers or other stakeholders. |
| 6) Integrated B-R assessment: analysis and visualization | Summarize data into tabular and graphical displays (e.g. effects table) to aid interpretation, identify and fill any information gaps, interpret summary information, potentially conduct sensitivity analyses to assess the impact of uncertainty on clinical or preference data. |
| 7) Expert judgment and communication | Render and communicate a decision. |

## Define Decision Context

The main role of the decision context is to ensure decision-makers are aligned on key elements of the assessment. Characterizing the severity of the disease and the medical need are particularly important, as the greater the severity or medical need, the more allowances typically may be made for treatment-related harms. These background elements are also an avenue for incorporating the patient perspective into B-R. The context forces up-front agreement on an appropriate comparator, dose and population, the choices of which are often not straightforward in post-approval contexts. For example, in post-approval settings, the most appropriate comparator may be the one used in recent clinical trials (e.g. placebo) or the standard of care or comparators available in claims or electronic health records.

Examples of decision contexts can be found in the FDA's "Voice of the Patient" reports and in recent drug approvals, searchable at https://www.accessdata.fda.gov/scripts/cder/daf.

## Identify and Define Outcomes

The second step of the BRAT B-R Framework is to identify and define the important outcomes; i.e. benefits, harms and other treatment properties. While studies measure many outcomes, some are highly correlated with each other or are causally dependent, some double-count events, and some have a wide range of clinical impacts. Generally, B-R requires identifying a smaller set of key outcomes that drive the assessment. A tool often used to select and depict the outcomes used in B-R is a value tree, a hierarchic graph in which outcomes are grouped by anatomic, functional or clinical impact (see Figure 23.1).

The value tree can be utilized to understand problems caused by the interrelationships between outcomes. Outcomes that are easily interpreted individually can be problematic when considered collectively for B-R. For example, in the Randomized Evaluation of Long-Term Anticoagulation Therapy (RE-LY) study, the pivotal trial of dabigatran for atrial

fibrillation, the primary efficacy outcome was stroke (ischemic or hemorrhagic) or systemic embolism, and the primary safety outcome was major bleeding. Major bleeding here was defined as the composite of fatal bleeding, symptomatic critical organ bleeding (e.g. hemorrhagic stroke, intracerebral hemorrhage), transfusions $\geq 2$ units packed red blood cells or whole blood, or hemoglobin drops $\geq 2$ g/dl. Fatal and non-fatal hemorrhagic stroke events are included in both the primary efficacy and safety outcomes. This double counting can lead to confusion, as some events will count as a both a benefit and a harm. Double counting also occurs between all-cause death and other efficacy outcomes, as strokes, myocardial infarctions and systemic emboli may be fatal. Counting these deaths twice can potentially distort the findings. Finally, major bleeding includes a mix of events that are fatal, cause irreversible harm or are transient without sequelae, yet each event is weighted equally in the composite outcome. This large range of clinical impacts under one outcome complicates the comparison between benefits and harm.

The value trees in Figure 23.1 show one way to resolve these issues. Figure 23.1a shows the key outcomes of a typical atrial fibrillation trial. Figure 23.1b includes the same events, but with ischemic events classified as benefits and hemorrhagic events classified as risks. This separation avoids double-counting occurring between benefits and harms. Additionally, efficacy outcomes are defined to avoid double-counting. Finally, benefits and harms are classified by whether they are fatal or generally result in irreversible harm. By separating the fatal and irreversible events from less impactful ones, a first pass at the B-R assessment can be made with clinically comparable benefits and harms, then less impactful events can be included (Figure 23.1b). In some cases, having multiple value trees can be helpful, particularly when different decision-makers have different views on which events are most important.

(a)

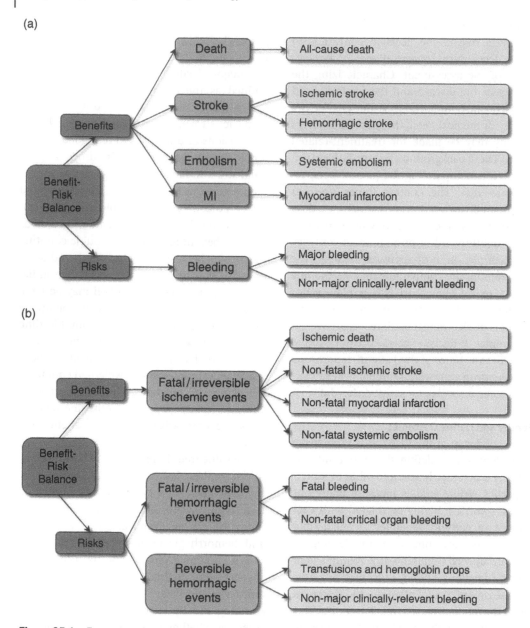

(b)

**Figure 23.1** Example value trees for treatment of atrial fibrillation. (a) Outcomes from a typical atrial fibrillation statistical analysis plan. (b) Modified value tree with one approach for benefit–risk assessment.

**Identify and Summarize Source Data**

Approaches for handling the choice of the database, study design, and analysis that apply to pharmacoepidemiology in general also apply to B-R assessment. The most robust data for B-R are from randomized controlled trials (see Chapter 17) and observational data sources (See Chapters 7–12), where the important outcomes from the value tree have been captured and where confounding and selection bias have been rigorously adjusted (see Chapter 22).

In medical product development, the main data sources are the pivotal clinical trials where the protocol and statistical analysis plan pre-specify the efficacy outcomes, populations and means for pooling data from multiple studies (see Chapter 17). Specific safety outcomes may be collected based on anticipated safety effects due to the mechanism of action (for example, bleeding events in an anticoagulant trial). Otherwise, there is passive collection and reporting of safety data (adverse events) by investigators.

Following a medical treatment's approval, data informing B-R accumulate in a larger sample of subjects in clinical practice and post-approval studies mainly through multiple observational sources. Post-approval studies are more likely to compare two or more active treatments and observational studies generally do not contain a placebo arm, unlike many randomized controlled trials for registration. Definitions of exposure and efficacy and safety outcomes in the observational settings are dependent upon the means of collection, and ascertainment may vary in quality and validity (See Chapter 13).

For the structured B-R assessment, the decisions on the inclusion or exclusion of studies should be based on a pre-specified analysis plan and documented for transparency in decision-making. If comparisons are made between effect estimates across studies or meta-analysis is considered (see Chapter 20), the extent to which study populations, definitions, study designs, and analysis approaches are comparable should be described including the potential for bias and confounding. This is particularly important in B-R given that multiple outcomes are assessed.

### Customize the Framework

After assessing source data, there may be a need to revisit the outcomes for B-R (Table 23.2, step 4). For example, new AEs may emerge or there may be differences between the outcomes of interest vs those available in the source data. In these cases, B-R assessment may require a revised set of outcomes.

Consider the value tree in Figure 23.1b. The outcomes in this tree require distinctions such as fatal vs non-fatal myocardial infarctions and

disabling vs transient major bleeds. If the available observational data sources cannot adequately measure these outcomes, the tree will need to be modified. In some cases, an algorithm can approximate a desired outcome. For example, principal hospital discharge diagnosis codes can be used to identify bleeding-related hospitalization and to differentiate upper and lower gastrointestinal bleeding. Another approach is to simplify the value tree to two composite outcomes, potential thromboembolic events and intracranial hemorrhage, both defined by ICD-10-CM or other medical codes. An advantage of this approach is a more intuitive interpretation of the study outcomes compared to a large value tree. Disadvantages are that the composite outcomes are mixtures of events with varying severity (ranging from fatal to transient with no sequelae) and there is the potential to miss important underlying differences between treatments.

### Assess Importance of Outcomes – Value Judgments and Patient Preferences

Step 5 of the BRAT framework (Table 23.2) is to assess the relative importance of the outcomes. Benefit–risk assessment is a combination of data-based probability assessment and value judgments. Statistical analyses provide the probability of events prevented and caused, but they do not indicate how important those events are to decision-makers, including patients. In B-R, these value judgments are typically called "weights" or "preferences."

Often, these value judgments are based on clinical judgment. FDA and EMA B-R assessments reflect this approach. For example, several FDA anticoagulant B-R assessments are similar to that described above, in which clinical judgment partitions events into two categories: events that are fatal or cause irreversible harm, and events that cause reversible harm. This partitioning gives two effective weights (roughly "high" and "low"). Similarly, the EMA's guidance on review of drug applications stresses the need to describe the value judgments used and notes that "a 'descriptive' approach with explicit considerations about the importance of the different effects and how trade-offs are weighed will generally be appropriate."

While most B-R problems can be assessed with clinical judgment, there are many that benefit from formal, rigorous studies to assess how patients weigh benefits and harms. These "patient preference studies" measure what attributes of a treatment are important to patients, the relative importance of these attributes, what tradeoffs between them patients would accept, and the heterogeneity of these results among patients. Preference studies are taking on increasing roles in pharmaceutical and medical device companies, patient groups and regulatory agencies. An increasing number of regulatory submissions include preference information, the FDA has issued guidance on roles for preference information in medical device reviews, and both the FDA and EMA are conducting preference studies. There are many methods to elicit patient preferences, ranging from qualitative interviews through quantitative surveys. Overviews of these methods are listed under Further Reading.

There have been numerous preference studies for anticoagulants, in both patients and other stakeholders. For example, in a preference survey for acute coronary syndrome, US patients regarded non-fatal disabling stroke as equal importance to death, or greater in importance to death in another survey, and they were willing to accept considerable probability of bleeding in exchange for reductions in the chance of death or disabling stroke. In addition to population averages, preference studies can measure heterogeneity in preferences. Some patients will be very tolerant of risks, while others will be very risk averse. Preference studies can measure how widely patients' preferences vary and whether there are distinct subgroups of patients with important difference in preferences.

While patient preference studies are increasingly popular for B-R applications, there are many unanswered questions on their use for regulatory applications. Ongoing initiatives to address them are described below.

### Putting it all Together – Integrated B-R Assessment

We discuss integrated B-R assessment and communicating the assessment, Steps 6 and 7 of the BRAT B-R framework (Figure 23.1), together.

There are numerous approaches to combining data on medical need, outcome data, uncertainty, clinical judgment, preferences, heterogeneity, etc. into a B-R assessment. Qualitative approaches use textual descriptive summaries to make a B-R argument. They are most applicable when the assessment is self-evident from the data, e.g. statistically significant benefit and no appreciable adverse events. Semi-quantitative approaches use a combination of tabular and graphical displays, potentially coupled with preference or weight information. Most B-R in regulatory applications is descriptive or semi-quantitative. Quantitative approaches compute summary metrics by combining the data and potentially preferences from multiple outcomes. These tend to be applied in the academic literature.

A common means to display B-R data is an effects table, which summarizes information on all key benefits and harms (Table 23.3). The columns vary, but may include the outcome name, a brief outcome definition and units, the outcome value for each treatment, estimates of between treatment differences (e.g. risk difference) with associated uncertainty (e.g. 95% confidence intervals), brief notes on strength of evidence and a link to data sources. While relative measures such as relative risk, odds ratio or hazards ratio can also be included, these measures are less useful for B-R. Because the baseline rates for outcomes may be disparate, a large relative risk may correspond to a very small absolute difference in the number of events when the baseline rate is low, while small relative risks may correspond to large

**Table 23.3** Effects table for atrial fibrillation (simulated data).

| Outcome | Event rate (/10 000 person-years) | | Rate difference / 10 000 person-years (95% CI) | NNT or NNH |
| --- | --- | --- | --- | --- |
| | Study drug | Comparator | | |
| **Efficacy** | | | | |
| Ischemic death, ischemic stroke, MI or systemic embolism | 430 | 512 | −87 (−143, −30) | −115 |
| Ischemic death | 189 | 221 | −34 (−72, 3) | −294 |
| Non-fatal ischemic stroke | 154 | 172 | −19 (−51, 13) | −526 |
| Non-fatal myocardial infarction | 83 | 100 | −17 (−43, 8) | −588 |
| Non-fatal systemic embolism | 4 | 20 | −16 (−26, −7) | −625 |
| **Safety** | | | | |
| Major bleeding | 398 | 345 | 49 (0, 99) | 204 |
| Fatal and critical organ bleeding | 119 | 125 | −6 (−33, 20) | −1667 |
| Fatal bleeding | 37 | 38 | −1 (−15, 13) | −10000 |
| Non-fatal critical site bleeding | 82 | 87 | −5 (−31, 21) | −2000 |
| Transfusions > = 2 units or Hbg drop >−2 gm/dl | 308 | 245 | 60 (17, 103) | 167 |
| Clinically relevant non-major bleeding | 1192 | 1137 | 44 (−50, 138) | 227 |

All outcomes are measured per 10 000 person-years. CI = confidence interval, MI = myocardial infarction, NNT = Number needed to treat, NNH = Number needed to harm. Positive NNTs or NNHs indicate more events on comparator. Negative NNTs or NNHs indicate more events on the study drug.

absolute differences when the baseline rate is high.

Table 23.3 shows an effects table for the atrial fibrillation value tree in Figure 23.1b. The data are simulated but realistic. All outcomes in the example presented are in person-year rates, though effects tables in general can include any type of risk or rate calculation and can show categorical or continuous outcomes. Because the incidence rate of most outcomes is low, the data are scaled to a hypothetical population (10 000 person-years) to simplify representation and comprehension of these data. The rate differences represent the additional number of events caused or prevented by using one treatment compared to another treatment with 10 000 person-years of exposure. With many outcomes considered in B-R, we generally show the 95% confidence interval as

a measure of uncertainty but not for statistical hypothesis testing. Number needed to treat (NNT) and number needed to harm (NNH) are also included in the table. NNT and NNH are calculated as the reciprocal of the corresponding rate differences. NNT (NNH) is interpreted as the number of person-years of exposure with a treatment vs the comparator needed to prevent (or cause) one additional harmful event. When comparing one benefit to one harm, NNT and NNH are often useful. However, when considering many outcomes at once, NNT and NNH are generally less helpful and can require complex mathematics and weights. Additionally, confidence intervals for NNT and NNH can be difficult to interpret when associations are not statistically significant. For these reasons, NNT and NNH have limited application in B-R assessment.

When considering the full set of outcomes, a forest plot of the rate differences in Table 23.3 is very helpful, particularly when communicating a B-R assessment (Figure 23.2). The interpretations of this effects table and forest plot are addressed in the case example.

### Weighting and the Patient Perspective

The integrated B-R approaches reviewed above used clinical judgment to make a defensible B-R decision. The example in Table 23.3 and Figure 23.2 lends itself to such approaches. When the B-R tradeoff is more complex; i.e. when some outcomes favor the study drug and other outcomes favor the comparator, weighting and preference assessments can be critical – both to incorporate the patient perspective and to make a B-R assessment.

There are numerous approaches by which the weighting or patient preferences can be incorporated into B-R. Graphic techniques show the clinical and preference data in unison. For example, the risk differences in

Figure 23.2 can sorted with the non-composite outcomes placed in order of decreasing weight. If the outcomes with largest weight all favor one treatment, benefits outweigh harms for that treatment. Another class of approaches are net clinical benefit (NCB) measures. While the terminology is not standard, we define NCB approaches as those that use a weighted sum of risk (or rate) differences between study drug and comparator to summarize the difference between treatments. Typically, beneficial events have positive weights and harmful events have negative weights. The larger the absolute value of the weight or the larger the risk difference for an outcome, the more that outcome contributes to NCB. Sensitivity analyses can be conducted on NCB measures, where distributions for the weights are propagated into uncertainty in the NCB result, allowing assessing more complex metrics such as the probability that benefit exceeds risk.

More general, and complex, approaches to B-R assessment include multi-criteria deci-

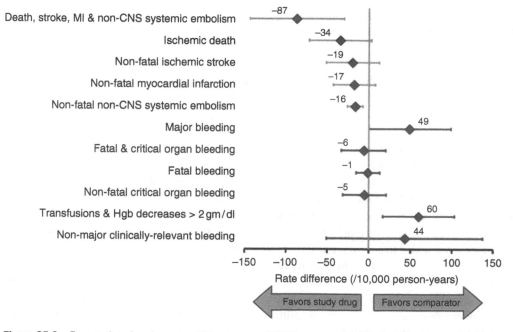

**Figure 23.2** Forest plot showing rate differences per 10 000 person-years for key benefits and harms in atrial fibrillation treatment (simulated data). Diamonds are points estimates. Bars show 95% confidence intervals. Efficacy outcomes are in orange. Safety outcomes are in green.

sion analysis and stochastic multi-criteria acceptability analysis, for which references are included under Further Reading. Finally, preference studies can be used to address the questions raised at the outset of this chapter– what probability of harm is acceptable in exchange for a given degree of benefit? A preference study can assess benefit–risk tradeoffs, such as the maximum acceptable risk, from the perspective of patients; i.e. the maximum probability or level of severity of a harm that a patient will accept in exchange for a given benefit. For example, in atrial fibrillation, in exchange for reducing the chance of non-fatal disabling stroke by one percentage point, US patients on average would accept over a 6.0% chance of non-major clinically relevant bleeding and up to about a 2.0% chance of extracranial major bleeding.

## The Future

### Initiatives, Guidances and Partnerships

There are many recent and on-going initiatives on B-R methods and policy. The FDA and EMA implemented structured approaches to communicating B-R assessment. New FDA guidance for drugs and biologics is forthcoming. Additional guidance will focus on systematic approaches to utilizing patient and caregiver input. The Council for International Organizations in the Medical Sciences has forthcoming updates to its publication on B-R evaluation. Public–private partnerships align stakeholders on methodology and policy. For example, the Innovative Medicines Initiative (IMI) developed recommendations for B-R methodology and communication (IMI PROTECT), and the Medical Device Innovation Consortium developed a framework on the use of patient preference studies in medical device development. The IMI PREFER project will generate recommendations on the use of patient preference studies. Other professional societies have developed innovative methods and standards for B-R decision making and

preference studies. The Quantitative Sciences in the Pharmaceutical Industry Benefit–Risk Working Group has developed novel statistical approaches. The International Society for Pharmacoeconomics and Outcomes Research, the Society for Medical Decision Making and the International Academy of Health Preference Research develop standards for B-R decision-making and the conduct of patient preference studies.

### Advanced Methods on the Horizon

Benefit–risk assessment is an evolving field in which assessments will become more structured and quantitative. Advances will include: (i) refinement of B-R and patient preference assessment tools, (ii) development of methodologies with greater clinical applicability, and (iii) transitioning B-R assessment from a *posthoc* exercise to a design and conduct issue having pre-specified plans. Communication of B-R will evolve with emphasis on risk (or rate) difference summaries and graphical communications.

A key goal of B-R is to contrast the benefits and harms of therapeutic alternatives as experienced by patients. Typical approaches analyze benefits and harms independently. B-R assessment based on combining the separate marginal effects of each outcome has limitations, failing to (i) account for outcome dependencies, (ii) systematically incorporate the relative importance of combinations of outcomes, (iii) summarize the cumulative nature of various outcomes, and (iv) effectively deal with competing risks.

For example, suppose 100 patients are treated with a new treatment vs placebo, and one efficacy outcome and one safety outcome are measured and considered equally important. Further suppose the efficacy and adverse event rates for the new treatment are both 50%, while the rates for both are zero for placebo. If the 50 patients who experience a treatment benefit are the same patients who experienced harm, then the net clinical benefit is zero for all patients (Figure 23.3a). However, if the 50 patients with benefit are different than the patients that experienced the harm, then the net clinical benefit is positive for half the patients and negative for half the patients (Figure 23.3b). Separate marginal summaries cannot distinguish these two scenarios.

One method that accounts for these dependencies is desirability of outcome ranking (DOOR). Conceptually, DOOR uses outcomes to analyze the patients rather than the patients to analyze the outcomes. A key to utilizing DOOR is to determine how to analyze one patient before analyzing many.

DOOR begins with construction of a global ordinal outcome, where a DOOR outcome is a composition of benefits and harms that occur in a single patient. In one approach to DOOR, one can estimate the probability that a randomly selected patient randomized to one treatment has a better DOOR than a randomly selected patient on the other treatment. This has an intuitive appeal from a clinical perspective given the connection to the clinical decision-making question of what is the probability that a patient will have a better overall response on one treatment relative to another. An alternate approach to DOOR assigns

"partial credit" to DOOR outcomes, ranging from the most desirable (100) to least desirable (0). The amount of partial credit may be obtained through patient preference studies or a survey of expert clinicians. Sensitivity analyses to varying partial credit scoring permits personalized analyses.

In the future, the bond between B-R assessment and precision medicine will grow. The goal in practice is not to identify who will benefit or who will be harmed, but who has a positive B-R profile. B-R assessment will transition from a post-hoc activity to one that begins in study design and proceeds through trial conduct, is pre-specified, systematic, and a primary focus. For example, structured B-R assessment may become a standard assessment of data monitoring committees. When formal B-R hypotheses cannot be prespecified, the planned methodology for assessing B-R can be prespecified. Patient preference studies and the collection of quality-of-life information will become more prevalent and will be included in clinical trials more often, rather than being evaluations in a separate population. Sensitivity analyses to patient preferences will become common, assessing the robustness of the results.

(a)

|        | Benefit | No benefit |
|--------|---------|------------|
| Harm    | 50%     | ...        |
| No harm | ...     | 50%        |
|        |         |            |

(b)

|        | Benefit | No benefit |
|--------|---------|------------|
| Harm    | ...     | 50%        |
| No harm | 50%     | ...        |
|        |         |            |

**Figure 23.3** Demonstration of the impact of dependencies between outcomes. Both tables show risk differences for an equally weighted benefit and risk. In Figure 23.3a the treatment benefits no one (NCB = 0 for all patients); In Figure 23.3b, the treatment benefits half of patients (NCB > 0 for 50 patients and NCB < 0 for 50 patients). However, the marginal distributions of benefit and harm of the two tables are identical.

---

## Case Example 23.8    For Benefit–Risk Assessment

*Background*

- A novel favor Xa inhibitor anticoagulant (study drug) was studied in a pivotal phase 3 randomized clinical trial, comparing the study drug to an active comparator in subjects with non-valvular atrial fibrillation (ECG-confirmed). 10 000 subjects age ≥ 18 years. Study duration was up to a maximum of four years.

- The primary efficacy outcome was the composite of stroke and non-central nervous system embolism (NCSE). The primary safety outcome was major bleeding, the composite of fatal bleeding, critical organ bleeding (e.g. hemorrhagic stroke, intracerebral hemorrhage), transfusions ≥ 2 units packed red blood cells or whole blood, or hemoglobin drops ≥ 2 g/dl.

*Question*

For the health authority submission, do benefits outweigh harms for the study drug vs active comparator?

*Approach*

- Utilize the BRAT framework to develop the decision context, value tree, consider the importance of outcomes and develop an integrated B-R assessment.

- The value tree based on clinical trial outcomes (Figure 23.1a) was modified for B-R assessment to remove double-counting and avoid composite outcomes that include events with a wide range of clinical impact (Figure 23.1b). The efficacy composite outcome is ischemic events that are generally fatal or cause irreversible harm. The safety composite outcome is hemorrhagic events that are generally fatal or cause irreversible harm. Additional hemorrhagic events are included under a composite outcome "reversible hemorrhagic events."

*Results*

- The decision context is to assess B-R of the study drug vs the comparator in subjects with non-valvular atrial fibrillation, over a period of up to four years from initial dose, for regulatory decision-makers.

- An effects table and a forest plots using exposure-time rates per 10 000 person-years were generated (Table 23.3, Figure 23.2). Focusing first on events that are fatal or cause irreversible harm, per 10 000 person-years, there are 87 (95% CI 30, 143) fewer events per 10 000 person-years in the efficacy composite of ischemic death, ischemic stroke, MI or systemic embolism; and there are 6 (95% CI -20, 33) fewer fatal and critical organ bleeding events on the study drug. The composite efficacy outcome is nominally statistically significant favoring the study drug, while the fatal and critical organ bleeding shows little difference; suggesting benefits outweigh harms.

- The forest plot makes clear visually that death, ischemic stroke, myocardial infarction and non-CNS systemic embolism each contribute meaningfully to efficacy. Major bleeding favors the comparator, but this difference is driven primarily by less impactful bleeds of transfusions and hemoglobin reductions. The B-R tradeoff is preventing 87 (95% CI 30, 143) fatal/irreversible harm ischemic events vs causing 60 (95% CI 17, 108) reversible bleeding events and 44 (−40, 13) clinically relevant non-major bleeds. Even without taking patient preferences into account, the benefits appear to outweigh the harms.

- This B-R analysis can also be performed with NNT and NNH. For example, one fatal/irreversible harm ischemic event is prevented for every 115 person-years of exposure to the study drug vs comparator

*(Continued)*

---

**Case Example 23.8    (Continued)**

(NNT), while 204 person-years exposure is needed to see an excess major bleeding event (NNH) on study drug, most of which are far less clinically impactful than the ischemic events, also strongly suggesting that benefit exceeds harm.

*Strengths*
- The use of outcomes that avoid double-counting, clearly distinguish between harmful events caused vs harmful events prevented, and the use of a pair of composite outcomes with similar clinical impact to simplify assessment of whether benefits outweigh harms.
- The use of risk differences to clearly indicate the number of events caused and prevented.
- Concise tabular and graphic depictions that clearly depict the B-R assessment.

*Limitations*
- The outcomes are considered independent. A more through B-R assessment would assess whether there is a dependency between key outcomes, especially between ischemic events and hemorrhagic events.
- While the transfusions, hemoglobin reductions and clinically relevant non-major bleeds are far less impactful than the benefits and harms in the primary B-R assessment, these less impactful bleeds may cause patients to discontinue treatment, indirectly favoring the comparator.

*Key points*
Use of a structured B-R framework enables a flexible, transparent and defensible approach to B-R assessment

---

**Key Points for Benefit-Risk Assessments of Medical Treatments**

- Assessing the B-R balance of medical treatments has always been an integral part of drug development, regulatory, and public health decisions.
- Methodology for B-R has advanced considerably, and health authorities worldwide have developed much more rigorous B-R regulatory policies relating to regulatory approval and post-approval decisions.
- These advances have led to transparent and rigorous systematic approaches to B-R which incorporate the patient perspective and can be communicated clearly and succinctly to clinical and patient audiences.

## Further Reading

## Studies of Drug Utilization

Beer, C., Hyde, Z., Almeida, O.P. et al. (2011). Quality use of medicines and health outcomes among a cohort of community dwelling older men: an observational study. *Br. J. Clin. Pharmacol.* 71: 592–599.

Brown, T.R. (ed.) (2006). *Handbook of Institutional Pharmacy Practice*, 4e. Bethesda, MD: American Society of Health System Pharmacists.

Dartnell, J.G.A. (2001). *Understanding, Influencing and Evaluating Drug Use.* Australia: Therapeutic Guidelines Limited.

Elseviers, M., Wettermark, B., Almarsdottir, A.B. et al. (eds.) (2016). *Drug Utilization Research: Methods and Applications.* Chichester, West Sussex: Hoboken NJ: Wiley.

Hennessy, S.M., Bilker, W.B., Zhou, L. et al. (2003). Retrospective drug utilization review, prescribing errors, and clinical outcomes. *JAMA* 290: 1494–1499.

Kauffman, D.W., Kelly, J.P., Rosenberg, L. et al. (2002). Recent patterns of medication use in the ambulatory adult population of the United States: the Slone survey. *JAMA* 287: 337–344.

Kidder, D. and Bae, J. (1999). Evaluation results from prospective drug utilization review: medicaid demonstrations. *Health Care Financ. Rev.* 20: 107–118.

World Health Organization (1993) How to Investigate Drug Use in Health Facilities: Selected Drug Use Indicators. WHO/DAP/93.1. Geneva: World Health Organization.

World Health Organization (2009) Medicines Use in Primary Care in Developing and Transitional Countries: Fact Book Summarizing Results from Studies Reported between 1990 and 2006. WHO/EMP/MAR/2009.3. Geneva, Switzerland: World Health Organization.

World Health Organization International Working Group for Drug Statistics Methodology, WHO Collaborating Centre for Drug Statistics Methodology, WHO Collaborating Centre for Drug Utilization Research and Clinical Pharmacology (2003). *Introduction to Drug Utilization Research*. Geneva: World Health Organization.

# Evaluating and Improving Prescribing

Arditi, C., Rege-Walther, M., Durieux, P., and Burnand, B. (2017). Computer-generated reminders delivered on paper to healthcare professionals: effects on professional practice and healthcare outcomes. *Cochrane Database Syst. Rev.* 7: CD001175.

Auerbach, A.D., Landefield, C.S., and Shojania, K.G. (2007). The tension between needing to improve care and knowing how to do it. *N. Engl. J. Med.* 357: 608–613.

Cabana, M.D., Rand, C.S., Power, N.R. et al. (1999). Why don't physicians follow clinical practice guidelines? *JAMA* 282: 1458–1465.

Christensen, M. and Lundh, A. (2016). Medication review in hospitalised patients to reduce morbidity and mortality. *Cochrane Database Syst. Rev.* 2: CD008986.

Cochrane Effective Practice and Organization of Care Group. What study designs should be included in an EPOC review and what should they be called? 2017; http://epoc.cochrane.org/sites/epoc.cochrane.org/files/public/uploads/Resources-for-authors2017/what_study_designs_should_be_included_in_an_epoc_review.pdf. Accessed November 29, 2017.

Davey, P., Marwick, C.A., Scott, C.L. et al. (2017). Interventions to improve antibiotic prescribing practices for hospital inpatients. *Cochrane Database Syst. Rev.* 2: CD003543.

Donner, A., Birkett, N., and Buck, C. (1981). Randomization by cluster – samples size requirements and analysis. *Am. J. Epidemiol.* 114: 906–914.

Flodgren, G., Parmelli, E., Doumit, G. et al. (2011). Local opinion leaders: effects on professional practice and health care outcomes. *Cochrane Database Syst. Rev.* 8: CD000125.

Giguere, A., Legare, F., Grimshaw, J. et al. (2012). Printed educational materials: effects on professional practice and healthcare outcomes. *Cochrane Database Syst. Rev.* 10: CD004398.

Gillaizeau, F., Chan, E., Trinquart, L. et al. (2013). Computerized advice on drug dosage to improve prescribing practice. *Cochrane Database Syst. Rev.* 11: CD002894.

Godin, G., Belanger-Gravel, A., Eccles, M., and Grimshaw, J. (2008). Healthcare professionals' intentions and behaviours: a systematic review of studies based on social cognitive theories. *Implement. Sci.* 3: 36–46.

Gonzales, R., Steiner, J.F., Lum, A., and Barrett, P.H. (1999). Decreasing antibiotic use in ambulatory practice: impact of a multidimensional intervention on the treatment of uncomplicated acute bronchitis in adults. *JAMA* 281: 1512–1519.

Greer, A.L. (1988). The state of the art versus the state of the science: the diffusion of new medical technologies into practice. *Int. J. Technol. Assess. Health Care* 4: 5–26.

Grimshaw, J.M., Shirran, L., Thomas, R. et al. (2001). Changing provider behavior: an overview of systematic reviews of interventions. *Med. Care* 39 (suppl 2): 2–45.

Grudniewicz, A., Kealy, R., Rodseth, R.N. et al. (2015). What is the effectiveness of printed educational materials on primary care physician knowledge, behaviour, and patient outcomes: a systematic review and meta-analyses. *Implement. Sci.* 10: 164.

Han, Y.Y., Carcillo, J.A., Venkataraman, S.T. et al. (2005). Unexpected increased mortality after implementation of a commercially sold computerized physician order entry system. *Pediatrics* 116: 1506–1512.

Isaac, T., Weissman, J.S., Davis, R.B. et al. (2009). Overrides of medication alerts in ambulatory care. *Arch. Intern. Med.* 169: 305–311.

Ivers, N., Jamtvedt, G., Flottorp, S. et al. (2012). Audit and feedback: effects on professional practice and healthcare outcomes. *Cochrane Database Syst. Rev.* 6: CD000259.

Johnson, M.J. and May, C.R. (2015). Promoting professional behaviour change in healthcare: what interventions work, and why? A theory-led overview of systematic reviews. *BMJ Open* 5: e008592.

Lu, C.Y., Ross-Degnan, D., Soumerai, S.B., and Pearson, S.A. (2008). Interventions designed to improve the quality and efficiency of medication use in managed care: a critical review of the literature – 2001-2007. *BMC Health Serv. Res.* 8: 75.

Luiza, V.L., Chaves, L.A., Silva, R.M. et al. (2015). Pharmaceutical policies: effects of cop and co-payment on rational use of medicines. *Cochrane Database Syst. Rev.* 2015: CD007017.

Majumdar, S.R., Guirguis, L.M., Toth, E.L. et al. (2003). Controlled trial of a multifaceted intervention for improving quality of care for rural patients with type 2 diabetes. *Diabetes Care* 26: 3061–3066.

Majumdar, S.R., McAlister, F.A., and Furberg, C.D. (2004). From knowledge to practice in chronic cardiovascular disease–a long and winding road. *J. Am. Coll. Cardiol.* 43: 1738–1742.

Majumdar, S.R., Tsuyuki, R.T., and McAlister, F.A. (2007). Impact of opinion leader-endorsed evidence summaries on the quality of prescribing for patients with cardiovascular disease: a randomized controlled trial. *Am. Heart J.* 153 (22): e21–e28.

Mason, J., Freemantle, N., Nazareth, I. et al. (2001). When is it cost-effective to change the behavior of health professionals? *JAMA* 286: 2988–2992.

Mostofian, F., Ruban, C., Simunovic, N., and Bhandari, M. (2015). Changing physician behavior: what works? *Am. J. Manag. Care* 21: 75–84.

Nanji, K.C., Slight, S.P., Seger, D.L. et al. (2014). Overrides of medication-related clinical decision support alerts in outpatients. *J. Am. Med. Inform. Assoc.* 21: 487–491.

O'Brien, M.A., Rogers, S., Jamtvedt, G. et al. (2007). Educational outreach visits: effects on professional practice and health care outcomes. *Cochrane Database Syst. Rev.* 4: CD000409.

Rousseau, N., McColl, E., Newton, J. et al. (2003). Practice based, longitudinal, qualitative interview study of computerized evidence based guidelines in primary care. *BMJ* 326: 314–322.

Serumaga, B., Ross-Degnan, R., Avery, A.J. et al. (2011). Has pay-for-performance improved the management and outcomes of hypertension in the United Kingdom? *BMJ* 342: 322–329.

Serumaga, B., Ross-Degnan, D., Avery, A.J. et al. (2011). Effect of pay for performance on the management and outcomes of hypertension in the United Kingdom: interrupted time series study. *BMJ* 342: d108.

Simon, S.R., Majumdar, S.R., Prosser, L.A. et al. (2005). Group versus individual academic detailing to improve the use of antihypertensive medications in primary care: a cluster-randomized controlled trial. *Am. J. Med.* 118: 521–528.

Soumerai, S.B., McLaughlin, T.J., and Avorn, J. (1989). Improving drug prescribing in primary care: a critical analysis of the experimental literature. *Milbank Q.* 62 (2): 268–317.

Soumerai, S.B., McLaughlin, T.J., Gurwitz, J.H. et al. (1998). Effect of local medical opinion leaders on quality of care for acute myocardial infarction: a randomized controlled trial. *JAMA* 279: 1358–1363.

## Special Methodological Issues in Pharmacoepidemiologic Studies of Vaccine Safety

Bate, A. and Evans, S.J.W. (2009). Quantitative signal detection using spontaneous ADR reporting. *Pharmacoepidemiol. Drug Saf.* 18: 427–436.

Cashman, P., Macartney, K., Khandaker, G. et al. (2017). Participant-centred active surveillance of adverse events following immunisation: a narrative review. *Int. Health* 9 (3): 164–176.

Centers for Disease Control and Prevention (1999). Intussusception among recipients of rotavirus vaccine– United States, 1998–1999. *MMWR Morb. Mortal. Wkly Rep.* 48: 577–581.

Fine, P.E. and Chen, R.T. (2001). Confounding in studies of adverse reactions to vaccines. *Am. J. Epidemiol.* 136: 121–135.

Glanz, J.M., McClure, D.L., Xu, S. et al. (2005). Four different study designs to evaluate vaccine safety were equally validated with contrasting limitations. *J. Clin. Epidemiol.* 59: 808–818.

Glanz, J.M., McClure, D.L., Magid, D.J. et al. (2009). Parental refusal of pertussis vaccination is associated with an increased risk of pertussis infection in children. *Pediatrics* 123: 1446–1451.

Gruber, M.F. and Marshall, V.B. (2018). Regulation and testing of vaccines. In: *Vaccines*, 7e (eds. S. Plotkin, W.A. Orenstein, P. Offit and K.M. Edward), 1547–1565. Philadelphia, PA: W.B. Saunders.

Halsell, J.S., Riddle, J.R., Atwood, J.E. et al. (2003). Myopericarditis following smallpox vaccination among vaccinia-naive US military personnel. *JAMA* 289: 3283–3289.

Howson, C.P., Howe, C.J., and Fineberg, H.V. (eds.) (1991). *Adverse Effects of Pertussis and Rubella Vaccines: A Report of the Committee to Review the Adverse Consequences of Pertussis and Rubella Vaccines. IOM (Institute of Medicine).* 1991 Washington, DC: National Academy Press.

Huang, W.T., Chen, R.T., Hsu, Y.C. et al. (2017). Vaccination and unexplained sudden death risk in Taiwanese infants. *Pharmacoepidemiol. Drug Saf.* 26 (1): 17–25.

Izurieta, H.S., Zuber, P., Bonhoeffer, J. et al. (2013). Roadmap for the international collaborative epidemiologic monitoring of safety and effectiveness of new high priority vaccines. *Vaccine* 31 (35): 3623–3627.

Kramarz, P., France, E.K., DeStefano, F. et al. (2001). Population-based study of rotavirus vaccination and intussusception. *Pediatr. Infect. Dis. J.* 20: 410–416.

Larson, H.J., Cooper, L.Z., Eskola, J. et al. (2011). Addressing the vaccine confidence gap. *Lancet* 378 (9790): 526–535.

McNeil, M.M., Gee, J., Weintraub, E.S. et al. (2014). The vaccine safety datalink: successes and challenges monitoring vaccine safety. *Vaccine* 32 (42): 5390–5398.

Murch, S.H., Anthony, A., Casson, D.H. et al. (2004). Retraction of an interpretation. *Lancet* 363: 750.

Murphy, T.V., Gargiullo, P.M., Massoudi, M.S. et al. (2001). Intussusception among infants given an oral rotavirus vaccine. *N. Engl. J. Med.* 344: 564–572.

Poland, G.A., Ovsyannikova, I.G., and Kennedy, R.B. (2018 Aug 28). Personalized vaccinology: a review. *Vaccine* 36 (36): 5350–5357.

Schonberger, L.B., Bregman, D.J., Sullivan-Bolyai, J.Z. et al. (1979). Guillain–Barre syndrome following vaccination in the National Influenza Immunization Program, United States, 1976–1977. *Am. J. Epidemiol.* 110: 105–123.

Stratton, K., Ford, A., Rusch, E., and Clayton, E.W. (eds.) (2011). *Adverse Effects of Vaccines: Evidence and Causality. IOM (Institute of Medicine).* Washington, DC: The National Academies Press.

Wang, S.V., Stefanini, K., Lewis, E. et al. (2020). Determining which of several simultaneously administered vaccines increase risk of an adverse event. *Drug Saf.* (in press).

Xu, S., Zhang, L., Nelson, J. et al. (2010). Identifying optimal risk windows for self-controlled case series studies of vaccine safety. *Stat. Med.* 30: 142–152.

Yih, W.K., Kulldorff, M., Dashevsky, I., and Maro, J.C. (2019 Jul 1). Using the self-controlled tree-temporal scan statistic to assess the safety of live attenuated herpes zoster vaccine. *Am. J. Epidemiol.* 188 (7): 1383–1388.

# Epidemiologic Studies of Implantable Medical Devices

Adhikari, S., Rose, S., and Normand, S.-L. (November 2019). Nonparametric Bayesian instrumental variable analysis: evaluating heterogeneous effects of coronary arterial access site strategies. *J. Am. Stat. Assoc.*: 1–14. https://doi.org/10.1080/01621459.2019.1688663.

Chughtai, B., Mao, J., Buck, J. et al. (2015). Use and risks of surgical mesh for pelvic organ prolapse surgery in women in New York state: population based cohort study. *BMJ* 350: h2685. https://doi.org/10.1136/bmj.h2685.

Fortune Business Insights. Medical Devices Market Size, Share and Industry Analysis By Type (Orthopedic Devices, Cardiovascular Devices, Diagnostic Imaging, IVD, MIS, Wound Management, Diabetes Care, Ophthalmic Devices, Dental & Nephrology), End User (Hospitals & Ambulatory Surgica. https://www.fortunebusinessinsights.com/industry-reports/medical-devices-market-100085. Published 2019. Accessed August 1, 2020.

Global News Wire. Global Medical Devices Market Report 2019–2022 - A $521+ Billion Opportunity Analysis. Research and Markets. https://www.globenewswire.com/news-release/2019/09/19/1918062/0/en/Global-Medical-Devices-Market-Report-2019-2022-A-521-Billion-Opportunity-Analysis.html. Published 2019. Accessed August 1, 2020.

International Medical Device Regulators Forum (IMDRF) Patient Registries Working Group. Principles of International System of Registries Linked to Other Data Sources and Tools. http://www.imdrf.org/docs/imdrf/final/technical/imdrf-tech-160930-principles-system-registries.pdf. Published 2016. Accessed May 1, 2018.

International Medical Device Regulators Forum (IMDRF) Patient Registries Working Group. Tools for Assessing the Usability of Registries in Support of Regulatory Decision-Making. http://www.imdrf.org/docs/imdrf/final/consultations/imdrf-cons-registries-n46-pd1-170817.pdf. Published 2017. Accessed May 1, 2018.

International Medical Device Regulators Forum (IMDRF) Patient Registries Working Group. Methodological Principles in the Use of International Medical Device Registry Data. http://www.imdrf.org/docs/imdrf/final/technical/imdrf-tech-170316-methodological-principles.pdf. Published 2016. Accessed May 1, 2018.

Rose, S. and Normand, S.-L. (2019). Double robust estimation for multiple unordered treatments and clustered observations: evaluating drug-eluting coronary artery stents. *Biometrics* 75 (1): 289–296. https://doi.org/10.1111/biom.12927.

Shuren, J. and Califf, R.M. (2016). Need for a National Evaluation System for Health Technology. *JAMA* 316 (23): 2429–2437.

Tsougranis, G., Eldrup-Jorgensen, J., Bertges, D. et al. (2020). The Vascular Implant Surveillance and Interventional Outcomes (VISION) Coordinated Registry Network: An effort to advance evidence evaluation for vascular devices. *J Vasc Surg.* 72 (6): 2153–2160.

# Research on the Effects of Medications in Pregnancy and in Children

de Bie, S., Coloma, P.M., Ferrajolo, C. et al. (2015). The role of electronic healthcare record databases in paediatric drug safety surveillance: a retrospective cohort study. *Br. J. Clin. Pharmacol.* 80 (2): 304–314.

Contopoulos-Ioannidis, D.G., Seto, I., Hamm, M.P. et al. (2012). Empirical evaluation of age groups and age-subgroup analyses in pediatric randomized trials and pediatric meta-analyses. *Pediatrics* 129 (Suppl 3): S161–S184.

Cooper, W., Hernandez-Diaz, S., Arbogast, P. et al. (2006). Major congenital malformations after first-trimester exposure to ACE inhibitors. *N. Engl. J. Med.* 354: 2443–2451.

D'Onofrio, B.M., Class, Q.A., Rickert, M.E. et al. (2016). Translational epidemiologic approaches to understanding the consequences of early-life exposures. *Behav. Genet.* 46 (3): 315–328.

Expert Panel on Therapeutic Products for Infants Children and Youth (2015). Chapter 3: children are not Small adults: considering variation in drug response. In: *Improving Medicines for Children in Canada*, 49–88.

Fiks, A.G., Grundmeier, R.W., Steffes, J. et al. (2015). Comparative effectiveness research through a collaborative electronic reporting consortium. *Pediatrics* 136 (1): e215–e224.

Forrest, C.B., Margolis, P.A., Bailey, L.C. et al. (2014). PEDSnet: a national pediatric learning health system. *J. Am. Med. Inform. Assoc.* 21 (4): 602–606.

Hales, C.M., Kit, B.K., Gu, Q., and Ogden, C.L. (2018). Trends in prescription medication use among children and adolescents-United States, 1999-2014. *JAMA* 319 (19): 2009–2020.

Hernan, M.A., Hernandez-Diaz, S., Werler, M.M., and Mitchell, A.A. (2002). Causal knowledge as a prerequisite for confounding evaluation: an application to birth defects epidemiology. *Am. J. Epidemiol.* 155 (2): 176.

Hernan, M.A., Hernandez-Diaz, S., and Robins, J.M. (2004). A structural approach to selection bias. *Epidemiology* 15 (5): 615–625.

Hernandez-Diaz, S., Werler, M.M., Walker, A.M., and Mitchell, A.A. (2000). Folic acid antagonists during pregnancy and the risk of birth defects. *N. Engl. J. Med.* 343 (22): 1608–1614.

Hernández-Díaz, S., Bateman, B.T., Palmsten, K. et al. (2019 Dec 20). Using nationally representative survey data for external adjustment of unmeasured confounders: an example using the NHANES data. *Pharmacoepidemiol. Drug Saf.* https://doi.org/10.1002/pds.4946. [Epub ahead of print].

Horton, D.B., Haynes, K., Denburg, M.R. et al. (2017). Oral glucocorticoid use and osteonecrosis in children and adults with chronic inflammatory diseases: a population-based cohort study. *BMJ Open* 7 (7): e016788.

Huybrechts, K.F., Palmsten, K., Avorn, J. et al. (2014). Antidepressant use in pregnancy and the risk of cardiac defects. *N. Engl. J. Med.* 370 (25): 2397–2407.

Huybrechts, K.F., Bröms, G., Christensen, L.B. et al. (2018 Feb 1). Association between methylphenidate and amphetamine use in pregnancy and risk of congenital malformations: a cohort study from the international pregnancy safety study consortium. *JAMA Psychiatry.* 75 (2): 167–175.

Huybrechts, K.F., Hernandez-Diaz, S., Straub, L. et al. (2018). Association of maternal first-trimester ondansetron use with cardiac malformations and oral clefts in offspring. *JAMA* 320 (23): 2429–2437.

Huybrechts, K.F., Bateman, B.T., and Hernandez-Diaz, S. (2019). Use of real-world evidence from healthcare utilization data to evaluate drug safety during pregnancy. *Pharmacoepidemiol. Drug Saf.* 28: 906–922. https://doi.org/10.1002/pds.4789pmid: 31074570.

Huybrechts, K.F., Hernandez-Diaz, S., and Bateman, B. (2020 Jun 1). Contextualizing potential risks of medications in pregnancy for the newborn: the case of ondansetron. *JAMA Pediatr.* https://doi.org/10.1001/jamapediatrics.2020.1325. Online ahead of print.

Khoury, M.J., Flanders, W.D., James, L.M., and Erickson, J.D. (1989). Human teratogens, prenatal mortality, and selection bias. *Am. J. Epidemiol.* 130: 361–370.

Kinlaw, A.C., Sturmer, T., Lund, J.L. et al. (2017). Trends in antibiotic use by birth season and birth year. *Pediatrics* 140 (3): e20170441. https://doi.org/10.1542/peds.2017-0441.

Lash, T.L., Schmidt, M., Jensen, A.O., and Engebjerg, M.C. (2010). Methods to apply probabilistic bias analysis to summary estimates of association. *Pharmacoepidemiol. Drug Saf.* 19 (6): 638–644.

Lash, T.L., Fox, M.P., MacLehose, R.F. et al. (2014). Good practices for quantitative bias analysis. *Int. J. Epidemiol.* 43 (6): 1969–1985.

Margulis, A.V., Mittleman, M.A., Glynn, R.J. et al. (2015). Effects of gestational age at enrollment in pregnancy exposure registries. *Pharmacoepidemiol. Drug Saf.* 24 (4): 343–352.

Mitchell, A.A. (2003). Systematic identification of drugs that cause birth defects – a new opportunity. *N. Engl. J. Med.* 349 (26): 2556–2559.

Mitchell, A.A., Gilboa, S.M., Werler, M.M. et al. (2011). Medication use during pregnancy, with particular focus on prescription drugs: 1976–2008. *Am. J. Obstet. Gynecol.* 205: 51. e1–51.e8.

Poulton, A.S., Bui, Q., Melzer, E., and Evans, R. (2016). Stimulant medication effects on growth and bone age in children with attention-deficit/hyperactivity disorder: a prospective cohort study. *Int. Clin. Psychopharmacol.* 31 (2): 93–99.

Rothman, K.J. (1990). No adjustments are needed for multiple comparisons. *Epidemiology* 1 (1): 43–46.

Rothman, K.J. (2014). Six persistent research misconceptions. *J. Gen. Intern. Med.* 29 (7): 1060–1064.

Schatz, M., Chambers, C.D., Jones, K.L. et al. (2011). The safety of influenza immunizations and treatment during pregnancy: the vaccines and medications in pregnancy surveillance system. *Am. J. Obstet. Gynecol.* 204: S64–S68.

Scott, F.I., Horton, D.B., Mamtani, R. et al. (2016). Administration of antibiotics to children before age 2 years increases risk for childhood obesity. *Gastroenterology* 151 (1): 120–129. e125.

Slaughter, J.L., Reagan, P.B., Newman, T.B., and Klebanoff, M.A. (2017). Comparative effectiveness of nonsteroidal anti-inflammatory drug treatment vs no treatment for patent ductus arteriosus in preterm infants. *JAMA Pediatr.* 171 (3): e164354.

Sturkenboom, M.C., Verhamme, K.M., Nicolosi, A. et al. (2008). Drug use in children: cohort study in three European countries. *BMJ* 337: a2245.

US Food and Drug Administration, US Department of Health and Human Services (2014). Content and format of labeling for human prescription drug and biological products; requirements for pregnancy and lactation labeling. Final rule. *Fed. Regist.* 79 (233): 72063–72103.

Werler, M.M., Louik, C., and Mitchell, A.A. (2011). Case-control studies for identifying novel teratogens. *Am. J. Med. Genet. C: Semin. Med. Genet.* 157C (3): 201–208.

Woolfenden, S., Eapen, V., Axelsson, E. et al. (2016). Who is our cohort: recruitment, representativeness, baseline risk and retention in the "watch me grow" study? *BMC Pediatr.* 16: 46.

## Risk Management

Directive (2001) 2001/83 EC, Article 1 (28b).

European Medicines Agency and Heads of Medicines Agencies (2012) Guideline on Good Pharmacovigilance Practices, Module V – Risk Management Systems (published July 2012. http://www.ema.europa.eu/docsen_GB/document_library/Scientific_guideline/2012/06/WC500129134.pdf

Institute of Medicine (2000). *To Err Is Human: Building a Safer Health System* (eds. L.T. Kohn, J.M. Corrigan and M.S. Donaldson). Institute of Medicine, Washington DC: National Academies Press.

National Coordinating Council for Medication Error Reporting and Prevention website, http://www. http://nccmerp.org/aboutMedErrors.html.

Ovation Pharmaceuticals, Inc. Advisory Committee Briefing Document. Sabril® (vigabatrin) Tablet and Powder for Oral Solution For Adjunctive Treatment of Refractory Complex Partial Seizures in Adults (NDA 20-427), For Monotherapy Treatment of Infantile Spasms (NDA 22-006). Peripheral and Central Nervous System Advisory Committee January 7–8, 2009. Available at http://www. http://fda.gov/downloads/Advisory Committees/Committees MeetingMaterials/ Drugs/PeripheralandCentralNervous System DrugsAdvisoryCommittee/UCM153780.pdf

US Department of Health and Human Services. Food and Drug Administration. Guidance. Drug Safety Information–FDA's Communication to the Public. March 2007. Available at http://www.fda.gov/downloads/ Drugs GuidanceComplianceRegulatory Information/Guidances/ UCM072281.pdf

US Food and Drug Administration. Guidance for Industry (2005) Development and Use of Risk Minimization Action Plans.

# The Pharmacoepidemiology of Medication Errors

Aronson, J.K. (2009). Medication errors: definitions and classification. *Br. J. Clin. Pharmacol.* 67: 599–604.

Bates, D.W., Boyle, D.L., Vander Vliet, M.B. et al. (1995). Relationship between medication errors and adverse drug events. *J. Gen. Intern. Med.* 10: 199–205.

Bates, D.W., Cullen, D., Laird, N. et al. (1995). Incidence of adverse drug events and potential adverse drug events: implications for prevention. *JAMA* 274: 29–34.

Bates, D.W., Leape, L.L., Cullen, D.J. et al. (1998). Effect of computerized physician order entry and a team intervention on prevention of serious medication errors. *JAMA* 280: 1311–1316.

Berwick, D.M. (1989). Continuous improvement as an ideal in health care. *N. Engl. J. Med.* 320: 53–56.

Chertow, G.M., Lee, J., Kuperman, G.J. et al. (2001). Guided medication dosing for inpatients with renal insufficiency. *JAMA* 286: 2839–2844.

Cypress BW (1982) *Drug Utilization in Office Visits to Primary Care Physicians: National Ambulatory Medical Care Survey, 1980.* Department of Health and Human Services publication (PHS) 82-1250. Public Health Service.

Falconnier, A.D., Haefeli, W.E., Schoenenberger, R.A. et al. (2001). Drug dosage in patients with renal failure optimized by immediate concurrent feedback. *J. Gen. Intern. Med.* 16: 369–375.

Forster, A.J., Murff, H.J., Peterson, J.F. et al. (2003). The incidence and severity of adverse events affecting patients after discharge from the hospital. *Ann. Intern. Med.* 138: 161–167.

Gandhi, T.K., Weingart, S.N., Borus, J. et al. (2003). Adverse drug events in ambulatory care. *N. Engl. J. Med.* 348: 1556–1564.

Hazlet, T.K., Lee, T.A., Hansten, P.D., and Horn, J.R. (2001). Performance of community pharmacy drug interaction software. *J. Am. Pharm. Assoc.* 41: 200–204.

Hennessy, S., Bilker, W.B., Zhou, L. et al. (2003). Retrospective drug utilization review, prescribing errors, and clinical outcomes. *JAMA* 290: 1494–1499.

Institute of Medicine (1999). *To Err Is Human: Building a Safer Health System* (eds. L.T. Kohn, J.M. Corrigan and M.S. Donaldson). Washington, DC: National Academy Press.

Kaushal, R., Bates, D.W., Landrigan, C. et al. (2001). Medication errors and adverse drug events in pediatric inpatients. *JAMA* 285: 2114–2120.

Kopp, B.J., Erstad, B.L., Allen, A.M. et al. (2006). Medication errors and adverse drug events in an intensive care unit: direct observation approach for detection. *Crit. Care Med.* 34: 415–425.

Koppel, R., Metlay, J.P., Cohen, A. et al. (2005). Role of computerized physician order entry systems in facilitating medication errors. *JAMA* 293: 1197–1203.

Krähenbühl-Melcher, A., Schlienger, R., Lampert, M. et al. (2007). Drug-related problems in hospitals: a review of the recent literature. *Drug Saf.* 30: 379–407.

Kuperman, G.J., Gandhi, T.K., and Bates, D.W. (2003). Effective drug-allergy checking: methodological and operational issues. *J. Biomed. Inform.* 36: 70–79.

Montesi, G. and Lechi, A. (2009). Prevention of medication errors: detection and audit. *Br. J. Clin. Pharmacol.* 67: 651–655.

Peterson, J.F. and Bates, D.W. (2001). Preventable medication errors: identifying and eliminating serious drug interactions. *J. Am. Pharm. Assoc.* 41: 159–160.

Potylycki, M.J., Kimmel, S.R., Ritter, M. et al. (2006). Nonputitive medication error reporting: 3-year findings from one hospital's primum non nocere initiative. *J. Nurs. Adm.* 36: 370–376.

Schiff, G.D., Klass, D., Peterson, J. et al. (2003). Linking laboratory and pharmacy: opportunities for reducing errors and improving care. *Arch. Intern. Med.* 163: 893–900.

Seidling, H.M., Storch, C.H., Bertsche, T. et al. (2009). Successful strategy to improve the specificity of electronic statin-drug interaction alerts. *Eur. J. Clin. Pharmacol.* 65: 1149–1157.

## Benefit-Risk Assessments of Medical Treatments

Coplan, P.M. et al. (2011). *Development of a framework for enhancing the transparency, reproducibility and communication of the benefit-risk balance of medicines. Clin. Pharmacol. Ther.* 89 (2): 312–315.

European Medicines Agency, Guidance document on the content of the <Co-> Rapporteur day <60><80> critical assessment report. 2011 Rev. 10.16]; Available from: http://www.ema.europa.eu/docs/en_GB/document_library/Regulatory_and_procedural_guideline/2016/05/WC500206989.pdf.

Evans, S.R. and Follmann, D. (2016). *Using outcomes to analyze patients rather than patients to analyze outcomes: a step toward pragmatism in benefit: risk evaluation. Stat. Biopharm. Res.* 8 (4): 386–393.

Evans, S.R. et al. (2015). *Desirability of outcome ranking (DOOR) and response adjusted for duration of antibiotic risk (RADAR). Clin. Infect. Dis.* 61 (5): 800–806.

Evans, S.R., Knutsson, M., Amarenco, P. et al. (2020). Methodologies for pragmatic and efficient assessment of benefits and harms: application to the SOCRATES trial. *Clinical Trials* 17 (6): 617–626.

Evans, S.R. et al. (2020). Presenting risks and benefits: helping the data monitoring committee do its job. *Ann. Intern. Med.* 172 (2): 119–125.

*Guidance for Industry and Food and Drug Administration Staff: Factors to Consider When Making Benefit-Risk Determinations in Medical Device Premarket Approval and De Novo Classifications.* 2016, FDA CDRH.

Food and Drug Administration, *Guidance for Industry and Food and Drug Administration Staff: Patient Preference Information – Voluntary Submission, Review in Premarket Approval Applications, Humanitarian Device Exemption Applications, and De Novo Requests, and Inclusion in Decision Summaries and Device Labeling* 2016, FDA CDRH.

Food and Drug Administration Benefit-Risk Assessment in Drug Regulatory Decision-Making. Draft PDUFA VI Implementation Plan 2018 March 30, 2018; Available from: https://www.fda.gov/downloads/ForIndustry/UserFees/PrescriptionDrugUserFee/UCM602885.pdf.

Hallgreen, C.E. et al. (2014). *Benefit-risk assessment in a post-market setting: a case study integrating real-life experience into benefit-risk methodology. Pharmacoepidemiol. Drug Saf.* 23 (9): 974–983.

Ho, M.P. et al. (2015). *Incorporating patient-preference evidence into regulatory decision making. Surg. Endosc.*

Lackey. L., Thompson, G., Eggers, S. (2021). FDA's Benefit-Risk Framework for Human Drugs and Biologics: Role in Benefit-Risk Assessment and Analysis of Use for Drug Approvals. *Ther Innov Regul Sci.* 55 (1): 170–179. doi: 10.1007/s43441-020-00203-6. Epub 2020 Aug 10.

Levitan, B.S. et al. (2011). *Application of the BRAT framework to case studies: observations and insights. Clin. Pharmacol. Ther.* 89 (2): 217–224.

MDUFA *Performance Goals And Procedures, Fiscal Years 2018 Through 2022.*

Medical Device Innovation Consortium, A framework for incorporating information on patient preferences regarding benefit and risk intro regulatory assessments of new medical technology. 2015; Available from: http://mdic.org/wp-content/uploads/2015/05/MDIC_PCBR_Framework_Web.pdf.

Muhlbacher, A. and Johnson, F.R. (2016). *Choice experiments to quantify preferences for health and healthcare: state of the practice. Appl. Health Econ. Health Policy* 14 (3): 253–266.

Pignatti, F. et al. (2015). *Structured frameworks to increase the transparency of the assessment of benefits and risks of medicines: current status and possible future directions. Clin. Pharmacol. Ther.* 98 (5): 522–533.

Soekhai, V., et al. *Compendium of Methods For Measuring Patient Preferences in Medical Treatment.* in *ISPOR 20th Annual European Congress.* 2017. Glasgow, Scotland.

**24**

# The Future of Pharmacoepidemiology

*Brian L. Strom[1], Stephen E. Kimmel[2], and Sean Hennessy[3]*

[1] Rutgers Biomedical and Health Sciences, Newark, NJ, USA
[2] University of Florida College of Public Health and Health Professions & College of Medicine, Gainesville, FL, USA
[3] University of Pennsylvania Perelman School of Medicine, Philadelphia, PA, USA

*We should all be concerned about the future because we will have to spend the rest of our lives there.*

Charles Franklin Kettering 1946

## Introduction

Speculating about the future is at least risky and possibly foolish. Nevertheless, the future of pharmacoepidemiology seems apparent in many ways, judging from past trends and recent events. Interest in the field by the pharmaceutical industry, government agencies, new trainees, and the public continues to grow, as is realization of what pharmacoepidemiology can contribute. Indeed, international attention on drug safety remains high, important safety questions involving widely used drugs continue to emerge, and questions concerning the effectiveness of systems of drug approval and drug safety monitoring remain.

As the functions of academia, industry, and government have become increasingly global, so has the field of pharmacoepidemiology. The number of individuals attending the annual International Conference on Pharmacoepidemiology has increased from approximately 50 in the early 1980s to over 1400 in 2017. The International Society for Pharmacoepidemiology (ISPE), established in 1991, has grown to approximately 1500 members from over 60 countries. It has developed a set of guidelines for Good Epidemiologic Practices for Drug, Device, and Vaccine Research in the United States in 1996, and updated these guidelines most recently in 2016 as the ISPE Guidelines for Good Pharmacoepidemiology Practices. Many national pharmacoepidemiologic societies have been formed as well. The journal, *Clinical Pharmacology and Therapeutics*, the major US academic clinical pharmacology journal, actively solicits pharmacoepidemiologic manuscripts, as did the *Journal of Clinical Epidemiology*. The major journal devoted to the field, *Pharmacoepidemiology and Drug Safety*, ISPE's official journal, is indexed on Medline and achieved an impact factor of 2.314 in 2018, remarkably high for a niche field. Other journals have been formed to publish pharmacoepidemiology research. The number of individuals seeking to enter the field continues to increase, as is their level of training. The number of programs of study in pharmacoepidemiology is increasing in schools of medicine, public health, and pharmacy. While in the 1980s the single summer short course in pharmacoepidemiology at the University of Minnesota was sometimes canceled because of insufficient interest, later the University of Michigan School of Public Health summer course in pharmacoepidemiology attracted 10% of all students in the entire summer program, and thereafter McGill University, Erasmus University Rotterdam, Utrecht University, and the Johns Hopkins Bloomberg School of Public Health all conduct summer short courses in pharmacoepidemiology. Several other short courses are given as well, including by ISPE itself which has seen a massive increase in pre-conference courses offered over the years. Regulatory bodies around the world have expanded their internal pharmacoepidemiologic programs. The number of pharmaceutical companies with their own pharmacoepidemiologic units has also increased, along with their support for academic units and their funding of external pharmacoepidemiologic studies. Requirements that a drug be shown to be cost-effective (see Chapter 18) have been added to many national health care systems, provincial health care systems, and managed care organizations, either to justify reimbursement or even to justify drug availability. Drug utilization review is being widely applied (see "Evaluating and Improving Prescribing" in Chapter 23), and many hospitals are becoming mini-pharmacoepidemiologic practice and research laboratories. The US Congress has recognized the importance of pharmacoepidemiology, requiring FDA to build a new data resource, containing at least 100 million lives, for evaluating potential adverse effects of medical products, and most recently passing the twenty-first Century Cures Act, encouraging the wide use of "real-world evidence." The latter has been deemed to range from traditional pharmacoepidemiology data sources like claims and medical record databases, and even ad hoc pharmacoepidemiology studies (see Part II), to novel data sources like e-health tools, m-health tools, and other wearable devices, as well as pragmatic trials using traditional pharmacoepidemiology databases to collect outcomes (see Chapter 17). The future is likely to see a marked expansion of these novel, technology-driven approaches.

Thus, from the perspective of those in the field, the trends in pharmacoepidemiology are remarkably positive, although many important challenges remain. In this chapter, we will briefly give our own view on the future of pharmacoepidemiology. Following the format of Part I of the book, we explore this future from the perspectives of academia, the pharmaceutical industry, regulatory agencies, and then the law.

## The View from Academia

### Scientific Developments

#### Methodologic Advances

Methodologically, the array of approaches available for performing pharmacoepidemiologic studies will continue to grow. Each of the methodologic issues discussed in Part III can be expected to be the subject of further research and development. The future is likely to see ever more advanced ways of performing and analyzing epidemiologic studies across all content areas, as the field of epidemiology continues to expand and develop. Some of these new techniques will, of course, be particularly useful to investigators in pharmacoepidemiology (see for example Chapter 22). The next few years will likely see continued expanded use of propensity scores, instrumental variables, the trend-in-trend design, sensitivity analysis, and novel methods to analyze time-varying exposures and confounders. In addition, we believe that we will see increasing application of pharmacoepidemiologic insight in the conduct of clinical trials, as well as increased use of the randomized trial design to examine questions traditionally addressed by observational pharmacoepidemiology (see Chapter 17), especially given the controversies resulting from inconsistencies between nonrandomized studies vs randomized trials, and given the emerging field of comparative effectiveness research.

Drug regulators have enthusiastically embraced therapeutic risk management (see "Risk Management" in chapter 23). Yet, this field is still very much in its infancy, with an enormous amount of work needed to develop new methods to measure, communicate, and manage the risks and benefits associated with medication use. Rigorous studies (i.e. program evaluations) of the effectiveness of risk management programs remain the exception rather than the rule. Development of this area will require considerable effort from pharmacoepidemiologists as well as those from other fields.

We may see developments in the processes used to assess causality from individual case reports (see Chapters 7 and 14). Data mining approaches will be used increasingly in spontaneous reporting databases to search for early signals of adverse reactions. Hopefully, we will see studies evaluating the utility of such approaches. The need for newer methods to screen for potential adverse drug effects, such as those using health care claims or medical record data and data from social media, is also clear.

We are likely to see increasing input from pharmacoepidemiologists into policy questions about drug approval (see "The View from Regulatory Agencies" in Chapter 6), with new attention to applying pharmacoepidemiology in the study of the growing opiate epidemic. We anticipate that emphasis will shift from studies evaluating whether a given drug is associated with an increased risk of a given event to those that examine as well patient-and regimen-specific factors that affect risk (see also Chapter 19 and "Risk Management" in Chapter 23). Such studies are crucial because, if risk factors for adverse reactions can be better understood before a safety crisis occurs, or early in the course of a crisis, then the clinical use of the drug may be able to be repositioned, avoiding the loss of useful drugs (see Chapter 15 as well as "Risk Management" and "Benefit-Risk Assessments of Medical Treatments in Chapter 23.).

With recent developments in molecular biology and bioinformatics, and their application to the study of pharmacogenetics, exciting developments have occurred in the ability of researchers to identify biologic factors that predispose patients to adverse drug reactions (see Chapter 15). However, relatively few of these discoveries have yet been shown useful in improving patient care, and new studies and methods must be pursued to determine the clinical utility of genetic testing. Pharmacogenetics has evolved from studies of measures of slow drug metabolism as a contributor to adverse reactions to the study of molecular genetic markers. This has been aided by the development of new, noninvasive methods to collect and analyze biosamples, making population-based genetic studies feasible. We believe that clinical measurement of biologic factors will ultimately complement existing approaches to tailoring therapeutic approaches for individual patients. However, it is unlikely that genotype will be the only, or even the major, factor that determines the optimal drug or dose for a given patient. Future years are likely to see much more of this cross-fertilization between pharmacoepidemiology and molecular biology, and newer forms of "-omics" such as the microbiome. From a research perspective, we can easily envision pharmacogenetic studies added to the process of evaluating potential adverse reactions. We also anticipate the availability of genotypic information for members of large patient cohorts for whom drug exposures and clinical outcomes are recorded electronically, and even for selected patients from electronic data systems, such as those described in Part II of this book.

### New Content Areas of Interest

In addition, there are a number of new content areas that are likely to be explored and developed more. Studies of drug utilization will continue and will continue to become more innovative (see "Studies of Drug Utilization" in Chapter 23). Particularly as the health care industry becomes more sensitive to the possibility of overutilization, underutilization, and inappropriate utilization of drugs, and the risks associated with each, one would expect to see an increased frequency of and sophistication in drug utilization review programs, which seek to improve care (see "Evaluating and Improving Prescribing" in Chapter 23), potentially incorporating techniques from molecular pharmacoepidemiology (see Chapter 15).

The US Joint Commission on Accreditation of Healthcare Organizations revolutionized US hospital pharmacoepidemiology through its standards requiring adverse drug reaction surveillance and drug use evaluation program in every hospital. Hospitals are also now experimenting with different methods of organizing their drug delivery systems to improve their use of drugs, e.g. use of computerized clinical decision support and the addition of pharmacists to patient care teams (see "The Pharmacoepidemiology of Medication Errors" in Chapter 23).

Interest in the field of pharmacoeconomics, i.e. the application of the principles of health economics to the study of drug effects, is continuing (see Chapter 18). Society is realizing that the acquisition cost of drugs is often a very minor part of their economic impact, and that their beneficial and harmful effects can be vastly more important. Further, more governments and insurance programs are increasingly requiring economic justification before permitting reimbursement for a drug. As a result, the number of studies exploring this is increasing. As the methods of pharmacoeconomics become increasingly sophisticated, and its applications clear, this could be expected to continue to be a popular field of inquiry.

More non-experimental studies of beneficial drug effects, particularly of drug effectiveness, can be expected, as the field becomes more aware that such studies are possible. This is being encouraged by the rapid increase in the use of propensity scores to adjust for measured covariates, although investigators using this method often place more confidence in that technique than is warranted, some not recognizing that its ability to control for confounding by indication remains dependent on one's ability to *measure* the true determinants of exposure (see Chapter 22). It is also being encouraged

by the development of comparative effectiveness research. Other approaches to controlling for confounding are similarly likely to become more common as they are further developed (see Chapter 22). New analytic approaches, like machine learning, artificial intelligence, and cognitive computing, are also likely to make their way into pharmacoepidemiology studies.

We will also see more use of pharmacoepidemiologic approaches prior to drug approval, e.g. to understand the baseline rate of adverse events that one can expect to see in patients who will eventually be treated with a new drug (see "The View from Industry" in Chapter 6).

Recent years have seen an explosion in the worldwide use of herbal and other complementary and alternative medications, including cannabis-based products. These are essentially pharmaceuticals sold without conventional standardization, and with no required premarketing testing of safety or efficacy. In a sense, for these products, this is a return to a pre-regulatory era. Therefore, it is quite likely that the next few years will see an analogous set of safety concerns associated with their use, and society will turn to pharmacoepidemiologists to help evaluate the use and effects of these products. Of course, if regulatory oversight is decreased in some countries, as has been suggested in the US, the same could occur with traditional medications.

Research interest in the entire topic of patient nonadherence with prescribed drug regimens goes back to about 1960, but little fruitful research could be done because methods for ascertaining drug exposure in individual ambulatory patients were grossly unsatisfactory. This problem has been mitigated greatly by advances in incorporating time-stamping microcircuitry into pharmaceutical containers, which records the date and time each time that the container is opened. Perhaps as a consequence of its inherent simplicity and economy, electronic monitoring is increasingly emerging as the de facto gold standard for compiling dosing histories of ambulatory patients, from which one can evaluate the extent of adherence to the prescribed drug regimen. Future years are likely to see a continuing increase in the use of this technique (see Chapter 21) in research, and perhaps in clinical practice. Perhaps equally importantly, new methods of measuring adherence that do not rely on purchasing and using alternative sources of drug dispensing, such as smartphone-based measures of pill taking, may expand our ability to measure adherence in real-world epidemiology studies.

The next few years are also likely to see the increasing ability to target drug therapy to the proper patients. This will involve both increasing use of statistical methods, and increasing use of laboratory techniques from other biological sciences, as described above. Statistical approaches will allow us to use predictive modeling to study, from a population perspective, who is most likely to derive benefit from a drug, and who is at greatest risk of an adverse outcome. Laboratory science will enable us to measure individuals' biomarkers to predict responses to drug therapy (i.e. molecular susceptibility). From the perspective of pre-approval testing, these developments may allow researchers to target specific patient-types for enrollment into their studies, those subjects most likely to succeed with a drug. From a clinical perspective, it will enable health care providers to incorporate biological factors in the individualization of choice of regimens.

The past few years have seen the increased use of surrogate markers, presumed to represent increased risk of rarer serious adverse effects when drugs are used in broader numbers of patients. These range from mild liver function test abnormalities, used as predictors of serious liver toxicity, to electrocardiographic QTc prolongation as a marker of risk of suffering the arrhythmia torsades des pointes, which can lead to death. Indeed, some drugs have been removed from the market, or from development, because of the presence of these surrogate markers. Yet, the utility of these markers as predictors of serious clinical outcomes is poorly studied. The next few years are likely to

see the increased use of both very large observational studies and large simple trials after marketing, to study important clinical outcomes (see Chapters 17 and 20).

In addition, with the growth of concerns about patient safety (see "The Pharmacoepidemiology of Medication Errors" in Chapter 23), there has been increasing attention to simultaneous use of pairs of drugs that have been shown in pharmacokinetic studies (see Chapter 4) to cause increased or decreased drug levels. Yet, population studies informing the clinical importance and pharmacologic aspects of drug–drug interactions have only been performed in the past few years. The next few years are likely to see the emergence of more studies to address such questions.

Finally, in the last few years, society has increasingly turned to pharmacoepidemiology for input into major policy decisions. For example, pharmacoepidemiology played a major role in the evaluations by the Institute of Medicine of the US National Academy of Sciences of the Anthrax Vaccine (deciding whether the existing vaccine was safe to use and, thereby, whether the military vaccine program should be restarted) and the Smallpox Vaccine program (deciding the shape of the program intended initially to vaccinate the entire US population). Pharmacoepidemiology is likely to contribute to future assessment of vaccine effectiveness and safety in the population (e.g. for the SARS-CoV-2 vaccine).

### Logistical Advances

Logistically, with the increased computerization of data in society in general and within health care in particular, and the increased emphasis on using electronic databases for pharmacoepidemiology (see Part II), some data resources will disappear (e.g. The Rhode Island Drug Use Reporting System and the inpatient databases discussed in prior editions of this book have disappeared, with new ones added) and a number of new computerized databases have emerged as major resources for pharmacoepidemiologic research (e.g.

commercial insurance databases [Chapter 9], inpatient databases, the databases from Ontario and Denmark [Chapter 9]). The importance of these databases to pharmacoepidemiology is now clear: they enable researchers to address, quickly and relatively inexpensively, questions about drug effects in different settings that require large sample sizes, with excellent quality data on drug exposures. Registries (Chapter 11) will also become increasingly important for pharmacoepidemiologic research. With the initiation of US Medicare Part D in 2006, which provides prescription drug coverage to US Medicare recipients, the availability of this data resource is advancing our ability to perform hypothesis testing studies, as it is so large relative to other resources; nearly 27 million Medicare beneficiaries were already subscribed to Part D coverage in 2009 (see Chapter 9). It has created an enormous new data resource for pharmacoepidemiology, as well as increased interest from the US government in what pharmacoepidemiology can do. The development of FDA's Sentinel Initiative has, similarly, provided a vast new data resource, initially intended for hypothesis generating, and more recently used for hypothesis strengthening and testing.

Nevertheless, even as the use of databases increases, it is important to keep in mind the importance of studies that collect data de novo (see Chapter 11). Each approach to pharmacoepidemiology has its advantages and its disadvantages, as described in Part II. No approach is ideal in all circumstances, and often a number of complementary approaches are needed to answer any given research question (see Chapter 12). To address some of the problems inherent in any database, we must maintain the ability to perform ad hoc studies, as well (see Chapter 11). Perhaps better, less expensive, and complementary approaches to ad hoc data collection in pharmacoepidemiology will be developed. For example, a potential approach that has not been widely used is the network of regional and national poison control centers. In particular, poison control centers would be expected to be a useful source of information about dose-dependent adverse drug effects. Others will undoubtedly be developed as well.

Of critical importance, there is increasing concern about patient privacy in many countries. The regulatory framework for human research is actively changing, in the process, e.g. Europe's new data protection law. As discussed in Chapter 16, this is already beginning to make pharmacoepidemiologic research more difficult, whether it is access to medical records in database studies, or access to a list of possible cases with a disease to enroll in ad hoc case–control studies. This will be an area of great interest and rapid activity over the next few years as electronic health records become much more commonplace, and one in which the field of pharmacoepidemiology will need to remain very active, or risk considerable interference with its activities.

It is likely that new types of research opportunities will emerge. For example, as the US finally implemented a drug benefit as part of Medicare, its health program for the elderly, US government drug expenditures suddenly increased by $49.5 billion in 2007. Outside the US, as well, many different opportunities to form databases are being developed. There is also an increased interest in the importance of pharmacoepidemiology in the developing world. Many developing world countries spend a disproportionate amount of their health care resources on drugs, yet these drugs are often used inappropriately. There have been a number of initiatives in response to this, including the World Health Organization's development of its list of "Essential Drugs."

## Funding

For a number of years, academic pharmacoepidemiology suffered from limited research funding opportunities. In the early 1980s, the only available US funding for the field was an extramural funding program from FDA with a total of $1 million/year. Industry interest and support were similarly limited. With the increasing interest in the field, this situation appears to be changing rapidly. FDA has expanded its internal pharmacoepidemiology program, and US National Institutes of Health (NIH) is funding pharmacoepidemiologic studies as well. In the US, other funding now comes from the Agency for Health Care Research and Quality (AHRQ), and from the Patient-Centered Outcomes Research Institute (PCORI), created as part of the Affordable Care Act. Much industry funding is available, as the perceived need for the field within industry grows (see below). This is likely to increase, especially as the FDA more often requires industry to perform postmarketing studies, and the legislative mandate for FDA to pay more attention to "real world evidence."

There is, of course, a risk associated with academic groups becoming too dependent on industry funding, both in terms of choice of study questions and credibility. Fortunately, in the US, AHRQ began to fund pharmacoepidemiologic research as well, as part of an initiative in pharmaceutical outcomes research. In particular, the AHRQ Centers for Education and Research on Therapeutics (CERTs) program provided federal support for ongoing pharmacoepidemiologic activities (see "The View from Academia" in Chapter 6). While still small relative to industry expenditures on research, it was large relative to the US federal funding previously available for pharmacoepidemiology. Similar programs have now been started in Europe and Canada. Unfortunately, the CERTs program has ended and periodically, the future of AHRQ itself is in question.

Even the US NIH now funds pharmacoepidemiologic projects more often. NIH is the logical major US source for such support, as it is the major funding source for most basic biomedical research in the US. Its funds are also accessible to investigators outside the US, via the same application procedures. However, NIH's current organizational structure represents an obstacle to pharmacoepidemiologic support. In general, the institutes within NIH are organized by organ system. Earlier in the development of pharmacoepidemiology, the National Institute of General Medical Sciences (NIGMS) provided most of the US government support for our field. It remains, conceptually, perhaps the most appropriate source of such support, since it is the institute that is intended to fund projects that are not specific to an organ system, and it is the institute that funds clinical pharmacologic research. However, over the past few years there has been limited funding from NIGMS for epidemiologic research. A notable exception was the NIGMS-funded Pharmacogenetics Research Network (PGRN), which has now been disbanded. In the meantime, NIH funding continues to be available if one tailors a project to fit an organ system or in some other way fits the priorities of one of the individual institutes, e.g. the National Institute on Aging or the National Institute of Child Health and Human Development.

## Personnel

With the major increase in interest in the field of pharmacoepidemiology, accompanied by an increased number of funding opportunities, a major remaining problem, aggravated by the other trends, is one of inadequate personnel resources. There is a desperate need for more well-trained people in the field, with employment opportunities available in academia, industry, and government agencies. Some early attempts were made to address this. The Burroughs Wellcome Foundation developed the Burroughs Wellcome Scholar Award in Pharmacoepidemiology, a faculty development award designed to bring new people into the field. This program, now discontinued, did not provide an opportunity for fellowship training of entry-level individuals, but was designed for more experienced investigators. Unfortunately, it is no longer an active program.

Outside of government, training opportunities are limited. In the US, the NIH is the major source of support for scientific training but as noted above, NIGMS, which funds training programs in clinical pharmacology, now supports one program in pharmacoepidemiology, while the National Heart, Lung and Blood Institute supports another. The National Institute of Child Health and Human Development also has funded limited training in pediatric pharmacoepidemiology. However, pharmacoepidemiologic training is still too dependent on non-federal sources of funds, especially at a time when such funding is becoming harder to obtain. There is a growing number of institutions now capable of carrying out such training, for example universities with faculty members interested in pharmacoepidemiology, including those with clinical research training programs supported by, for example, an NIH Clinical and Translational Science Award and organ system-specific training grants. Young scientists interested in undergoing training in pharmacoepidemiology, however, can only do so if they happen to qualify for support from such programs. No ongoing support is normally available from these programs for training in pharmacoepidemiology per se. This was addressed in the past, primarily through the leadership and generosity of some pharmaceutical companies. Much more is needed, however. Fortunately, with the rapid rise in interest in comparative effectiveness research, additional training support emerged from both NIH and AHRQ/PCORI, but this too is now in question going forward.

## The View from Industry

It appears that the role of pharmacoepidemiology in industry is and will continue to be expanding rapidly. All that was said above about the future of pharmacoepidemiology scientifically, as it relates to academia (see Chapter 6), obviously relates to industry, as well (see again Chapter 6). The necessity of pharmacoepidemiology for industry has become apparent to many of those in industry.

In addition to being useful for exploring the effects of their drugs, manufacturers are beginning to realize that the field can contribute not only to identifying problems, but also to documenting drug safety and developing and evaluating risk management programs. An increasing number of manufacturers are mounting pharmacoepidemiologic studies "prophylactically," to have safety data available in advance of when crises may occur. Proper practice would argue for postmarketing studies for all newly marketed drugs used for chronic diseases, and all drugs expected to be either pharmacologically novel or sales blockbusters, because of the unique risks that these situations present. Pharmacoepidemiology also can be used for measuring beneficial drug effects and even for marketing purposes, in the form of descriptive market research and analyses of the effects of marketing efforts. Perhaps most importantly for the industry's financial bottom line, pharmacoepidemiologic studies can be used to protect the major investment made in developing a new drug against false allegations of adverse effects and protecting good drugs for a public that needs them. Further, even if a drug is found to have a safety problem, the legal liability of the company may be diminished if the company has, from the outset, been forthright in its efforts to learn about that drug's risks. Finally, as noted in Chapter 1 and above, FDA now has new authority to require postmarketing pharmacoepidemiologic studies, and a new charge to focus on "real world evidence," so one can expect to see many more required of industry by regulators.

Industry is always interested in predictability. With that, there is increased interest in developing a formulaic approach to benefit–risk assessment (see "Benefit-Risk Assessments of Medical Treatments" in Chapter 23). The next few years are likely to see considerable additional work in this area.

In light of these advantages, most major pharmaceutical firms have formed their own pharmacoepidemiologic units. Of course, this then means that industry confronts and, in fact, aggravates the problem of an insufficient number of well-trained personnel described above. Many pharmaceutical companies increased their investment in external pharmacoepidemiologic data resources, so that they will be available for research when crises arise. This has been declining, however. A risk of the growth in the number of pharmacoepidemiologic studies for industry is the generation of an increased number of false signals about harmful drug effects. This is best addressed by having adequately trained individuals in the field, and by having personnel and data resources available to address these questions quickly, responsibly, and effectively, when they are raised.

## The View from Regulatory Agencies

It appears that the role of pharmacoepidemiology in regulatory agencies is also expanding (see Chapter 6). Again, all of what was said above about the future of pharmacoepidemiology scientifically, as it relates to academia, obviously relates to regulatory agencies, as well. In addition, there have been a large number of major drug crises, many described throughout this book. Many of these crises resulted in the removal of the drugs from the market. The need for and importance of pharmacoepidemiologic studies have become clear. Again, this can be expected to continue in the future. It has even been suggested that postmarketing pharmacoepidemiologic studies might replace some premarketing Phase III studies in selected situations, as was done with zidovudine. As noted, regulatory agencies are being given increased authority to require such studies after marketing. Regulatory bodies are also expanding their pharmacoepidemiologic staffing and seeking training in pharmacoepidemiology for those already employed by the agencies.

We are also seeing increasing governmental activity and interest in pharmacoepidemiology, outside the traditional realm of regulatory bodies. For example, in the US, pharmacoepidemiology used to play an important role within the AHRQ, the Centers for Disease Control and Prevention, PCORI, and the NIH, and there has been for over 40 years intermittent debate about the wisdom of developing an independent new Center for Drug Surveillance.

As noted above, the use of therapeutic risk management approaches (see "Risk Management" in Chapter 23) has been aggressively embraced by regulatory bodies around the world, and there has been considerable discussion about benefit–risk assessments of medical products (see "Benefit-Risk Assessments of Medical Treatments" in Chapter 23). This will continue to change regulation as more experience with it is gained.

There is considerable regulatory interest in getting important new drugs onto the market quickly, using mechanisms such as FDA's initiatives on orphan drugs, expanded access programs, compassionate use programs, fast track regulations, accelerated approval, priority review, breakthrough drug designation, and use of "real-world evidence," and analogous initiatives elsewhere. On the other hand, efforts like the Right to Try Act may compromise the scientific rigor of the normal regulatory approach. The future is likely to see continued creative regulatory initiatives toward maintaining this balance.

There is also increased interest in encouraging the use of generic drugs, reducing costs, and reducing regulatory obstacles to the availability of generically equivalent drugs, once patents expire.

Finally, there is an enormous increase in attention to drug safety, e.g. driven by drug safety issues identified with COX-2 inhibitors and even traditional nonsteroidal anti-inflammatory drugs, and then by the thiazolidinediones, used for treatment of diabetes. The net result has been major regulatory change, and even new legislation. Between 2009 and 2012, for example, FDA approved 110 new drugs and biologics for 120 indications, and only 13 of them did not have any postmarketing requirements.

## The View from the Law

Finally, the importance of pharmacoepidemiology to the law has also been increasing. The potential financial risk to drug manufacturers posed by lawsuits related to adverse drug effects is very large. Some financial payments have been enormous, and indeed put large multinational companies at risk. It is clear that the interest in the field and the need for more true experts in the field will, therefore, increase accordingly.

## Conclusion

*There are no really "safe" biologically active drugs. There are only "safe" physicians.*
Harold A. Kaminetzsky 1963

All drugs have adverse effects. Pharmacoepidemiology will never succeed in preventing them. It can only detect them, hopefully early, and thereby educate health care providers and the public, which will lead to better medication use. Pharmacoepidemiology can also lead to safer use of medications through a better understanding of the factors that alter the risk: benefit balance of medications. The net results of increased activity in pharmacoepidemiology will be better for industry and academia but, most importantly, for the public's health. The next drug disaster cannot be prevented by pharmacoepidemiology. However, pharmacoepidemiology can minimize its adverse public health impact by detecting it early. At the same time, it can improve the use of drugs that have a genuine role, protecting against the loss of useful drugs. The past few decades have demonstrated the utility of this new field. They also have pointed out some of its problems. With luck, the next few years will see the utility accentuated and the problems ameliorated.

## Key Points

- The discipline of pharmacoepidemiology has been growing and will likely continue to grow within academia, industry, and government.
- Methodological advances are expected to continue in order to support pharmacoepidemiologic studies as well as newer approaches such as risk management programs and molecular pharmacoepidemiology.
- Content areas such as pharmacoeconomics, medication adherence, risk management, and intermediate surrogate markers will grow as interest and need for these foci increases.
- Both automated databases and de novo studies will continue to be important to the field and will serve as important complements to each other.
- Challenges faced by pharmacoepidemiology include limited funding opportunities, regulatory restrictions and privacy concerns surrounding human research, limited training opportunities, and inadequate personnel resources.
- All sectors responsible for the public health, including academia, industry, and government, must address the challenges facing pharmacoepidemiology, and must support its continued development in order to maximize the benefit and minimize the risk inherent in all medications and medical devices.

## Further Reading

Andrews, E.B., Avorn, J., Bortnichak, E.A. et al. (1996). Guidelines for good epidemiology practices for drug, device, and vaccine research in the United States. *Pharmacoepidemiol. Drug Saf.* 5: 333–338.

Bates, D.W., Leape, L.L., Cullen, D.J. et al. (1998). Effect of computerized physician order entry and a team intervention on prevention of serious medication errors. *JAMA* 280: 1311–1316.

Classen, D.C., Pestotnik, S.L., Evans, R.S., and Burke, J.P. (1991). Computerized surveillance of adverse drug events in hospital patients. *JAMA* 266: 2847–2851.

Committee on Smallpox Vaccination Program Implementation, Board on Health Promotion and Disease Prevention (2005). *The Smallpox Vaccination Program: Public Health in an Age of Terrorism* (eds. A. Baciu, A.P. Anason, K. Stratton and B. Strom). Washington, DC: The National Academies Press.

Food and Drug Administration, eHealth Foundation, and the Brookings Institute (2008) Sentinel Initiative: structure, function and scope. Washington, D.C. December 16, 2008. http://www.fda.gov/oc/initiatives/criticalpath/transcript121608.pdf

Howard, N.J. and Laing, R.O. (1991). Changes in the World Health Organization essential drug list. *Lancet* 338: 743–745.

Institute of Medicine (2005). *The Smallpox Vaccination Program: Public Health in an Age of Terrorism*. Washington, DC: National Academies Press.

ISPE (2008). Guidelines for good pharmacoepidemiology practices (GPP). *Pharmacoepidemiol. Drug Saf.* 17: 200–208.

Joellenbeck, L.M., Zwanziger, L.L., Durch, J.S., and Strom, B.L. (eds.) (2002). *The Anthrax Vaccine: Is It Safe? Does It Work?* Washington, DC: National Academies Press.

Kettering, C.F. (January 1946). *Picturesque Speech and Patter, Reader's Digest*, vol. 48, 102. Pleasantville, New York: The Reader's Digest Association.

Leeder, J.S., Riley, R.J., Cook, V.A., and Spielberg, S.P. (1992). Human anti-cytochrome P450 antibodies in aromatic anticonvulsant-induced hypersensitivity reactions. *J. Pharmacol. Exp. Ther.* 263: 360–367.

Lunde, P.K.M. (1984). WHOs programme on essential drugs. Background, implementation, present state and prospectives. *Dan. Med. Bull.* 31 (suppl 1): 23–27.

Pullar, T. and Feely, M. (1990). Problems of compliance with drug treatment: new solutions? *Pharm. J.* 245: 213–215.

Spielberg, S.P. (1992). Idiosyncratic drug reactions: interaction of development and genetics. *Semin. Perinatol.* 16: 58–62.

Strom, B.L. and Carson, J.L. (1990). Use of automated databases for pharmacoepidemiology research. *Epidemiol. Rev.* 12: 87–107.

Strom, B.L. and Gibson, G.A. (1993). A systematic integrated approach to improving drug prescribing in an acute care hospital: a potential model for applied hospital pharmacoepidemiology. *Clin. Pharmacol. Ther.* 54: 126–133.

Strom, B.L., West, S.L., Sim, E., and Carson, J.L. (1989). The epidemiology of the acute flank pain syndrome from suprofen. *Clin. Pharmacol. Ther.* 46: 693–699.

Urquhart, J. (1997). The electronic medication event monitor–lessons for pharmacotherapy. *Clin. Pharmacokinet.* 32: 345–356.

Woosley, R.L., Drayer, D.E., Reidenberg, M.M. et al. (1978). Effect of acetylator phenotype on the rate at which procainamide induces antinuclear antibodies and the lupus syndrome. *N. Engl. J. Med.* 298: 1157–1159.

Young, F.E. (1988). The role of the FDA in the effort against AIDS. *Public Health Rep.* 103: 242–245.

Yudkin, J.S. (1980). The economics of pharmaceutical supply in Tanzania. *Int. J. Health Serv.* 10: 455–477.

Yudkin, J.S. (1984). Use and misuse of drugs in the third world. *Dan. Med. Bull.* 31 (suppl 1): 11–17.

# Sample Size Tables

**Table A1** Sample sizes for cohort studies[a].

| Incidence in control group | Relative risk to be detected | | | | | | | | | | | | | | | |
|---|---|---|---|---|---|---|---|---|---|---|---|---|---|---|---|---|
| | 0.2 | 0.3 | 0.5 | 0.75 | 1.25 | 1.5 | 2.0 | 2.5 | 3.0 | 3.5 | 4.0 | 5.0 | 7.5 | 10.0 | 20.0 | 50.0 |
| 0.00001 | 1970717 | 2788497 | 6306290 | 29429320 | 37837603 | 10510431 | 3153120 | 1634946 | 1051034 | 756742 | 583904 | 394133 | 211445 | 142727 | 61134 | 22318 |
| 0.00005 | 394133 | 557684 | 1261219 | 5885657 | 7567179 | 2101980 | 630585 | 326965 | 210189 | 151334 | 116768 | 78816 | 42280 | 28538 | 12220 | 4458 |
| 0.0001 | 197060 | 278832 | 630585 | 2942699 | 3783376 | 1050923 | 315268 | 163467 | 105083 | 75657 | 58376 | 39401 | 21135 | 14264 | 6106 | 2225 |
| 0.0005 | 39401 | 55751 | 126078 | 588332 | 756333 | 210078 | 63015 | 32669 | 20999 | 15117 | 11662 | 7870 | 4219 | 2845 | 1215 | 439 |
| 0.001 | 19694 | 27865 | 63015 | 294037 | 377953 | 104973 | 31483 | 16320 | 10488 | 7549 | 5823 | 3928 | 2104 | 1418 | 603 | 216 |
| 0.005 | 3928 | 5557 | 12564 | 58600 | 75249 | 20888 | 6257 | 3240 | 2080 | 1495 | 1152 | 775 | 412 | 276 | 114 | 37 |
| 0.01 | 1957 | 2769 | 6257 | 29170 | 37411 | 10378 | 3104 | 1605 | 1028 | 738 | 568 | 381 | 201 | 133 | 53 | 15 |
| 0.05 | 381 | 538 | 1212 | 5627 | 7140 | 1969 | 582 | 297 | 188 | 133 | 101 | 65 | 32 | 19 | 4 | – |
| 0.10 | 184 | 259 | 582 | 2684 | 3357 | 918 | 266 | 133 | 82 | 57 | 42 | 26 | 10 | 4 | – | – |
| 0.15 | 118 | 166 | 372 | 1703 | 2095 | 568 | 161 | 79 | 47 | 32 | 23 | 13 | – | – | – | – |
| 0.20 | 85 | 120 | 266 | 1212 | 1465 | 393 | 109 | 52 | 30 | 19 | 13 | 6 | – | – | – | – |
| 0.25 | 65 | 92 | 203 | 918 | 1086 | 287 | 77 | 35 | 19 | 12 | 7 | – | – | – | – | – |
| 0.30 | 52 | 73 | 161 | 722 | 834 | 217 | 56 | 24 | 12 | 6 | – | – | – | – | – | – |
| 0.35 | 43 | 60 | 131 | 582 | 654 | 167 | 41 | 16 | 7 | – | – | – | – | – | – | – |
| 0.40 | 36 | 50 | 109 | 477 | 519 | 130 | 30 | 11 | – | – | – | – | – | – | – | – |
| 0.45 | 30 | 42 | 91 | 395 | 414 | 101 | 21 | 6 | – | – | – | – | – | – | – | – |
| 0.50 | 26 | 36 | 77 | 329 | 329 | 77 | 14 | – | – | – | – | – | – | – | – | – |
| 0.55 | 22 | 31 | 66 | 276 | 261 | 58 | 8 | – | – | – | – | – | – | – | – | – |
| 0.60 | 19 | 27 | 56 | 231 | 203 | 42 | 2 | – | – | – | – | – | – | – | – | – |
| 0.65 | 17 | 23 | 48 | 194 | 155 | 29 | – | – | – | – | – | – | – | – | – | – |
| 0.70 | 15 | 20 | 41 | 161 | 113 | 17 | – | – | – | – | – | – | – | – | – | – |
| 0.75 | 13 | 17 | 35 | 133 | 77 | 7 | – | – | – | – | – | – | – | – | – | – |
| 0.80 | 11 | 15 | 30 | 109 | 46 | – | – | – | – | – | – | – | – | – | – | – |
| 0.85 | 10 | 13 | 25 | 87 | 18 | – | – | – | – | – | – | – | – | – | – | – |
| 0.90 | 8 | 11 | 21 | 68 | – | – | – | – | – | – | – | – | – | – | – | – |
| 0.95 | 7 | 9 | 17 | 51 | – | – | – | – | – | – | – | – | – | – | – | – |

[a] $\alpha = 0.05$ (two-tailed), $\beta = 0.10$ (power = 90%), control: exposed ratio = 1:1. The sample size listed is the number of subjects needed in the exposed group. An equivalent number would be included in the control group.

**Table A2** Sample size for cohort studies[a].

| Incidence in control group | Relative risk to be detected | | | | | | | | | | | | | | | |
|---|---|---|---|---|---|---|---|---|---|---|---|---|---|---|---|---|
| | 0.2 | 0.3 | 0.5 | 0.75 | 1.25 | 1.5 | 2.0 | 2.5 | 3.0 | 3.5 | 4.0 | 5.0 | 7.5 | 10.0 | 20.0 | 50.0 |
| 0.00001 | 1529057 | 2153636 | 4825616 | 22279822 | 28149090 | 7764537 | 2302889 | 1183563 | 755529 | 540883 | 415381 | 278329 | 147626 | 99000 | 41938 | 15197 |
| 0.0001 | 152896 | 215349 | 482527 | 2227804 | 2814625 | 776367 | 230258 | 118337 | 151093 | 108167 | 83068 | 55659 | 29520 | 19795 | 8384 | 3036 |
| 0.0005 | 30570 | 43057 | 96475 | 445402 | 562673 | 155196 | 46024 | 23651 | 75539 | 54077 | 41528 | 27825 | 14756 | 9895 | 4189 | 1516 |
| 0.001 | 15280 | 21521 | 48218 | 222602 | 281179 | 77550 | 22994 | 11815 | 15095 | 10805 | 8297 | 5558 | 2946 | 1974 | 834 | 300 |
| 0.005 | 3047 | 4292 | 9613 | 44362 | 55984 | 15433 | 4571 | 2346 | 7540 | 5396 | 4143 | 2774 | 1469 | 984 | 414 | 148 |
| 0.01 | 1518 | 2138 | 4787 | 22082 | 27834 | 7668 | 2268 | 1163 | 1496 | 1069 | 820 | 548 | 288 | 192 | 79 | 26 |
| 0.05 | 295 | 415 | 927 | 4258 | 5315 | 1456 | 426 | 216 | 740 | 528 | 404 | 269 | 141 | 93 | 37 | 11 |
| 0.10 | 142 | 200 | 444 | 2030 | 2500 | 680 | 196 | 97 | 136 | 95 | 72 | 47 | 23 | 14 | 3 | – |
| 0.15 | 91 | 128 | 283 | 1287 | 1561 | 421 | 119 | 58 | 60 | 41 | 31 | 19 | 8 | 3 | – | – |
| 0.20 | 66 | 92 | 203 | 916 | 1092 | 291 | 80 | 38 | 35 | 23 | 17 | 9 | – | – | – | – |
| 0.25 | 50 | 70 | 155 | 693 | 811 | 214 | 57 | 26 | 22 | 14 | 10 | 4 | – | – | – | – |
| 0.30 | 40 | 56 | 123 | 545 | 623 | 162 | 42 | 18 | 14 | 9 | 5 | – | – | – | – | – |
| 0.35 | 33 | 46 | 100 | 439 | 489 | 125 | 31 | 12 | 9 | 4 | – | – | – | – | – | – |
| 0.40 | 27 | 38 | 82 | 359 | 388 | 97 | 22 | 8 | 5 | – | – | – | – | – | – | – |
| 0.45 | 23 | 32 | 69 | 297 | 310 | 76 | 16 | – | – | – | – | – | – | – | – | – |
| 0.50 | 20 | 27 | 58 | 248 | 248 | 58 | 11 | – | – | – | – | – | – | – | – | – |
| 0.55 | 17 | 23 | 49 | 207 | 196 | 44 | 5 | – | – | – | – | – | – | – | – | – |
| 0.60 | 15 | 20 | 42 | 173 | 154 | 32 | – | – | – | – | – | – | – | – | – | – |
| 0.65 | 13 | 17 | 36 | 145 | 117 | 22 | – | – | – | – | – | – | – | – | – | – |
| 0.70 | 11 | 15 | 31 | 120 | 86 | 13 | – | – | – | – | – | – | – | – | – | – |
| 0.75 | 9 | 13 | 26 | 99 | 59 | – | – | – | – | – | – | – | – | – | – | – |
| 0.80 | 8 | 11 | 22 | 80 | 35 | – | – | – | – | – | – | – | – | – | – | – |
| 0.85 | 7 | 10 | 18 | 64 | – | – | – | – | – | – | – | – | – | – | – | – |
| 0.90 | 6 | 8 | 15 | 49 | – | – | – | – | – | – | – | – | – | – | – | – |
| 0.95 | 5 | 7 | 12 | 36 | – | – | – | – | – | – | – | – | – | – | – | – |

[a] $\alpha = 0.05$ (two-tailed), $\beta = 0.10$ (power = 90%), control: exposed ratio = 2:1. The sample size listed is the number of subjects needed in the exposed group. Double this number would be included in the control group.

**Table A3** Sample sizes for cohort studies[a].

| Incidence in control group | Relative risk to be detected | | | | | | | | | | | | | | | |
|---|---|---|---|---|---|---|---|---|---|---|---|---|---|---|---|---|
| | 0.2 | 0.3 | 0.5 | 0.75 | 1.25 | 1.5 | 2.0 | 2.5 | 3.0 | 3.5 | 4.0 | 5.0 | 7.5 | 10.0 | 20.0 | 50.0 |
| 0.00001 | 1369471 | 1930847 | 4322614 | 19888657 | 24913372 | 6843626 | 2014756 | 1029014 | 653418 | 465696 | 356275 | 237254 | 124571 | 83030 | 34793 | 12510 |
| 0.00005 | 273886 | 386158 | 864495 | 3977589 | 4982452 | 1368657 | 402927 | 205788 | 130673 | 93131 | 71248 | 47445 | 24910 | 16602 | 6955 | 2499 |
| 0.0001 | 136938 | 193072 | 432230 | 1988706 | 2491087 | 684286 | 201449 | 102885 | 65330 | 46560 | 35619 | 23719 | 12452 | 8299 | 3476 | 1248 |
| 0.0005 | 27380 | 38603 | 86418 | 397599 | 497995 | 136790 | 40266 | 20563 | 13055 | 9303 | 7117 | 4738 | 2486 | 1656 | 692 | 247 |
| 0.001 | 13685 | 19294 | 43192 | 198711 | 248859 | 68352 | 20118 | 10272 | 6521 | 4646 | 3554 | 2365 | 1240 | 825 | 344 | 122 |
| 0.005 | 2729 | 3847 | 8611 | 39600 | 49549 | 13603 | 4000 | 2040 | 1294 | 921 | 703 | 467 | 244 | 161 | 66 | 21 |
| 0.01 | 1359 | 1916 | 4288 | 19711 | 24636 | 6759 | 1985 | 1011 | 640 | 455 | 347 | 230 | 119 | 78 | 31 | 9 |
| 0.05 | 264 | 372 | 830 | 3800 | 4705 | 1284 | 373 | 188 | 117 | 82 | 62 | 40 | 19 | 12 | 2 | – |
| 0.10 | 127 | 179 | 398 | 1811 | 2213 | 600 | 171 | 85 | 52 | 36 | 26 | 16 | 7 | 3 | – | – |
| 0.15 | 81 | 114 | 254 | 1148 | 1383 | 372 | 104 | 50 | 30 | 20 | 14 | 8 | – | – | – | – |
| 0.20 | 58 | 82 | 181 | 817 | 968 | 257 | 71 | 33 | 19 | 12 | 8 | 4 | – | – | – | – |
| 0.25 | 45 | 63 | 138 | 618 | 719 | 189 | 50 | 23 | 13 | 7 | 4 | – | – | – | – | – |
| 0.30 | 36 | 50 | 109 | 485 | 552 | 143 | 37 | 16 | 8 | 4 | – | – | – | – | – | – |
| 0.35 | 29 | 41 | 89 | 391 | 434 | 111 | 27 | 11 | 4 | – | – | – | – | – | – | – |
| 0.40 | 24 | 34 | 73 | 319 | 345 | 86 | 20 | 7 | – | – | – | – | – | – | – | – |
| 0.45 | 20 | 28 | 61 | 264 | 275 | 67 | 14 | – | – | – | – | – | – | – | – | – |
| 0.50 | 17 | 24 | 52 | 220 | 220 | 52 | 9 | – | – | – | – | – | – | – | – | – |
| 0.55 | 15 | 21 | 44 | 184 | 175 | 39 | – | – | – | – | – | – | – | – | – | – |
| 0.60 | 13 | 18 | 37 | 154 | 137 | 29 | – | – | – | – | – | – | – | – | – | – |
| 0.65 | 11 | 15 | 32 | 128 | 105 | 19 | – | – | – | – | – | – | – | – | – | – |
| 0.70 | 10 | 13 | 27 | 106 | 77 | 10 | – | – | – | – | – | – | – | – | – | – |
| 0.75 | 8 | 11 | 23 | 87 | 53 | – | – | – | – | – | – | – | – | – | – | – |
| 0.80 | 7 | 10 | 19 | 71 | 31 | – | – | – | – | – | – | – | – | – | – | – |
| 0.85 | 6 | 8 | 16 | 56 | – | – | – | – | – | – | – | – | – | – | – | – |
| 0.90 | 5 | 7 | 13 | 43 | – | – | – | – | – | – | – | – | – | – | – | – |
| 0.95 | 4 | 6 | 11 | 31 | – | – | – | – | – | – | – | – | – | – | – | – |

[a] $\alpha = 0.05$ (two-tailed), $\beta = 0.10$ (power $= 90\%$), control : exposed ratio $= 3:1$. The sample size listed is the number of subjects needed in the exposed group. Triple this number would be included in the control group.

**Table A4** Sample sizes for cohort studies[a].

| Incidence in control group | Relative risk to be detected | | | | | | | | | | | | | | | |
|---|---|---|---|---|---|---|---|---|---|---|---|---|---|---|---|---|
| | 0.2 | 0.3 | 0.5 | 0.75 | 1.25 | 1.5 | 2.0 | 2.5 | 3.0 | 3.5 | 4.0 | 5.0 | 7.5 | 10.0 | 20.0 | 50.0 |
| 0.00001 | 1 285 566 | 1 815 876 | 4 068 209 | 18 690 665 | 23 293 643 | 6 381 472 | 1 869 238 | 950 463 | 601 217 | 427 061 | 325 766 | 215 895 | 112 429 | 74 554 | 30 945 | 11 048 |
| 0.00005 | 257 106 | 363 164 | 813 616 | 3 737 999 | 4 658 521 | 1 276 231 | 373 825 | 190 079 | 120 234 | 85 404 | 65 147 | 43 174 | 22 482 | 14 907 | 6186 | 2207 |
| 0.0001 | 128 548 | 181 575 | 406 791 | 1 868 916 | 2 329 131 | 638 076 | 186 899 | 95 031 | 60 111 | 42 697 | 32 569 | 21 583 | 11 238 | 7451 | 3091 | 1102 |
| 0.0005 | 25 702 | 36 304 | 81 332 | 373 649 | 465 619 | 127 552 | 37 358 | 18 993 | 12 013 | 8532 | 6507 | 4311 | 2244 | 1487 | 615 | 218 |
| 0.001 | 12 846 | 18 145 | 40 650 | 186 741 | 232 680 | 63 737 | 18 665 | 9488 | 6000 | 4261 | 3249 | 2152 | 1119 | 741 | 306 | 107 |
| 0.005 | 2562 | 3618 | 8104 | 37 214 | 46 329 | 12 684 | 3711 | 1884 | 1190 | 844 | 643 | 425 | 220 | 145 | 58 | 19 |
| 0.01 | 1276 | 1802 | 4035 | 18 523 | 23 035 | 6303 | 1842 | 934 | 589 | 417 | 318 | 209 | 107 | 70 | 27 | 8 |
| 0.05 | 248 | 349 | 781 | 3571 | 4399 | 1198 | 346 | 174 | 108 | 76 | 57 | 36 | 17 | 10 | 2 | – |
| 0.10 | 119 | 168 | 374 | 1702 | 2070 | 560 | 159 | 78 | 48 | 33 | 24 | 15 | 6 | 2 | – | – |
| 0.15 | 76 | 107 | 238 | 1079 | 1294 | 347 | 97 | 47 | 28 | 19 | 13 | 7 | – | – | – | – |
| 0.20 | 55 | 77 | 171 | 767 | 905 | 240 | 66 | 31 | 18 | 11 | 8 | 3 | – | – | – | – |
| 0.25 | 42 | 59 | 130 | 580 | 672 | 177 | 47 | 21 | 12 | 7 | 4 | – | – | – | – | – |
| 0.30 | 33 | 47 | 103 | 456 | 517 | 134 | 34 | 15 | 7 | – | – | – | – | – | – | – |
| 0.35 | 27 | 38 | 83 | 366 | 406 | 103 | 25 | 10 | 3 | – | – | – | – | – | – | – |
| 0.40 | 23 | 32 | 69 | 300 | 323 | 81 | 18 | 6 | – | – | – | – | – | – | – | – |
| 0.45 | 19 | 27 | 58 | 248 | 258 | 63 | 13 | – | – | – | – | – | – | – | – | – |
| 0.50 | 16 | 23 | 48 | 206 | 206 | 48 | 8 | – | – | – | – | – | – | – | – | – |
| 0.55 | 14 | 19 | 41 | 172 | 164 | 37 | – | – | – | – | – | – | – | – | – | – |
| 0.60 | 12 | 16 | 35 | 144 | 128 | 27 | – | – | – | – | – | – | – | – | – | – |
| 0.65 | 10 | 14 | 30 | 120 | 98 | 18 | – | – | – | – | – | – | – | – | – | – |
| 0.70 | 9 | 12 | 25 | 99 | 72 | 7 | – | – | – | – | – | – | – | – | – | – |
| 0.75 | 8 | 10 | 21 | 81 | 50 | – | – | – | – | – | – | – | – | – | – | – |
| 0.80 | 6 | 9 | 18 | 66 | 29 | – | – | – | – | – | – | – | – | – | – | – |
| 0.85 | 6 | 8 | 15 | 52 | – | – | – | – | – | – | – | – | – | – | – | – |
| 0.90 | 5 | 6 | 12 | 39 | – | – | – | – | – | – | – | – | – | – | – | – |
| 0.95 | 4 | 5 | 10 | 28 | – | – | – | – | – | – | – | – | – | – | – | – |

[a] $\alpha = 0.05$ (two-tailed), $\beta = 0.10$ (power = 90%), control : exposed ratio = 4 : 1. The sample size listed is the number of subjects needed in the exposed group. Quadruple this number would be included in the control group.

**Table A5**  Sample sizes for cohort studies[a].

| Incidence in control group | Relative risk to be detected | | | | | | | | | | | | | | | |
|---|---|---|---|---|---|---|---|---|---|---|---|---|---|---|---|---|
| | 0.2 | 0.3 | 0.5 | 0.75 | 1.25 | 1.5 | 2.0 | 2.5 | 3.0 | 3.5 | 4.0 | 5.0 | 7.5 | 10.0 | 20.0 | 50.0 |
| 0.00001 | 1472091 | 2082958 | 4710686 | 21983178 | 28264016 | 7851105 | 2355325 | 1221276 | 785104 | 565273 | 436166 | 294411 | 157946 | 106615 | 45666 | 16672 |
| 0.00005 | 294411 | 416580 | 942108 | 4396481 | 5652548 | 1570142 | 471036 | 244238 | 157008 | 113044 | 87224 | 58875 | 31583 | 21318 | 9129 | 3330 |
| 0.0001 | 147201 | 208283 | 471036 | 2198144 | 2826115 | 785022 | 235500 | 122108 | 78496 | 56515 | 43606 | 29433 | 15788 | 10656 | 4562 | 1663 |
| 0.0005 | 29433 | 41645 | 94178 | 439474 | 564968 | 156925 | 47071 | 24404 | 15686 | 11292 | 8712 | 5879 | 3152 | 2126 | 908 | 329 |
| 0.001 | 14711 | 20816 | 47071 | 219641 | 282325 | 78413 | 23518 | 12191 | 7835 | 5639 | 4350 | 2935 | 1572 | 1060 | 451 | 162 |
| 0.005 | 2935 | 4152 | 9385 | 43774 | 56210 | 15604 | 4675 | 2421 | 1554 | 1117 | 861 | 579 | 309 | 207 | 86 | 28 |
| 0.01 | 1463 | 2069 | 4675 | 21790 | 27946 | 7752 | 2319 | 1199 | 769 | 552 | 425 | 285 | 151 | 100 | 40 | 12 |
| 0.05 | 285 | 402 | 906 | 4204 | 5334 | 1471 | 435 | 222 | 141 | 100 | 76 | 49 | 24 | 15 | 3 | – |
| 0.10 | 138 | 194 | 435 | 2005 | 2508 | 686 | 200 | 100 | 62 | 43 | 32 | 20 | 8 | 4 | – | – |
| 0.15 | 89 | 125 | 278 | 1273 | 1566 | 425 | 121 | 59 | 36 | 24 | 17 | 10 | – | – | – | – |
| 0.20 | 64 | 90 | 200 | 906 | 1095 | 294 | 82 | 39 | 24 | 15 | 10 | 5 | – | – | – | – |
| 0.25 | 49 | 69 | 152 | 686 | 812 | 215 | 58 | 27 | 15 | 9 | 6 | – | – | – | – | – |
| 0.30 | 40 | 55 | 121 | 540 | 623 | 163 | 42 | 19 | 10 | 5 | – | – | – | – | – | – |
| 0.35 | 33 | 45 | 99 | 435 | 489 | 125 | 31 | 13 | 6 | – | – | – | – | – | – | – |
| 0.40 | 27 | 38 | 82 | 357 | 388 | 97 | 23 | 8 | 5 | – | – | – | – | – | – | – |
| 0.45 | 23 | 32 | 69 | 295 | 309 | 76 | 16 | 5 | – | – | – | – | – | – | – | – |
| 0.50 | 20 | 27 | 58 | 247 | 247 | 58 | 11 | – | – | – | – | – | – | – | – | – |
| 0.55 | 17 | 24 | 50 | 207 | 195 | 44 | 7 | – | – | – | – | – | – | – | – | – |
| 0.60 | 15 | 20 | 42 | 173 | 152 | 32 | 2 | – | – | – | – | – | – | – | – | – |
| 0.65 | 13 | 18 | 36 | 145 | 116 | 22 | – | – | – | – | – | – | – | – | – | – |
| 0.70 | 11 | 15 | 31 | 121 | 85 | 13 | – | – | – | – | – | – | – | – | – | – |
| 0.75 | 10 | 13 | 27 | 100 | 58 | 6 | – | – | – | – | – | – | – | – | – | – |
| 0.80 | 9 | 12 | 23 | 82 | 35 | – | – | – | – | – | – | – | – | – | – | – |
| 0.85 | 8 | 10 | 19 | 66 | 14 | – | – | – | – | – | – | – | – | – | – | – |
| 0.90 | 7 | 9 | 16 | 51 | – | – | – | – | – | – | – | – | – | – | – | – |
| 0.95 | 6 | 8 | 14 | 38 | – | – | – | – | – | – | – | – | – | – | – | – |

[a] $\alpha = 0.05$ (two-tailed), $\beta = 0.20$ (power = 80%), control : exposed ratio = 1:1. The sample size listed is the number of subjects needed in the exposed group. An equivalent number would be included in the control group.

**Table A6** Sample sizes for cohort studies[a].

| Incidence in control group | Relative risk to be detected | | | | | | | | | | | | | | | |
|---|---|---|---|---|---|---|---|---|---|---|---|---|---|---|---|---|
| | 0.2 | 0.3 | 0.5 | 0.75 | 1.25 | 1.5 | 2.0 | 2.5 | 3.0 | 3.5 | 4.0 | 5.0 | 7.5 | 10.0 | 20.0 | 50.0 |
| 0.00001 | 1190356 | 1663432 | 3680447 | 16792779 | 20878641 | 5726194 | 1683582 | 859799 | 546209 | 389547 | 298242 | 198909 | 104767 | 69986 | 29458 | 10630 |
| 0.00005 | 238065 | 332677 | 736066 | 3358436 | 4175543 | 1145183 | 336697 | 171948 | 109233 | 77903 | 59643 | 39777 | 20950 | 13994 | 5889 | 2124 |
| 0.0001 | 119028 | 166332 | 368018 | 1679143 | 2087655 | 572556 | 168336 | 85967 | 54611 | 38947 | 29818 | 19886 | 10473 | 6995 | 2943 | 1061 |
| 0.0005 | 23799 | 33257 | 73580 | 335708 | 417346 | 114455 | 33648 | 17182 | 10914 | 7783 | 5958 | 3973 | 2091 | 1396 | 586 | 210 |
| 0.001 | 11895 | 16622 | 36775 | 167779 | 208557 | 57193 | 16812 | 8584 | 5452 | 3887 | 2975 | 1983 | 1043 | 696 | 292 | 104 |
| 0.005 | 2372 | 3315 | 7332 | 33436 | 41526 | 11382 | 3343 | 1705 | 1082 | 771 | 589 | 392 | 205 | 136 | 56 | 19 |
| 0.01 | 1182 | 1651 | 3651 | 16643 | 20647 | 5656 | 1659 | 845 | 536 | 381 | 291 | 193 | 100 | 66 | 26 | 8 |
| 0.05 | 230 | 321 | 707 | 3208 | 3944 | 1075 | 312 | 157 | 99 | 69 | 52 | 34 | 17 | 10 | 2 | – |
| 0.10 | 111 | 154 | 339 | 1529 | 1856 | 503 | 144 | 71 | 44 | 30 | 23 | 14 | 6 | 3 | – | – |
| 0.15 | 71 | 99 | 216 | 969 | 1160 | 312 | 88 | 43 | 26 | 17 | 13 | 7 | – | – | – | – |
| 0.20 | 51 | 71 | 155 | 689 | 812 | 216 | 60 | 28 | 17 | 11 | 8 | 4 | – | – | – | – |
| 0.25 | 39 | 54 | 118 | 522 | 603 | 159 | 43 | 20 | 11 | 7 | 4 | – | – | – | – | – |
| 0.30 | 31 | 43 | 93 | 410 | 464 | 121 | 32 | 14 | 7 | 4 | – | – | – | – | – | – |
| 0.35 | 26 | 35 | 76 | 330 | 365 | 93 | 23 | 10 | 4 | – | – | – | – | – | – | – |
| 0.40 | 21 | 29 | 63 | 270 | 290 | 73 | 17 | 6 | – | – | – | – | – | – | – | – |
| 0.45 | 18 | 25 | 52 | 223 | 232 | 57 | 13 | – | – | – | – | – | – | – | – | – |
| 0.50 | 15 | 21 | 44 | 186 | 186 | 44 | 9 | – | – | – | – | – | – | – | – | – |
| 0.55 | 13 | 18 | 38 | 155 | 148 | 34 | 5 | – | – | – | – | – | – | – | – | – |
| 0.60 | 11 | 16 | 32 | 130 | 116 | 25 | – | – | – | – | – | – | – | – | – | – |
| 0.65 | 10 | 13 | 27 | 108 | 89 | 18 | – | – | – | – | – | – | – | – | – | – |
| 0.70 | 9 | 12 | 23 | 90 | 66 | 11 | – | – | – | – | – | – | – | – | – | – |
| 0.75 | 8 | 10 | 20 | 74 | 46 | – | – | – | – | – | – | – | – | – | – | – |
| 0.80 | 7 | 9 | 17 | 60 | 28 | – | – | – | – | – | – | – | – | – | – | – |
| 0.85 | 6 | 7 | 14 | 47 | – | – | – | – | – | – | – | – | – | – | – | – |
| 0.90 | 5 | 6 | 12 | 36 | – | – | – | – | – | – | – | – | – | – | – | – |
| 0.95 | 4 | 5 | 9 | 26 | – | – | – | – | – | – | – | – | – | – | – | – |

[a] $\alpha = 0.05$ (two-tailed), $\beta = 0.20$ (power = 80%), control: exposed ratio = 2:1. The sample size listed is the number of subjects needed in the exposed group. Double this number would be included in the control group.

**Table A7** Sample sizes for cohort studies[a].

| Incidence in control group | Relative risk to be detected | | | | | | | | | | | | | | | |
|---|---|---|---|---|---|---|---|---|---|---|---|---|---|---|---|---|
| | 0.2 | 0.3 | 0.5 | 0.75 | 1.25 | 1.5 | 2.0 | 2.5 | 3.0 | 3.5 | 4.0 | 5.0 | 7.5 | 10.0 | 20.0 | 50.0 |
| 0.00001 | 1088323 | 1516254 | 3330831 | 15057392 | 18412768 | 5014203 | 1456566 | 736622 | 464207 | 328848 | 250342 | 165451 | 85870 | 56861 | 23565 | 8410 |
| 0.00005 | 217658 | 303242 | 666145 | 3011370 | 3682391 | 1002792 | 291297 | 147315 | 92835 | 65764 | 50064 | 33087 | 17171 | 11370 | 4711 | 1681 |
| 0.0001 | 108825 | 151615 | 333059 | 1505617 | 1841094 | 501366 | 145638 | 73651 | 46413 | 32879 | 25029 | 16541 | 8584 | 5684 | 2355 | 839 |
| 0.0005 | 21759 | 30314 | 66590 | 301015 | 368057 | 100225 | 29111 | 14721 | 9276 | 6570 | 5001 | 3305 | 1714 | 1134 | 469 | 166 |
| 0.001 | 10875 | 15151 | 33281 | 150439 | 183927 | 50082 | 14545 | 7354 | 4634 | 3282 | 2498 | 1650 | 855 | 566 | 233 | 82 |
| 0.005 | 2169 | 3021 | 6635 | 29979 | 36623 | 9968 | 2892 | 1461 | 920 | 651 | 495 | 326 | 168 | 111 | 45 | 15 |
| 0.01 | 1080 | 1505 | 3304 | 14922 | 18210 | 4954 | 1436 | 725 | 456 | 322 | 245 | 161 | 83 | 54 | 21 | 6 |
| 0.05 | 210 | 292 | 639 | 2876 | 3480 | 942 | 271 | 135 | 84 | 59 | 44 | 29 | 14 | 8 | 2 | – |
| 0.10 | 101 | 140 | 306 | 1370 | 1638 | 441 | 125 | 62 | 38 | 26 | 19 | 12 | 5 | 2 | – | – |
| 0.15 | 65 | 90 | 195 | 868 | 1025 | 274 | 76 | 37 | 22 | 15 | 11 | 6 | – | – | – | – |
| 0.20 | 46 | 64 | 139 | 617 | 718 | 190 | 52 | 25 | 14 | 9 | 6 | 3 | – | – | – | – |
| 0.25 | 36 | 49 | 106 | 466 | 534 | 140 | 37 | 17 | 10 | 6 | 4 | – | – | – | – | – |
| 0.30 | 28 | 39 | 84 | 366 | 411 | 107 | 28 | 12 | 6 | 3 | – | – | – | – | – | – |
| 0.35 | 23 | 32 | 68 | 294 | 323 | 83 | 21 | 9 | 4 | – | – | – | – | – | – | – |
| 0.40 | 19 | 26 | 56 | 240 | 257 | 65 | 15 | 6 | – | – | – | – | – | – | – | – |
| 0.45 | 16 | 22 | 47 | 199 | 206 | 51 | 11 | – | – | – | – | – | – | – | – | – |
| 0.50 | 14 | 19 | 39 | 165 | 165 | 39 | 8 | – | – | – | – | – | – | – | – | – |
| 0.55 | 12 | 16 | 33 | 138 | 132 | 30 | – | – | – | – | – | – | – | – | – | – |
| 0.60 | 10 | 14 | 28 | 115 | 104 | 23 | – | – | – | – | – | – | – | – | – | – |
| 0.65 | 9 | 12 | 24 | 96 | 80 | 16 | – | – | – | – | – | – | – | – | – | – |
| 0.70 | 8 | 10 | 20 | 79 | 60 | 9 | – | – | – | – | – | – | – | – | – | – |
| 0.75 | 7 | 9 | 17 | 65 | 42 | – | – | – | – | – | – | – | – | – | – | – |
| 0.80 | 6 | 7 | 14 | 52 | 26 | – | – | – | – | – | – | – | – | – | – | – |
| 0.85 | 5 | 6 | 12 | 41 | – | – | – | – | – | – | – | – | – | – | – | – |
| 0.90 | 4 | 5 | 10 | 31 | – | – | – | – | – | – | – | – | – | – | – | – |
| 0.95 | 3 | 4 | 8 | 22 | – | – | – | – | – | – | – | – | – | – | – | – |

[a] $\alpha = 0.05$ (two-tailed), $\beta = 0.20$ (power = 80%), control: exposed ratio = $3:1$. The sample size listed is the number of subjects needed in the exposed group. Triple this number would be included in the control group.

**Table A8** Sample sizes for cohort studies[a].

| Incidence in control group | Relative risk to be detected | | | | | | | | | | | | | | | |
|---|---|---|---|---|---|---|---|---|---|---|---|---|---|---|---|---|
| | 0.2 | 0.3 | 0.5 | 0.75 | 1.25 | 1.5 | 2.0 | 2.5 | 3.0 | 3.5 | 4.0 | 5.0 | 7.5 | 10.0 | 20.0 | 50.0 |
| 0.00001 | 1034606 | 1440316 | 3154116 | 14188116 | 17178604 | 4657092 | 1342104 | 674194 | 422454 | 297814 | 225764 | 148182 | 76019 | 49975 | 20438 | 7223 |
| 0.00005 | 206915 | 288054 | 630802 | 2837520 | 3435570 | 931374 | 268406 | 134830 | 84485 | 59558 | 45149 | 29633 | 15201 | 9993 | 4086 | 1443 |
| 0.0001 | 103454 | 144022 | 315388 | 1418696 | 1717691 | 465659 | 134194 | 67410 | 42238 | 29776 | 22572 | 14815 | 7599 | 4995 | 2042 | 721 |
| 0.0005 | 20685 | 28795 | 63057 | 283636 | 343387 | 93087 | 26824 | 13473 | 8442 | 5950 | 4510 | 2960 | 1518 | 997 | 407 | 143 |
| 0.001 | 10338 | 14392 | 31515 | 141754 | 171599 | 46516 | 13402 | 6731 | 4217 | 2972 | 2253 | 1478 | 757 | 497 | 203 | 71 |
| 0.005 | 2061 | 2870 | 6282 | 28248 | 34169 | 9259 | 2665 | 1338 | 837 | 590 | 446 | 292 | 149 | 98 | 39 | 13 |
| 0.01 | 1027 | 1429 | 3128 | 14059 | 16990 | 4601 | 1323 | 663 | 415 | 292 | 221 | 144 | 73 | 48 | 19 | 6 |
| 0.05 | 199 | 277 | 605 | 2709 | 3247 | 876 | 250 | 124 | 77 | 53 | 40 | 26 | 12 | 8 | 2 | – |
| 0.10 | 96 | 133 | 289 | 1290 | 1529 | 410 | 115 | 57 | 35 | 24 | 17 | 11 | 5 | 2 | – | – |
| 0.15 | 61 | 85 | 184 | 817 | 957 | 255 | 71 | 34 | 20 | 14 | 10 | 6 | – | – | – | – |
| 0.20 | 44 | 61 | 132 | 581 | 670 | 177 | 48 | 23 | 13 | 9 | 6 | 3 | – | – | – | – |
| 0.25 | 34 | 47 | 100 | 439 | 499 | 130 | 35 | 16 | 9 | 5 | 3 | – | – | – | – | – |
| 0.30 | 27 | 37 | 79 | 344 | 384 | 99 | 26 | 11 | 6 | – | – | – | – | – | – | – |
| 0.35 | 22 | 30 | 64 | 277 | 302 | 77 | 19 | 8 | 3 | – | – | – | – | – | – | – |
| 0.40 | 18 | 25 | 53 | 226 | 241 | 60 | 14 | 5 | – | – | – | – | – | – | – | – |
| 0.45 | 15 | 21 | 44 | 186 | 193 | 47 | 10 | – | – | – | – | – | – | – | – | – |
| 0.50 | 13 | 18 | 37 | 155 | 155 | 37 | 7 | – | – | – | – | – | – | – | – | – |
| 0.55 | 11 | 15 | 31 | 129 | 124 | 28 | – | – | – | – | – | – | – | – | – | – |
| 0.60 | 9 | 13 | 26 | 108 | 97 | 21 | – | – | – | – | – | – | – | – | – | – |
| 0.65 | 8 | 11 | 22 | 89 | 75 | 15 | – | – | – | – | – | – | – | – | – | – |
| 0.70 | 7 | 9 | 19 | 74 | 56 | 7 | – | – | – | – | – | – | – | – | – | – |
| 0.75 | 6 | 8 | 16 | 60 | 39 | – | – | – | – | – | – | – | – | – | – | – |
| 0.80 | 5 | 7 | 13 | 48 | 24 | – | – | – | – | – | – | – | – | – | – | – |
| 0.85 | 4 | 6 | 11 | 38 | – | – | – | – | – | – | – | – | – | – | – | – |
| 0.90 | 4 | 5 | 9 | 28 | – | – | – | – | – | – | – | – | – | – | – | – |
| 0.95 | 3 | 4 | 7 | 20 | – | – | – | – | – | – | – | – | – | – | – | – |

[a] $\alpha = 0.05$ (two-tailed), $\beta = 0.20$ (power = 80%), control: exposed ratio = 4:1. The sample size listed is the number of subjects needed in the exposed group. Quadruple this number would be included in the control group.

Table A9  Sample sizes for case–control studies[a].

| Prevalence in control group | Odds ratio to be detected | | | | | | | | | | | | | | | |
|---|---|---|---|---|---|---|---|---|---|---|---|---|---|---|---|---|
| | 0.2 | 0.3 | 0.5 | 0.75 | 1.25 | 1.5 | 2.0 | 2.5 | 3.0 | 3.5 | 4.0 | 5.0 | 7.5 | 10.0 | 20.0 | 50.0 |
| 0.00001 | 1970728 | 2788519 | 6306363 | 29429793 | 37838497 | 10510715 | 3153225 | 1635011 | 1051081 | 756780 | 583937 | 394159 | 211464 | 142743 | 61147 | 22330 |
| 0.00005 | 394143 | 557705 | 1261292 | 5886130 | 7568072 | 2102264 | 630690 | 327029 | 210236 | 151372 | 116801 | 78842 | 42300 | 28555 | 12234 | 4469 |
| 0.0001 | 197070 | 278853 | 630659 | 2943172 | 3784269 | 1051207 | 315373 | 163532 | 105130 | 75696 | 58409 | 39427 | 21155 | 14281 | 6120 | 2237 |
| 0.0005 | 39412 | 55772 | 126151 | 588806 | 757227 | 210362 | 63120 | 32734 | 21046 | 15155 | 11695 | 7896 | 4238 | 2862 | 1228 | 451 |
| 0.001 | 19704 | 27887 | 63088 | 294510 | 378847 | 105257 | 31588 | 16384 | 10535 | 7587 | 5856 | 3954 | 2124 | 1435 | 617 | 228 |
| 0.005 | 3939 | 5579 | 12638 | 59074 | 76145 | 21173 | 6363 | 3304 | 2127 | 1533 | 1184 | 801 | 432 | 293 | 128 | 49 |
| 0.01 | 1968 | 2790 | 6331 | 29646 | 38309 | 10663 | 3210 | 1669 | 1076 | 777 | 601 | 407 | 221 | 150 | 67 | 27 |
| 0.05 | 391 | 560 | 1288 | 6111 | 8059 | 2261 | 690 | 363 | 237 | 172 | 135 | 93 | 52 | 37 | 18 | 9 |
| 0.10 | 195 | 281 | 659 | 3181 | 4302 | 1219 | 379 | 202 | 133 | 98 | 77 | 54 | 32 | 23 | 13 | 8 |
| 0.15 | 129 | 189 | 451 | 2215 | 3072 | 879 | 278 | 150 | 100 | 75 | 60 | 43 | 26 | 19 | 11 | 8 |
| 0.20 | 97 | 143 | 348 | 1741 | 2476 | 716 | 230 | 126 | 85 | 64 | 52 | 37 | 23 | 18 | 11 | 8 |
| 0.25 | 77 | 116 | 287 | 1465 | 2137 | 624 | 203 | 113 | 77 | 59 | 48 | 35 | 23 | 18 | 12 | 9 |
| 0.30 | 64 | 98 | 248 | 1289 | 1930 | 569 | 188 | 106 | 73 | 56 | 46 | 34 | 23 | 18 | 13 | 10 |
| 0.35 | 56 | 86 | 222 | 1174 | 1802 | 536 | 180 | 103 | 72 | 56 | 46 | 35 | 24 | 19 | 14 | 11 |
| 0.40 | 49 | 77 | 203 | 1097 | 1727 | 519 | 177 | 102 | 72 | 56 | 47 | 36 | 25 | 20 | 15 | 12 |
| 0.45 | 44 | 70 | 191 | 1048 | 1694 | 513 | 178 | 104 | 74 | 58 | 49 | 38 | 27 | 22 | 17 | 14 |
| 0.50 | 40 | 66 | 182 | 1023 | 1696 | 519 | 182 | 108 | 77 | 61 | 52 | 40 | 29 | 24 | 19 | 16 |
| 0.55 | 38 | 62 | 178 | 1019 | 1732 | 535 | 191 | 114 | 82 | 66 | 56 | 44 | 32 | 27 | 21 | 18 |
| 0.60 | 36 | 61 | 177 | 1035 | 1806 | 562 | 203 | 123 | 89 | 72 | 61 | 49 | 36 | 31 | 25 | 21 |
| 0.65 | 35 | 60 | 180 | 1077 | 1927 | 605 | 222 | 135 | 99 | 80 | 69 | 56 | 42 | 36 | 29 | 25 |
| 0.70 | 34 | 61 | 188 | 1149 | 2110 | 669 | 248 | 153 | 113 | 92 | 79 | 64 | 49 | 43 | 35 | 31 |
| 0.75 | 35 | 64 | 203 | 1268 | 2390 | 764 | 287 | 178 | 133 | 109 | 94 | 77 | 59 | 52 | 43 | 38 |
| 0.80 | 37 | 70 | 230 | 1465 | 2831 | 913 | 348 | 218 | 164 | 135 | 117 | 97 | 75 | 66 | 55 | 49 |
| 0.85 | 43 | 82 | 278 | 1811 | 3591 | 1168 | 451 | 285 | 216 | 179 | 156 | 129 | 101 | 90 | 75 | 68 |
| 0.90 | 54 | 108 | 379 | 2527 | 5143 | 1687 | 659 | 420 | 320 | 266 | 233 | 195 | 154 | 137 | 116 | 105 |
| 0.95 | 93 | 190 | 690 | 4717 | 9851 | 3257 | 1288 | 828 | 635 | 531 | 466 | 391 | 313 | 280 | 238 | 217 |

[a] $\alpha = 0.05$ (two-tailed), $\beta = 0.10$ (power = 90%), control: case ratio = 1:1. The sample size listed is the number of subjects needed in the case group. An equivalent number would be included in the control group.

**Table A10** Sample sizes for case–control studies[a].

| Prevalence in control group | Odds ratio to be detected | | | | | | | | | | | | | | | |
|---|---|---|---|---|---|---|---|---|---|---|---|---|---|---|---|---|
| | 0.2 | 0.3 | 0.5 | 0.75 | 1.25 | 1.5 | 2.0 | 2.5 | 3.0 | 3.5 | 4.0 | 5.0 | 7.5 | 10.0 | 20.0 | 50.0 |
| 0.00001 | 1529065 | 2153652 | 4825672 | 22280178 | 28149758 | 7764749 | 2302966 | 1183610 | 755564 | 540911 | 415405 | 278348 | 147639 | 99012 | 41948 | 15205 |
| 0.00005 | 305811 | 430731 | 965148 | 4456162 | 5630233 | 1553041 | 460628 | 236743 | 151128 | 108194 | 83091 | 55678 | 29534 | 19807 | 8393 | 3044 |
| 0.0001 | 152904 | 215366 | 482583 | 2228160 | 2815293 | 776578 | 230335 | 118385 | 75573 | 54105 | 41552 | 27844 | 14770 | 9906 | 4199 | 1524 |
| 0.0005 | 30578 | 43073 | 96531 | 445759 | 563340 | 155407 | 46101 | 23698 | 15130 | 10833 | 8321 | 5577 | 2960 | 1986 | 843 | 307 |
| 0.001 | 15288 | 21537 | 48274 | 222959 | 281846 | 77761 | 23072 | 11862 | 7574 | 5424 | 4167 | 2793 | 1483 | 996 | 424 | 155 |
| 0.005 | 3055 | 4308 | 9669 | 44719 | 56653 | 15644 | 4649 | 2393 | 1530 | 1097 | 844 | 567 | 302 | 204 | 88 | 34 |
| 0.01 | 1526 | 2154 | 4843 | 22440 | 28505 | 7880 | 2346 | 1210 | 775 | 556 | 428 | 289 | 155 | 105 | 46 | 19 |
| 0.05 | 303 | 431 | 984 | 4623 | 6001 | 1674 | 506 | 264 | 171 | 124 | 97 | 66 | 37 | 26 | 13 | 7 |
| 0.10 | 150 | 216 | 503 | 2405 | 3207 | 904 | 279 | 148 | 97 | 71 | 56 | 39 | 23 | 17 | 9 | 6 |
| 0.15 | 100 | 145 | 343 | 1673 | 2292 | 653 | 205 | 111 | 74 | 55 | 44 | 31 | 19 | 14 | 8 | 6 |
| 0.20 | 74 | 110 | 265 | 1313 | 1849 | 533 | 170 | 93 | 63 | 47 | 38 | 28 | 17 | 13 | 8 | 6 |
| 0.25 | 59 | 89 | 218 | 1104 | 1597 | 465 | 151 | 84 | 57 | 44 | 35 | 26 | 17 | 13 | 9 | 6 |
| 0.30 | 49 | 75 | 188 | 971 | 1443 | 425 | 140 | 79 | 55 | 42 | 34 | 26 | 17 | 14 | 9 | 7 |
| 0.35 | 42 | 65 | 168 | 883 | 1349 | 401 | 135 | 77 | 54 | 42 | 34 | 26 | 18 | 14 | 10 | 8 |
| 0.40 | 37 | 58 | 154 | 825 | 1294 | 388 | 133 | 77 | 54 | 42 | 35 | 27 | 19 | 15 | 11 | 9 |
| 0.45 | 33 | 53 | 144 | 788 | 1270 | 385 | 133 | 78 | 56 | 44 | 37 | 28 | 20 | 17 | 13 | 10 |
| 0.50 | 31 | 50 | 137 | 768 | 1272 | 389 | 137 | 81 | 58 | 46 | 39 | 31 | 22 | 19 | 14 | 12 |
| 0.55 | 28 | 47 | 133 | 764 | 1301 | 402 | 144 | 86 | 62 | 50 | 42 | 33 | 24 | 21 | 16 | 14 |
| 0.60 | 27 | 45 | 133 | 775 | 1357 | 423 | 154 | 93 | 68 | 55 | 47 | 37 | 28 | 24 | 19 | 16 |
| 0.65 | 26 | 45 | 135 | 805 | 1449 | 456 | 168 | 103 | 76 | 61 | 52 | 42 | 32 | 28 | 22 | 19 |
| 0.70 | 26 | 45 | 140 | 859 | 1588 | 505 | 188 | 116 | 86 | 70 | 61 | 49 | 38 | 33 | 27 | 23 |
| 0.75 | 26 | 47 | 151 | 947 | 1799 | 577 | 218 | 136 | 102 | 84 | 72 | 59 | 46 | 40 | 33 | 29 |
| 0.80 | 28 | 51 | 170 | 1092 | 2133 | 690 | 265 | 166 | 125 | 104 | 90 | 74 | 58 | 51 | 42 | 38 |
| 0.85 | 31 | 60 | 205 | 1349 | 2708 | 884 | 343 | 218 | 165 | 137 | 120 | 100 | 78 | 70 | 58 | 53 |
| 0.90 | 39 | 78 | 279 | 1880 | 3881 | 1278 | 503 | 322 | 246 | 205 | 180 | 150 | 119 | 107 | 90 | 82 |
| 0.95 | 66 | 137 | 506 | 3505 | 7438 | 2472 | 984 | 635 | 489 | 410 | 360 | 303 | 243 | 218 | 186 | 169 |

[a] $\alpha = 0.05$ (two-tailed), $\beta = 0.10$ (power = 90%), control: case ratio = 2:1. The sample size listed is the number of subjects needed in the case group. Double this number would be included in the control group.

**Table A11** Sample size for case–control studies.[a]

| Prevalence in control group | Odds ratio to be detected | | | | | | | | | | | | | | | |
|---|---|---|---|---|---|---|---|---|---|---|---|---|---|---|---|---|
| | 0.2 | 0.3 | 0.5 | 0.75 | 1.25 | 1.5 | 2.0 | 2.5 | 3.0 | 3.5 | 4.0 | 5.0 | 7.5 | 10.0 | 20.0 | 50.0 |
| 0.00001 | 1369478 | 1930861 | 4322663 | 19888975 | 24913964 | 6843813 | 2014824 | 1029056 | 653448 | 465720 | 356295 | 237271 | 124583 | 83040 | 34800 | 12517 |
| 0.00005 | 273893 | 386172 | 864545 | 3977907 | 4983044 | 1368844 | 402996 | 205830 | 130703 | 93155 | 71268 | 47461 | 24922 | 16612 | 6963 | 2506 |
| 0.0001 | 136945 | 193086 | 432280 | 1989023 | 2491679 | 684473 | 201517 | 102927 | 65360 | 46584 | 35640 | 23735 | 12464 | 8309 | 3483 | 1254 |
| 0.0005 | 27387 | 38617 | 86468 | 397917 | 498587 | 136977 | 40334 | 20604 | 13086 | 9328 | 7137 | 4754 | 2498 | 1666 | 700 | 253 |
| 0.001 | 13692 | 19309 | 43242 | 199028 | 249451 | 68540 | 20186 | 10314 | 6551 | 4671 | 3574 | 2382 | 1252 | 836 | 352 | 128 |
| 0.005 | 2736 | 3862 | 8661 | 39918 | 50143 | 13790 | 4068 | 2082 | 1324 | 945 | 724 | 484 | 256 | 171 | 73 | 28 |
| 0.01 | 1367 | 1931 | 4338 | 20030 | 25231 | 6947 | 2054 | 1053 | 671 | 480 | 368 | 246 | 131 | 88 | 39 | 16 |
| 0.05 | 271 | 387 | 881 | 4125 | 5313 | 1477 | 444 | 231 | 149 | 108 | 84 | 57 | 32 | 22 | 11 | 6 |
| 0.10 | 134 | 194 | 450 | 2145 | 2841 | 799 | 245 | 129 | 85 | 62 | 49 | 34 | 20 | 14 | 8 | 5 |
| 0.15 | 89 | 130 | 307 | 1491 | 2031 | 577 | 180 | 97 | 64 | 48 | 38 | 27 | 16 | 12 | 7 | 5 |
| 0.20 | 66 | 98 | 236 | 1171 | 1639 | 471 | 150 | 82 | 55 | 41 | 33 | 24 | 15 | 12 | 7 | 5 |
| 0.25 | 53 | 79 | 195 | 984 | 1417 | 412 | 133 | 74 | 50 | 38 | 31 | 23 | 15 | 12 | 8 | 6 |
| 0.30 | 44 | 67 | 168 | 865 | 1281 | 376 | 124 | 70 | 48 | 37 | 30 | 23 | 15 | 12 | 8 | 6 |
| 0.35 | 38 | 58 | 150 | 786 | 1197 | 355 | 119 | 68 | 47 | 37 | 30 | 23 | 16 | 13 | 9 | 7 |
| 0.40 | 33 | 52 | 137 | 734 | 1149 | 345 | 118 | 68 | 48 | 37 | 31 | 24 | 16 | 14 | 10 | 8 |
| 0.45 | 30 | 47 | 128 | 700 | 1128 | 342 | 119 | 69 | 49 | 39 | 32 | 25 | 18 | 15 | 11 | 9 |
| 0.50 | 27 | 44 | 122 | 682 | 1131 | 346 | 122 | 72 | 52 | 41 | 35 | 27 | 19 | 16 | 12 | 10 |
| 0.55 | 25 | 42 | 119 | 679 | 1156 | 357 | 128 | 76 | 55 | 44 | 38 | 30 | 22 | 18 | 14 | 12 |
| 0.60 | 24 | 40 | 118 | 689 | 1207 | 377 | 137 | 83 | 60 | 49 | 41 | 33 | 25 | 21 | 17 | 14 |
| 0.65 | 23 | 40 | 119 | 715 | 1289 | 406 | 150 | 91 | 67 | 55 | 47 | 38 | 28 | 24 | 20 | 17 |
| 0.70 | 23 | 40 | 124 | 762 | 1414 | 450 | 168 | 104 | 77 | 63 | 54 | 44 | 33 | 29 | 24 | 21 |
| 0.75 | 23 | 42 | 133 | 839 | 1602 | 515 | 195 | 121 | 91 | 75 | 65 | 53 | 41 | 36 | 29 | 26 |
| 0.80 | 24 | 45 | 150 | 968 | 1900 | 616 | 236 | 149 | 112 | 93 | 80 | 66 | 52 | 45 | 38 | 34 |
| 0.85 | 27 | 52 | 180 | 1194 | 2413 | 789 | 307 | 195 | 148 | 123 | 107 | 89 | 70 | 62 | 52 | 46 |
| 0.90 | 34 | 68 | 245 | 1664 | 3459 | 1142 | 450 | 288 | 220 | 184 | 161 | 134 | 107 | 95 | 80 | 72 |
| 0.95 | 57 | 119 | 444 | 3100 | 6632 | 2208 | 881 | 569 | 438 | 367 | 323 | 271 | 217 | 194 | 165 | 150 |

[a] $\alpha = 0.05$ (two-tailed), $\beta = 0.10$ (power = 90%), control : case ratio = 3 : 1. The sample size listed is the number of subjects needed in the case group. Triple this number would be included in the control group.

**Table A12** Sample sizes for case–control studies[a].

| Prevalence in control group | Odds ratio to be detected | | | | | | | | | | | | | | | |
|---|---|---|---|---|---|---|---|---|---|---|---|---|---|---|---|---|
| | 0.2 | 0.3 | 0.5 | 0.75 | 1.25 | 1.5 | 2.0 | 2.5 | 3.0 | 3.5 | 4.0 | 5.0 | 7.5 | 10.0 | 20.0 | 50.0 |
| 0.00001 | 1285573 | 1815890 | 4068256 | 18690963 | 23294197 | 6381647 | 1869301 | 950501 | 601245 | 427084 | 325786 | 215910 | 112440 | 74563 | 30952 | 11054 |
| 0.00005 | 257112 | 363178 | 813662 | 3738297 | 4659075 | 1276406 | 373889 | 190118 | 120262 | 85427 | 65166 | 43189 | 22493 | 14916 | 6193 | 2213 |
| 0.0001 | 128555 | 181589 | 406838 | 1869214 | 2329685 | 638251 | 186963 | 95070 | 60139 | 42720 | 32588 | 21599 | 11249 | 7461 | 3098 | 1108 |
| 0.0005 | 25709 | 36318 | 81379 | 373947 | 466173 | 127727 | 37422 | 19032 | 12041 | 8554 | 6526 | 4326 | 2255 | 1496 | 622 | 224 |
| 0.001 | 12853 | 18159 | 40697 | 187039 | 233234 | 63912 | 18729 | 9527 | 6028 | 4284 | 3269 | 2167 | 1130 | 750 | 313 | 113 |
| 0.005 | 2568 | 3632 | 8151 | 37513 | 46884 | 12860 | 3775 | 1923 | 1219 | 867 | 662 | 440 | 231 | 154 | 65 | 25 |
| 0.01 | 1283 | 1816 | 4082 | 18823 | 23592 | 6479 | 1906 | 973 | 618 | 440 | 337 | 224 | 118 | 79 | 34 | 14 |
| 0.05 | 255 | 363 | 829 | 3876 | 4969 | 1378 | 412 | 214 | 137 | 99 | 77 | 52 | 29 | 20 | 10 | 5 |
| 0.10 | 126 | 182 | 423 | 2015 | 2658 | 746 | 228 | 120 | 78 | 57 | 45 | 31 | 18 | 13 | 7 | 4 |
| 0.15 | 83 | 122 | 289 | 1401 | 1901 | 539 | 168 | 90 | 60 | 44 | 35 | 25 | 15 | 11 | 7 | 4 |
| 0.20 | 62 | 92 | 222 | 1099 | 1534 | 440 | 140 | 76 | 51 | 38 | 31 | 22 | 14 | 11 | 7 | 5 |
| 0.25 | 50 | 74 | 183 | 923 | 1326 | 385 | 125 | 69 | 47 | 36 | 29 | 21 | 14 | 11 | 7 | 5 |
| 0.30 | 41 | 63 | 158 | 812 | 1200 | 352 | 116 | 65 | 45 | 34 | 28 | 21 | 14 | 11 | 7 | 6 |
| 0.35 | 35 | 55 | 140 | 738 | 1122 | 333 | 111 | 63 | 44 | 34 | 28 | 21 | 14 | 12 | 8 | 6 |
| 0.40 | 31 | 49 | 128 | 688 | 1077 | 323 | 110 | 63 | 45 | 35 | 29 | 22 | 15 | 13 | 9 | 7 |
| 0.45 | 28 | 44 | 120 | 657 | 1058 | 320 | 111 | 65 | 46 | 36 | 30 | 23 | 17 | 14 | 10 | 8 |
| 0.50 | 25 | 41 | 114 | 640 | 1060 | 324 | 114 | 67 | 48 | 38 | 32 | 25 | 18 | 15 | 11 | 10 |
| 0.55 | 23 | 39 | 111 | 636 | 1084 | 335 | 120 | 72 | 52 | 41 | 35 | 28 | 20 | 17 | 13 | 11 |
| 0.60 | 22 | 38 | 110 | 645 | 1132 | 354 | 128 | 78 | 57 | 46 | 39 | 31 | 23 | 20 | 15 | 13 |
| 0.65 | 21 | 37 | 111 | 669 | 1209 | 381 | 140 | 86 | 63 | 51 | 44 | 35 | 26 | 23 | 18 | 16 |
| 0.70 | 21 | 37 | 116 | 713 | 1326 | 422 | 158 | 97 | 72 | 59 | 51 | 41 | 31 | 27 | 22 | 19 |
| 0.75 | 21 | 39 | 125 | 786 | 1504 | 483 | 183 | 114 | 85 | 70 | 61 | 50 | 38 | 33 | 27 | 24 |
| 0.80 | 22 | 42 | 140 | 905 | 1784 | 579 | 222 | 140 | 105 | 87 | 75 | 62 | 48 | 42 | 35 | 31 |
| 0.85 | 25 | 48 | 168 | 1117 | 2266 | 742 | 289 | 183 | 139 | 115 | 101 | 83 | 65 | 58 | 48 | 43 |
| 0.90 | 31 | 63 | 228 | 1556 | 3248 | 1073 | 423 | 271 | 207 | 173 | 151 | 126 | 100 | 89 | 75 | 67 |
| 0.95 | 52 | 110 | 412 | 2897 | 6229 | 2076 | 829 | 536 | 412 | 345 | 303 | 255 | 203 | 182 | 154 | 139 |

[a] $\alpha = 0.05$ (two-tailed), $\beta = 0.10$ (power $= 90\%$), control: case ratio $= 4:1$. The sample size listed is the number of subjects needed in the case group. Quadruple this number would be included in the control group.

**Table A13** Sample sizes for case–control studies[a].

| Prevalence in control group | Odds ratio to be detected | | | | | | | | | | | | | | | |
|---|---|---|---|---|---|---|---|---|---|---|---|---|---|---|---|---|
| | 0.2 | 0.3 | 0.5 | 0.75 | 1.25 | 1.5 | 2.0 | 2.5 | 3.0 | 3.5 | 4.0 | 5.0 | 7.5 | 10.0 | 20.0 | 50.0 |
| 0.00001 | 1472099 | 2082974 | 4710741 | 21983531 | 28264683 | 7851317 | 2355404 | 1221324 | 785139 | 565302 | 436191 | 294430 | 157960 | 106627 | 45676 | 16681 |
| 0.00005 | 294418 | 416596 | 942163 | 4396835 | 5653216 | 1570354 | 471115 | 244286 | 157043 | 113073 | 87248 | 58894 | 31598 | 21330 | 9139 | 3339 |
| 0.0001 | 147208 | 208299 | 471091 | 2198497 | 2826782 | 785234 | 235579 | 122156 | 78531 | 56544 | 43631 | 29452 | 15803 | 10668 | 4572 | 1671 |
| 0.0005 | 29440 | 41661 | 94233 | 439828 | 565636 | 157137 | 47150 | 24452 | 15721 | 11321 | 8736 | 5899 | 3166 | 2138 | 918 | 337 |
| 0.001 | 14719 | 20831 | 47126 | 219994 | 282992 | 78625 | 23596 | 12239 | 7870 | 5668 | 4375 | 2954 | 1587 | 1072 | 461 | 171 |
| 0.005 | 2943 | 4168 | 9441 | 44128 | 56879 | 15816 | 4753 | 2469 | 1589 | 1146 | 885 | 599 | 323 | 219 | 96 | 37 |
| 0.01 | 1470 | 2085 | 4730 | 22145 | 28617 | 7966 | 2398 | 1248 | 804 | 581 | 449 | 305 | 165 | 113 | 50 | 20 |
| 0.05 | 293 | 419 | 962 | 4566 | 6020 | 1690 | 516 | 272 | 177 | 129 | 101 | 70 | 39 | 28 | 14 | 7 |
| 0.10 | 146 | 211 | 493 | 2377 | 3214 | 911 | 283 | 151 | 100 | 74 | 58 | 41 | 24 | 18 | 10 | 6 |
| 0.15 | 97 | 142 | 337 | 1655 | 2295 | 657 | 208 | 113 | 75 | 56 | 45 | 32 | 20 | 15 | 9 | 6 |
| 0.20 | 73 | 107 | 260 | 1301 | 1850 | 535 | 172 | 95 | 64 | 48 | 39 | 28 | 18 | 14 | 9 | 6 |
| 0.25 | 58 | 87 | 215 | 1095 | 1597 | 466 | 152 | 85 | 58 | 44 | 36 | 27 | 17 | 14 | 9 | 7 |
| 0.30 | 49 | 74 | 186 | 964 | 1442 | 425 | 141 | 80 | 55 | 42 | 35 | 26 | 18 | 14 | 10 | 8 |
| 0.35 | 42 | 65 | 166 | 877 | 1346 | 401 | 135 | 77 | 54 | 42 | 35 | 26 | 18 | 15 | 11 | 9 |
| 0.40 | 37 | 58 | 152 | 820 | 1291 | 388 | 133 | 77 | 54 | 42 | 35 | 27 | 19 | 16 | 12 | 10 |
| 0.45 | 33 | 53 | 143 | 784 | 1266 | 384 | 133 | 78 | 56 | 44 | 37 | 29 | 20 | 17 | 13 | 11 |
| 0.50 | 31 | 50 | 137 | 765 | 1267 | 388 | 137 | 81 | 58 | 46 | 39 | 31 | 22 | 19 | 15 | 12 |
| 0.55 | 29 | 47 | 133 | 761 | 1294 | 400 | 143 | 85 | 62 | 50 | 42 | 33 | 25 | 21 | 16 | 14 |
| 0.60 | 27 | 46 | 133 | 774 | 1350 | 421 | 152 | 92 | 67 | 54 | 46 | 37 | 28 | 24 | 19 | 16 |
| 0.65 | 26 | 45 | 135 | 805 | 1440 | 453 | 166 | 101 | 75 | 61 | 52 | 42 | 32 | 27 | 22 | 19 |
| 0.70 | 26 | 46 | 141 | 859 | 1577 | 500 | 186 | 115 | 85 | 69 | 60 | 49 | 37 | 32 | 26 | 23 |
| 0.75 | 27 | 48 | 152 | 948 | 1785 | 571 | 215 | 134 | 100 | 82 | 71 | 58 | 45 | 39 | 33 | 29 |
| 0.80 | 28 | 53 | 172 | 1095 | 2115 | 682 | 260 | 163 | 123 | 101 | 88 | 73 | 57 | 50 | 42 | 37 |
| 0.85 | 32 | 62 | 208 | 1353 | 2683 | 873 | 337 | 213 | 162 | 134 | 117 | 97 | 76 | 68 | 57 | 51 |
| 0.90 | 41 | 81 | 283 | 1888 | 3842 | 1260 | 493 | 314 | 240 | 200 | 175 | 146 | 116 | 103 | 87 | 79 |
| 0.95 | 70 | 142 | 516 | 3524 | 7359 | 2433 | 962 | 619 | 475 | 397 | 349 | 293 | 234 | 210 | 179 | 162 |

[a] $\alpha = 0.05$ (two-tailed), $\beta = 0.20$ (power = 80%), control: case ratio = 1:1. The sample size listed is the number of subjects needed in the case group. An equivalent number would be included in the control group.

**Table A14** Sample sizes for case–control studies[a].

| Prevalence in control group | Odds ratio to be detected | | | | | | | | | | | | | | | |
|---|---|---|---|---|---|---|---|---|---|---|---|---|---|---|---|---|
| | 0.2 | 0.3 | 0.5 | 0.75 | 1.25 | 1.5 | 2.0 | 2.5 | 3.0 | 3.5 | 4.0 | 5.0 | 7.5 | 10.0 | 20.0 | 50.0 |
| 0.00001 | 1190363 | 1663444 | 3680489 | 16793046 | 20879138 | 5726351 | 1683639 | 859834 | 546235 | 389568 | 298260 | 198923 | 104777 | 69995 | 29465 | 10635 |
| 0.00005 | 238071 | 332689 | 736108 | 3358703 | 4176039 | 1145339 | 336754 | 171983 | 109259 | 77923 | 59660 | 39791 | 20960 | 14003 | 5896 | 2129 |
| 0.0001 | 119034 | 166344 | 368060 | 1679410 | 2088152 | 572713 | 168393 | 86001 | 54637 | 38967 | 29835 | 19899 | 10483 | 7004 | 2950 | 1066 |
| 0.0005 | 23805 | 33269 | 73622 | 335976 | 417842 | 114612 | 33705 | 17216 | 10939 | 7803 | 5975 | 3986 | 2101 | 1405 | 593 | 216 |
| 0.001 | 11901 | 16635 | 36817 | 168047 | 209054 | 57349 | 16869 | 8618 | 5477 | 3907 | 2993 | 1997 | 1053 | 705 | 298 | 109 |
| 0.005 | 2378 | 3327 | 7374 | 33704 | 42024 | 11540 | 3400 | 1740 | 1107 | 791 | 607 | 406 | 215 | 145 | 63 | 24 |
| 0.01 | 1188 | 1664 | 3693 | 16911 | 21146 | 5814 | 1717 | 880 | 561 | 402 | 308 | 207 | 211 | 75 | 33 | 14 |
| 0.05 | 236 | 333 | 750 | 3482 | 4455 | 1237 | 371 | 193 | 125 | 91 | 70 | 48 | 27 | 19 | 10 | 5 |
| 0.10 | 117 | 167 | 383 | 1810 | 2383 | 669 | 205 | 109 | 71 | 53 | 41 | 29 | 17 | 13 | 7 | 5 |
| 0.15 | 77 | 112 | 261 | 1258 | 1704 | 484 | 152 | 82 | 54 | 41 | 32 | 23 | 14 | 11 | 7 | 5 |
| 0.20 | 58 | 84 | 201 | 987 | 1376 | 396 | 126 | 69 | 47 | 35 | 28 | 21 | 13 | 10 | 7 | 5 |
| 0.25 | 46 | 68 | 166 | 829 | 1190 | 346 | 112 | 62 | 43 | 33 | 27 | 20 | 13 | 10 | 7 | 5 |
| 0.30 | 38 | 57 | 143 | 729 | 1076 | 316 | 105 | 59 | 41 | 32 | 26 | 20 | 13 | 10 | 7 | 6 |
| 0.35 | 33 | 50 | 127 | 662 | 1006 | 299 | 101 | 58 | 40 | 31 | 26 | 20 | 14 | 11 | 8 | 7 |
| 0.40 | 29 | 45 | 116 | 618 | 966 | 290 | 99 | 58 | 41 | 32 | 27 | 21 | 15 | 12 | 9 | 7 |
| 0.45 | 26 | 41 | 108 | 590 | 949 | 288 | 100 | 59 | 42 | 33 | 28 | 22 | 16 | 13 | 10 | 8 |
| 0.50 | 24 | 38 | 103 | 574 | 951 | 292 | 103 | 61 | 44 | 35 | 30 | 24 | 17 | 15 | 11 | 10 |
| 0.55 | 22 | 36 | 100 | 571 | 973 | 301 | 108 | 65 | 47 | 38 | 32 | 26 | 19 | 16 | 13 | 11 |
| 0.60 | 21 | 34 | 99 | 579 | 1016 | 318 | 116 | 70 | 52 | 42 | 36 | 29 | 22 | 19 | 15 | 13 |
| 0.65 | 20 | 34 | 101 | 601 | 1085 | 343 | 127 | 78 | 58 | 47 | 40 | 33 | 25 | 22 | 18 | 16 |
| 0.70 | 20 | 34 | 105 | 640 | 1190 | 380 | 143 | 89 | 66 | 54 | 47 | 38 | 29 | 26 | 21 | 19 |
| 0.75 | 20 | 35 | 112 | 705 | 1350 | 435 | 166 | 104 | 78 | 64 | 56 | 46 | 36 | 32 | 26 | 23 |
| 0.80 | 21 | 38 | 126 | 812 | 1601 | 520 | 201 | 127 | 96 | 80 | 70 | 58 | 45 | 40 | 34 | 30 |
| 0.85 | 23 | 44 | 152 | 1002 | 2034 | 667 | 261 | 167 | 127 | 106 | 93 | 77 | 61 | 55 | 46 | 42 |
| 0.90 | 29 | 58 | 205 | 1395 | 2916 | 965 | 383 | 246 | 189 | 158 | 139 | 117 | 94 | 84 | 71 | 65 |
| 0.95 | 48 | 100 | 371 | 2598 | 5592 | 1868 | 750 | 487 | 376 | 316 | 279 | 236 | 190 | 171 | 147 | 134 |

[a] $\alpha = 0.05$ (two-tailed), $\beta = 0.20$ (power = 80%), control: case ratio = 2 : 1. The sample size listed is the number of subjects needed in the case group. Double this number would be included in the control group.

**Table A15** Sample sizes for case–control studies[a].

| Prevalence in control group | Odds ratio to be detected | | | | | | | | | | | | | | | |
|---|---|---|---|---|---|---|---|---|---|---|---|---|---|---|---|---|
| | 0.2 | 0.3 | 0.5 | 0.75 | 1.25 | 1.5 | 2.0 | 2.5 | 3.0 | 3.5 | 4.0 | 5.0 | 7.5 | 10.0 | 20.0 | 50.0 |
| 0.00001 | 1088 329 | 1516 265 | 3330 869 | 15057 631 | 18413 208 | 5014 341 | 1456 616 | 736 652 | 464 229 | 328 865 | 250 357 | 165 463 | 85 879 | 56 868 | 23 570 | 8 415 |
| 0.00005 | 217 664 | 303 253 | 666 182 | 3011 608 | 3682 831 | 1002 930 | 291 347 | 147 345 | 92 856 | 65 782 | 50 079 | 33 098 | 17 180 | 11 377 | 4717 | 1 685 |
| 0.0001 | 108 831 | 151 626 | 333 096 | 1505 856 | 1841 534 | 501 504 | 145 688 | 73 681 | 46 435 | 32 896 | 25 044 | 16 553 | 8592 | 5691 | 2360 | 844 |
| 0.0005 | 21 764 | 30 325 | 66 628 | 301 253 | 368 496 | 100 363 | 29 161 | 14 751 | 9298 | 6588 | 5016 | 3316 | 1723 | 1141 | 474 | 171 |
| 0.001 | 10 881 | 15 162 | 33 319 | 150 678 | 184 367 | 50 220 | 14 595 | 7384 | 4655 | 3299 | 2513 | 1662 | 864 | 573 | 239 | 87 |
| 0.005 | 2174 | 3032 | 6672 | 30 218 | 37 064 | 10 107 | 2943 | 1491 | 942 | 668 | 510 | 338 | 177 | 118 | 50 | 19 |
| 0.01 | 1086 | 1516 | 3342 | 15 161 | 18 652 | 5093 | 1486 | 755 | 478 | 340 | 259 | 173 | 91 | 61 | 27 | 11 |
| 0.05 | 215 | 303 | 678 | 3120 | 3932 | 1085 | 323 | 167 | 107 | 77 | 60 | 41 | 23 | 16 | 8 | 4 |
| 0.10 | 107 | 152 | 345 | 1620 | 2105 | 588 | 179 | 94 | 62 | 45 | 35 | 25 | 15 | 11 | 6 | 4 |
| 0.15 | 70 | 101 | 235 | 1125 | 1507 | 426 | 132 | 71 | 47 | 35 | 28 | 20 | 12 | 9 | 6 | 4 |
| 0.20 | 52 | 76 | 181 | 882 | 1218 | 349 | 111 | 60 | 41 | 31 | 25 | 18 | 11 | 9 | 6 | 4 |
| 0.25 | 42 | 62 | 149 | 741 | 1053 | 305 | 99 | 55 | 37 | 29 | 23 | 17 | 11 | 9 | 6 | 5 |
| 0.30 | 35 | 52 | 128 | 650 | 954 | 280 | 92 | 52 | 36 | 28 | 23 | 17 | 12 | 9 | 7 | 5 |
| 0.35 | 30 | 45 | 114 | 590 | 892 | 265 | 89 | 51 | 36 | 28 | 23 | 18 | 12 | 10 | 7 | 5 |
| 0.40 | 26 | 40 | 104 | 550 | 857 | 257 | 88 | 51 | 36 | 28 | 24 | 18 | 13 | 11 | 7 | 6 |
| 0.45 | 23 | 36 | 97 | 525 | 843 | 256 | 89 | 52 | 37 | 30 | 25 | 19 | 14 | 12 | 8 | 7 |
| 0.50 | 21 | 34 | 92 | 511 | 846 | 259 | 92 | 55 | 39 | 32 | 27 | 21 | 15 | 13 | 9 | 7 |
| 0.55 | 19 | 32 | 89 | 507 | 866 | 268 | 97 | 58 | 42 | 34 | 29 | 23 | 17 | 15 | 10 | 9 |
| 0.60 | 18 | 30 | 88 | 514 | 905 | 283 | 104 | 63 | 46 | 38 | 32 | 26 | 19 | 17 | 12 | 10 |
| 0.65 | 18 | 30 | 89 | 533 | 967 | 306 | 114 | 70 | 52 | 42 | 36 | 30 | 23 | 20 | 13 | 12 |
| 0.70 | 17 | 30 | 92 | 567 | 1061 | 339 | 128 | 80 | 60 | 49 | 42 | 35 | 27 | 23 | 16 | 14 |
| 0.75 | 17 | 31 | 99 | 624 | 1204 | 389 | 149 | 93 | 70 | 58 | 51 | 42 | 32 | 29 | 19 | 17 |
| 0.80 | 18 | 33 | 111 | 718 | 1429 | 466 | 181 | 115 | 87 | 72 | 63 | 52 | 41 | 37 | 24 | 21 |
| 0.85 | 20 | 38 | 132 | 884 | 1817 | 598 | 235 | 151 | 115 | 96 | 84 | 70 | 56 | 50 | 31 | 28 |
| 0.90 | 25 | 50 | 179 | 1230 | 2607 | 867 | 345 | 223 | 172 | 144 | 127 | 107 | 85 | 77 | 42 | 38 |
| 0.95 | 41 | 85 | 323 | 2288 | 5002 | 1678 | 678 | 442 | 342 | 288 | 255 | 215 | 174 | 157 | 65 | 59 |
| | | | | | | | | | | | | | | | 134 | 123 |

[a] $\alpha = 0.05$ (two-tailed), $\beta = 0.20$ (power = 80%), control: case ratio = 3: 1. The sample size listed is the number of subjects needed in the case group. Triple this number would be included in the control group.

**Table A16** Sample sizes for case–control studies[a].

| Prevalence in control group | Odds ratio to be detected | | | | | | | | | | | | | | | |
|---|---|---|---|---|---|---|---|---|---|---|---|---|---|---|---|---|
| | 0.2 | 0.3 | 0.5 | 0.75 | 1.25 | 1.5 | 2.0 | 2.5 | 3.0 | 3.5 | 4.0 | 5.0 | 7.5 | 10.0 | 20.0 | 50.0 |
| 0.00001 | 1034611 | 1440327 | 3154151 | 14188340 | 17179015 | 4657221 | 1342151 | 674222 | 422474 | 297830 | 225778 | 148193 | 76026 | 49982 | 20443 | 7227 |
| 0.00005 | 206920 | 288065 | 630838 | 2837745 | 3435981 | 931503 | 268452 | 134858 | 84505 | 59574 | 45162 | 29644 | 15209 | 9999 | 4091 | 1447 |
| 0.0001 | 103459 | 144032 | 315424 | 1418920 | 1718102 | 465788 | 134240 | 67438 | 42259 | 29792 | 22585 | 14825 | 7607 | 5002 | 2047 | 725 |
| 0.0005 | 20690 | 28806 | 63092 | 283861 | 343799 | 93216 | 26870 | 13501 | 8462 | 5966 | 4524 | 2970 | 1525 | 1003 | 412 | 147 |
| 0.001 | 10344 | 14403 | 31551 | 141978 | 172011 | 46645 | 13449 | 6759 | 4237 | 2988 | 2266 | 1489 | 765 | 504 | 207 | 75 |
| 0.005 | 2067 | 2880 | 6318 | 28473 | 34581 | 9388 | 2712 | 1366 | 858 | 606 | 460 | 303 | 157 | 104 | 44 | 17 |
| 0.01 | 1032 | 1440 | 3164 | 14285 | 17404 | 4731 | 1370 | 691 | 435 | 308 | 234 | 155 | 81 | 54 | 23 | 10 |
| 0.05 | 205 | 288 | 641 | 2938 | 3670 | 1009 | 298 | 153 | 98 | 70 | 54 | 37 | 20 | 14 | 7 | 4 |
| 0.10 | 101 | 144 | 327 | 1525 | 1966 | 547 | 166 | 87 | 57 | 41 | 32 | 23 | 13 | 10 | 5 | 3 |
| 0.15 | 67 | 96 | 222 | 1059 | 1408 | 397 | 123 | 66 | 43 | 32 | 26 | 18 | 11 | 8 | 5 | 4 |
| 0.20 | 50 | 72 | 171 | 830 | 1138 | 325 | 103 | 56 | 38 | 28 | 23 | 17 | 10 | 8 | 5 | 4 |
| 0.25 | 39 | 58 | 140 | 696 | 985 | 285 | 92 | 51 | 35 | 26 | 21 | 16 | 10 | 8 | 6 | 4 |
| 0.30 | 33 | 49 | 121 | 611 | 892 | 261 | 86 | 48 | 33 | 26 | 21 | 16 | 11 | 9 | 6 | 5 |
| 0.35 | 28 | 42 | 107 | 554 | 836 | 248 | 83 | 47 | 33 | 26 | 21 | 16 | 11 | 9 | 7 | 5 |
| 0.40 | 24 | 38 | 97 | 517 | 803 | 241 | 82 | 48 | 34 | 26 | 22 | 17 | 12 | 10 | 7 | 6 |
| 0.45 | 22 | 34 | 91 | 492 | 790 | 240 | 83 | 49 | 35 | 28 | 23 | 18 | 13 | 11 | 8 | 7 |
| 0.50 | 20 | 32 | 86 | 479 | 793 | 243 | 86 | 51 | 37 | 30 | 25 | 20 | 14 | 12 | 9 | 8 |
| 0.55 | 18 | 30 | 83 | 475 | 812 | 252 | 91 | 55 | 40 | 32 | 27 | 22 | 16 | 14 | 11 | 9 |
| 0.60 | 17 | 28 | 82 | 481 | 849 | 266 | 97 | 59 | 44 | 35 | 30 | 24 | 18 | 16 | 13 | 11 |
| 0.65 | 16 | 28 | 83 | 498 | 908 | 288 | 107 | 66 | 49 | 40 | 34 | 28 | 21 | 18 | 15 | 13 |
| 0.70 | 16 | 28 | 86 | 530 | 997 | 319 | 121 | 75 | 56 | 46 | 40 | 33 | 25 | 22 | 18 | 16 |
| 0.75 | 16 | 29 | 92 | 583 | 1131 | 366 | 140 | 88 | 67 | 55 | 48 | 39 | 31 | 27 | 22 | 20 |
| 0.80 | 17 | 31 | 103 | 670 | 1343 | 439 | 171 | 108 | 82 | 68 | 60 | 50 | 39 | 35 | 29 | 26 |
| 0.85 | 18 | 35 | 123 | 826 | 1708 | 564 | 222 | 143 | 109 | 91 | 80 | 67 | 53 | 47 | 40 | 36 |
| 0.90 | 23 | 45 | 166 | 1148 | 2452 | 817 | 327 | 211 | 163 | 137 | 120 | 101 | 81 | 73 | 62 | 56 |
| 0.95 | 37 | 78 | 298 | 2133 | 4707 | 1583 | 641 | 419 | 325 | 273 | 242 | 205 | 165 | 149 | 127 | 116 |

[a] $\alpha = 0.05$ (two-tailed), $\beta = 0.20$ (power = 80%), control: case ratio = 4 : 1. The sample size listed is the number of subjects needed in the case group. Quadruple this number would be included in the control group.

**Table A17** Tabular values of 95% confidence limit factors for estimates of a poisson-distributed variable.

| Observed number on which estimate is based (n) | Lower limit factor (L) | Upper limit factor (U) | Observed number on which estimate is based (n) | Lower limit factor (L) | Upper limit factor (U) | Observed number on which estimate is based (n) | Lower limit factor (L) | Upper limit factor (U) |
|---|---|---|---|---|---|---|---|---|
| 1 | 0.0253 | 5.57 | 21 | 0.619 | 1.53 | 120 | 0.833 | 1.200 |
| 2 | 0.121 | 3.61 | 22 | 0.627 | 1.51 | 140 | 0.844 | 1.184 |
| 3 | 0.206 | 2.92 | 23 | 0.634 | 1.50 | 160 | 0.854 | 1.171 |
| 4 | 0.272 | 2.56 | 24 | 0.641 | 1.49 | 180 | 0.862 | 1.160 |
| 5 | 0.324 | 2.33 | 25 | 0.647 | 1.48 | 200 | 0.868 | 1.151 |
| 6 | 0.367 | 2.18 | 26 | 0.653 | 1.47 | 250 | 0.882 | 1.134 |
| 7 | 0.401 | 2.06 | 27 | 0.659 | 1.46 | 300 | 0.892 | 1.121 |
| 8 | 0.431 | 1.97 | 28 | 0.665 | 1.45 | 350 | 0.899 | 1.112 |
| 9 | 0.458 | 1.90 | 29 | 0.670 | 1.44 | 400 | 0.906 | 1.104 |
| 10 | 0.480 | 1.84 | 30 | 0.675 | 1.43 | 450 | 0.911 | 1.098 |
| 11 | 0.499 | 1.79 | 35 | 0.697 | 1.39 | 500 | 0.915 | 1.093 |
| 12 | 0.517 | 1.75 | 40 | 0.714 | 1.36 | 600 | 0.922 | 1.084 |
| 13 | 0.532 | 1.71 | 45 | 0.729 | 1.34 | 700 | 0.928 | 1.078 |
| 14 | 0.546 | 1.68 | 50 | 0.742 | 1.32 | 800 | 0.932 | 1.072 |
| 15 | 0.560 | 1.65 | 60 | 0.770 | 1.30 | 900 | 0.936 | 1.068 |
| 16 | 0.572 | 1.62 | 70 | 0.785 | 1.27 | 1000 | 0.939 | 1.064 |
| 17 | 0.583 | 1.60 | 80 | 0.798 | 1.25 | | | |
| 18 | 0.593 | 1.58 | 90 | 0.809 | 1.24 | | | |
| 19 | 0.602 | 1.56 | 100 | 0.818 | 1.22 | | | |
| 20 | 0.611 | 1.54 | | | | | | |

# Glossary

The *accuracy* of a measurement is the degree to which the measurement approximates the truth.

Ad hoc *studies* are studies that require primary data collection.

*Active surveillance* is surveillance carried out via a continuous, defined process in a specific population, using one of several approaches. Active surveillance can be medical product-based, identifying adverse events in patients taking certain products; setting-based, identifying adverse events in certain healthcare settings where patients are likely to present for treatment (e.g. emergency departments); or event-based, identifying adverse events likely to be associated with medical products (e.g. acute liver failure).

*Actual knowledge*, in a legal sense, is defined as literal awareness of a fact. Actual knowledge can be demonstrated by showing that the manufacturer was cognizant of reasonable information suggesting, for example, a particular risk.

An *adverse drug event, adverse drug experience, adverse event,* or *adverse experience* is an untoward outcome that occurs during or following clinical use of a drug. It does not necessarily have a causal relationship with this treatment. It may or may not be preventable.

An *adverse drug reaction* is an adverse drug event that is judged to be caused by the drug.

Studies of *adverse effects* examine case reports of adverse drug reactions, attempting to judge subjectively whether the adverse events were indeed caused by the antecedent drug exposure.

*Adverseomics* is the study of vaccine adverse reactions using immunogenomics and systems biology approaches.

*Agreement* is the degree to which different methods or sources of information give the same answers. Agreement between two sources or methods does not imply that either is valid or reliable.

*Analyses of secular trends* examine trends in disease events over time and/or across different geographic locations, and correlate them with trends in putative exposures, such as rates of drug utilization. The unit of observation is usually a subgroup of a population, rather than individuals. Also called ecological studies.

*Analytic studies* are studies with control groups, such as case–control studies, cohort studies, and randomized clinical trials.

*Anticipated beneficial effects* of drugs are desirable effects that are presumed to be caused by the drug. They usually represent the reason for prescribing or ingesting the drug.

*Anticipated harmful effects* of drugs are unwanted effects that could have been predicted on the basis of existing knowledge.

*Textbook of Pharmacoepidemiology*, Third Edition. Edited by Brian L. Strom, Stephen E. Kimmel, and Sean Hennessy.
© 2022 John Wiley & Sons Ltd. Published 2022 by John Wiley & Sons Ltd.

An *association* is when two events occur together more often than one would expect by chance.

*Autocorrelation* is where any individual observation is to some extent a function of the previous observation.

*Bias* is any systematic (rather than random) error in a study.

*Biological inference* is the process of generalizing from a statement about an association seen in a population to a causal statement about biological relationships.

*Case-cohort studies* are studies that compare cases with a disease to a sample of subjects randomly selected from the parent cohort.

*Case–control studies* are studies that compare cases with a disease to controls without the disease, looking for differences in antecedent exposures.

*Case-crossover studies* are studies that compare cases at the time of disease occurrence to different time periods in the same individuals, looking for differences in antecedent exposures.

*Case reports* are reports of the experience of individual patients. As used in pharmacoepidemiology, a case report usually describes a patient who was exposed to a drug and experienced a particular outcome, usually an adverse event.

*Case series* are reports of collections of patients, all of whom have a common exposure, examining what their clinical outcomes were. Alternatively, case series can be reports of patients who have a common disease, examining what their antecedent exposures were. No control group is present.

An exposure *causes* a health event when it truly increases the probability of that event in some individuals. That is, there are at least some individuals who would experience the event given the exposure who would not experience the event absent the exposure.

*Changeability* is the ability of an instrument to measure a difference in score in patients who have improved or deteriorated.

*Channeling bias* is a type of selection bias, which occurs when a drug is claimed to be safe and therefore is used in high-risk patients who did not tolerate other drugs for that indication. It is sometimes used synonymously with *confounding by indication*.

*Clearance* is the proportion of the apparent volume of distribution that is cleared of drug in a specified time. Its units are volume per time, such as liters per hour. The total body clearance is the sum of clearances by different routes, e.g. renal, hepatic, pulmonary.

*Clinical pharmacology* is the study of the effects of drugs in humans.

*Cohort studies* are studies that identify defined populations and follow them forward in time, examining their frequencies (e.g. incidence rate, cumulative incidence) of disease. Cohort studies generally identify and compare exposed patients to unexposed patients or to patients who receive a different exposure.

*Combination-triggered drug–drug interaction* is, in a potential drug–drug interaction, the scenario in which both the object drug and precipitant drugs are initiated simultaneously.

*Confidence interval* can be conceptualized to represent a range of values within which the true population value lies, with some probability.

*Confidentiality* is the right of patients to limit the transfer and disclosure of private information.

A *confounding variable*, or *confounder*, is a variable other than the risk factor and outcome variable under study that is related independently both to the risk factor and to the outcome. A confounder can artificially inflate or reduce the magnitude of association between and exposure and outcome.

*Confounding by indication* can occur when the underlying diagnosis or other clinical features that affect the use of a certain drug are also related to the outcome under study.

*Construct validity* refers to the extent to which results from a given instrument are consistent with those from other measures in a manner consistent with theoretical hypotheses.

*Constructive knowledge*, from a legal perspective, is knowledge that a person did not have, but could have acquired by the exercise of reasonable care.

A *cost* is the consumption of a resource that could otherwise be used for another purpose.

*Cost–benefit analysis* of medical care compares the cost of a medical intervention to its benefit. Both costs and benefits must be measured in the same monetary units (e.g. dollars).

*Cost-effectiveness analysis* of medical care compares the cost of a medical intervention to its effectiveness. Costs are expressed in monetary units, while effectiveness is determined independently and may be measured in terms of any clinically meaningful unit. Cost-effectiveness analyses usually examine the additional cost per unit of additional effectiveness.

*Cost-identification analysis* enumerates the costs involved in medical care, ignoring the outcomes that result from that care.

*Criterion validity* refers to the ability of an instrument to measure what it is supposed to measure, as judged by agreement with a reference (gold) standard.

*Cross-sectional studies* examine exposures and outcomes in populations at one point in time; they have no time sense.

*Data mining* is exploratory data analysis for hypothesis generation. As part of a knowledge discovery process, data mining looks to uncover patterns or correlations in the data set with no or limited presupposition, with the intent of more rigorous testing of any emerging hypothesis tailored to the issue at hand.

The *defined daily dose* (DDD) is the usual daily maintenance dose for a drug for its main indication in adults.

*Descriptive studies* are studies that do not have control groups, namely case reports, case series, and analyses of secular trends. They are in contrast with analytic studies.

*Detection bias* is an error in the results of a study due to a systematic difference between the study groups in the procedures used for ascertainment, diagnosis, or verification of disease.

*Differential misclassification* occurs when the degree of misclassification of one variable (e.g. drug usage) varies according to the level of another variable (e.g. disease status).

The *direct medical costs* of medical care are the costs that are incurred in providing the care.

*Direct non-medical costs* are non-medical care costs incurred because of an illness or the need to seek medical care. They can include the cost of transportation to the hospital or physician's office, the cost of special clothing needed because of the illness, and the cost of hotel stays and special housing (e.g. modification of the home to accommodate the ill individual).

*Discriminative instruments* are those that measure differences among people at a single point in time.

*Disease registries* are registries characterized by inclusion of subjects based on diagnosis of a common disease or condition.

A *drug* is any exogenously administered substance that exerts a physiologic effect.

*Drug–drug interaction* is the phenomenon in which one or more drugs affects the pharmacokinetics and/or pharmacodynamics of one or more other drugs.

*Drug utilization*, as defined by the World Health Organization (WHO), is the "marketing, distribution, prescription and use of drugs in a society, with special emphasis on the resulting medical, social, and economic consequences."

*Drug utilization evaluation (DUE) programs* are ongoing structured systems designed to improve drug use by intervening when inappropriate drug use is detected. See also drug utilization review programs.

*Drug utilization evaluation studies* are ad hoc investigations that assess the appropriateness of drug use. They are designed to detect and quantify the frequency of drug use problems.

*Drug utilization review programs* are ongoing structured systems designed to improve drug use by intervening when inappropriate drug use is detected.

*Drug utilization review studies* are ad hoc investigations that assess the appropriateness of drug use. They are designed to detect and quantify any drug use problems. See also drug utilization evaluation programs.

*Drug utilization studies* are descriptive studies that quantify the use of a drug. Their objective is to quantify the present state, the developmental trends, and the time course of drug usage at various levels of the health care system, whether national, regional, local, or institutional.

*Ecological studies* examine trends in disease events over time or across different geographic locations and correlate them with trends in putative exposures, such as rates of drug utilization. The unit of observation is a subgroup of a population, rather than individuals. See also analyses of secular trends.

*Effect modification* occurs when the magnitude of effect of a drug in causing an outcome differs according to the levels of a variable other than the drug or the outcome (e.g. sex, age group). Effect modification can be assessed on an additive and/or multiplicative scale. See interaction.

A study of drug *effectiveness* is a study of whether, in the usual clinical setting, a drug in fact achieves the effect intended when prescribing it.

A study of drug *efficacy* is a study of whether, *under ideal conditions*, a drug has the ability to bring about the effect intended when prescribing it.

A study of drug *efficiency* is a study of whether a drug can bring about its desired effect at an acceptable cost.

*Enriched* or hybrid study designs draw upon both primary and secondary data, with some data collected de novo, specifically for the purposes of the study and other study-specific data collected via probabilistic or deterministic linkage with other data sources, such as electronic health records, administrative claims and billing data, vital records and genetic information.

*Epidemiology* is the study of the distribution and determinants of disease or health-related states in populations.

*Evaluative instruments* are those designed to measure changes within individuals over time.

*Experimental studies* are studies in which the investigator controls the therapy that is to be received by each participant, generally using that control to randomly allocate participants among the study groups.

*Face validity* is a judgment about the validity of an instrument, based on an intuitive assessment of the extent to which an instrument meets a number of criteria including applicability, clarity and simplicity, likelihood of bias, comprehensiveness, and whether redundant items have been included.

*Fixed costs* are costs that are incurred regardless of the volume of activity.

*General causation,* from a legal perspective, addresses whether a product is capable of causing a particular injury in the population of patients like the plaintiff.

*Generic quality-of-life instruments* aim to cover the complete spectrum of function, disability, and distress of the patient, and are applicable to a variety of populations.

*Half-life* ($T_{1/2}$) is the time taken for the drug concentration to decline by half. Half-life is a function of both the apparent volume of distribution and clearance of the drug.

*Hawthorne Effect* is when study subjects alter their behavior simply because of their participation in a study, unrelated to the study procedures or intervention.

*Health profiles* are single instruments that measure multiple different aspects of quality-of-life.

*Health-related quality-of-life* is a multifactorial concept which, from the patient's perspective, represents the end-result of all the physiological, psychological, and social influences of the disease and the therapeutic process. Health-related quality-of-life may be considered on different levels: overall assessment of well-being; several broad domains—physiological, functional, psychological, social, and economic status; and subcomponents of each domain—for example pain, sleep, activities of daily living, and sexual function within physical and functional domains.

A *human research subject*, as defined in US regulation, is "a living individual, about whom an investigator (whether professional or student) conducting research obtains either: 1) data through intervention or interaction with the individual, or 2) identifiable private information." (Title 45 US Code of Federal Regulations Part 46.102 (f)).

*Hybrid* or enriched study designs draw upon both primary and secondary data, with some data collected de novo, specifically for the purposes of the study and other study-specific data collected via probabilistic or deterministic linkage with other data sources, such as electronic health records, administrative claims and billing data, vital records and genetic information.

*Hypothesis-generating studies* are studies that give rise to new questions about drug effects to be explored further in subsequent analytical studies.

*Hypothesis-strengthening studies* are studies that reinforce, although do not provide definitive evidence for, existing hypotheses.

*Hypothesis-testing studies* are studies that evaluate in detail hypotheses raised elsewhere.

*Inception cohort design* is a cohort study that is restricted to new users of the exposure(s) of interest.

*Incidence/prevalence bias*, a type of selection bias, may occur in studies when prevalent cases rather than new cases of a condition are selected for a study. A strong association with prevalence may be related to the duration of the disease rather than to its incidence, because prevalence is proportional to both incidence and duration of the disease.

The *incidence rate* of a disease is a measure of how frequently the disease occurs. Specifically, it is the number of new cases of the disease which develop over a defined time period in a defined population at risk, divided by the number of people in that population at risk.

*Indirect costs* are costs that do not stem directly from transactions for goods or services, but represent the loss of opportunities to use a valuable resource in alternative ways. They include costs due to morbidity (e.g. time lost from work) and mortality (e.g. premature death leading to removal from the work force).

*Information bias* is an error in the results of a study due to a systematic difference between the study groups in the accuracy of the measurements being made of their exposure or outcome.

*Instrumental variable* is a variable used to adjust for confounding that meets certain specific criteria: it should affect treatment or be associated with treatment choice by sharing a common cause; should be a factor that is as good as randomly assigned, so that it is unrelated to patient characteristics; and should not be related to the outcome other than through its association with treatment.

*Intangible costs* are those of pain, suffering, and grief.

*Interaction*, see effect modification.

*Interrupted time-series designs* include multiple observations of study populations before and after an intervention.

*Knowledge*, as used in court cases, can be actual or constructive; see those terms.

*Large simple trials* are randomized trials characterized by large sample sizes, broad entry criteria consistent with the approved medication label, randomization based on equipoise, minimal data requirements, objectively-measured endpoints, follow-up that minimizes interventions or interference with normal clinical practice, follow-up of all patients regardless of whether they discontinue randomized medication; and intent-to-treat analysis.

*Medication errors* are any error in the process of prescribing, transcribing, dispensing, administering, or monitoring a drug, regardless of whether an injury occurred or the potential for injury was present.

*Meta-analysis* is a systematic, structured review of the literature and formal statistical analysis of a collection of analytic results for the purpose of integrating the findings. Meta-analysis is used to identify sources of variation among study findings and, when appropriate, to provide an overall measure of effect as a summary of those findings.

*Microbiome* includes the microorganisms, primarily bacteria in the gut, and their genes, harbored within each person.

*Misclassification bias* is the error resulting from classifying study subjects as exposed when they truly are unexposed, or vice versa. Alternatively, misclassification bias can result from classifying study subjects as diseased when they truly are not diseased, or vice versa.

*Molecular pharmacoepidemiology* is the study of the manner in which molecular biomarkers alter the clinical effects of medications.

An *N-of-1 RCT* is a randomized controlled trial within an individual patient, using repeated assignments to the experimental or control arms.

*Near misses* are medication errors that have high potential for causing harm but did not, either because they were intercepted prior to reaching a patient or because the error reached the patient who fortuitously did not have any observable untoward sequelae.

*Negative control precipitant drug* is, in a study of a potential drug–drug interaction, a drug that is used in similar clinical circumstances as the potential precipitant under study, yet by virtue of the control precipitant's pharmacology is not believed to interact with the study object

*Negative control object drug* is, in a study of a potential drug–drug interaction, a drug that is used for similar indications as the object under study, but is not believed to interact pharmacologically with the study precipitant

*Non-differential misclassification* occurs when the misclassification of one variable does not vary by the level of another variable. Non-differential misclassification usually results in bias toward the null.

*Non-experimental studies* are studies in which the investigator does not control the therapy, but observes and evaluates the results of ongoing medical care. The study designs that are used are those that do not involve random allocation, such as case reports, case series, analyses of secular trends, case–control studies, and cohort studies.

*Object drug* is, in a drug–drug interaction, the drug(s) whose pharmacokinetics or pharmacodynamics are affected by the other drug(s).

*Object-triggered drug–drug interaction* is, in a study of a potential drug–drug interaction, the scenario in which the object drug is started in a person already taking the precipitant drug.

*Observational studies* (or nonexperimental studies) are studies in which the investigator does not control the therapy, but observes and evaluates the results of ongoing medical care. The study designs that are used are those that do not involve randomization, such as case reports, case series, analyses of secular trends, case–control studies, and cohort studies.

The *odds ratio* is the odds of exposure in the diseased group divided by the odds of exposure in the non-diseased group. When the underlying risk of disease is low (about 10% or lower) it is an unbiased estimator of the relative risk. It is also an unbiased estimate of the rate ratio in a nested or population-based case–control study in which controls are selected at random from the population at risk of disease at the time that the case occurred.

*One-group, post-only study design* consists of making only one observation on a single group which has already been exposed to a treatment.

An *opportunity cost* is the value of a resource's next best use, a use that is no longer possible once the resource has been used.

A *p-value* is the probability that a difference as large as or larger than the one observed in the study could have occurred purely by chance if no association truly existed.

*Patient reported outcomes* are any report of the status of a patient's health condition that comes directly from the patient, without interpretation of the patient's response by a clinician or anyone else.

*Pharmacodynamics* is the study of the relationship between drug level and drug effect. It involves the study of the response of the target tissues in the body to a given concentration of drug.

*Pharmacoeconomics* is the study of how the price of pharmaceutical products and their economic impact health and the health care system.

*Pharmacogenetic epidemiology* is the study of the effects of genetic determinants of drug response on outcomes in large numbers of people.

*Pharmacoepidemiology* is the study of the use of and the effects of drugs in large numbers of people. It is also the application of the research methods of clinical epidemiology to the content area of clinical pharmacology, and the primary science underlying the public health practice of drug safety surveillance.

*Pharmacogenetics* is the study of genetic determinants of responses to drugs. Although it is sometimes used synonymously with pharmacogenomics, it often refers to a candidate-gene approach as opposed to a genome-wide approach.

*Pharmacogenomics* is the study of genetic determinants of responses to drugs. Although it is sometimes used synonymously with pharmacogenetics, it often refers to a genome-wide approach as opposed to a candidate-gene approach.

A *pharmacokinetic compartment* is a theoretical space into which drug molecules are said to distribute, and is represented by a given linear component of the log-concentration versus time curve. It is not an actual anatomic or physiologic space, but is sometimes thought of as a tissue or group of tissues that have similar blood flow and drug affinity.

*Pharmacokinetics* is the study of the relationship between the dose administered of a drug and the concentration achieved in the blood, in the serum, or at the site of action. It includes the study of the processes of drug absorption, distribution, metabolism, and excretion.

*Pharmacovigilance* is the identification and evaluation of drug safety signals. More recently, some have also used the term as synonymous with pharmacoepidemiology. WHO defines *pharmacovigilance* as the science and activities relating to the detection, assessment, understanding and prevention of adverse effects or any other possible drug-related problems (WHO. Safety monitoring of medicinal products. *The importance of pharmacovigilance*. Geneva, World Health Organization, 2002). Mann defines *pharmacovigilance* as "the study of the safety of marketed drugs under the practical conditions of clinical usage in large communities" (*Pharmacovigilance.* R.D. Mann and E.B. Andrews, eds. John Wiley & Sons Ltd., Chichester, 2002).

*Pharmacology* is the study of the effects of drugs in a living system.

*Pharmacotherapeutics* is the application of the principles of clinical pharmacology to rational prescribing, the conduct of clinical trials, and the assessment of outcomes during real-life clinical practice.

*Pharmionics* is the study of how patients use or misuse prescription drugs in ambulatory care.

*Population-based databases or studies* refers to whether there is an identifiable population (which is not necessarily based in geography), all of whose medical care would be included in that database, regardless of the provider. This allows one to determine incidence rates of diseases, as well as being more certain that one knows of all medical care that any given patient receives.

*Positive control precipitant drug* is, in a study of a potential drug–drug interaction, a precipitant drug known to produce an association with an outcome in patients receiving the object drug of interest.

*Postmarketing surveillance* is the study of drug use and drug effects after release onto the market. This term is sometimes used synonymously with "pharmacoepi-demiology," but the latter can be relevant to premarketing studies, as well. Conversely, the term "postmarketing surveillance" is sometimes felt to apply to only those studies conducted after drug marketing that systematically screen for adverse drug effects. However, this is a more restricted use of the term than that used in this book.

*Potency* refers to the amount of drug that is required to elicit a given response. A more potent drug requires a smaller milligram quantity to exert the same response as a less

potent drug, although it is not necessarily more effective.

*Potential adverse drug events* are medication errors that have high potential for causing harm but did not, either because they were intercepted prior to reaching a patient or because the error reached the patient who fortuitously did not have any observable untoward sequelae.

The *power (statistical power)* of a study is the probability of detecting a difference in the study if a difference really exists (either between study groups or between treatment periods).

*Pragmatic clinical trials* typically fall somewhere in between a typical randomized trial and a simple and a large simple trial, where the goal is to introduce one or more pragmatic elements into the design but with substantial protocol-required follow-up and testing outside of usual care practice.

*Precipitant drug* is, in a drug–drug interaction, the drug that affects the pharmacokinetics or pharmacodynamics of the other drug(s).

*Precipitant-triggered drug–drug interaction* is, in a study of a potential drug–drug interaction, the scenario in which the precipitant drug is started in a person already taking the object drug.

*Precision* is the degree of absence of random error. Precise estimates have narrow confidence intervals.

*Precision medicine* has been defined by the National Institutes of Health (NIH) in the United States as an "approach to disease prevention and treatment based on people's individual differences in environment, genes and lifestyle."

*Pre-post with comparison group design* includes a single observation both before and after treatment in a non-randomly selected group exposed to a treatment (e.g. physicians receiving feedback on specific prescribing practices), as well as simultaneous before and after observations of a similar (comparison) group not receiving treatment.

*Prescribing errors* refer to issues related to underuse, overuse, and misuse of prescribed drugs, all of which contribute to the suboptimal utilization of pharmaceutical therapies.

The *prevalence* of a disease is a measurement of how common the disease is. Specifically, it is the number of existing cases of the disease in a defined population at a given point in time or over a defined time period, divided by the number of people in that population.

*Prevalence study bias*, a type of selection bias that may occur in studies when prevalent cases rather than new cases of a condition are selected for a study. A strong association with prevalence may be related to the duration of the disease rather than to its incidence, because prevalence is proportional to both incidence and duration of the disease.

*Privacy*, in the setting of research, refers to each individual's right to be free from unwanted inspection of, or access to, personal information by unauthorized persons.

*Procedure registries* are registries characterized by inclusion of subjects based on receipt of specific services, such as procedures, or based on hospitalizations.

*Product registries* are registries characterized by inclusion of subjects based on use of a specific product (drug or device) or related products in a given therapeutic area.

*Propensity scores* are an approach to controlling for confounding that uses mathematical modeling to predict exposure based on observed variables, and uses the predicted probability of exposure as the basis for matching or adjustment.

*Prospective drug utilization review* is designed to detect drug-therapy problems before an individual patient receives the drug.

*Prospective studies* are studies performed simultaneously with the events under study; namely, patient outcomes have not yet occurred as of the outset of the study.

*Proteomics* is, within the context of pharmacoepidemiology, the study of how proteins are responsible for variability in medication response.

*Protopathic bias* is interpreting a factor to be a result of an exposure when it is in fact a determinant of the exposure, and can occur when an early sign of the disease under study led to the prescription of the drug under study.

*Publication bias* occurs when publication of a study's results is related to the study's findings, such that study results are not published or publication is delayed because of the results.

*Qualitative drug utilization studies* are studies that assess the *appropriateness* of drug use.

*Quality-of-life* is the description of aspects (domains) of physical, social, and emotional health that are relevant and important to the patient.

*Quantitative drug utilization studies* are descriptive studies of *frequency* of drug use.

*Random allocation* is the assignment of subjects who are enrolled in a study into study groups in a manner determined by chance.

*Random error* is error due to chance.

*Random selection* is the selection of subjects into a study from among those eligible in a manner determined by chance.

*Randomized clinical trials* are studies in which the investigator randomly assigns patients to different therapies, one of which may be a control therapy.

*Recall bias* is an error in the results of a study due to a systematic difference between the study groups in the accuracy or completeness of their memory of their past exposures or health events.

*Referral bias* is error in the results of a study that occurs when the reasons for referring a patient for medical care are related to the exposure status, e.g. when the use of the drug contributes to the diagnostic process.

*Registries* are organized systems that use observational study methods to collect uniform data (clinical and other) to evaluate specified outcomes for a population defined by a particular disease, condition, or exposure, and that serves one or more predetermined scientific, clinical, or policy purposes. Registries can be thought of as both the process for collecting data from which studies are derived, as well as referring to the actual database.

*Regression to the mean* is the tendency for observations on populations selected on the basis of an abnormality to approach normality on subsequent observations.

The *relative rate* is the ratio of the incidence rate of an outcome in the exposed group to the incidence rate of the outcome in the unexposed group. It is synonymous with the terms *rate ratio* and *incidence rate ratio*.

The *relative risk* is the ratio of the cumulative incidence of an outcome in the exposed group to the cumulative incidence of the outcome in the unexposed group. It is synonymous with the term *cumulative incidence ratio*.

*Reliability* is the degree to which the results obtained by a measurement procedure can be replicated. The measurement of reliability does not require a gold standard, since it assesses only the concordance between two or more measures.

A *reporting rate* in a spontaneous reporting system is the number of reported cases of an adverse event of interest divided by some measure of the suspect drug's utilization, usually the number of dispensed prescriptions. This is perhaps better referred to as a *rate of reported cases*.

*Reproducibility* is the ability of an instrument to obtain more or less the same scores upon repeated measurements of patients who have not changed.

*Research*, as defined in US regulation, is any activity designed to "develop or contribute to generalizable knowledge". (Title 45 US Code of Federal Regulations Part 46.102 (d))

A *research subject* is "a living individual, about whom an investigator (whether professional or student) conducting research obtains either: 1) data through intervention or interaction with the individual, or 2) identifiable private information" (US Code of Federal Regulations 46.102f).

*Responsiveness* is an instrument's ability to detect change.

*Retrospective drug utilization review* compares past drug use against predetermined criteria to identify aberrant prescribing patterns or patient-specific deviations from explicit criteria.

*Retrospective studies* are studies conducted after the events under study have occurred. Both exposure and outcome have already occurred as of the outset of the study.

*Risk* is the cumulative probability that something will happen.

*Risk evaluation and mitigation strategy (REMS)* is a pharmacovigilance assessment plan in the United States, approved by regulators in advance of implementation, to ensure that the benefits of a drug or biological product outweigh its risks. In the EU, pharmacovigilance legislation explicitly requires the active monitoring of the outcome of risk minimization activities contained in the *risk management plan*, placing the obligation on manufacturers and regulatory authorities for this activity.

A judgment about *safety* is a personal and/or social judgment about the degree to which a given risk is acceptable.

*Safety signal* is a concern about an excess of adverse events compared to what is expected to be associated with a product's (drug or device) use.

*Service registries* are registries characterized by inclusion of subjects based on receipt of specific services, such as procedures, or based on hospitalizations.

*Sample distortion bias* is another name for selection bias.

*Scientific inference* is the process of generalizing from a statement about a population, which is an association, to a causal statement about scientific theory.

*Selection bias* is error in a study that is due to systematic differences in characteristics between those who are selected for the study and those who are not.

*Self-controlled designs* are studies that include only persons who experienced the outcome, using each person as her/his own control, and include self-controlled case series and case-crossover designs.

*Self-controlled case series (SCCS) design* is a self-controlled design that is analogous to the cohort design. It includes only individuals who experienced the outcome, and examines the rate of the outcome during exposed vs. unexposed periods within those individuals.

*Sensibility* is a judgment about the validity of an instrument, based on an intuitive assessment of the extent to which an instrument meets a number of criteria including applicability, clarity and simplicity, likelihood of bias, comprehensiveness, and whether redundant items have been included.

*Sensitivity* is the proportion of persons who truly have a characteristic, who are correctly classified by a diagnostic test as having it.

*Sensitivity analysis* is a set of procedures in which the results of a study are recalculated using alternate values for some of the study's variables, in order to test the sensitivity of the conclusions to altered specifications.

A *serious adverse experience* is any adverse experience occurring at any dose that results in any of the following outcomes: death, a life-threatening adverse experience, inpatient hospitalization or prolongation of existing hospitalization, a persistent or significant disability/incapacity, or congenital anomaly/birth defect.

*Signal* is a hypothesis that calls for further work to be performed to evaluate that hypothesis.

*Signal detection* is the process of looking for or identifying signals from any source.

*Signal generation,* sometimes referred to as data mining, is an approach that uses statistical methods to identify a safety signal. No particular medical product exposure or adverse outcome is prespecified.

*Signal refinement* is a process by which an identified safety signal is further evaluated to determine whether evidence exists to support a relationship between the exposure and the outcome.

*Specific causation*, from a legal perspective, addresses whether the product in question actually caused an alleged injury in the individual plaintiff.

*Specific quality-of-life instruments* are focused on disease or treatment issues specifically relevant to the question at hand.

*Specificity* is the proportion of persons who truly do **not** have a characteristic, who are correctly classified by a diagnostic test as not having it.

*Spontaneous reporting systems* are maintained by regulatory bodies throughout the world and collect unsolicited clinical observations that originate outside of a formal study.

*Statistical inference* is the process of generalizing from a sample of study subjects to the entire population from which those subjects are theoretically drawn.

*Statistical interaction*, see effect modification.

A *statistically significant difference* is a difference between two study groups that is unlikely to have occurred purely by chance.

*Steady state*, within pharmacokinetics, is the situation when the amount of drug being administered equals the amount of drug being eliminated from the body.

*Systematic error* is any error in study results other than that due to random variation.

The *therapeutic ratio* is the ratio of the drug concentration that produces toxicity to the concentration that produces the desired therapeutic effect.

*Therapeutics* is the application of the principles of clinical pharmacology to rational prescribing, the conduct of clinical trials, and the assessment of outcomes during real-life clinical practice.

*Type A adverse reactions* are those that are the result of an exaggerated but otherwise predictable pharmacological effect of the drug. They tend to be common and dose-related.

*Type B adverse reactions* are those that are aberrant effects of the drug. They tend to be uncommon, not dose-related, and unpredictable.

A *type I statistical error* is concluding there is an association when in fact one does not exist, i.e. erroneously rejecting the null hypothesis.

A *type II statistical error* is concluding there is no association when in fact one does exist, i.e. erroneously accepting the null hypothesis.

*Unanticipated beneficial effects* of drugs are desirable effects that could not have been predicted on the basis of existing knowledge.

*Unanticipated harmful effects* of drugs are unwanted effects that could not have been predicted on the basis of existing knowledge.

*Uncontrolled studies* refer to studies without a comparison group.

An *unexpected adverse experience* means any adverse experience that is not listed in the current labeling for the product. This includes an event that may be symptomatically and pathophysiologically related to an event listed in the labeling, but differs from the event because of greater severity or specificity.

*Utility measures* of quality-of-life are measured holistically as a single number along a continuum, e.g. from death (0.0) to full health (1.0). The key element of a utility instrument is that it is preference-based.

*Validity* is the degree to which an assessment (e.g. questionnaire or other instrument) measures what it purports to measure.

*Variable costs* are costs that increase with increasing volume of activity.

Apparent *volume of distribution* ($V_D$) is the apparent volume that a drug is distributed in after complete absorption. It is usually calculated from the theoretical plasma concentration at a time when all of the drug was assumed to be present in the body and uniformly distributed. This is calculated from back extrapolation to time zero of the plasma concentration time curve after intravenous administration.

*Vaccinovigilance* is the identification and evaluation of adverse events following immunizations.

*Voluntariness* is the concept in research ethics, that investigators must tell subjects that participation in the research study is voluntary, and that subjects have the right to discontinue participation at any time.

# Index

*Textbook of Pharmacoepidemiology*, Third Edition. Edited by Brian L. Strom, Stephen E. Kimmel, and Sean Hennessy.
© 2022 John Wiley & Sons Ltd. Published 2022 by John Wiley & Sons Ltd.